High-Resolution CT of the Lung

SECOND EDITION

High-Resolution CT of the Lung

SECOND EDITION

W. Richard Webb, M.D.
Professor of Radiology
University of California, San Francisco
Director of Thoracic Imaging
University of California, San Francisco Medical Center
San Francisco, California

Nestor L. Müller, M.D., Ph.D.
Professor of Radiology
University of British Columbia
Director of Thoracic Imaging
Vancouver Hospital and Health Sciences Centre
Vancouver, British Columbia, Canada

David P. Naidich, M.D.
Professor of Radiology
New York University Medical Center
Director of Body Computed Tomography
Bellevue Hospital
New York, New York

Property of U S Army

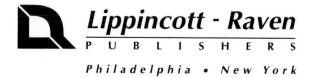

Lippincott - Raven
P U B L I S H E R S

Philadelphia • New York

**Lippincott-Raven Publishers, 227 East Washington Square,
Philadelphia, Pennsylvania 19106**

Made in the United States of America

Library of Congress Cataloging-in-Publication Data

Webb, W. Richard (Wayne Richard), 1945–
    High-resolution CT of the lung / W. Richard Webb, Nestor L.
Müller, David P. Naidich. — 2nd ed.
        p.   cm.
    Includes bibliographical references and index.
    ISBN 0-7817-0217-8
    1. Lungs—Tomography   I. Müller, Nestor Luiz, 1948–
II. Naidich, David P.   III. Title.
    [DNLM: 1. Lung—radiography.   2. Tomography, X-Ray Computed.
3. Lung Diseases—pathology.   WF 600 W368h 1996]
RC734.T64W43   1996
616.2′407572—dc20
DNLM/DLC
for Library of Congress   95–16591

9   8   7   6   5   4

To
our wives and children,
Teresa, Emma, Clifford, and Andy
Ruth, Alison, and Phillip
Jocelyn and Zachary

To
Roberta (Bobby) Miller
whose vitality and scholarly contributions
in the field of HRCT-pathologic correlation
were a constant inspiration for us all.

Contents

Foreword

As a surgical pathologist, it is an honor to be asked to write the foreword to this book. During my years of association with one of the authors, it has become increasingly clear to me how complementary and interdependent are the disciplines of pathology and radiology.

The goal of both radiologists and pathologists is to assess anatomy, although radiologists generally assess black, white, and grey images, whereas anatomic pathologists need color. On the other hand, although gross anatomy is the focus of radiological diagnosis, this technique is sometimes short-changed in the pathology laboratory in favor of detailed microscopic descriptions of slides that are made using dozens of special stains. The opportunity to work with colleagues in chest radiology, particularly high-resolution CT (HRCT) of the lungs, has helped me focus on the gross anatomy from which our microscopic samples are taken, and on its potential value in diagnosis, since some diseases have characteristic appearances on gross inspection.

In the introduction to this book, the authors list five specific ways in which HRCT can guide the diagnostic and clinical approach to a patient with lung disease. HRCT can: 1) detect gross pathology that is not apparent by less sensitive means, such as the chest radiograph; 2) delineate the characteristics of the abnormality, thus allowing for a reasonable differential diagnosis or, in some cases, a specific diagnosis; 3) detect whether a process is active or burnt out; 4) be used as a guide to the appropriate biopsy site and technique; and 5) function as a follow-up technique to determine the efficacy of treatment. In my practice of surgical lung pathology, these five principles have been put to use many times. For example, biopsies are often performed in patients with normal or nonspecific radiographs and particular HRCT abnormalities. Also, in cases with subtle lung disease, biopsies of palpably normal lungs are performed using HRCT guidance only, and in cases with gross disease, HRCT can help the surgeon avoid areas of nonspecific fibrosis.

I would like to suggest two additional uses of HRCT that I find valuable: First, in the event that biopsies from two sites are dissimilar in terms of disease activity, HRCT best determines which site is representative of the patient's lung disease as a whole. Second, before issuing a final diagnosis, HRCT can provide a surgical pathologist with the clinical and "gross-in-black-and-white" findings to answer the question, "Is my diagnosis reasonable?". The microscopic appearances of some very different diseases can be quite similar, while their gross appearances are quite distinct.

High-Resolution CT of the Lung, written by three well-known experts in the field, illustrates how HRCT can be applied to greatest advantage in the overall care of patients with lung disease. It was a pleasure to read this book, as it is a pleasure to work with the people who wrote it.

Roberta R. Miller, M.D.
Consultant Pathologist
Vancouver General Hospital

Preface to the First Edition

In his paper "A New Look at Pattern Recognition of Diffuse Pulmonary Disease," Ben Felson (1) reviewed the many problems that are inherent in any attempt to precisely characterize diffuse lung disease on the basis of plain radiographic findings. Although he was a great proponent of pattern recognition and an accomplished master of this technique, he stated in the first sentence of this paper that the "the common practice of describing the histologic distribution of pulmonary lesions from their radiographic patterns is often inaccurate." He continued:

> After many years of trying and testing, I have convinced myself that certain patterns of diffuse pulmonary shadows can be distinguished in most patients. Nevertheless I have had considerable difficulty in teaching others how to do it. In fact, a number of respected colleagues who also claim success in pattern recognition often differ with me when viewing the same films. Others even feel that the pattern approach to chest radiography is so unreliable it should be abandoned altogether.
> Why the problems?

As indicated by Dr. Felson, and as we review in the introduction to this book, chest radiographs are limited in their ability to characterize lung morphology precisely and to represent the pathological alterations in morphology that occur in the presence of lung disease. High-resolution CT (HRCT), on the other hand, provides the radiologist and clinician with a tool capable of accurately demonstrating gross lung anatomy and accurately characterizing abnormal findings. The correlation between HRCT findings and pathologic findings is excellent and certainly exceeds that possible with plain radiographs. As discussed by Roberta Miller in the Foreword to this book, to the extent that gross pathology can be used to diagnose lung disease, HRCT can as well. In the last five years, HRCT has revolutionized the radiological approach to diagnosing lung disease.

A further advantage of HRCT is that the interpretation of HRCT scans is easier to teach than is the interpretation of chest radiographs. Because of the clarity and precision with which HRCT represents lung anatomy, there is much less individual variation in interpreting HRCT than there is with chest radiographs. It is much easier to recognize HRCT findings as something one has seen before (e.g., a thick-walled bronchus always looks like a thick-walled bronchus), and to understand what they represent. Far fewer HRCT cases must be classified as belonging to the "'I don't know' pattern" (1) than is necessary when interpreting plain films.

In this book, we have limited our discussion of HRCT findings, both normal and abnormal, and the HRCT descriptions of diseases to what is known and described. We have avoided *speculating* as to what the HRCT might look like in patients with one disease or another based on the plain film findings. As indicated above, the notable inaccuracy of plain films would make this a hazardous endeavor.

In answering his own question, "Why the problems?" with plain radiographs, Dr. Felson replied, "I believe inconsistent terminology and certain misconceptions in respect to pathologic alterations are responsible for many of the difficulties" (1). This is a problem we hope to avoid. In this book we will define and name HRCT findings, whenever possible, in relation to specific anatomic structures.

REFERENCE

1. Felson B. A new look at pattern recognition of diffuse pulmonary disease. *AJR* 1979;133:183–189.

Preface

During the 4 years since we wrote the First Edition of this book, the use of high-resolution CT (HRCT) as a method of diagnosing lung disease has been extensively studied, and this technique has become firmly established in a number of clinical settings. While the First Edition was written during the development of HRCT, the Second Edition finds this technique to be a maturing modality. Although more research in evaluating this technique and its uses remains to be done, a great deal has been learned.

We now have a much more detailed understanding of the correlations between HRCT abnormalities and clinical and pathologic findings, the HRCT features characteristic of a number of lung diseases, the differential diagnosis of specific HRCT findings, and the utility of HRCT in diagnosing patients with acute as well as chronic lung diseases. Although the organization of this volume remains largely the same as that of the First Edition, it has been extensively revised to incorporate recent advances. Following a review and update of HRCT techniques, and normal lung anatomy as shown on HRCT, we discuss basic HRCT findings and the HRCT features of specific lung diseases. As in the First Edition, lung diseases are grouped in relation to their predominant HRCT appearance, be it linear or reticular, nodular, associated with increased lung opacity, or associated with decreased lung opacity, cysts, or abnormal airways. It is our feeling that this approach best allows an understanding of the differential diagnosis of HRCT abnormalities.

Sections reviewing the appearances of lung disease as shown on HRCT, their pathologic correlates, and the differential diagnosis of specific HRCT findings have been greatly expanded, and tables of differential diagnosis of HRCT findings are presented (tinted gray) for easy reference. As understanding the utility of HRCT in different clinical situations is of great importance, the usefulness of HRCT in diagnosing specific diseases is emphasized, along with its overall utility. Although the First Edition primarily discussed the use of HRCT in patients with chronic infiltrative lung disease, the use of HRCT in assessing patients with acute diseases, and particularly infectious diseases, is discussed in greater detail in this edition.

Acknowledgments

We acknowledge Drs. Roberta Miller, Vancouver General Hospital; Martha Warnock, University of California, San Francisco; and Jaishree Jagirdar, New York University Medical Center/Bellevue Hospital for providing some of the illustrations of pathologic and histologic specimens that appear in this book.

Numerous new illustrations have been provided, and a number of these have been furnished to us by colleagues from around the world. We wish to take this opportunity to thank them for their cooperation and gracious assistance. They are listed alphabetically below:

Denise Aberle, M.D., Los Angeles, California
Masanori Akira, M.D., Osaka, Japan
Minnie Bhalla, M.D., Boston, Massachusetts
M. Joseph Cherian, M.D., Kuwait City, Kuwait
Jung-Gi Im, M.D., Seoul, Korea
Harumi Itoh, M.D., Kyoto, Japan
Shin-Ho Kook, M.D., Seoul, Korea
Peter Kullnig, M.D., Graz, Austria
Edward Lubat, M.D., Englewood, New Jersey
Koichi Nishimura, Kyoto, Japan
Raymond Glyn Thomas, M.D., Johannesburg, South Africa

Introduction

Plain chest radiographs are indispensable in the diagnostic evaluation of patients suspected of having diffuse lung disease. Indeed, in some patients, radiographs can provide information which is sufficiently diagnostic for patient management. However, in patients with acute or chronic diffuse lung disease, chest radiographs are limited in their sensitivity, specificity, and diagnostic accuracy (1). Because many parenchymal structures, both normal and abnormal, are superimposed on the chest radiographic image, it can sometimes be extremely difficult to decide whether or not a radiograph is abnormal, and if abnormal, what the abnormality may represent anatomically. Although a pattern recognition approach to the diagnosis of lung disease can be helpful, it has limitations, and correlation with histologic findings is often poor (2–4).

High-resolution computed tomography (HRCT) has proven to be of great value in assessing patients with diffuse lung disease, and it is often used in problematic patients as a supplement to plain radiographs and clinical studies (5–7). Generally, in patients with suspected diffuse lung disease, HRCT is used in an attempt to answer 5 questions. It will be helpful to keep these in mind when reading subsequent chapters in this book, as the utility of HRCT will be discussed in detail in relation to individual disease entities, and is summarized in Chapter 8.

1. Is there lung disease?

   HRCT is often used to detect morphologic lung disease in patients with symptoms of respiratory distress or abnormal pulmonary function tests who have normal chest radiographs or questionable radiographic abnormalities; in this setting, HRCT findings of disease can indicate the need for further diagnostic evaluation. Although not all patients with respiratory symptoms and a significant lung disease will show HRCT abnormalities, in the large majority, HRCT evidence of disease will be visible. On the other hand, in some patients who have symptoms and pulmonary function abnormalities suggesting the presence of lung disease, HRCT will show that these abnormalities are the result of emphysema, which is not diagnosable on the basis of plain radiographic or functional findings; in such patients no further evaluation is usually needed.

2. What is it?

   HRCT is used to characterize lung disease when clinical and chest radiographic findings are nonspecific. Based on morphologic findings visible on HRCT, a specific diagnosis can sometimes be made, or the differential diagnosis can be limited to a few possibilities, thus influencing the subsequent diagnostic evaluation or treatment.

3. Is there acute or active disease?

   HRCT is used to help determine the presence or absence, and extent, of reversible (acute or active) and irreversible (fibrotic) lung disease. If HRCT findings suggest that the lung disease is active or reversible, a lung biopsy or other appropriate studies are usually performed in order to make a histologic diagnosis, and determine appropriate treatment. On the other hand, if HRCT findings suggest the presence of inactive or "end-stage" lung, it can indicate that no biopsy need be done.

4. Where should a biopsy be performed?

   HRCT is often used as a guide for lung biopsy, determining which lung regions should be sampled histologically. Many "diffuse" lung diseases are quite patchy in distribution, with different lung regions showing differing degrees or types of abnormality. Since both active and fibrotic disease can be present in the same lung, HRCT can be used to target the specific lung regions which are most likely to contain active (and diagnostic) lesions. Furthermore, depending on the appearance and location of abnormalities on HRCT, it can sometimes be suggested whether open biopsy, bronchoscopy with transbronchial biopsy, or bronchoalveolar lavage will be needed to provide a diagnosis.

5. Has there been a change?

Because HRCT can more accurately identify subtle or "active" lung disease, it can be used to follow patients who are being treated, in order to monitor the success or failure of the treatment which is being employed.

REFERENCES

1. Naidich DP. Pulmonary parenchymal high-resolution CT: to be or not to be. *Radiology* 1989;171:22–24.
2. Heitzman ER. Pattern recognition in pulmonary radiology. In: *The Lung: Radiologic-Pathologic Correlations, 2nd Ed.* St. Louis: C. V. Mosby, 1984, 70–105.
3. Felson B. A new look at pattern recognition of diffuse pulmonary disease. *AJR* 1979;133:183–189.
4. Genereux GP. Pattern recognition in diffuse lung disease: a review of theory and practice. *Med Radiogr Photog* 1985; 61:2–31.
5. Müller NL. Clinical value of high resolution CT in chronic diffuse lung disease. *AJR* 1991;157:1163–1170.
6. Padley SPG, Adler B, Müller NL. High-resolution computed tomography of the chest: current indications. *J Thorac Imag* 1993;8:189–199.
7. Primack SL, Müller NL. High-resolution computed tomography in acute diffuse lung disease in the immunocompromised patient. *Rad Clin N Am* 1994;32:731–744.

High-Resolution CT of the Lung

SECOND EDITION

ONE

Technical Aspects of HRCT

Although the introduction of computed tomography (CT) revolutionized the radiologic diagnosis of chest diseases, the ability of early CT scanners to evaluate pulmonary parenchymal diseases was limited by the resolving power of the scanners employed (1). Specifically, CT obtained with long scan times (18 sec) and using 1-cm collimation, provided insufficient anatomic detail to allow a precise evaluation of normal and abnormal pulmonary anatomy, at least to the degree that it would surpass the information available on plain radiographs.

Attempts to improve the resolution of CT for diagnosing lung abnormalities were first described relative to the assessment of focal lung disease and lung nodules. In 1980, Siegelman et al. (2) emphasized the necessity of using 5-mm collimation for the detection of calcification in lung nodules. As thinner collimation became available on commercial scanners, simultaneous with other developments in CT technology, the use of CT for the precise anatomic definition of diffuse lung diseases became possible, and was reported by several authors. The first use of the term "high-resolution" CT (HRCT) has been attributed to Todo et al. (3), who, in 1982, described the potential use of this technique for assessing lung disease. The first reports of HRCT in English date to 1985, including landmark descriptions of HRCT findings by Nakata, Naidich, and Zerhouni (4–6).

HRCT techniques developed over the last 10 years are capable of imaging the lung with excellent spatial resolution, providing anatomic detail similar to that available from gross pathologic specimens or lung slices (7–10). HRCT can demonstrate both the normal and abnormal lung interstitium, and morphologic characteristics of both localized and diffuse parenchymal abnormalities; in this regard, HRCT is clearly superior to plain radiographs and conventional CT. This technique has led to a renaissance of interest in the use of CT for diagnosing lung disease, and has become established as an important diagnostic modality in both the radiologic and pulmonary medicine communities (7–10). In this chapter, we will review the modifications in CT technique that are appropriate in obtaining HRCT, the radiation dose associated with HRCT, the spatial resolution of this technique, common HRCT artifacts, and the scan protocols recommended in specific clinical settings.

SCAN TECHNIQUE

HRCT technique attempts to optimize the demonstration of lung anatomy. There is no general agreement among investigators as to what constitutes a "high-resolution" CT study, and each of the three of us performs HRCT in a slightly different manner. However, most chest radiologists agree as to which technical adaptations are essential for performing HRCT of the lung parenchyma. This section reviews the effect of various technical factors on the appearance of HRCT, and summarizes our compromise recommendations as to what techniques are necessary when performing HRCT and what techniques are optional and can be tailored to suit an individual case or an individual institution.

A number of technical modifications are possible in obtaining an optimal lung CT. The most important modifications of CT technique, that make it "high-resolution" are: (i) the use of thin collimation, (ii) image reconstruction with a high-spatial frequency (sharp) algorithm, (iii) increased kVp or mA technique, (iv) the use of a large matrix size, and (v) targeted image reconstruction (Table 1-1) (7–13). However, not all of these are performed on a routine basis.

The first three technical adaptations, namely the use of thin collimation, a sharp reconstruction algorithm, and increased kVp and mA technique, are accomplished prospectively. The last two involve postprocessing of the scan data, or image reconstruction.

1

TABLE 1-1. *Summary of recommended HRCT technique*

Essential

1. Collimation: Thinnest available collimation (1–1.5 mm).
2. Reconstruction algorithm: High-spatial frequency or "sharp" algorithm (i.e., GE "bone").
3. Scan time: As short as possible (1–2 seconds).
4. kVp; mA; mAs: kVp 120–140; mA 140–240; mAs 240–400
5. Matrix size: Largest available (512 × 512).
6. Windows: At least one consistent lung window setting is necessary. Window mean/width values of −600 HU to −700 HU/1,000 HU to 1,500 HU are appropriate. −700/1,000 HU or −600/1,500 HU are good combinations. Soft-tissue windows of approximately 50/350 HU should also be used for the mediastinum, hila, and pleura.

Recommended

1. Windows: Windows may need to be customized; a low-window mean (−800 to −900 HU) is optimal for diagnosing emphysema. 50/350 HU is recommended for viewing the mediastinum. −600/2,000 HU is recommended for viewing pleuro-parenchymal disease.
2. Photography: 6 on 1 (14 × 17) for lung parenchyma; 12 on 1 for soft-tissue windows.

Optional

1. kVp/mA:

   Increased kVp/mAs (i.e., 140/340). Recommended in large patients. Otherwise optional.
   Reduced mAs (low-dose HRCT). 40–80 mAs
2. Targeted reconstruction: (15–25 cm field of view).

Scan Collimation

With 1-cm collimation, volume averaging within the plane of scan significantly reduces the ability of CT to resolve small structures. Therefore, scanning with the thinnest possible collimation (1–1.5 mm) is essential if spatial resolution is to be optimized (4,6,10,11). The use of 5-mm collimation should not be considered HRCT. We recommend using 1- or 1.5-mm collimation as routine for HRCT (Table 1-1).

Clearly, the thinnest collimation available with any scanner provides the best resolution. However, in one study of HRCT techniques (14), the differences between 1.5-mm collimation and 3-mm collimation in allowing the resolution of certain features of lung architecture were felt to be small.

Murata et al. (14), compared the ability of HRCT with 1.5-mm collimation to that of HRCT with 3-mm collimation in identifying small vessels, bronchi, interlobular septa, and some pathologic findings. With 1.5-mm collimation, there was greater contrast between vessels and surrounding lung parenchyma, more branches of small vessels were sometimes seen, and small bronchi were more often recognizable, but the differences were considered to be insignificant (14). The authors of this study also concluded that certain pathologic findings such as thickened interlobular septa were similarly visible on images with 1.5- and 3-mm collimation (14). However, slight increases in lung attenuation (as in early interstitial disease, or decreases

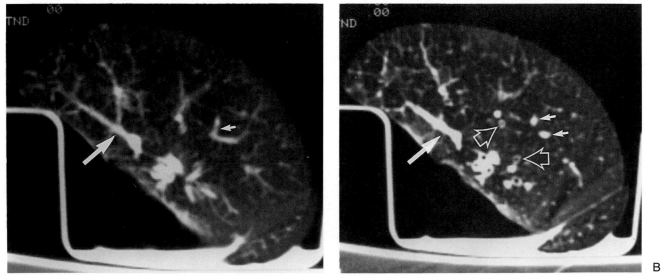

A   B

FIG. 1-1. Effects of collimation on resolution. **A:** Conventional CT of a fresh inflated human lung obtained with 1-cm collimation and reconstructed with the standard algorithm. Several cylindrical or branching pulmonary arteries (*small arrow*) are visible. A large pulmonary artery branch (*large arrow*) lies in the plane of scan. **B:** CT at the same level with 1.5-mm collimation; technical parameters and reconstructed algorithm are otherwise identical. Pulmonary arteries seen as branching or cylindrical on the scan obtained using 1-cm collimation appear "nodular" on the scan with 1.5-mm collimation (*small arrows*). Small bronchi (*open arrows*) are much better seen with thin collimation. Note that the large pulmonary vessel that lies in the plane of scan appears to have a greater diameter with thin collimation (*large arrow*) than it does with 1-cm collimation.

in attenuation (as in emphysema) were better resolved with 1.5-mm collimation.

There are several differences as to how lung structures are visualized on scans performed with thin collimation, as compared with 1-cm collimation scans. With thin collimation, it is more difficult to follow the courses of vessels and bronchi than it is with 1-cm collimation. With 1-cm collimation, for example, vessels that lie in the plane of scan look like vessels (i.e., they appear cylindrical), and can be clearly identified as such. With thin collimation, vessels can appear "nodular" because only short segments may lie in the plane of scan; this finding sometimes leads to confusion (Fig. 1-1), but with experience, this difficulty can be easily avoided.

Also, with thin collimation, the diameter of a vessel that lies in or near the plane of scan can appear larger than it does with 1-cm collimation, because less volume averaging is occurring between the rounded edge of the vessel and the adjacent air-filled lung (Fig. 1-1); thin collimation scans more accurately reflect vessel diameter in this setting. This is quite analogous to the better estimation of the diameter of a lung nodule that is possible with thin collimation. Furthermore, with 1.5-mm collimation, bronchi that are oriented obliquely relative to the scan plane are much better

defined than they are with 1-cm collimation, and their wall thickness and luminal diameter are more accurately assessed (15). The diameter of vessels or bronchi that lie perpendicular to the scan plane appear the same with both thin and thick collimation.

Reconstruction Algorithm

The inherent or maximum spatial resolution of a CT scanner is determined by the geometry of the data collecting system and the frequency at which scan data are sampled during the scan sequence (11). The spatial resolution of the image produced is less than the inherent resolution of the scan system, depending on the reconstruction algorithm that is used, and the matrix size and the field of view (FOV) which, in turn, determine pixel size. In HRCT, these parameters are optimized to increase the spatial resolution of the image as much as possible.

With conventional body CT, scan data are usually reconstructed with a relatively low-spatial frequency algorithm (i.e., GE "standard" or "soft-tissue" algorithms), that smoothes the image, reduces visible image noise, and improves the contrast resolution to some degree (12,13). "Low-spatial frequency" simply means that the frequency of information recorded in

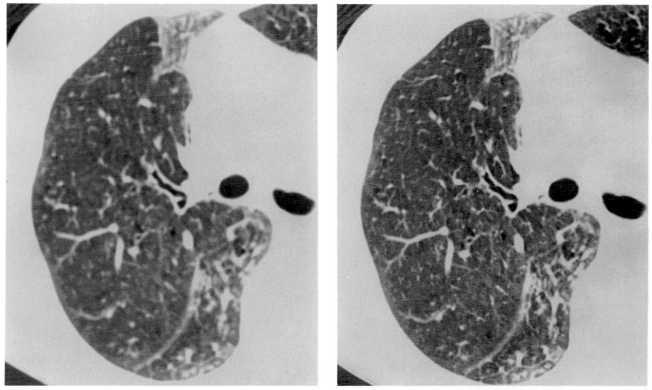

A B

FIG. 1-2. Effect of reconstruction algorithm on resolution. A CT scan obtained with 1.5-mm collimation has been reconstructed using a smoothing ("standard") algorithm (**A**) and a sharp ("bone") algorithm (**B**). Lung structures appear much sharper with the "bone" algorithm.

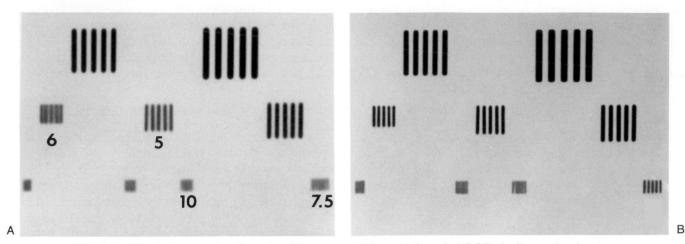

A   B

FIG. 1-3. Effect of reconstruction algorithm on spatial resolution. **A:** HRCT of a line-pair phantom obtained with 1.5-mm collimation and reconstructed with the standard algorithm. Numbers indicate the resolution in line pairs per centimeter. The resolution with this technique is 6-line pairs per cm. **B:** When the same scan is reconstructed using the bone algorithm, spatial resolution improves. 7.5-line pairs (*arrow*) are easily resolved, and edges are considerably sharper than on the scan reconstructed using the standard algorithm. (From Mayo et al., ref. 11, with permission.)

the final image is relatively low; this is the same thing as saying that the algorithm is "low- resolution" rather than high-resolution.

Reconstruction of the image using a high-spatial frequency algorithm, or in other words a high-resolution algorithm (i.e., GE "bone" algorithm), reduces image smoothing and increases spatial resolution, making structures appear sharper (Fig. 1-2) (4,11,14). In one study of HRCT techniques (11), a quantitative improvement in spatial resolution was found when the bone algorithm was used instead of the standard algorithm to reconstruct scan data (Fig. 1-3); in this study, subjective image quality was also rated more highly with the bone algorithm. In another study of HRCT (14), small vessels and bronchi were better seen with the bone algorithm than the standard algorithm. Recently, the use of a sharp algorithm has also been recommended for routine chest CT performed using 1-cm collimation, in order to improve spatial resolution (16).

Using a sharp, or high-resolution algorithm is a critical element in performing HRCT (Table 1-1) (12,13).

kVp, mA (mAs), and Scan Time

In HRCT, image noise is more apparent than with standard CT. This noise usually appears as a graininess or mottle that can be distracting and may obscure anatomic detail (Fig. 1-4) (11).

High-resolution techniques, such as the use of a sharp reconstruction algorithm, in addition to increasing image sharpness, increases the visibility of noise in the CT image (12,13) (Fig. 1-3). Since much of this noise is quantum related and thus decreases with in-

creased technique (number of photons), increasing the kilovolt peak (kVp) or milliamperes (mA) used during scanning, or increasing scan time can reduce noise and improve scan quality (Fig. 1-5) (11); noise is inversely proportional to the number of photons absorbed (precisely, it is inversely proportional to the square root of the product of the mA and scan time).

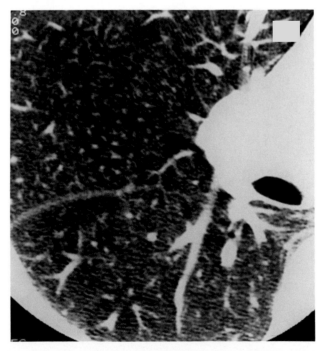

FIG. 1-4. Image noise. Detailed view of an HRCT image of the right lung. The mottled appearance, which is most evident posteriorly, represents image noise. Very thin linear streaks best seen in the anterior part of the image represent "aliasing" artifacts.

Increasing scan time is not generally desirable with lung CT. Because of patient motion, increased scan times can result in an increase in motion-related artifacts. Scans times of 1 to 2 sec are most appropriate for HRCT, and recommended (Table 1-1).

However, kVp and mA can be easily increased when obtaining HRCT, and this increase in technique can result in a reduction in visible image noise. In one study (11), a measure of image noise was reduced by about 30% when kVp/mA were increased from 120/100 to 140/170 (Fig. 1-5), and the scans with increased kVp and mA settings were rated by observers as being of better quality 80% of the time (Fig. 1-6) (11). It should also be kept in mind, however, that increasing scan technique also increases the patient's radiation dose (17), although with HRCT, radiation is limited to a few thin scan levels (as is discussed below).

Although increasing kVp and mA reduce image noise, it is somewhat subjective as to whether it is necessary to use increased kVp and mA settings for HRCT (Fig. 1-6). Some investigators scan most patients with kVp/mA settings of 140/170 and a scan time of 2 sec (9), a technique that exceeds what is routinely used for chest CT in their institution (120 kVp, 100 mA). Nonetheless, adequate diagnostic scans can also be obtained in patients with the techniques that are routine for chest CT (18), although image quality may not be quite as good as when technique is increased. Using

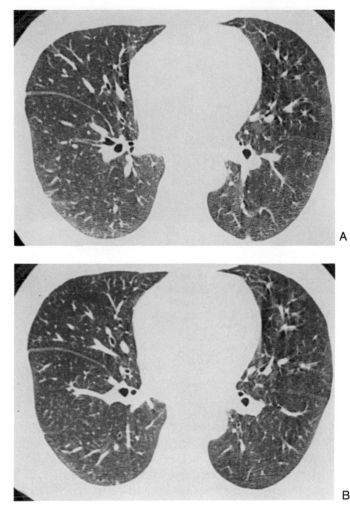

FIG. 1-6. Effect of kVp and mA on image noise. HRCT scans obtained with kVp/mA settings of 120/100 (**A**), and 140/170 (**B**). Noise is most evident posteriorly and in the paravertebral regions. Although noise is greater in A, the difference is probably not significant clinically. Nonetheless, increasing the kVp/mA is optimal. Also note pulsation ("star") artifacts in the left lung on both images and a "double" left major fissure. (From Mayo et al., ref. 11, with permission.)

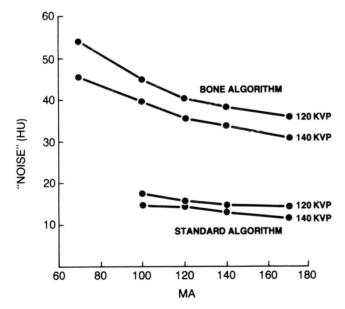

FIG. 1-5. Effect of algorithm, kVp, and mA on image noise. Graph of HRCT image noise (standard deviation of Hounsfield unit measurements in an anthropomorphic CT phantom (21) as related to the reconstruction algorithm and scan technique. Noise increases when the "bone" algorithm is used instead of the "standard" algorithm. With the bone algorithm, noise decreases about 30% with increased kVp and mA settings. (From Mayo et al., ref. 11, with permission.)

current scanners capable of a 1-sec scan time, scan techniques of 120 to 140 kVp and mA values of approximately 240 (mAs = 240) have proven quite satisfactory (19).

Furthermore the efficacy of "low-dose high-resolution CT" has been assessed in two recent studies (20–22). In a study by Zwirewich et al. (20), scans with 1.5-mm collimation, 2-sec scan time, and at 120 kVp, were obtained using both 20 mA (low-dose HRCT) and 200 mA (conventional-dose HRCT) at selected levels in the chest in 31 patients. Observers evaluated the visibility of normal structures, various parenchymal abnormalities, and artifacts using both techniques. The low-dose and conventional-dose HRCT were equivalent for the demonstration of vessels, lobar and seg-

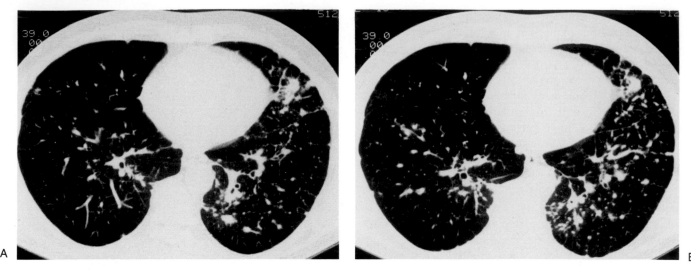

FIG. 1-7. Low-dose (**A**) and conventional-dose (**B**) HRCT in a patient with sarcoidosis. Both techniques demonstrate the presence of small peribronchovascular, septal, and subpleural nodules typical of this disease. Despite the increased noise on the low-dose image, the pattern and extent of abnormalities are equally well seen with both techniques. (From Lee et al., ref. 21, with permission.)

mental bronchi, structures of the secondary pulmonary lobule, and in characterizing the extent and distribution of reticular abnormalities, honeycomb cysts, and thickened interlobular septa. However, the low-dose technique failed to demonstrate ground-glass opacity in 2 of 10 cases, and emphysema in 1 of 9 cases, in which they were evident but subtle on the usual-dose HRCT. Linear streak artifacts were also more prominent on images acquired with the low-dose technique, but the two techniques were judged equally diagnostic in 97% of cases. The authors concluded that HRCT images acquired at 20 mA yield anatomic information equivalent to that obtained with 200 mA scans in the majority of patients, without significant loss of spatial resolution or image degradation due to streak artifacts.

In a subsequent study (21), the diagnostic accuracy of chest radiographs, low-dose HRCT (80 mAs; 120 kVp, 40 mA, 2 sec), and conventional-dose HRCT (340 mAs; 120 kVp, 170 mA, 2 sec) were compared in 50 patients with chronic infiltrative lung disease and 10 normal controls. For each HRCT technique, only three images were used, obtained at the levels of the aortic arch, tracheal carina, and 1-cm above the right hemidiaphragm. A correct first choice diagnosis was made significantly more often with either HRCT technique than with radiography; the correct diagnosis was made in 65% of cases using radiographs, 74% of cases with low-dose HRCT ($p < 0.02$), and 80% of conventional

HRCT ($p < 0.005$). A high confidence level in making a diagnosis was reached in 42% of radiographic examinations, 61% of the low-dose ($p < 0.01$), and 63% of the conventional-dose HRCT examinations ($p < 0.005$), which were correct in 92%, 90%, and 96% of the studies, respectively. Although conventional-dose HRCT was more accurate than low-dose HRCT, this difference was not significant, and both techniques provided quite similar anatomic information (Figs. 1-7, 1-8) (21).

Majurin et al. (22) compared a variety of low-dose techniques in 45 patients with suspected asbestos-related lung disease. Of the 37 patients with CT evidence of lung fibrosis, HRCT images obtained with mAs as low as 120 (60 mA/2 sec) clearly showed parenchymal bands, curvilinear opacities, and honeycombing. However, reliable identification of interstitial lines or areas of ground-glass opacity required a minimum technique of 160 mAs (80 mA/2 sec). Furthermore, these authors showed that using the lowest possible dosage (30 mA/2 sec) HRCT was sufficient only for detecting marked pleural thickening and areas of gross lung fibrosis.

Although optimizing resolution would require the use of increased kVp and mA, we feel that this is optional (Table 1-1). In the large majority of patients, diagnostic scans will be obtained without increasing scan technique. Since noise is usually a bigger problem in large patients (Fig. 1-9) (because more x-ray photons

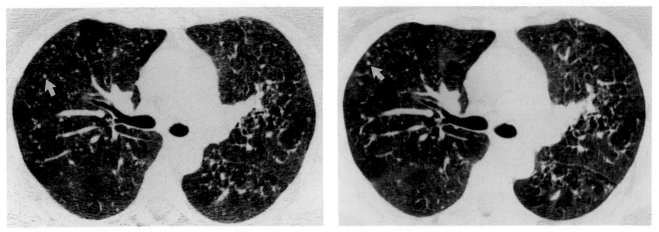

A   B

FIG. 1-8. Low-dose (**A**) and conventional-dose (**B**) HRCT in a patient with hypersensitivity pneumonitis. Although noise is much more obvious on the low-dose image, areas of ground-glass opacity and ill-defined nodules (*arrows*) are visible with both techniques. (From Lee et al., ref. 21, with permission.)

are absorbed by the patient) and in the posterior part of the scan image (because of photon absorption by the spine), it would be most important to use increased technical factors when studying large patients or patients with suspected posterior lung disease (11). Low-dose HRCT technique should not be routinely employed for the initial evaluation of patients with lung disease, although it would be valuable in following patients with a known lung abnormality, or in screening large populations at risk for lung disease. Optimal low-dose techniques will likely vary with the clinical setting, and remain to be established.

Matrix Size

The largest matrix available should be used routinely in image reconstruction, in order to reduce pixel size (4,11,14). The largest available matrix is usually 512 × 512.

Field of View and the Use of Targeted Reconstruction

Scanning should be performed using a field of view large enough to encompass the patient (i.e., 35 cm).

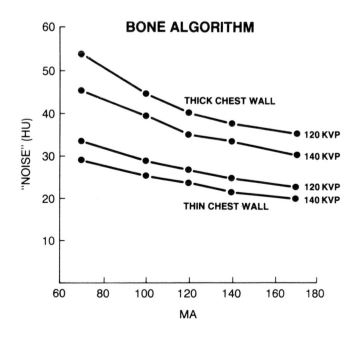

FIG. 1-9. Relationship of noise to patient size. Graph of image noise measured using an anthropomorphic chest phantom (21), with simulated thick and thin chest walls. Noise significantly increases with the thick chest wall. (From Mayo et al., ref. 11, with permission.)

Retrospectively targeting image reconstruction to a single lung instead of the entire thorax, using a smaller field of view, significantly reduces the image pixel size and thus, increases spatial resolution (Fig. 1-10) (11,18). For example, with a 40-cm reconstruction circle (field of view or FOV) and a 512 × 512 matrix, pixel size measures 0.78 mm. With targeted image reconstruction using a 25-cm FOV, pixel size is reduced to 0.49 mm, and the spatial resolution is correspondingly increased (Fig. 1-11). Using a 15-cm FOV further reduces pixel size to 0.29 mm, but this FOV is usually insufficient to view an entire lung, and is not often used clinically. With the GE 9800 system, optimal matching of the inherent spatial resolution of the scanner and pixel size occurs at a reconstruction diameter of approximately 13 cm and a pixel size of 0.25 mm (11–13); thus, further reduction in the FOV is of no benefit in improving spatial resolution.

In actual clinical practice, image targeting is uncommonly done because it requires a significant amount of time, the raw scan data must be saved, and because targeting usually requires a radiologist's input. Gener-

ally, using thin collimation and reconstruction with the bone algorithm produce most of the improvement in spatial resolution that is possible, and the ability to see both lungs on the same image with a non-targeted reconstruction is often preferred.

Image targeting is considered to be optional (Table 1-1), and is recommended only when optimal resolution is desired.

Image Photography

Although the manner in which the images are photographed does not affect the actual spatial resolution of the image, proper photography is important in allowing the images to be interpreted accurately. The window mean and width used for photography have a significant impact on the appearance of the lung parenchyma, and the dimensions of visualized structures (Fig. 1-12) (15). Subtle abnormalities are difficult to detect if the photographic technique used is not appropriate, and normal structures can be made to look abnormal.

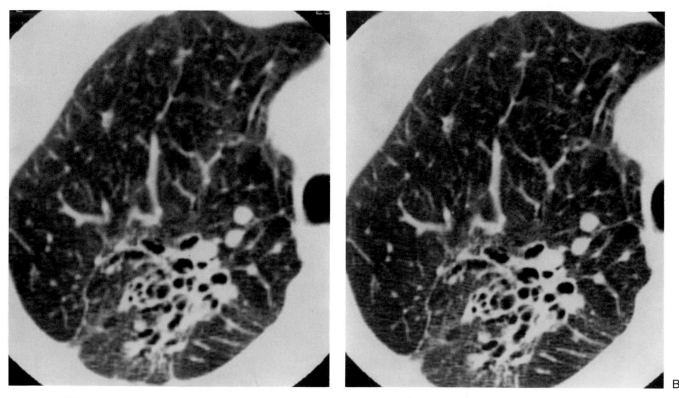

FIG. 1-10. Effect of targeted reconstruction on resolution. **A:** CT image in a patient with end-stage sarcoidosis obtained with a 38-cm FOV and 1.5-mm collimation, and reconstructed using the bone algorithm and a 38-cm reconstruction circle. **B:** The same CT scan has been reconstructed using a targeted field of view (15 cm), reducing image-pixel diameter. Image sharpness is improved as compared to A.

It should be emphasized that there are no "correct" or ideal window settings for the demonstration of lung anatomy, to be used when photographing a HRCT study. Often the precise window width and levels chosen are a matter of personal preference; the techniques indicated below should serve only as guidelines. However, it is important that at least one lung window setting be used consistently in all patients. Unless this is done, it is difficult to compare one case to another, develop an understanding of what appearances are normal and abnormal, and compare sequential examinations in the same patient. Although it is not inappropriate to use some different window settings in specific cases, depending on what is being sought, the effects of the variations in window settings on the appearance of the resulting images must be kept in mind.

The most important window setting to use in photography is the so-called lung window. Level and width settings of approximately −700/1000 Hounsfield Units (HU) would be appropriate for routine lung windows (Fig. 1-12). Some authors prefer using an extended window width of 1500 to 2000 HU when viewing the lung, but this reduces contrast between lung parenchymal structures such as vessels and bronchi, and the air-containing alveoli. On the other hand, extended windows can be of value in detecting abnormalities of overall lung attenuation (23,24), and are also useful in evaluating the relationship of peripheral parenchymal abnormalities to the pleural surfaces. Images with a window mean of −600 to −700 HU and an extended window width of 1500 HU are appropriate for routine lung windows. A window of −500 to −700/2000 HU could also be employed, and is particularly useful when pleuro-parenchymal abnormalities are being evaluated (Fig. 1-12H,I) (9,18). Window level/width settings of 50/350 are best for evaluating of the mediastinum, hila, and pleura, information sometimes of value in interpreting HRCT of the lung (Table 1-1).

As stated above, choosing different window levels can be advantageous in individual cases, but the effects of different windows on the appearance of the lung must be kept in mind (Fig. 1-12). Low-window settings (−800 to −900) with narrow-window widths (500) can be valuable in contrasting emphysema or air-filled cystic lesions with normal lung parenchyma. Quite simply, with such a low-window mean, normal lung parenchyma looks gray, while areas of emphysema remain black. On the other hand, using this same window to image the lung interstitium would be improper. Such a low-window mean, particularly combined with a narrow-window width, would make the lung interstitium appear much more prominent than it really is, and could make a normal case appear abnormal. This window would also result in an overestimation of the size of vessels, and an overestimation of bronchial wall thickness.

The use of an electronic workstation to view HRCT images has both advantages and disadvantages. Although it would seem that being able to vary window settings would be of value in diagnosis, this does not seem to be the case. In a recent study, viewing HRCT studies with a fixed-window (−500/2000 HU) setting proved to be more accurate than viewing them with operator-varied window settings (23).

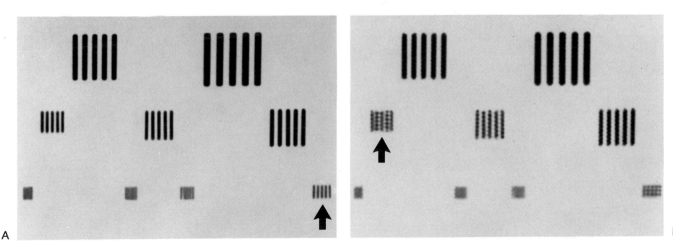

FIG. 1-11. Effect of targeted reconstruction on spatial resolution. **A:** HRCT of a line-pain phantom. The scan was obtained with a 40-cm FOV, and reconstructed using a targeted FOV of 25 cm. The resolution with this technique is 7.5-line pairs (*arrow*). **B:** The same scan viewed without targeting shows the effects of larger pixel size. Only 6-line pairs can be resolved (*arrow*) and the margins of the lines appear jagged or wavy. (From Mayo et al., ref. 11, with permission.)

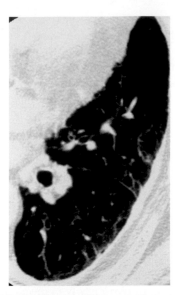

A. −500/1000 HU (window mean/window width)

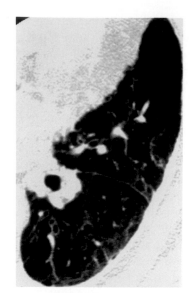

B. −600/1000 HU

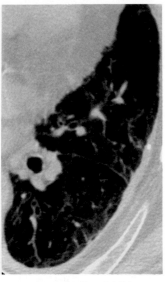

E. −500/1500 HU

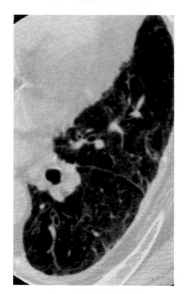

F. −600/1500 HU

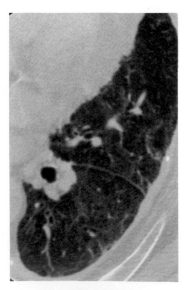

H. −500/2000 HU

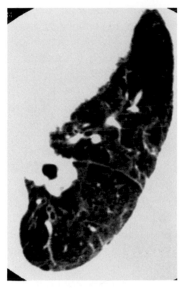

C. −700/1000 HU

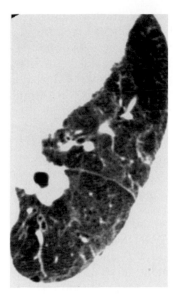

D. −800/1000 HU

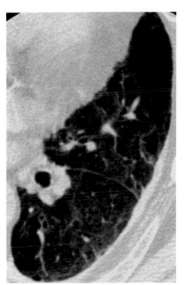

G. −700/1500 HU

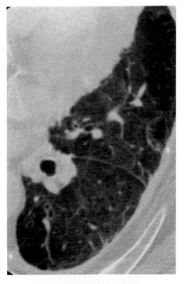

I. −700/2000 HU

FIG. 1-12. Effects of window mean and width on the appearance of lung and soft tissues in a patient with asbestosis. Window means decrease from left to right. Window widths increase from top to bottom. **A–D:** A window width of 1000 HU and a window mean of −700 HU (Fig. 1-10C) provides good contrast between soft tissue structures in the lung (vessels and interstitial abnormalities) and lung parenchyma, allows areas of lung with varying attenuation to be distinguished, and allows air-filled structures (bronchi, cysts, etc.) to be contrasted with lung parenchyma. Abnormal reticular opacities and areas of increased lung and decreased lung attenuation are all visible in Fig. 1-10C. Higher window means (Fig. 1-10A) make lung opacities more difficult to see or make them appear smaller. A lower window mean (Fig. 1-10D) accentuates the visibility of lung opacities and allows air-filled structures to be contrasted with lung parenchyma, but can also make normal lung appear abnormally dense. **E–G:** Wider window settings result in less contrast between soft tissue lung structures and lung parenchyma. Those images with window levels of −600 and −700 (Fig. 1-10F,G) and a width of 1500 HU provide information comparable to −700/1000 HU. **H,I:** With a window width of 2000 HU, much less contrast between normal and abnormal lung regions is visible. However, with this window setting, pleural thickening and calcification are visible.

Large images are much easier to read. A 6 on 1 format using 14 × 17 film is recommended for photography of lung window images in order to make the images large enough to view easily, particularly if both lungs are shown on the same slice. On smaller images subtle findings can be missed. A 12 on 1 format may be satisfactory for photography of images reconstructed with a small field of view, and are satisfactory for photographing soft-tissue window images.

Use of Spiral CT

The use of spiral or helical technique is not recommended for HRCT in patients with suspected diffuse lung disease. In most instances, HRCT obtained with a scanner capable of spiral or helical imaging should be performed without table motion, using thin (1 mm) collimation, a 1-sec scan time, and a high-resolution reconstruction algorithm. Obtaining scans with a spiral technique results in an increase in effective slice thickness, as compared to scans obtained without table motion, thus resulting in some loss of spatial resolution (25,26), although this effect may be minimal with proper technique (27). The ability to obtain contiguous slices during a single breath hold, as is possible using spiral CT, is not a major advantage in assessing most patients with diffuse lung disease; HRCT in patients with suspected diffuse lung disease involves a sampling of lung anatomy in different lung regions, and obtaining contiguous scans in a single lung region is not usually of diagnostic value.

The use of spiral HRCT is likely to be of more value in assessing patients with focal lung disease or lung nodules than it is in patients with diffuse lung disease (26). Obtaining a volumetric HRCT, with 1 or 2 cm being scanned using 1-mm collimation and a pitch of 1, would be of potential value in demonstrating the secondary lobular distribution of abnormalities in patients with diffuse lung disease, but this would seem to be of limited clinical utility (26). A recent study (28), assessed the utility of volumetric HRCT, obtained without helical technique. In this study, four contiguous HRCT scans were obtained at each of three locations (the aortic arch, carina, and 2-cm above the right hemidiaphragm) in 50 consecutive patients with interstitial lung disease or bronchiectasis. Each individual scan was analyzed for the presence of motion-induced artifacts or blurring, and the diagnostic information obtainable from each set of four scans was compared to that obtainable from the first scan in the set of 4. When the full set of 4 scans was considered instead of the first scan only, the number of scan levels having at least one motion-free scan increased 40%.

Although more findings of disease were identified

when the contiguous scans were used (28), it is likely that this improvement in sensitivity more likely reflects the number of scans viewed than the fact that they were obtained in contiguity. The sensitivity of the first scan as compared to the set of 4 was 84% for the detection of bronchiectasis, 97% for ground-glass opacity, 88% for honeycombing, 88% for septal thickening, and 86% for nodular opacities.

RADIATION DOSE ASSOCIATED WITH HRCT

One of the concerns often expressed regarding HRCT is the radiation dose involved. However, it has been made clear that HRCT as routinely performed results in a low-radiation dose as compared to conventional CT obtained with contiguous 1-cm collimation (29). Radiation doses at the breast skin surface for patients undergoing conventional chest CT with contiguous 10-mm collimation (140 kVp, 200 mAs) are approximately 20 mGy (milliGray) (30).

Initially, a study of contiguous HRCT scans reported the "upper limit" of the radiation dose that could be expected using this technique, as measured in the center of a 16-cm plastic phantom (11). In this study, contiguous HRCT scans resulted in a higher dose than contiguous scans with 10-mm collimation—1.5 mm scans (120 kVp, 300 mAs) resulted in a dose of 61 mGy, as compared to 55 mGy for contiguous 10-mm collimated scans obtained using the same technique. However, it is important to recognize that the measured radiation dose is affected by scatter and penumbra effects (30). These are greater with contiguous scans than with spaced scans, and it must be kept in mind that HRCT is normally performed using scans spaced at 1- or 2-cm intervals.

In a more recent study (29) the radiation dose to the chest associated with spaced HRCT scans was compared to the radiation dose produced by conventional CT. In this study, using a scan technique of 120 kVp, 200 mA, 2 sec, the mean skin radiation dose was 4.4 mGy for 1.5-mm HRCT scans at 10 mm-intervals, 2.1 mGy for scans at 20-mm intervals, and 36.3 mGy for conventional 10-mm scans at 10-mm intervals. Thus, HRCT scanning at 10- and 20-mm intervals, which is done in clinical imaging, results in 12% and 6%, respectively, of the radiation dose associated with conventional CT. It has also been pointed out, that obtaining low-dose HRCT (20 mA, 2 sec) (20) at 20-mm intervals would result in an average skin dose comparable to that administered with chest radiography (29). This has subsequently been confirmed by Lee et al. (21); the effective radiation dose of low-dose HRCT obtained at three levels, with 80 mAs is quite similar to that of chest radiographs (31,32).

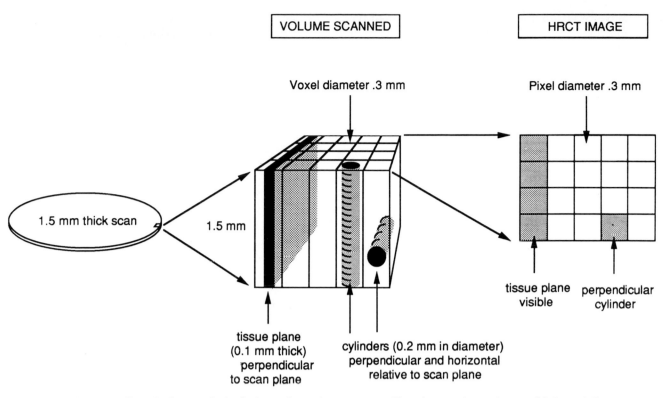

FIG. 1-13. Resolution and size/orientation of structures. The tissue plane, 1-mm thick and the perpendicular cylinder, 0.2 mm in diameter, are visible on the HRCT scan because they extend through the thickness of the scan volume or voxel. The horizontal cylinder cannot be seen.

SPATIAL RESOLUTION OF HRCT

There is a fundamental relationship between pixel size and the size of structures that can be resolved using CT. For optimal matching of image display to the attainable spatial resolution of the scanner, there should be two pixels for the smallest structure resolved (12). Current scanners are capable of providing scan data with a spatial resolution of 0.5 mm, equivalent to 10-line pairs per cm, with a FOV of 12.8 cm and a pixel size of 0.25 mm (11). Reducing pixel size further does not improve spatial resolution.

Structures smaller than the pixel size should be difficult to resolve on HRCT; however, this is sometimes possible. Interlobular septa as thin as 0.1 mm and arteries with a diameter of 0.3 mm are sometimes visible on HRCT using a small FOV. The reasons such small structures are visible include the large differences in attenuation between the soft tissue structures present in the lung and the air-filled alveoli surrounding them, and the use of a high-spatial frequency algorithm for reconstruction, which often results in some edge enhancement.

The ability of HRCT to resolve fine lung structures depends on their orientation relative to the scan plane (Fig. 1-13). Structures measuring 0.1 to 0.2 mm in thickness can be seen if they are largely oriented perpendicular to the scan plane, and extend through the thickness of the scan plane or voxel[1] (i.e., 1.5 mm) (10,11,33,34). Similarly sized structures (0.1 to 0.2 mm) that are oriented horizontally within the scan plane will not be visible because of volume averaging with the air-filled lung, which occupies most of the thickness of the voxel.

These limitations explain the visibility of various lung structures on HRCT. For example, HRCT can allow us to resolve some normal interlobular septa, which represent a plane of tissue approximately 100 to 200 μm or 0.1 to 0.2 mm in thickness, or small vessels, that are oriented perpendicular to the scan plane (Fig. 1-13) (10,33,34), whereas, vessels or septa lying in the plane of scan are usually visible as discrete structures only if they are larger or thicker than 0.3 to 0.5 mm. Bronchi or bronchioles measuring less than 2 to 3 cm in diameter and having a wall thickness of approximately 0.3 mm are usually invisible in peripheral lung because they have courses that lie roughly in the plane of scan. Bronchi or bronchioles of similar size are

---

[1]voxel = "volume element," or the volume of the patient that is represented by a specific pixel in the final image. In other words, it is equal to the pixel size multiplied by the scan thickness.

sometimes visible when oriented perpendicular to the plane of scan.

It should be kept in mind, that although soft tissue structures can be resolved when they are thinner or smaller than the pixel size, their apparent size in the final HRCT image will be determined by the pixel size and not by their actual dimensions. This can make the measurement of such small structures difficult on HRCT, and prone to inaccuracies.

ARTIFACTS ON HRCT

Several confusing artifacts can be seen on HRCT. However, familiarity with their appearances should eliminate potential misdiagnoses (9,11,35,36).

Streak Artifacts

Fine streak artifacts that radiate from the edges of sharply marginated, high-contrast structures such as bronchial walls, ribs, or vertebral bodies are common on HRCT. On HRCT, streak artifacts are often visible as fine, linear, or net-like opacities (Figs. 1-4,1-14,1-15), that can be seen anywhere, but are most common overlying the posterior lung, paralleling the pleural surface and posterior chest wall (11). Although streak artifacts degrade the image, they do not usually mimic pathology or cause confusion in image interpretation.

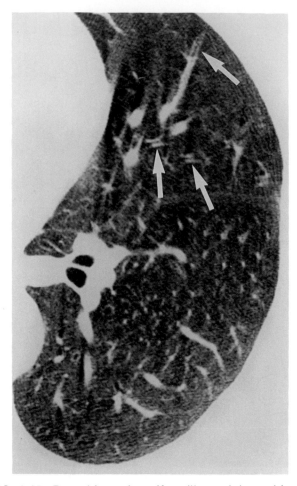

FIG. 1-15. Bronchiectasis artifact ("pseudobronchiectasis"). Several linear structures (*arrows*) appear double, mimicking bronchiectasis.

Streak artifacts are thinner and less dense than the normal or abnormal interstitium (interlobular septa) visible in this region, and have a different appearance. Streak artifacts can result from two separate mechanisms, "aliasing" and "correlated noise."

Aliasing is a geometric phenomenon that occurs because of undersampling of spatial information, and is related to detector spacing and scan collimation (12). As it is independent of radiation dose, increasing scan technique is of no value in reducing this type of artifact.

Correlated noise has a similar appearance and is most notable in the paravertebral regions, adjacent to the highly attenuating vertebral bodies (12). This type of artifact is strongly related to radiation dose, and can be minimized by increasing kVp and mAs.

Motion Artifacts

Pulsation or "star" artifacts are commonly visible, particularly at the left lung base, adjacent to the heart (Figs. 1-6,1-14,1-15). With pulsation artifacts, thin

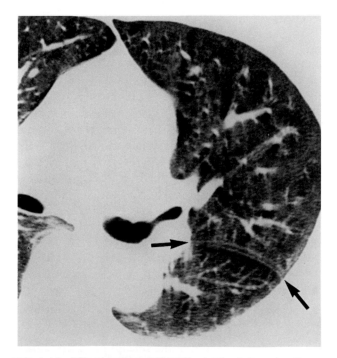

FIG. 1-14. "Double fissure" artifact. The left major fissure (*arrows*) appears to be double. Fine aliasing artifacts are visible posteriorly. Pulsation artifacts are also visible adjacent to the left heart border.

streaks radiate from the edges of vessels or other visible structures, which therefore resemble stars, and small areas of apparent lucency may be seen between these streaks. These lucent areas, if not recognized as artifactual, may be mistaken for dilated bronchi (36).

Also, the major fissure, usually on the left (Fig. 1-14), or other parenchymal structures such as vessels and bronchi, may be seen as double because of cardiac pulsation (35). This appearance can mimic bronchiectasis (Fig. 1-15). It results when a linear structure, such as the fissure or vessel, is in slightly different positions when scanned by the gantry from opposite directions (180 degrees apart) (Fig. 1-16). As with image noise, these artifacts are much more conspicuous when high-resolution techniques are used simply because they are more sharply resolved.

HRCT SCAN PROTOCOLS

In obtaining clinical studies, the inspiratory level, patient position, and scan spacing can be varied. This may be determined by the clinical setting. Scans obtained with thicker collimation (5 mm) and expiratory scans may also be of value in certain situations.

Inspiratory Level

Routine HRCT is obtained during suspended full inspiration. Selected scans obtained following or during forced expiration may also be valuable in diagnosing patients with obstructive lung disease or airway abnormalities. The use of expiratory HRCT will be discussed below, and in Chapter 3.

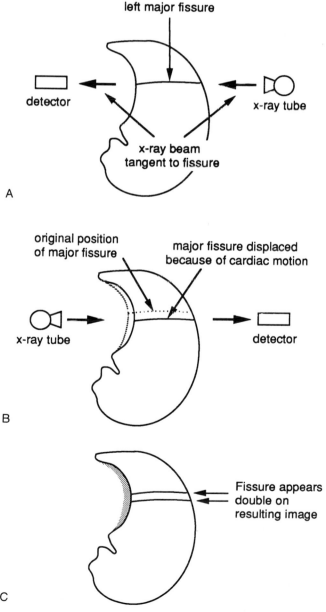

FIG. 1-16. Mechanism of "double fissure" artifact. The major fissure is "seen" by the scanner only when the x-ray beam is tangent to it. If the position of the fissure is slightly altered by cardiac pulsation during the period in which the gantry has rotated 180 degrees (**A,B**), it appears to be seen in two different locations on the resulting image (**C**).

Patient Position

Scans obtained with the patient supine are adequate in most instances. However, scans obtained with the patient prone are sometimes necessary for diagnosing subtle lung disease. Atelectasis is commonly seen in the dependent lung in both normal and abnormal subjects, resulting in a so-called dependent density or subpleural line (37). These normal findings can closely mimic the appearance of early lung fibrosis, and they can be impossible to distinguish from true pathology on supine scans alone. However, if scans are obtained in both supine and prone positions, "dependent density" can be easily differentiated from true pathology (Fig. 1-17); a true abnormality remains unchanged re-

gardless of whether it is dependent or nondependent. Normal "dependent density" disappears in the prone position.

Some investigators (18,38) obtain HRCT in the prone position only when dependent lung collapse is problematic (39); however, this approach requires that the scans be closely monitored, or that the patient be called back for additional scans. Others use prone scanning routinely; this approach has proven particularly valuable in detecting early lung fibrosis in patients with asbestos exposure (37,40).

It should be pointed out that dependent density results in a diagnostic dilemma only in patients who are normal or have subtle lung abnormalities. In patients with obvious abnormalities, such as honeycombing, or

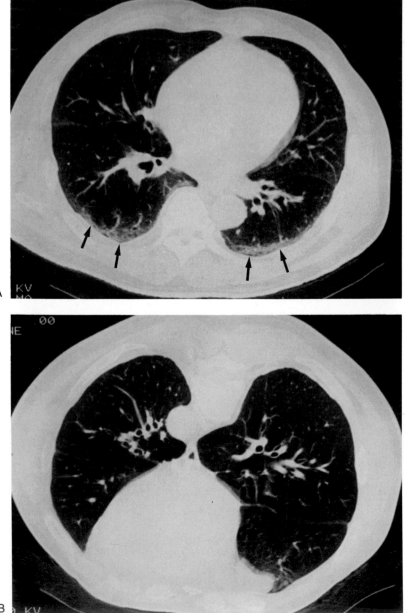

FIG. 1-17. Supine and prone scans with normal "dependent density." **A:** Supine scan in a normal patient shows an ill-defined opacity in the posterior aspect of both lungs (*arrows*). It is impossible to know whether this represents lung disease or is normal atelectasis. **B:** Prone scan done at this same level shows no evidence of an abnormality.

who have diffuse lung disease, dependent density is not a diagnostic problem. Thus, if the patient being studied has evidence of moderate to severe lung disease on plain radiographs, prone scans are likely to be unnecessary. On the other hand, if the patient is suspected of having an interstitial abnormality, and the plain radiograph is normal or near normal, or the results of chest radiographs are unknown, either the supine scan sequence must be closely monitored or prone scans should be obtained.

In patients who are suspected of having airways disease, such as bronchiectasis, or other obstructive lung diseases, dependent atelectasis is not usually a problem, and prone scans are not usually needed. It has been further suggested that, in patients with bronchiectasis, angling the gantry 20 degrees caudally (with the scan plane angled anteriorly and toward the feet) improves visibility of the segmental and subsegmental bronchi, by aligning them parallel to the plane of scan (41). This technique can prove valuable in assessing patients with bronchiectasis (42). However, in the vast majority of patients with bronchiectasis, HRCT without gantry angulation is sufficient for diagnosis.

Scan Spacing

Two fundamentally different approaches to HRCT have been used, at least partially determined by the indications for the scan. The first approach is to obtain HRCT at a few preselected levels, combined with a conventional CT study in which the entire thorax is imaged using contiguous 8- to 10-mm collimation scans (12,18,38). This technique is most appropriate when the primary indication for the study is an evaluation of the entire thorax; examples would include the detection of pulmonary metastases, the diagnosis of complex pleuro-parenchymal processes, or the staging of lung cancer. In these cases, the addition of a few HRCT scans may provide significant additional information. This technique has also been applied to patients with suspected diffuse lung disease, and has been shown to be clinically efficacious (38); HRCT scans obtained at the levels of the aortic arch, carina, and at a level 2-cm above the right hemidiaphragm allow the assessment of the lung regions in which lung biopsies are most frequently performed (12). Combining a few selected HRCT images with a conventional CT examination has also been recommended when first gaining experience with this technique (12).

The second approach is to obtain HRCT images only, in lieu of performing a conventional CT examination. Because HRCT is most often obtained to evaluate a patient suspected of having diffuse lung disease (9), scanning at a number of levels is desirable. With this approach, scans can be obtained at more levels, and

more of the lung can thus be imaged. The great majority of HRCT studies obtained in current clinical practice are obtained in this manner.

There has been no consensus as to how many scans are necessary for an adequate HRCT examination of the lung parenchyma. Different investigators have obtained HRCT scans at 1-cm, 2-cm, 3-cm , and even 4-cm intervals (9,39), at three preselected levels (38), or at one or two levels through the lower lungs (18). HRCT is performed for a variety of reasons, and to some extent, the number of scans obtained and their levels can vary depending on the clinical indications for the study. We wish to emphasize that there is no single *correct* HRCT protocol that should be used.

In choosing a sequence of HRCT scans to use in an individual patient, it is important to recognize that HRCT is usually intended to "sample" lung anatomy, with the presumptions being that a diffuse lung disease will be visible at one of the levels sampled, and that the findings seen at the levels scanned will be representative of what is present throughout the lung. We consider scans obtained at 1-cm intervals from the lung apices to bases to be the most appropriate routine scanning protocol, allowing a complete sampling of the lung and lung disease, regardless of its distribution. Obtaining scans at smaller intervals or obtaining contiguous scans is not necessary for diagnosis and would not be desirable because of the radiation dose involved.

In patients who are likely to require prone images, several prone scans can be added to the routine supine sequence obtained with 1-cm scan spacing; a reasonable protocol would include additional prone scans at 4-cm intervals. Alternatively, scans can be obtained at 2-cm intervals from lung apices to bases, in both supine and prone positions. Since the prone and supine images will be slightly different, even if obtained at the same level, the number of images obtained will be equivalent to a supine position scan protocol using 1-cm spacing.

It may sometimes be appropriate to customize the number or location of scans, depending on the patient's suspected disease, clinical findings, or the location of plain radiographic abnormalities. For example, if the lung disease being studied predominates in a certain region of lung, as determined by chest radiographs, conventional CT (18), or other imaging studies, it makes sense that more scans should be obtained in the most abnormal area. In patients with suspected asbestosis, it has been recommended that more scans be performed near the diaphragm than in the upper lobes, because of the typical basal distribution of this disease, even if the chest radiograph does not suggest an abnormality in this region (37,40).

Some support for this approach has been lent by a recent paper (43) describing theoretical methods useful in selecting the appropriate number of HRCT images necessary for estimating any quantitative parameter of lung disease; a marked reduction in the number of images necessary for quantification of a desired parameter can be achieved by using a stratified sampling technique based on prior knowledge of the disease distribution.

Recommended Protocols

The following protocols are provided as guides. At least to some extent, the scan protocol should be determined by the indications for the HRCT study. In patients suspected of having a fibrotic or restrictive lung disease on the basis of clinical, pulmonary function, or plain radiographic findings, it is appropriate to obtain HRCT scans at 1-cm intervals, with the patient supine. If the plain radiograph shows a distinct abnormality, prone scans will not likely be needed. However, if the chest radiograph appears normal or subtle lung disease is present, the scans should be monitored for the presence of problematic dependent opacity, or additional prone scans should be obtained. In patients suspected of having restrictive or fibrotic lung disease, or having a diffuse lung disease of unknown type, scans at 2-cm intervals, in both supine and prone positions can be obtained routinely, and monitoring scans will not be necessary (Table 1-2).

In patients suspected of having airways or obstructive disease on the basis of clinical, pulmonary function, or plain radiographic findings, HRCT should be obtained at full inspiration, at 1-cm intervals from lung apices to bases, and with the patient supine (Table 1-2); prone scans are not usually needed. This protocol has been recommended by Grenier for studying patients with suspected bronchiectasis (44). Scans following forced expiration can also be valuable in such patients.

In patients who present with hemoptysis, possibly related to airway abnormalities or an endobronchial lesion, it has been recommended that CT be obtained with 5-mm collimated scans at 5-mm intervals through the hila, in order to allow evaluation of the central bronchi, with HRCT at 1-cm intervals through the remainder of the lung parenchyma to look for bronchiectasis or other airway abnormalities (45,46).

Use of Expiratory CT

Recently, CT scans performed during or following expiration have been used to demonstrate air trapping in patients with diseases associated with airway abnormalities or findings of obstruction on pulmonary function tests. The use of expiratory CT has been reported in patients with emphysema (47), asthma, the Swyer-James syndrome (48,49), the cystic lung diseases associated with histiocytosis X and tuberous sclerosis (50),

TABLE 1-2. *Summary of recommended HRCT technique: scan protocols*

Suspected Restrictive or Fibrotic Lung Disease, or Diffuse Lung Disease of Unknown Type

Chest Radiograph Abnormal
Full inspiration.
Supine scans with 1-cm spacing from lung apices to bases.

Chest Radiograph Normal or Minimally Abnormal
Option 1: Full inspiration.
Supine scans with 1-cm spacing from lung apices to bases; monitor scans for "dependent density," or obtain additional prone scans with 4-cm spacing or at three levels (aortic arch, carina, 2-cm above right hemidiaphragm).

Option 2: Full inspiration.
Scans with 2-cm spacing in both prone and supine positions.

Suspected Airways Disease or Obstructive Lung Disease

Full inspiration.
Supine scans with 1-cm spacing from lung apices to bases.
Option 1: Expiratory scans at three levels (aortic arch, carina, 2-cm above right hemidiaphragm).
Option 2: 20° gantry angulation.

Patients with Hemoptysis

Full inspiration.
Supine scans with contiguous 5-mm collimation through the hila and HRCT with 1-cm spacing at other levels.

and in patients with a variety of causes of large and small airway obstruction (51,52). In normal subjects, in most lung regions, lung parenchyma increases uniformly in attenuation during expiration (6,53–57), but in the presence of air trapping, lung parenchyma remains lucent on expiration and shows little change in volume. On expiratory scans visible differences in attenuation between normal and obstructed lung regions are visible using standard lung window settings, and can be quantitated using regions of interest (ROI). Differences in attenuation between normal lung regions and regions that show air trapping often measure more than 100 HU (51,56). The use of expiratory HRCT is discussed in detail in Chapter 3.

In patients with obstructive lung disease, airways disease, or emphysema, HRCT scans obtained during suspended respiration, following forced expiration, can show evidence of air trapping in the absence of morphologic abnormalities recognizable on inspiratory HRCT scans. Expiratory scans at three selected levels (aortic arch, hila, lower lobes) are generally sufficient for showing significant air trapping when present, and are used routinely by one of us, in addition to an inspiratory scan series in patients with suspected airways

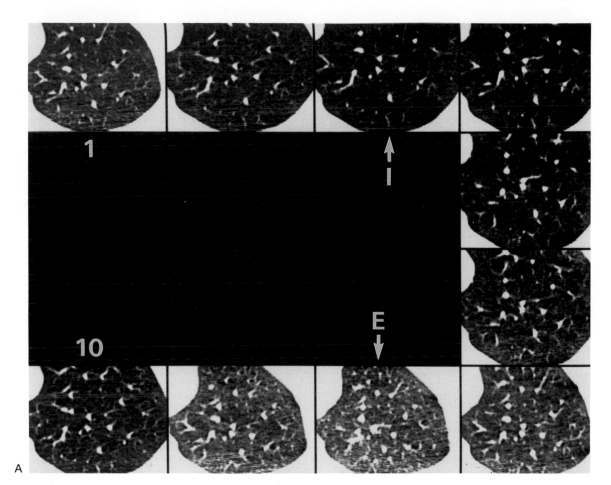

A

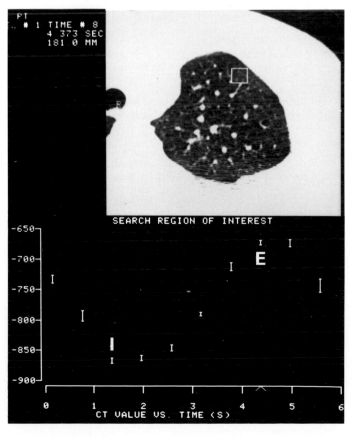

B

FIG. 1-18. DUHRCT during expiration in a normal subject. **A:** The 10-image DUHRCT sequence acquired during a single forced vital capacity maneuver is shown, with the field of view is limited to the left upper lobe. These ten 100 msec images were obtained at 600 msec intervals. They are shown in sequence, in a clockwise fashion, from the left upper corner (1) to the lower left corner (10). Images at full inspiration (I) and full expiration (E) are visible. Note the increase in lung attenuation and decrease in lung volume that occurs as the subject exhales. As in most normal subjects, lung attenuation increase on expiration is relatively homogeneous. **B:** A time-attenuation curve is produced by measuring the mean lung attenuation (HU) for a specific ROI. In this subject, for an ROI in the anterior lung, attenuation decreases to approximately −870 HU at maximum inspiration (I) and increases in attenuation to −670 HU at maximum expiration (E) for an overall attenuation increase of approximately 200 HU. Each point on the time-attenuation curve represents one image from the dynamic sequence. (From Webb et al., ref. 56, with permission.)

or obstructive lung diseases. In obtaining expiratory HRCT, the patient is instructed to forcefully exhale and then hold his or her breath for the duration of the single scan obtained. This maneuver is practiced with the patient before the scans are obtained, to ensure an adequate level of expiration.

It is not necessary to measure or control lung volume when obtaining expiratory scans if patient compliance has been assured. However, some investigators have used CT scans gated to spirometry (58,59). With this method, the patient breathes through a microcomputer-controlled pocket spirometer during the CT examination. At a user-selected respiratory level, the CT scan is triggered and air flow is mechanically inhibited (58,59). With this method, reproducible measurements of lung attenuation are possible at varying lung volumes (58,59).

A technique termed dynamic ultrafast high-resolution CT (DUHRCT) has also been shown to be valuable in the diagnosis of air-trapping (50,51,60). With DUHRCT, a series of fast HRCT scans are rapidly obtained as the patient forcefully exhales, in order to demonstrate dynamic abnormalities of lung attenuation and morphology that result from air-trapping (52). DUHRCT studies have been performed using an ultrafast electron-beam CT scanner that is capable of obtaining HRCT images with a 100 msec scan time (3-mm collimation, 150 kVp, 650 mA) (50,61). In general, when performing DUHRCT using this machine, the imaging sequence consists of 10 slices obtained during a 6-sec period, as the patient performs a forced inspiratory and expiratory vital capacity maneuver (Fig. 1-18). Little motion-related image degradation is visible because of the very rapid scan time employed (50,61). It may also be possible to adapt cine helical HRCT techniques to performing dynamic expiratory CT.

As with static expiratory scans, the dynamic scan sequence is viewed with attention to changes in lung attenuation and regional lung volume during the forced expiration. Air trapping is considered to be present when the lung fails to increase normally in attenuation during exhalation (50–52). The image sequence can be analyzed quantitatively as well as qualitatively. The mean HU attenuation for a specific ROI in the lung can be measured and plotted for each scan, producing a time-attenuation curve graphically demonstrating the changes in lung attenuation that have occurred during the single expiration and inspiration (Fig. 1-18B) (50). This use of DUHRCT is discussed further in Chapters 2 and 3.

REFERENCES

1. Naidich DP. Pulmonary parenchymal high-resolution CT: to be or not to be. *Radiology* 1989;171:22–24.
2. Siegelman SS, Zerhouni EA, Leo FP, Khouri NF, Stitik FP. CT of the solitary pulmonary nodule. *AJR* 1980;135:1–13.
3. Todo G, Itoh H, Nakano Y, et al. High-resolution CT for the evaluation of pulmonary peripheral disorders. *Jpn J Clin Radiol* 1982;27:1319–1326.
4. Nakata H, Kimoto T, Nakayama T, Kido M, Miyazaki N, Harada S. Diffuse peripheral lung disease: evaluation by high-resolution computed tomography. *Radiology* 1985;157:181–185.
5. Naidich DP, Zerhouni EA, Hutchins GM, Genieser NB, McCauley DI, Siegelman SS. Computed tomography of the pulmonary parenchyma. Part 1: distal air-space disease. *J Thorac Imaging* 1985;1(1):39–53.
6. Zerhouni EA, Naidich DP, Stitik FP, Khouri NF, Siegelman SS. Computed tomography of the pulmonary parenchyma. Part 2: interstitial disease. *J Thorac Imaging* 1985;1(1):54–64.
7. Müller NL, Miller RR. Computed tomography of chronic diffuse infiltrative lung disease: part 1. *Am Rev Respir Dis* 1990;142:1206–1215.
8. Müller NL, Miller RR. Computed tomography of chronic diffuse infiltrative lung disease: part 2. *Am Rev Respir Dis* 1990;142:1440–1448.
9. Webb WR. High-resolution CT of the lung parenchyma. *Radiol Clin North Am* 1989;27:1085–1097.
10. Zerhouni E. Computed tomography of the pulmonary parenchyma: an overview. *Chest* 1989;95:901–907.
11. Mayo JR, Webb WR, Gould R, et al. High-resolution CT of the lungs: an optimal approach. *Radiology* 1987;163:507–510.
12. Mayo JR. High resolution computed tomography: technical aspects. *Radiol Clin North Am* 1991;29:1043–1049.
13. Mayo JR. The high-resolution computed tomography technique. *Semin Roentgenol* 1991;26:104–109.
14. Murata K, Khan A, Rojas KA, Herman PG. Optimization of computed tomography technique to demonstrate the fine structure of the lung. *Invest Radiol* 1988;23:170–175.
15. Webb WR, Gamsu G, Wall SD, Cann CE, Proctor E. CT of a bronchial phantom: factors affecting appearance and size measurements. *Invest Radiol* 1984;19:394–398.
16. Zwirewich CV, Terriff B, Müller NL. High-spatial-frequency (bone) algorithm improves quality of standard CT of the thorax. *AJR* 1989;153:1169–1173.
17. Naidich DP, Marshall CH, Gribbin C, Arams RS, McCauley DI. Low-dose CT of the lungs: preliminary observations. *Radiology* 1990;175:729–731.
18. Murata K, Khan A, Herman PG. Pulmonary parenchymal disease: evaluation with high-resolution CT. *Radiology* 1989;170:629–635.
19. Remy-Jardin M, Giraud F, Remy J, Wattinne L, Wallaert B, Duhamel A. Pulmonary sarcoidosis: role of CT in the evaluation of disease activity and functional impairment and in prognosis assessment. *Radiology* 1994;191:675–680.
20. Zwirewich CV, Mayo JR, Müller NL. Low-dose high-resolution CT of lung parenchyma. *Radiology* 1991;180:413–417.
21. Lee KS, Primack SL, Staples CA, Mayo JR, Aldrich JE, Müller NL. Chronic infiltrative lung disease: comparison of diagnostic accuracies of radiography and low- and conventional-dose thin-section CT. *Radiology* 1994;191:669–673.
22. Majorin ML, Varpula M, Kurki T, Pakkala L. High-resolution CT of the lung in asbestos-exposed subjects. Comparison of low-dose and high-dose HRCT. *Acta Radiologica* 1994;35:473–477.
23. Maguire WM, Herman PG, Khan A, et al. Comparison of fixed and adjustable window width and level settings in the CT evaluation of diffuse lung disease. *J Comput Assist Tomogr* 1993;17:847–852.
24. Remy-Jardin M, Remy J, Giraud F, Wattinne L, Gosselin B. Computed tomography assessment of ground-glass opacity: semiology and significance. *J Thorac Imaging* 1993;8:249–264.
25. Kalender WA, Seissler W, Klotz E, Vock P. Spiral volumetric CT with single-breath-hold technique, continuous transport, and continuous scanner rotation. *Radiology* 1990;176:181–183.
26. Vock P, Soucek M. Spiral computed tomography in the assessment of focal and diffuse lung disease. *J Thorac Imaging* 1993; 8:283–290.
27. Paranjpe DV, Bergin CJ. Spiral CT of the lungs: optimal tech-

nique and resolution compared with conventional CT. *AJR* 1994; 162:561–567.

28. Engeler CE, Tashjian JH, Engeler SCM, Giese RA, Holm JC, Ritenour ER. Volumetric high-resolution CT in the diagnosis of interstitial lung disease and bronchiectasis: diagnostic accuracy and radiation dose. *AJR* 1994;163:31–35.

29. Mayo JR, Jackson SA, Müller NL. High-resolution CT of the chest: radiation dose. *AJR* 1993;160:479–481.

30. Evans SH, Davis R, Cooke J, Anderson W. A comparison of radiation doses to the breast in computed tomographic chest examinations for two scanning protocols. *Clin Radiol* 1989;40: 45–46.

31. Reuter FG, Conway BJ, McCrohan ML, Suleiman OH. Average radiation exposure values for three diagnostic radiographic examinations. *Radiology* 1990;177:341–345.

32. Müller NL. Clinical value of high-resolution CT in chronic diffuse lung disease. *AJR* 1991;157:1163–1170.

33. Webb WR, Stein MG, Finkbeiner WE, Im JG, Lynch D, Gamsu G. Normal and diseased isolated lungs: high-resolution CT. *Radiology* 1988;166:81–87.

34. Murata K, Itoh H, Todo G, et al. Centrilobular lesions of the lung: demonstration by high-resolution CT and pathologic correlation. *Radiology* 1986;161:641–645.

35. Mayo JR, Müller NL, Henkelman RM. The double-fissure sign: a motion artifact on thin-section CT scans. *Radiology* 1987;165: 580–581.

36. Tarver RD, Conces DJ, Godwin JD. Motion artifacts on CT simulate bronchiectasis. *AJR* 1988;151:1117–1119.

37. Aberle DR, Gamsu G, Ray CS, Feuerstein IM. Asbestos-related pleural and parenchymal fibrosis: detection with high-resolution CT. *Radiology* 1988;166:729–734.

38. Mathieson JR, Mayo JR, Staples CA, Müller NL. Chronic diffuse infiltrative lung disease: comparison of diagnostic accuracy of CT and chest radiography. *Radiology* 1989;171:111– 116.

39. Swensen SJ, Aughenbaugh GL, Brown LR. High-resolution computed tomography of the lung. *Mayo Clin Proc* 1989;64: 1284–1294.

40. Aberle DR, Gamsu G, Ray CS. High-resolution CT of benign asbestos-related diseases: clinical and radiographic correlation. *AJR* 1988;151:883–891.

41. Remy-Jardin M, Remy J. Comparison of vertical and oblique CT in evaluation of the bronchial tree. *J Comput Assist Tomogr* 1988;12:956–962.

42. Grenier P, Cordeau MP, Beigelman C. High-resolution computed tomography of the airways. *J Thorac Imaging* 1993;8: 213–229.

43. Henschke CI. Image selection for computed tomography of the chest: a sampling approach. *Invest Radiol* 1992;27:908–911.

44. Grenier P, Maurice F, Musset D, Menu Y, Nahum H. Bronchiectasis: assessment by thin-section CT. *Radiology* 1986;161: 95–99.

45. Naidich DP, Funt S, Ettenger NA, Arranda C. Hemoptysis: CT-bronchoscopic correlations in 58 cases. *Radiology* 1990;177: 357– 362.

46. Set PAK, Flower CDR, Smith IE, Cahn AP, Twentyman OP, Shneerson JM. Hemoptysis: comparative study of the role of CT and fiberoptic bronchoscopy. *Radiology* 1993;189:677–680.

47. Knudson RJ, Standen JR, Kaltenborn WT, et al. Expiratory computed tomography for assessment of suspected pulmonary emphysema. *Chest* 1991;99:1357–1366.

48. Marti-Bonmati L, Ruiz PF, Catala F, Mata JM, Calonge E. CT findings in Swyer-James syndrome. *Radiology* 1989;172: 477–480.

49. Moore ADA, Godwin JD, Dietrich PA, Verschakelen JA, Henderson WR. Swyer-James syndrome: CT findings in eight patients. *AJR* 1992;158:1211–1215.

50. Stern EJ, Webb WR, Golden JA, Gamsu G. Cystic lung disease associated with eosinophilic granuloma and tuberous sclerosis: air trapping at dynamic ultrafast high-resolution CT. *Radiology* 1992;182:325–329.

51. Stern EJ, Webb WR, Gamsu G. Dynamic quantitative computed tomography: a predictor of pulmonary function in obstructive lung diseases. *Invest Radiol* 1994;29:564–569.

52. Stern EJ, Webb WR. Dynamic imaging of lung morphology with ultrafast high-resolution computed tomography. *J Thorac Imaging* 1993;8:273–282.

53. Vock P, Malanowski D, Tschaeppeler H, Kirks DR, Hedlund LW, Effmann EL. Computed tomographic lung density in children. *Invest Radiol* 1987;22:627–631.

54. Robinson PJ, Kreel L. Pulmonary tissue attenuation with computed tomography: comparison of inspiration and expiration scans. *J Comput Assist Tomogr* 1979;3:740–748.

55. Millar AB, Denison DM. Vertical gradients of lung density in healthy supine men. *Thorax* 1989;44:485–490.

56. Webb WR, Stern EJ, Kanth N, Gamsu G. Dynamic pulmonary CT: findings in normal adult men. *Radiology* 1993;186:117–124.

57. Verschakelen JA, Van Fraeyenhoven L, Laureys G, Demedts M, Baert AL. Differences in CT density between dependent and nondependent portions of the lung: influence of lung volume. *AJR* 1993;161:713–717.

58. Kalender WA, Rienmuller R, Seissler W, Behr J, Welke M, Fichte H. Measurement of pulmonary parenchymal attenuation: use of spirometric gating with quantitative CT. *Radiology* 1990; 175:265–268.

59. Kalender WA, Fichte H, Bautz W, Skalej M. Semiautomatic evaluation procedures for quantitative CT of the lung. *J Comput Assist Tomogr* 1991;15:248–255.

60. Stern EJ, Webb WR, Warnock ML, Salmon CJ. Bronchopulmonary sequestration: dynamic, ultrafast, high-resolution CT evidence of air trapping. *AJR* 1991;157:947–949.

61. Lynch DA, Brasch RC, Hardy KA, Webb WR. Pediatric pulmonary disease: assessment with high-resolution ultrafast CT. *Radiology* 1990;176:243–248.

TWO

Normal Lung Anatomy

The accurate interpretation of high-resolution CT (HRCT) images requires a detailed understanding of normal lung anatomy and of the pathologic alterations in normal lung anatomy that occur in the presence of disease (1–4). In this chapter, only those aspects of lung anatomy that are important in using and interpreting HRCT will be reviewed.

THE LUNG INTERSTITIUM

The lung is supported by a network of connective tissue fibers, called the lung interstitium. Although the lung interstitium is not generally visible on HRCT in normal subjects, interstitial thickening is often recognizable. For the purpose of interpretation of HRCT and the identification of abnormal findings, the interstitium can be thought of as having several components (Fig. 2-1) (5).

The *peribronchovascular interstitium* is a system of fibers that invests bronchi and pulmonary arteries (Fig. 2-1). In the parahilar regions the peribronchovascular interstitium forms a strong connective tissue sheath that surrounds large bronchi and arteries. The more peripheral continuum of this interstitial fiber system, associated with small centrilobular bronchioles and arteries, is usually termed the *centrilobular interstitium*, although the term *centrilobular peribronchovascular interstitium* would also be appropriate (Fig. 2-1). Taken together, the peribronchovascular interstitium and centrilobular interstitium correspond to the "axial fiber system" described by Weibel, which extends peripherally from the pulmonary hila to the level of the alveolar ducts and sacs (5).

The *subpleural interstitium*, is located beneath the visceral pleura, and envelopes the lung in a fibrous sac from which connective tissue septa penetrate into the

THE LUNG INTERSTITIUM

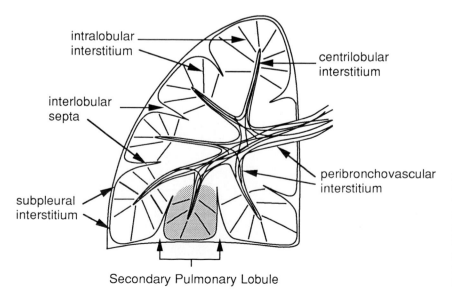

Secondary Pulmonary Lobule

FIG. 2-1. Components of the lung interstitium. Taken together, the peribronchovascular interstitium and centrilobular interstitium correspond to the "axial fiber system" described by Weibel (5). The subpleural interstitium and interlobular septa correspond to Weibel's "peripheral fiber system." The intralobular interstitium is roughly equivalent to the "septal fibers" described by Weibel.

lung parenchyma (Fig. 2-1). These septa include the *interlobular septa*, which are described in detail below. The subpleural interstitium and interlobular septa are both parts of the "peripheral fiber system" described by Weibel (5).

The *intralobular interstitium* is a network of thin fibers that forms a fine connective tissue mesh in the walls of alveoli, and thus bridges the gap between the centrilobular interstitium in the center of lobules, and the interlobular septa and subpleural interstitium in the lobular periphery (Fig. 2-1). Together, the intralobular interstitium, peribronchovascular interstitium, centrilobular interstitium, subpleural interstitium, and interlobular septa form a continuous fiber skeleton for the

lung (Fig. 2-1). The intralobular interstitium corresponds to the "septal fibers" described by Weibel (5).

LARGE BRONCHI AND ARTERIES

Within the lung parenchyma, the bronchi and pulmonary artery branches are closely associated and branch in parallel. As indicated above, they are encased by the peribronchovascular interstitium, which extends from the pulmonary hila into the peripheral lung. Since some lung diseases produce thickening of the peribronchovascular interstitium in the central or parahilar lung, in relation to large bronchi and pulmonary vessels, it

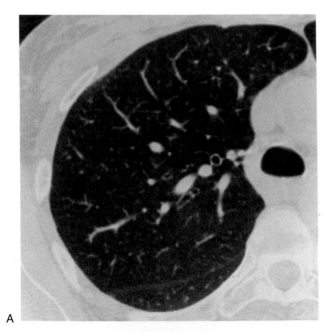

A

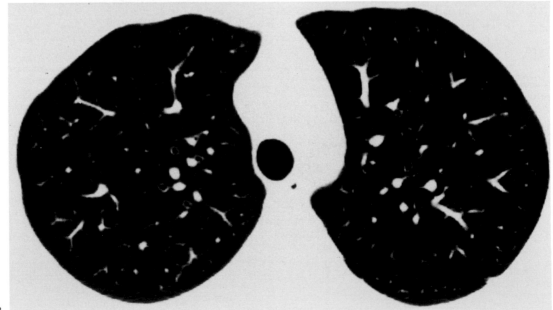

B

FIG. 2-2. Normal appearances of large bronchi and arteries photographed with window settings of −600/2000 HU (**A**) and −700/1000 HU (**B**). The diameters of vessels and their neighboring bronchi are approximately equal. The outer walls of bronchi and pulmonary vessels are smooth and sharply defined. Bronchi are invisible within the peripheral 2 cm of lung despite the fact that vessels are well seen in this region.

TABLE 2-1. *Relation of airway diameter to wall thickness*

	Diameter (mm)	Wall thickness (mm)
Lobar and segmental bronchi	5–8	1.5
Subsegmental bronchi/ bronchiole	1.5–3	0.2–0.3
Lobular bronchiole	1	0.15
Terminal bronchiole	0.7	0.1
Acinar bronchiole	0.5	0.05

From Weibel, ref. 9.

is important to be aware of the normal HRCT appearances of the parahilar bronchi and pulmonary vessels.

When imaged at an angle to their longitudinal axis, central pulmonary arteries normally appear as rounded or elliptic opacities on HRCT, accompanied by uniformly thin-walled bronchi of similar shape (Fig. 2-2). When imaged along their axis, bronchi and vessels should appear roughly cylindric, or show slight tapering as they branch, depending on the length of the segment that is visible; tapering of a vessel or bronchus is most easily seen when a long segment is visible.

The diameter of an artery and its neighboring bronchus should be approximately equal, although vessels may appear slightly larger than their accompanying bronchus, particularly in dependent lung regions. Although the presence of bronchi larger than their adjacent arteries is often assumed to indicate bronchial dilatation, or bronchiectasis, bronchi may appear larger than adjacent arteries in a significant number of normal subjects. In a HRCT study of normal subjects, Lynch et al. (6) compared the internal diameters of lobar, segmental, subsegmental, and smaller bronchi to those of adjacent artery branches. Nineteen percent of bronchi had an internal bronchial diameter greater than the artery diameter, and 59% of normal subjects showed at least one such bronchus.

The outer walls of visible pulmonary artery branches form a smooth and sharply defined interface with the surrounding lung, whether they are seen in cross-section or along their length. The walls of large bronchi, outlined by lung on one side, and air in the bronchial lumen on the other, should appear to be smooth and of uniform thickness. Thickening of the peribronchial and perivascular interstitium can result in irregularity of the interface between arteries and bronchi and the adjacent lung (4,7).

Assessment of bronchial wall thickness on HRCT is quite subjective, and is dependent on the window settings used (6). Also, since the apparent thickness of

the bronchial wall represents not only the wall itself, but the surrounding peribronchovascular interstitium as well, peribronchovascular interstitial thickening can result in apparent bronchial wall thickening (so-called peribronchial cuffing) on HRCT.

The wall thickness of conducting bronchi and bronchioles is approximately proportional to their diameter, at least for bronchi distal to the segmental level. In general, the thickness of the wall of a bronchus or bronchiole less than 5 mm in diameter should measure from $\frac{1}{6}$ to $\frac{1}{10}$ of its diameter (Table 2-1) (8); however, precise measurement of the wall thickness of small bronchi or bronchioles is difficult as wall thickness approximates pixel size.

Because bronchi taper and become thinner walled as they branch, and thus become more difficult to see as they become more peripheral. Bronchi less than 2 mm in diameter, and closer than 2 cm to the pleural surface are not normally visible on HRCT (Figs. 2-2, 2-3) (10,11).

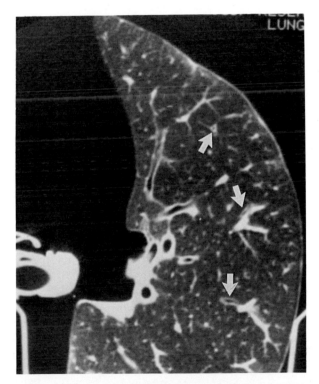

FIG. 2-3. Normal appearances of large bronchi and arteries. In an isolated lung, the smallest bronchi visible (*arrows*) measures approximately 2 to 3 mm in diameter. Thus, bronchi are not visible within the peripheral 2 to 3 cm of lung, although the artery branches that accompany these bronchi are sharply seen. [Note: The "isolated" lungs illustrated in this volume are fresh lungs obtained at autopsy and scanned while inflated with air at a pressure of approximately 30 cm of water (10).]

THE SECONDARY PULMONARY LOBULE

The *secondary pulmonary lobule*, as defined by Miller, refers to the smallest unit of lung structure marginated by connective tissue septa (8,12). Secondary lobules are easily visible on the surface of the lung because of these septa (Fig. 2-4) (8,13). The terms *secondary pulmonary lobule, secondary lobule*, and *pulmonary lobule* are often used interchangeably, and are used as synonymous in this book. The term *primary pulmonary lobule* has also been used by Miller to describe a much smaller lung unit associated with a single alveolar duct (13,14), but this designation is not in common use.

Secondary pulmonary lobules are irregularly polyhedral in shape and somewhat variable in size, measuring approximately 1 to 2.5 cm in diameter in most locations (Fig. 2-5A,B) (5,8,13,15,16). In one study, the average diameter of pulmonary lobules measured in several adults ranged from 11 to 17 mm (15). Each secondary lobule is supplied by a small bronchiole and pulmonary artery, and is variably marginated, in different lung regions, by connective tissue interlobular septa that contain pulmonary vein and lymphatic branches (13).

Secondary pulmonary lobules are made up of a limited number of pulmonary acini, usually a dozen or fewer, although the reported number varies considerably in different studies (Fig. 2-5A) (9,17); in a study by

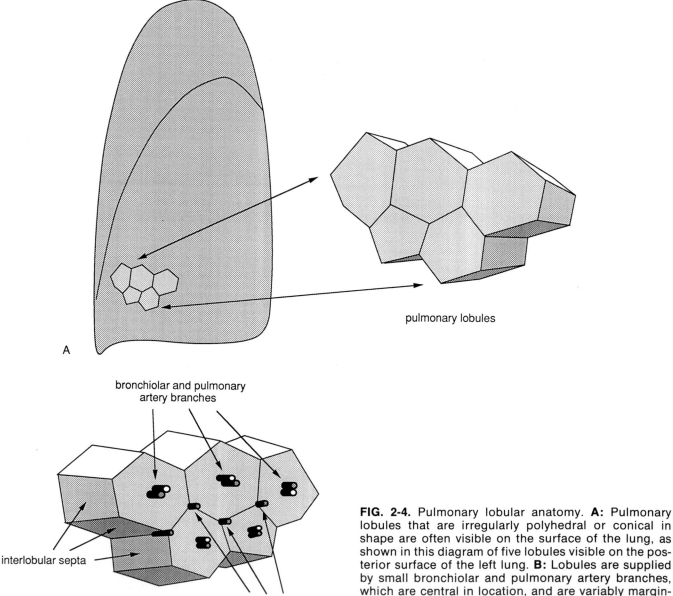

pulmonary lobules

bronchiolar and pulmonary artery branches

interlobular septa

pulmonary vein branches

FIG. 2-4. Pulmonary lobular anatomy. **A:** Pulmonary lobules that are irregularly polyhedral or conical in shape are often visible on the surface of the lung, as shown in this diagram of five lobules visible on the posterior surface of the left lung. **B:** Lobules are supplied by small bronchiolar and pulmonary artery branches, which are central in location, and are variably marginated by connective tissue interlobular septa that contain pulmonary vein and lymphatic branches.

Nishimura and Itoh (18), the number of acini counted in lobules of varying sizes ranged from 3 to 24. A pulmonary acinus is defined as the portion of the lung parenchyma distal to a terminal bronchiole and supplied by a first order respiratory bronchiole or bronchioles (17). Since respiratory bronchioles are the largest airways that have alveoli in their walls, an acinus is the largest lung unit in which all airways participate in gas exchange. Acini are usually described as ranging from 6 to 10 mm in diameter (15,19).

As indicated above, Miller has defined the secondary lobule as the smallest lung unit marginated by connective tissue septa. Reid has suggested an alternate definition of the secondary pulmonary lobule, based on the branching pattern of peripheral bronchioles, rather than the presence and location of connective tissue

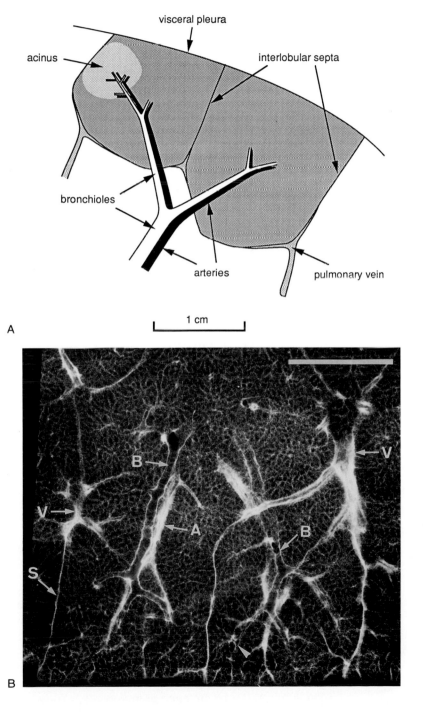

FIG. 2-5. **A:** Anatomy of the secondary pulmonary lobule, as defined by Miller. Two adjacent lobules are shown in this diagram. **B:** Radiographic anatomy of the secondary pulmonary lobule. Radiograph of a 1-mm lung slice taken from the lower lobe. Two well-defined secondary pulmonary lobules are visible. Lobules are marginated by thin interlobular septa (*S*) containing pulmonary vein (*V*) branches. Bronchioles (*B*) and pulmonary arteries (*A*) are centrilobular. Bar = 1 cm. (Courtesy of Harumi Itoh, M.D., Chest Research Institute, Kyoto University, Kyoto, Japan. Reprinted from Itoh et al., ref. 18, with permission.)

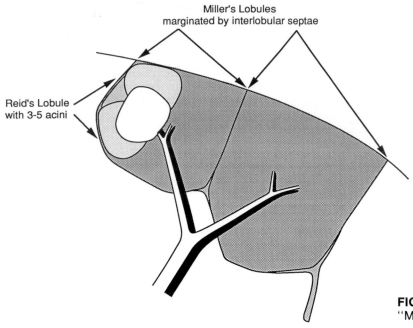

Miller's Lobules
marginated by interlobular septae

Reid's Lobule
with 3-5 acini

FIG. 2-6. Relative size and relationships of "Miller's lobule" and "Reid's lobule."

septa (Fig. 2-6) (13,17,20). On bronchograms, small bronchioles can be seen to arise at intervals of 5 to 10 mm from larger airways, the so-called centimeter pattern of branching; these small bronchioles then show branching at approximately 2-mm intervals, the "millimeter pattern" (20). Airways showing the millimeter pattern of branching are considered by Reid to be intralobular, with each branch corresponding to a terminal bronchiole (17). Lobules are considered to be the lung units supplied by 3 to 5 "millimeter pattern" bronchioles. Although Reid's criteria delineate lung units of approximately equal size, about 1 cm in diameter and containing 3 to 5 acini, it should be noted, that this definition does not necessarily describe lung units equivalent to secondary lobules as defined by Miller and marginated by interlobular septa (Fig. 2-6) (17,18), although a small Miller's lobule can be the same as a Reid's lobule. Miller's definition is most applicable to the interpretation of HRCT, and is widely accepted by pathologists because interlobular septa are visible on histologic sections (18). In this book, we use the term *secondary pulmonary lobule* to refer to a lobule as defined by Miller.

Anatomy of the Secondary Lobule and Its Components

An understanding of secondary lobular anatomy, and the appearances of lobular structures, are key to the interpretation of HRCT. HRCT can show many features of the secondary pulmonary lobule in both normal and abnormal lungs, and, many lung diseases, particularly interstitial diseases, produce some characteristic changes in lobular structures (3,4,7,10,11, 21,22). Heitzman has been instrumental in emphasizing the importance of the secondary pulmonary lobule in the radiologic diagnosis of lung disease (13,23,24).

As discussed in Chapter 1, the visibility of normal lobular structures on HRCT is related to their size and orientation relative to the plane of scan, although size is most important (Fig. 2-7). Generally, the smallest structures visible on HRCT range from 0.3 to 0.5 mm in thickness; thinner structures, measuring 0.1 to 0.2 mm, are occasionally seen.

For the purposes of the interpretation of HRCT, the secondary lobule is most appropriately conceptualized as having three principal parts or components:

1. the interlobular septa and contiguous subpleural interstitium,
2. the centrilobular or lobular core structures, and
3. the lobular parenchyma and acini.

Interlobular Septa

Anatomically, secondary lobules are marginated by connective tissue interlobular septa, which extend inward from the pleural surface (Figs. 2-4,2-5). These septa are part of the peripheral interstitial fiber system described by Weibel (Fig. 2-1) (5), which extends over the surface of the lung beneath the visceral pleura. Pulmonary veins and lymphatics lie within the connective tissue interlobular septa that marginate the lobule.

It should be emphasized that not all interlobular septa are equally well defined. The interlobular septa are thickest and most numerous in the apical, anterior, and lateral aspects of the upper lobes, the anterior and lateral aspects of the middle lobe and lingula, the anterior and diaphragmatic surfaces of the lower lobes, and along the mediastinal pleural surfaces (25); thus, secondary lobules are best defined in these regions. Septa measure about 100 μm (0.1 mm) in thickness in a subpleural location (3,5,10,11). Within the central lung,

interlobular septa are thinner and less well defined than peripherally, and lobules are more difficult to identify in this location.

Peripherally, interlobular septa measuring 100 μm or 0.1 mm in thickness are at the lower limit of HRCT resolution (11), but nonetheless they are sometimes visible on HRCT scans performed in vitro (10). On in vitro HRCT, interlobular septa are often visible as very thin, straight lines of uniform thickness that are usually 1 to 2.5 cm in length and perpendicular to the pleural

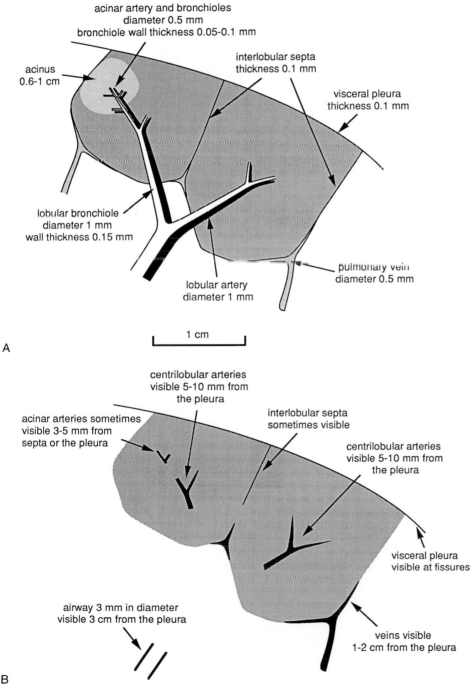

FIG. 2-7. Dimensions of secondary lobular structures (**A**), and their visibility on HRCT (**B**).

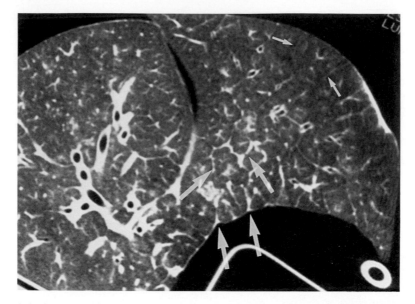

FIG. 2-8. Interlobular septa in an isolated lung. Some thin, normal interlobular septa (*small arrows*) are faintly visible in the peripheral lung. Interlobular septa along the mediastinal pleural surface (*large arrows*) are slightly thickened by edema fluid and are more easily seen. Note that a very thin line is visible at the pleural surfaces and in the lung fissure, similar in appearance and thickness to the normal interlobular septa. This line represents the subpleural interstitial compartment and visceral pleura. (From Webb et al., ref. 10, with permission of *Radiology*.)

surface (Figs. 2-7, 2-8). Several septa in continuity can be seen as a linear opacity measuring up to 4 cm in length (Fig. 2-9) (10).

On clinical scans in normal patients, interlobular septa are less commonly seen, and are seen less well, than they are in studies of isolated lungs. A few septa are often visible in the lung periphery in normal subjects, but they tend to be inconspicuous (Fig. 2-10); normal septa are most often seen anteriorly and along the mediastinal pleural surfaces (4,26). When visible, they are usually seen extending to the pleural surface. In the central lung, septa are thinner than they are pe-

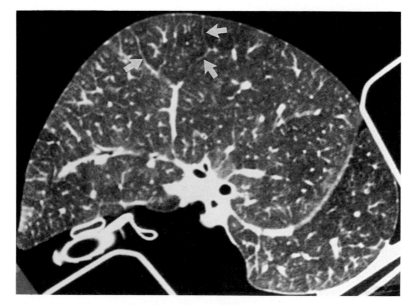

FIG. 2-9. Interlobular septa in continuity in an isolated lung. On HRCT, long interlobular septa (*arrows*) can be seen marginating several secondary lobules. The septa in this lung are slightly thickened by fluid. Septa are well seen peripherally, but note that the septa and, therefore, secondary lobules are less well defined in the central lung. (From Webb et al., ref. 10, with permission of *Radiology*.)

ripherally and are infrequently seen in normal subjects (Fig. 2-9); often interlobular septa that are clearly defined in this region are abnormally thickened. Occasionally, when interlobular septa are not clearly visible, their locations can be inferred by locating septal pulmonary vein branches, approximately 0.5 mm in diameter. Veins can sometimes be seen as linear (Fig. 2-10B), arcuate, or branching structures (Fig. 2-10C), or as a row or chain of dots, surrounding centrilobular arteries, and approximately 5 to 10 mm from them.

The Centrilobular Region and Lobular Core Structures

The central portion of the lobule, referred to as the centrilobular region or lobular core (13), contains the pulmonary artery and bronchiolar branches that supply the lobule, as well as some supporting connective tissue (the centrilobular interstitium described above) (3,5,8,10,11). It is difficult to precisely define lobules in relation to the bronchial or arterial trees; lobules do not arise at a specific branching generation or from a specific type of bronchiole or artery (8).

The branching of the lobular bronchiole and artery are irregularly dichotomous (18). In other words, when they divide, they divide into two branches that are usually of different sizes; one branch is nearly the same size as the one it arose from, and the other is smaller (Fig. 2-5B). Thus, on bronchograms or arteriograms (or HRCT), there often appears to be a single dominant bronchiole and artery in the center of the lobule, which give off smaller branches at intervals along their length.

The HRCT appearances and visibility of structures in the lobular core are determined primarily by their size (Fig. 2-7). Secondary lobules are supplied by arteries and bronchioles measuring approximately 1 mm in diameter, while intralobular terminal bronchioles and arteries measure about 0.7 mm in diameter, and acinar bronchioles and arteries range from 0.3 mm to 0.5 mm in diameter. Arteries of this size can be easily resolved using HRCT technique (10,11).

On clinical scans, a linear, branching, or dot-like opacity frequently seen within the center of a lobule, or within a centimeter of the pleural surface, represents the intralobular artery branch or its divisions (Figs. 2-

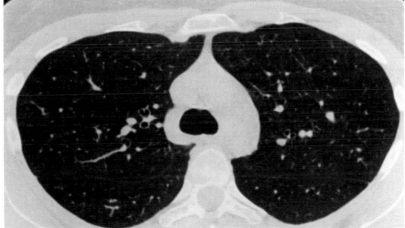

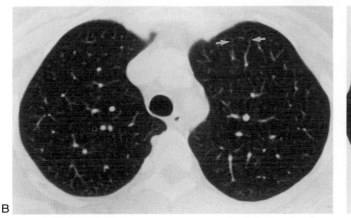

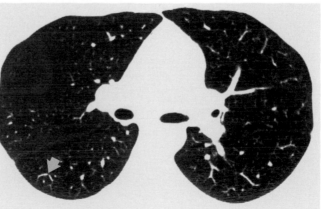

FIG. 2-10. A: HRCT in a normal subject; window mean/width—600/2000 HU. Interlobular septa are inconspicuous, and those few that are visible are very thin. The major fissures appear as thin, sharply defined lines. **B:** Two pulmonary vein branches (*arrows*) marginate a pulmonary lobule in the anterior lung, but the interlobular septa surrounding this lobule are very thin and difficult to see. The centrilobular artery lies equidistant between the veins. **C:** HRCT in a normal subject (−700/100 HU) shows few interlobular septa. A venous arcade (*arrow*) is visible in the lower lobe, with the centrilobular artery visible as a dot, centered within the arcade.

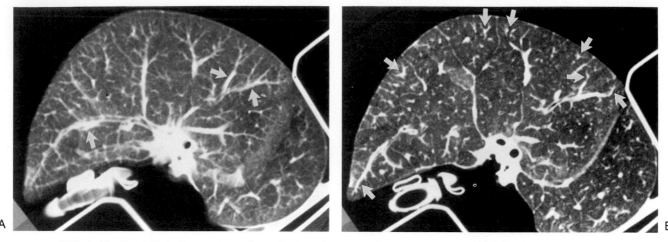

FIG. 2-11. Centrilobular anatomy in an isolated lung. **A:** On a CT scan obtained with 1-cm collimation, pulmonary artery branches (*arrows*) with their accompanying bronchi can be identified. **B:** On an HRCT scan at the same level, interlobular septa can be seen marginating one or more lobules (see Fig. 2-9). Pulmonary artery branches (*arrows*) can be seen extending into the centers of pulmonary lobuies, but intralobular bronchioles are not visible. The last visible branching point of pulmonary arteries is about 1 cm from the pleural surface. Bronchi are invisible within 2 or 3 cm of the pleural surface. (From Webb et al., ref. 10, with permission of *Radiology*.)

10C,2-11,2-12) (3,10,11). The smallest arteries resolved extend to within 3 to 5 mm of the pleural surface or lobular margin and are as small as 0.2 mm in diameter (3,10,11). The visible centrilobular arteries are not seen to extend to the pleural surface in the absence of atelectasis (Fig. 2-13).

Regarding the visibility of bronchioles in normals, it is necessary to consider bronchiolar wall thickness rather than bronchiolar diameter. For a 1-mm bronchiole supplying a secondary lobule, the thickness of its wall measures approximately 0.15 mm; this is at the lower limit of HRCT resolution. The wall of a terminal bronchiole measures only 0.1 mm in thickness, and that of an acinar bronchiole only 0.05 mm, both of which are below the resolution of HRCT technique for a tubular structure (Fig. 2-7). In one in vitro study, only bronchioles having a diameter of 2 mm or more or having a wall thickness of more than 100 μm (0.1 mm) were visible using HRCT (11); and resolution is certainly less than this on clinical scans. It is important to remember that on clinical HRCT, intralobular bronchioles are not normally visible, and bronchi or bronchioles are not normally seen within 2 cm of the pleural surface (Figs. 2-11,2-12).

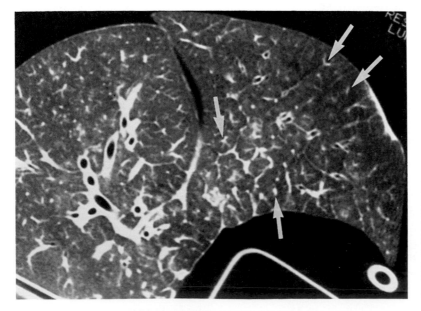

FIG. 2-12. Centrilobular anatomy in an isolated lung. Lobular core anatomy in an isolated lung. Branching pulmonary arteries (*arrows*) are visible within 1 cm of the pleural surface, but intralobular bronchioles are invisible. Within the central lung, centrilobular arteries (*arrows*) appear dot-like or as a branching structure. (From Webb et al., ref. 10, with permission of *Radiology*.)

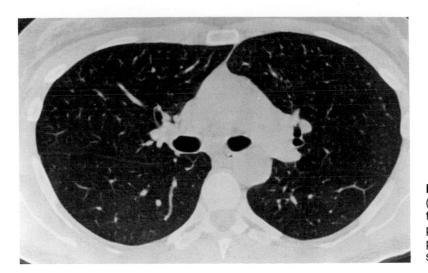

FIG. 2-13. Normal lobular anatomy. HRCT (−600/2000 HU) in a normal subject shows artery branches extending to within 1 cm of the pleural surface, but they do not reach the pleura. (From Webb et al., ref. 10, with permission of *Radiology*.)

The Lobular Parenchyma

The substance of the secondary lobule, surrounding the lobular core and contained within the interlobular septa, consists of functioning lung parenchyma, namely alveoli and the associated pulmonary capillary bed, supplied by small airways and branches of the pulmonary arteries and veins. This parenchyma is supported by a connective tissue stroma, a fine network of very thin fibers within the alveolar septa called the *intralobular interstitium* (Fig. 2-1) (5,8), which are normally invisible. On HRCT, the lobular parenchyma should be of greater opacity than air (Fig. 2-14), but this difference may vary with window settings (see Chapter 1). Some small intralobular vascular branches are often visible.

It should be emphasized that all three interstitial fiber systems described by Weibel (axial, peripheral, and septal) are represented at the level of the pulmonary lobule (Fig. 2-1), and abnormalities in any can produce recognizable lobular abnormalities on HRCT (10). Axial (centrilobular) fibers surround the artery and bronchiole in the lobular core, peripheral fibers making up the interlobular septa marginate the lobule, and septal fibers (the intralobular interstitium) extend throughout the substance of the lobule in relation to the alveolar walls.

The Pulmonary Acinus

Pulmonary acini are not normally visible on HRCT (18). As with lobules, acini vary in size. They are usually described as ranging from 6 to 10 mm in diameter, and have been measured as averaging approximately 7 to 8 mm in diameter in adults (15,19). As indicated

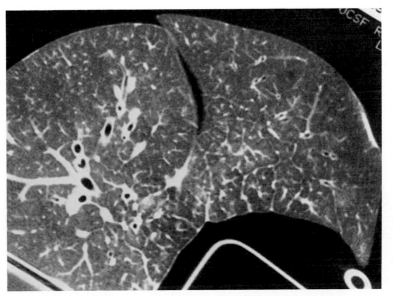

FIG. 2-14. Normal appearance of the lobular parenchyma. The lung parenchyma should appear to be homogeneously denser than air in the bronchi, or as in this isolated lung, denser than room air surrounding the specimen. The relative opacities of lung and air will depend on the window settings.

above, secondary pulmonary lobules defined by the presence of connective tissue interlobular septa usually consist of a dozen or fewer pulmonary acini (Fig. 2-5A) (8,9,15,16).

First order respiratory bronchioles and the acinar artery branch measure about 0.5 mm in diameter (Fig. 2-7A); thus, intralobular acinar arteries are large enough to be seen on HRCT in some normal subjects (5,8,15,16). Murata (11) has shown that pulmonary artery branches as small as 0.2 mm, associated with a respiratory bronchiole, and thus acinar in nature, are visible on HRCT, and extend to within 3 to 5 mm of the lobular margins or pleural surface (Fig. 2-7).

Lobular Anatomy and the Concept of "Cortical" and "Medullary" Lung

At least partially based on differences in lobular anatomy, it has been suggested that the lung can be divided into a peripheral "cortex" and a central "medulla" (13,27). Although these terms are not in general use, the concept of cortical and medullary lung regions is useful in highlighting differences in lung anatomy, and the varying appearances of secondary pulmonary lobules in the peripheral and central lung regions (28). It also serves to emphasize some anatomic (and perhaps physiologic) differences between the peripheral and central lung that are useful in predicting the HRCT distribution of some lung diseases (29).

Peripheral or "Cortical" Lung

Cortical lung can be conceived of as consisting of two or three rows or tiers of well-organized and well-defined secondary pulmonary lobules, which together form a layer about 3 to 4 cm in thickness at the lung periphery and along the lung surfaces adjacent to fissures (Fig. 2-15) (13,27). The pulmonary lobules in the lung cortex are relatively large in size, and are marginated by interlobular septa that are thicker and better defined than in other parts of the lung; thus cortical lobules tend to be better defined than those in the central or medullary lung. Bronchi and pulmonary vessels in the lung cortex are relatively small; although cortical arteries and veins are visible on HRCT, bronchi and bronchioles are uncommonly visible. This contrasts with the anatomy of medullary lung, in which large vessels and bronchi are visible.

Lobules in the lung cortex tend to be relatively uniform in appearance, and can be conceived of as being similar to the stones in a Roman arch—all of similar size and shape (Fig. 2-15) (27). They can appear cuboidal, or be shaped like a truncated cone or pyramid (13). However, it should be kept in mind that the size, shape, and appearance of pulmonary lobules as seen on HRCT

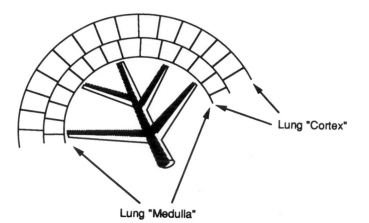

FIG. 2-15. Cortico-medullary differentiation in the lung. The lung cortex is composed of one or two rows or tiers of well-organized and well-defined secondary pulmonary lobules about 3 to 4 cm in thickness. The pulmonary lobules in the lung cortex tend to be well defined and relatively large, and can be conceived of as being similar to the stones in a Roman arch—all of similar size and shape. The cortical airways and vessels are small, usually being less than 2 to 3 mm in diameter.

are significantly affected by the orientation of the scan plane relative to the central and longitudinal axes of the lobules. A single scan will typically traverse different parts of adjacent lobules (Figs. 2-8,2-9), resulting in widely varying appearances of the lobules, despite the fact that they are all of similar size and shape.

Central or "Medullary" Lung

Pulmonary lobules in the central or medullary lung are smaller and more irregular in shape than in the cortical lung, and are marginated by interlobular septa that are thinner and less well defined. When visible, medullary lobules may appear hexagonal or polygonal in shape, but well-defined lobules are uncommonly seen in normals. In contrast with the peripheral lung, parahilar vessels and bronchi in the lung medulla are large and easily seen on HRCT.

THE SUBPLEURAL INTERSTITIUM AND PLEURAL SURFACES

Diffuse infiltrative lung diseases involving the subpleural interstitium or pleura can result in abnormalities visible at the pleural surfaces.

The Subpleural Interstitium and Visceral Pleura

The visceral pleura consists of a single layer of flattened mesothelial cells, subtended by layers of fibroelastic connective tissue; it measures 0.1 to 0.2 mm in thickness (30,31). The connective tissue component of

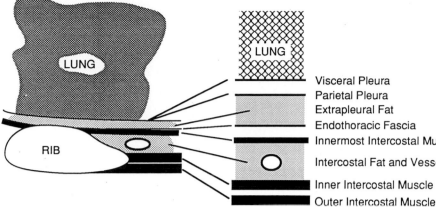

Visceral Pleura
Parietal Pleura
Extrapleural Fat
Endothoracic Fascia
Innermost Intercostal Muscle
Intercostal Fat and Vessels
Inner Intercostal Muscle
Outer Intercostal Muscle

FIG. 2-16. Anatomy of the pleural surfaces and chest wall.

the visceral pleura, is generally referred to on HRCT as the *subpleural interstitium*, and is part of the "peripheral" interstitial fiber network described by Weibel (Fig. 2-1) (5). The subpleural interstitium contains small vessels, which are involved in the formation of pleural fluid, and lymphatic branches. Interstitial lung diseases that affect the interlobular septa, or result in lung fibrosis, often result in abnormalities of the subpleural interstitium.

Abnormalities of the subpleural interstitium can be recognized over the costal surfaces of the lung, but are more easily seen in relation to the major fissures, where two layers of the visceral pleura and subpleural interstitium come in contact. In contrast to conventional CT, in which the obliquely oriented major fissures are usually seen as broad bands of increased or decreased opacity, these fissures are consistently visualized on HRCT as continuous, smooth, very thin, linear opacities. Normal fissures are less than 1-mm thick, smooth in contour, uniform in thickness, and sharply defined (Figs. 2-2A,2-10A,2-13). The visceral pleura and subpleural interstitium along the costal surfaces of lung are not visible on HRCT in normal subjects.

The Parietal Pleura

The parietal pleura, as with the visceral pleura, consists of a mesothelial cell membrane in association with a thin layer of connective tissue. The parietal pleura is somewhat thinner than the visceral pleura, measuring about 0.1 mm (30,31). External to the parietal pleura is a thin layer of loose areolar connective tissue or extrapleural fat, which separates the pleura from the fibroelastic endothoracic fascia and lines the thoracic cavity (Fig. 2-16); the endothoracic fascia is about 0.25 mm in thickness (31,32). External to the endothoracic fascia are the innermost intercostal muscles and ribs. The innermost intercostal muscles pass between adjacent ribs, but do not extend into the paravertebral regions.

As stated in Chapter 1, window level/width settings

of 50/350 HU are best for evaluating the parietal pleura and adjacent chest wall. Images at a level of −600, with an extended window width of 2000 are also useful in evaluating the relationship of peripheral parenchymal abnormalities to the pleural surfaces (3,33).

On HRCT in normal patients, the innermost intercostal muscles are often visible as 1- to 2-mm thick stripes (the intercostal stripes) of soft tissue opacity at the lung–chest wall interface, passing between adjacent rib segments in the anterolateral, lateral, and posterolateral thorax (Fig. 2-17). The parietal pleura is too

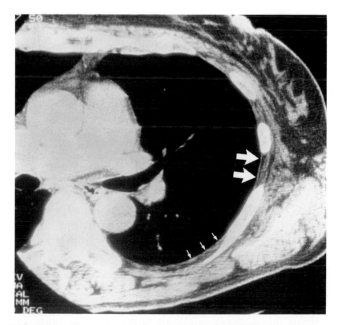

FIG. 2-17. Normal intercostal stripe. On HRCT in a normal subject, the intercostal stripe is visible as a thin white line (*large arrows*). Although it represents the combined thicknesses of visceral and parietal pleurae, the fluid-filled pleural space, endothoracic fascia, and innermost intercostal muscle, it primarily represents the innermost intercostal muscle. The intercostal stripe is seen as separate from the more external layers of the intercostal muscles because of a layer of intercostal fat. Posteriorly, the intercostal stripe (*small arrow*) is visible anterior to the lower edge of a rib.

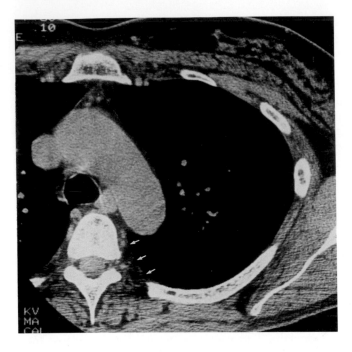

FIG. 2-18. The paravertebral line. In the paravertebral regions (*arrows*), the innermost intercostal muscle is absent, and at most, a very thin line (the "paravertebral line") is present at the lung–chest wall interface. As in this case, a distinct line may not be seen.

thin to see on HRCT along the costal pleural surfaces, even in combination with the visceral pleura and endothoracic fascia (34). However, in the paravertebral regions, the innermost intercostal muscle is anatomically absent, and a very thin line (the paravertebral line) is sometimes visible at the interface between lung and paravertebral fat or rib (Fig. 2-18) (34). This line probably represents the combined thicknesses (approximately 0.2 to 0.4 mm) of the normal pleural layers and endothoracic fascia.

HRCT MEASUREMENTS OF LUNG ATTENUATION

Generally speaking, lung attenuation as seen on HRCT scans obtained at full inspiration appears relatively homogeneous. Measurements of lung attenuation in normal subjects can range from −700 to −900 HU, corresponding to lung densities of approximately 0.300 to 0.100 g/mL, respectively (35,36). However, an attenuation gradient is normally present, if measurements are made, with the most dependent lung regions being the densest, and the most nondependent lung regions being the least dense. This gradient is largely due to regional differences in blood volume and gas volume that, in turn, are determined by gravity, mechanical stresses on the lung, and intrapleural pressures (33,35). Differences in attenuation between anterior and posterior lung have been measured in supine patients, and values generally range from 50 to 100 HU

(35,37,38), although gradients of more than 200 HU have been reported (37). The anteroposterior attenuation gradient was found to be nearly linear, and was present regardless of whether the subject was supine or prone (37).

Genereaux measured anteroposterior attenuation gradients at three levels (at the aortic arch, the carina, and above the right hemidiaphragm) in normal subjects (38). An anteroposterior attenuation gradient was found at all levels, although the gradient was larger at the lung bases than in the upper lung; the anteroposterior gradient averaged 36 HU at the aortic arch, 65 HU at the carina, and 88 HU at the lung bases. The attenuation gradient was even larger if only cortical lung was considered. Within cortical lung, the attenuation differences at the three levels studied are, respectively, 45, 81, and 113 HU.

Vock et al. (35) analyzed CT measured pulmonary attenuation in children. In general, lung attenuation in children is greater than that in adults (35,37), but anteroposterior attenuation gradients were similar to those found in adults, averaging 56 HU at the subcarinal level.

Although most authors have reported that normal anteroposterior lung attenuation gradients are linear, with attenuation increasing gradually from anterior to posterior lung, the lingula and superior segments of the lower lobes can appear relatively lucent in some normal subjects (39); focal lucency in these segments should be considered a normal finding. Although the reason for this is unclear, these slender segments may be less well ventilated than adjacent lung and therefore less well perfused, or some air-trapping may be present.

NORMAL EXPIRATORY HRCT

A number of studies have shown that lung parenchyma normally increases in CT attenuation as lung volume is reduced during expiration. This change can generally be recognized on HRCT as an increase in lung opacity (Figs. 1-18–1-20) (7,35–37,40,41). Robinson and Kreel (40) found significant inverse correlations between lung volume determined spirometrically, and CT measured lung attenuation, for the whole lung ($r = -0.680$, $p > 0.0005$) and for anterior, middle, and posterior lung zones considered individually. In other studies of both adults and children (7,35,37,41), lung attenuation was found to increase by 150 to 300 HU during exhalation, depending on the region of lung studied. In a recent study (39) of ten normal subjects using dynamic expiratory HRCT, an increase in lung attenuation averaging 200 HU was consistently seen during expiration, but the increase was variable, and ranged from 84 to 372 HU.

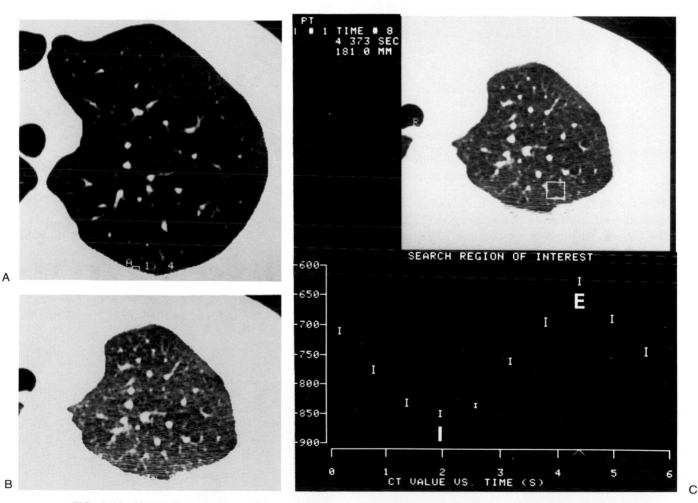

FIG. 2-19. Normal dynamic expiratory HRCT. Inspiratory (**A**) and expiratory (**B**) images from a sequence of 10 scans obtained during forced expiration in a normal subject. Lung attenuation increases and cross-sectional lung area decreases on the expiratory scan. **C:** A region of interest has been positioned in the posterior lung, and a time-attenuation curve calculated for this region of interest shows an increase in attenuation from −850 HU to −625 HU from maximal inspiration (*I*) to maximal expiration (*E*). Each point on the time density curve represents one image from the dynamic sequence.

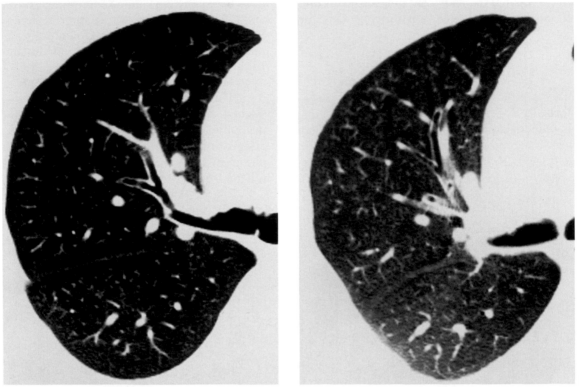

FIG. 2-20. Inspiratory (**A**) and post-expiratory (**B**) HRCT in a normal subject. On the expiratory scan, lung increases in attenuation. Posterior dependent lung increases in attenuation to a greater degree than anterior nondependent lung.

In some normal subjects, small areas of focal lucency are visible on expiratory scans (Figs. 2-21,2-22); in these regions, lung does not increase normally in attenuation, probably as a result of focal air trapping. This appearance is most typical in the superior segments of the lower lobes, or in the anterior middle lobe or lingula (39), and is limited to a small proportion of lung volume.

Changes in lung attenuation during expiration can be related to changes in cross-sectional lung area as shown on HRCT. Simply stated, cross-sectional lung area decreases during expiration at the same time attenuation increases (Fig. 2-19). For example, Robinson and Kreel (39) found a significant inverse correlation between the expiratory change in cross-sectional lung area measured on CT and changes in CT measured lung

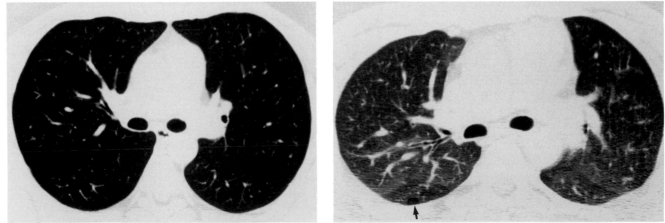

FIG. 2-21. Inspiratory (**A**) and post-expiratory (**B**) HRCT in a normal subject. On the expiratory scan, there is relative lucency in the superior segments of the lower lobes, posterior to the major fissures. This appearance is normal. Also, focal air trapping is present in a single lobule (*arrow*) in the posterior right lung.

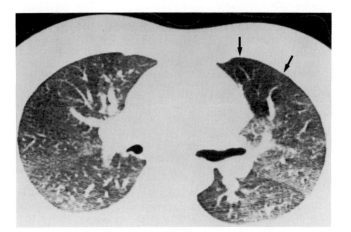

FIG. 2-22. Dynamic expiratory HRCT in a normal subject showing air trapping in the anterior lingula (*arrows*), and relative lucency posterior to the left major fissure. Pulmonary lobules in the lung medulla are smaller and less well defined than in the periphery. However, vessels and bronchi in the lung medulla are large and easily seen on HRCT.

attenuation ($r = -0.793$, $p > 0.0005$). In a study using dynamic expiratory HRCT (39) a correlation between cross-sectional lung area and lung attenuation was found for each of three lung regions evaluated (upper lung, $r = 0.51$, $p = 0.03$; midlung, $r = 0.58$, $p = 0.01$; lower lung, $r = 0.51$, $p = 0.05$). The lower lung zone showed a greater attenuation increase for a given area change; this phenomenon likely reflects the much greater effect of diaphragmatic elevation on basal lung attenuation than occurs in the upper lungs. Normal morphologic changes that can be seen on expiratory CT also includes a decrease in tracheal diameter associated with anterior bowing of the posterior tracheal membrane (42), and a small decrease in the diameter of the bronchi. Pulmonary vessels may appear somewhat increased in diameter on expiration.

As indicated above, lung attenuation is greater in dependent lung than it is in nondependent lung; differences in attenuation between anterior and posterior lung have been measured in supine patients, and values generally range from 50 to 100 HU (35,37,38). Following expiration, dependent lung regions increase more in attenuation than do nondependent lung regions (Fig. 2-20). This results in an accentuation of the normal anterior to posterior lung attenuation gradient; the increase in the anterior to posterior attenuation gradient following expiration has been reported to range from 47 to 130 HU in different studies (7,35,39,41). Although measurements of attenuation gradients on inspiration and expiration have been investigated as a method of diagnosing lung disease (7,36,43), this technique has not assumed a clinical role.

REFERENCES

1. Müller NL, Miller RR. Computed tomography of chronic diffuse infiltrative lung disease: part 1. *Am Rev Respir Dis* 1990;142: 1206–1215.
2. Müller NL, Miller RR. Computed tomography of chronic diffuse infiltrative lung disease: part 2. *Am Rev Respir Dis* 1990;142: 1440–1448.
3. Webb WR. High-resolution CT of the lung parenchyma. *Radiol Clin North Am* 1989;27:1085–1097.
4. Zerhouni E. Computed tomography of the pulmonary parenchyma: an overview. *Chest* 1989;95:901–907.
5. Weibel ER. Looking into the lung: what can it tell us? *AJR* 1979; 133:1021–1031.
6. Lynch DA, Newell JD, Tschomper BA, Cink TM, Newman LS, Bethel R. Uncomplicated asthma in adults: comparison of CT appearance of the lungs in asthmatic and healthy subjects. *Radiology* 1993;188:829–833.
7. Zerhouni EA, Naidich DP, Stitik FP, Khouri NF, Siegelman SS. Computed tomography of the pulmonary parenchyma. Part 2: interstitial disease. *J Thorac Imaging* 1985;1:54–64.
8. Weibel ER, Taylor CR. Design and structure of the human lung. In: *Pulmonary Diseases and Disorders*. New York: McGraw-Hill; 1988:11–60.
9. Weibel ER. High resolution computed tomography of the pulmonary parenchyma: anatomical background. Presented at the Fleischner Society Symposium on Chest Disease, Scottsdale, Arizona, 1990.
10. Webb WR, Stein MG, Finkbeiner WE, Im JG, Lynch D, Gamsu G. Normal and diseased isolated lungs: high-resolution CT. *Radiology* 1988;166:81–87.
11. Murata K, Itoh H, Todo G, et al. Centrilobular lesions of the lung: demonstration by high-resolution CT and pathologic correlation. *Radiology* 1986;161:641–645.
12. Miller WS. *The Lung*. Springfield, IL: Charles C Thomas; 1947: 203.
13. Heitzman ER, Markarian B, Berger I, Dailey E. The secondary pulmonary lobule: a practical concept for interpretation of radiographs. I. Roentgen anatomy of the normal secondary pulmonary lobule. *Radiology* 1969;93:508–513.
14. Miller WS. *The Lung*. Springfield, IL:Charles C Thomas; 1947: 39–42.
15. Osborne DR, Effmann EL, Hedlund LW. Postnatal growth and size of the pulmonary acinus and secondary lobule in man. *AJR* 1983;140:449–454.
16. Raskin SP. The pulmonary acinus: historical notes. *Radiology* 1982;144:31–34.
17. Reid L. The secondary pulmonary lobule in the adult human lung, with special reference to its appearance in bronchograms. *Thorax* 1958;13:110–115.
18. Itoh H, Murata K, Konishi J, Nishimura K, Kitaichi M, Izumi T. Diffuse lung disease: pathologic basis for the high-resolution computed tomography findings. *J Thorac Imaging* 1993;8: 176–188.
19. Gamsu G, Thurlbeck WM, T. MP, Fraser RG. Peripheral bronchographic morphology in the normal human lung. *Invest Radiol* 1971;6:161–170.
20. Reid L, Simon G. The peripheral pattern in the normal bronchogram and its relation to peripheral pulmonary anatomy. *Thorax* 1958;13:103–109.
21. Bergin C, Roggli V, Coblentz C, Chiles C. The secondary pulmonary lobule: normal and abnormal CT appearances. *AJR* 1988; 151:21–25.
22. Hruban RH, Meziane MA, Zerhouni EA, et al. High resolution computed tomography of inflation fixed lungs: pathologic-radiologic correlation of centrilobular emphysema. *Am Rev Respir Dis* 1987;136:935–940.
23. Heitzman ER, Markarian B, Berger I, Dailey E. The secondary pulmonary lobule: a practical concept for interpretation of radiographs. II. Application of the anatomic concept to an understanding of roentgen pattern of disease states. *Radiology* 1969; 93:514–520.
24. Heitzman ER. Subsegmental anatomy of the lung. In: *The Lung:*

Radiologic-Pathologic Correlations, 2nd ed. St. Louis: Mosby; 1984:42–49.

25. Reid L, Rubino M. The connective tissue septa in the foetal human lung. *Thorax* 1959;14:3–13.

26. Aberle DR, Gamsu G, Ray CS, Feuerstein IM. Asbestos-related pleural and parenchymal fibrosis: detection with high-resolution CT. *Radiology* 1988;166:729–734.

27. Fleischner FG. The butterfly pattern of pulmonary edema. In: *Frontiers of Pulmonary Radiology*. New York: Grune & Stratton; 1969:360–379.

28. Genereux GP. The Fleischner lecture: computed tomography of diffuse pulmonary disease. *J Thorac Imaging* 1989;4:50–87.

29. Gurney JW. Cross-sectional physiology of the lung. *Radiology* 1991;178:1–10.

30. Agostoni E, Miserocchi G, Bonanni MV. Thickness and pressure of the pleural liquid in some mammals. *Respir Phys* 1969; 6:245– 256.

31. Bernaudin J-F, Fleury J. Anatomy of the blood and lymphatic circulation of the pleural serosa. In: *The Pleura in Health and Disease*. New York: Marcel Dekker; 1985:101–124.

32. Policard A, Galy P. *La Plevre*. Paris: Masson; 1942:23– 33.

33. Murata K, Khan A, Herman PG. Pulmonary parenchymal disease: evaluation with high-resolution CT. *Radiology* 1989;170: 629–635.

34. Im JG, Webb WR, Rosen A, Gamsu G. Costal pleura: appearances at high-resolution CT. *Radiology* 1989;171:125–131.

35. Vock P, Malanowski D, Tschaeppeler H, Kirks DR, Hedlund LW, Effmann EL. Computed tomographic lung density in children. *Invest Radiol* 1987;22:627–631.

36. Millar AB, Denison DM. Vertical gradients of lung density in healthy supine men. *Thorax* 1989;44:485–490.

37. Rosenblum LJ, Mauceri RA, Wellenstein DE, et al. Density patterns in the normal lung as determined by computed tomography. *Radiology* 1980;137:409–416.

38. Genereux GP. Computed tomography and the lung: review of anatomic and densitometric features with their clinical application. *J Can Assoc Radiol* 1985;36:88–102.

39. Webb WR, Stern EJ, Kanth N, Gamsu G. Dynamic pulmonary CT: findings in normal adult men. *Radiology* 1993;186:117–124.

40. Robinson PJ, Kreel L. Pulmonary tissue attenuation with computed tomography: comparison of inspiration and expiration scans. *J Comput Assist Tomogr* 1979;3:740–748.

41. Verschakelen JA, Van Fraeyenhoven L, Laureys G, Demedts M, Baert AL. Differences in CT density between dependent and nondependent portions of the lung: influence of lung volume. *AJR* 1993;161:713–717.

42. Stern EJ, Graham CM, Webb WR, Gamsu G. Normal trachea during forced expiration: dynamic CT measurements. *Radiology* 1993;187:27–31.

43. Millar AB, Denison DM. Vertical gradients of lung density in supine subjects with fibrosing alveolitis or pulmonary emphysema. *Thorax* 1990;45:602–605.

THREE

HRCT Findings of Lung Disease

On HRCT, lung diseases can produce recognizable alterations in parenchymal anatomy in each of the regions described in Chapter 2 (1–4). In this chapter, we will review the HRCT findings commonly seen in patients with diffuse or chronic lung diseases, and the various distributions of abnormalities helpful in the differential diagnosis of lung disease.

First, a word about terminology. During the past 10 years, different terms have often been used by different authors to describe similar or identical HRCT abnormalities; this has lead to some confusion, and has made it difficult to compare one study to another (5). In this book, whenever possible, we will name and define HRCT findings on the basis of their specific corresponding anatomic abnormalities; there is a close correlation in many instances between HRCT findings and pathologic or histologic lung abnormalities. We will avoid nonspecific, descriptive, or nonanatomic terms, unless the HRCT findings themselves are nonspecific and cannot be related to particular anatomic abnormalities, or unless a descriptive term is particularly helpful in understanding and recognizing the abnormality. For easy reference, an illustrated glossary of many of these terms is provided at the end of this book.

Generally, HRCT findings of lung disease can be classified into four large categories, based on their appearances. These are (i) linear and reticular opacities, (ii) nodules and nodular opacities, (iii) increased lung opacity, and (iv) abnormalities associated with decreased lung opacity, including cystic lesions, emphysema, and airway abnormalities.

LINEAR AND RETICULAR OPACITIES

Thickening of the interstitial fiber network of the lung by fluid, fibrous tissue, or because of interstitial infiltration by cells or other material, primarily results in an increase in linear or reticular lung opacities as seen on HRCT. Linear or reticular opacities can be manifested by the interface sign, peribronchovascular interstitial thickening, interlobular septal thickening, intralobular interstitial thickening, honeycombing, subpleural lines, centrilobular or lobular core abnormalities, and airway abnormalities (Fig. 3-1).

The Interface Sign

The presence of irregular interfaces between the aerated lung parenchyma and bronchi, vessels, or the visceral pleural surfaces, has been termed the *interface sign* by Zerhouni et al. (4,6) (Fig. 3-2). The interface sign is commonly seen in patients with an interstitial abnormality, regardless of its cause. In the original description of the interface sign, this finding was visible in 89% of patients with interstitial lung disease (6).

The interface sign is generally associated with an increase in lung reticulation; the presence of thin linear opacities contacting the bronchi, vessels, or pleural surfaces is responsible for their having an irregular or spiculated appearance on HRCT. These linear opacities generally represent thickened interlobular septa or thickened intralobular interstitial fibers (Fig. 3-1). The interface sign is most frequently visible in patients with fibrotic lung disease, and Nishimura et al. (7) reported the presence of irregular pleural surfaces and irregular vessel margins in 94% and 98%, respectively, of patients with idiopathic pulmonary fibrosis. In virtually all cases showing the interface sign, other more specific abnormal findings will also be visible on HRCT.

Peribronchovascular Interstitial Thickening

Central bronchi and pulmonary arteries are surrounded by a strong connective tissue sheath, termed the *peribronchovascular interstitium*, that extends from the level of the pulmonary hila into the peripheral lung, in relation to alveolar ducts and alveoli (Fig. 3-

41

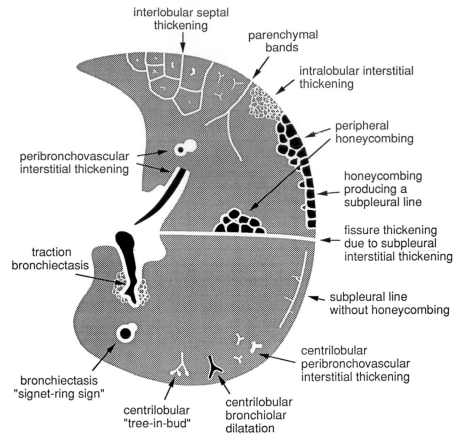

FIG. 3-1. Linear and reticular opacities visible on HRCT.

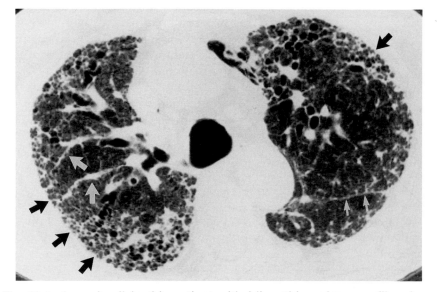

FIG. 3-2. The "interface sign." In this patient with idiopathic pulmonary fibrosis and honeycombing, irregular interfaces are visible between the aerated lung parenchyma and structures such as vessels (*large white arrows*), fissures (*small white arrows*), and the visceral pleural surfaces (*black arrows*). This finding is commonly seen in patients with an interstitial abnormality, regardless of its cause, but is most frequent in patients with abnormal reticular opacities and fibrosis.

TABLE 3-1. *Differential diagnosis of peribronchovascular interstitial thickening*

Diagnosis	Comments
Lymphangitic carcinomatosis, Lymphoma	Common: smooth or nodular; may be the only abnormality
Pulmonary edema	Common; smooth
Sarcoidosis	Common; usually nodular or irregular; conglomerate masses of fibrous tissue with bronchiectasis typical in end-stage
Idiopathic pulmonary fibrosis (IPF) or other cause of Usual interstitial pneumonia (UIP)	Common; often irregular; associated with traction bronchiectasis; however, other findings of fibrosis predominate
Silicosis/Coal worker's pneumoconiosis, talcosis	Conglomerate masses
Hypersensitivity pneumonitis (chronic)	Sometimes visible; often irregular; associated with traction bronchiectasis

1); this is termed the *axial interstitium* by Weibel (8). Thickening of the parahilar peribronchovascular interstitium occurs in many diseases that cause a generalized interstitial abnormality (3,9,10,11). Peribronchovascular interstitial thickening is common in patients with lymphangitic spread of carcinoma (9,10,12) or interstitial pulmonary edema, and can be seen in many diseases that result in pulmonary fibrosis, particularly sarcoidosis (13), which has a propensity to involve the peribronchovascular interstitium (Table 3-1) (14). Peribronchovascular interstitial thickening has also been reported in as many as 19% of patients with chronic hypersensitivity pneumonitis (13).

Since the thickened peribronchovascular interstitium cannot be distinguished from the underlying opacity of the bronchial wall or pulmonary artery, this abnormality is usually perceived on HRCT as (i) an increase in bronchial wall thickness and (ii) an increase in diameter of pulmonary artery branches (Fig. 3-3) (9). Apparent bronchial wall thickening is the easiest of these two findings to recognize, and is exactly equivalent to "peribronchial cuffing" seen on plain chest radiographs in patients with an interstitial abnormality.

Thickening of the peribronchovascular interstitium can appear smooth, nodular, or irregular in different diseases (Fig. 3-3) (Table 3-1). Smooth peribroncho-

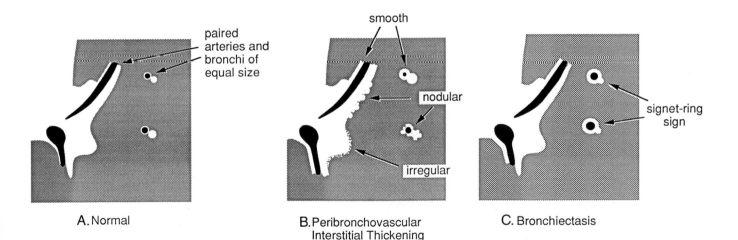

A. Normal   B. Peribronchovascular Interstitial Thickening   C. Bronchiectasis

FIG. 3-3. Differentiation of peribronchovascular interstitial thickening and bronchiectasis. **A:** In a normal subject, bronchi are uniformly thin-walled, and appear approximately equal in diameter to adjacent pulmonary arteries. **B:** In the presence of peribronchovascular interstitial thickening, there appears to be an increase in bronchial wall thickness and a corresponding increase in diameter of pulmonary artery branches. The contours of the bronchi and vessels can appear smooth, nodular, or irregular in different diseases. **C:** In bronchiectasis, bronchi are usually thick-walled and appear larger than adjacent pulmonary arteries. This can result in the so-called signet-ring sign.

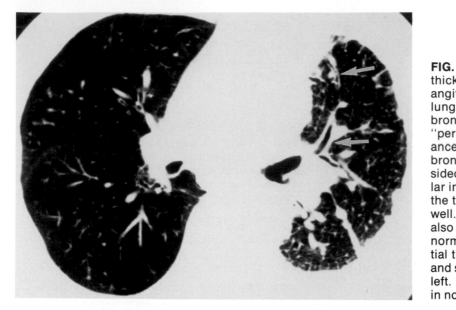

FIG. 3-4. Peribronchovascular interstitial thickening. In a patient with unilateral lymphangitic spread of carcinoma involving the left lung, there is smooth thickening of the peribronchovascular interstitium manifested by "peribronchial cuffing" (*arrows*); this appearance is easily contrasted with that of normal bronchi in the right lung. Note that the left-sided pulmonary artery branches appear similar in diameter to the cuffed bronchi because the thickened interstitium surrounds them as well. Small intrapulmonary vessels on the left also appear more prominent than those on the normal side, because of perivascular interstitial thickening. Interlobular septal thickening and subpleural nodules are also visible on the left. Subpleural interstitial thickening results in nodular thickening of the left major fissure.

vascular interstitial thickening is most typical of patients with lymphangitic spread of carcinoma (Fig. 3-4) and interstitial pulmonary edema (15), but can be seen in patients with fibrotic lung disease as well. Nodular thickening of the peribronchovascular interstitium is particularly common in sarcoidosis (Fig. 3-5) and lymphangitic spread of carcinoma. The presence of irregular peribronchovascular interstitial thickening, as an example of the interface sign, is most frequently seen in patients with peribronchovascular and adjacent lung fibrosis. Extensive peribronchovascular fibrosis can result in the presence of large conglomerate masses of fibrous tissue (Fig. 3-6). This can occur in patients

with sarcoidosis, silicosis, tuberculosis, and talcosis, and is discussed in greater detail below.

Peribronchovascular interstitial thickening is easy to diagnose if it is of a marked degree, and bronchial walls appear several millimeters in thickness, or bronchovascular structures show evidence of the interface sign or nodules. However, the diagnosis of minimal peribronchovascular thickening can be difficult and quite subjective, particularly if the abnormality is diffuse and symmetric. Although the thickness of the wall of a normal bronchus should measure from $\frac{1}{6}$ to $\frac{1}{10}$ of its diameter (16), there are no reliable criteria as to what represents the upper limit of normal for the combined

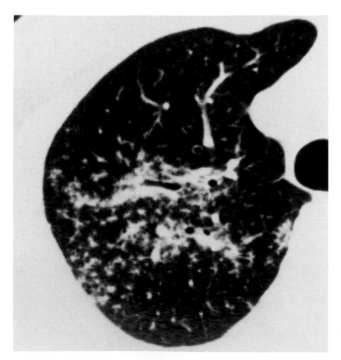

FIG. 3-5. Nodular peribronchovascular interstitial thickening in a patient with sarcoidosis. Numerous small nodules surround central bronchi and vessels.

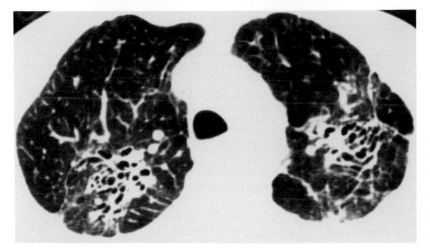

FIG. 3-6. Peribronchovascular interstitial thickening in end-stage sarcoidosis, with conglomerate masses of fibrous tissue surrounding central vessels and bronchi. Bronchi appear dilated and thick walled because of surrounding fibrosis and traction bronchiectasis. Note that vessels and bronchi appear to be of similar diameter.

thicknesses of bronchial wall and the surrounding interstitium. Furthermore, these measurements vary depending on the lung window chosen, and too low a window mean can make normal bronchi or vessels appear abnormal. Fortunately, however, in many patients with peribronchovascular interstitial thickening, and particularly in patients with lymphangitic spread of carcinoma and sarcoidosis, this abnormality is unilateral or patchy, sparing some areas of lung. In such patients, normal and abnormal lung regions can be easily contrasted (Fig. 3-4). As a rule, bronchial walls in

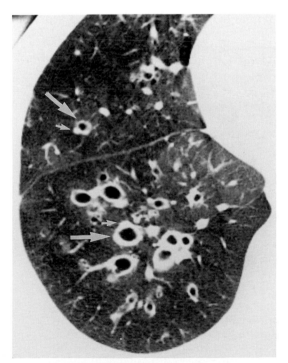

FIG. 3-7. Bronchiectasis with the "signet-ring sign." Thick-walled and dilated bronchi (*large arrows*) appear larger than the adjacent pulmonary artery branches (*small arrows*). This appearance is termed the signet-ring sign, and is typical of bronchiectasis.

corresponding regions of one or both lungs should be quite similar in thickness.

In patients with lung fibrosis and peribronchovascular interstitial thickening, bronchial dilatation is commonly present, resulting from traction by fibrous tissue on the bronchi walls. This is termed *traction bronchiectasis* (Figs. 3-1,3-6); it typically results in irregular bronchial dilatation that appears "varicose" (17,18). Traction bronchiectasis usually involves the segmental and subsegmental bronchi, and is most commonly visible in the parahilar regions in patients with significant lung fibrosis. It can also affect small peripheral bronchi or bronchioles, an occurrence termed *traction bronchiolectasis*.

Bronchial wall thickening, which occurs in patients with true bronchiectasis, produces an abnormality that closely mimics the HRCT appearance of peribronchovascular interstitial thickening. However, airway diseases and interstitial diseases can usually be distinguished on the basis of symptoms or pulmonary function abnormalities, and confusion between these two is not often a problem in clinical diagnosis. In addition, some HRCT findings also allow these two entities to be distinguished (Fig. 3-3). First, peribronchovascular interstitial thickening is often associated with other findings of interstitial disease, such as septal thickening, honeycombing, or the interface sign, while bronchiectasis usually is not. Second, in patients with bronchiectasis, the abnormal thick-walled and dilated bronchi often appear much larger than the adjacent pulmonary artery branches (Fig. 3-7). This results in the appearance of large ring shadows, each associated with a small, rounded opacity, a finding that has been termed the *signet-ring sign*, and is considered to be diagnostic of bronchiectasis (19–23). In patients with peribronchovascular interstitial thickening, on the other hand, the size relationship between the bronchus and artery is maintained, and they appear of approximately equal size. The diagnosis and appearances of

TABLE 3-2. *Differential diagnosis of interlobular septal thickening*

Diagnosis	Comments
Lymphangitic carcinomatosis, Lymphoma	Common; predominant finding in most; smooth or nodular
Pulmonary edema	Common; predominant finding in most; smooth; ground-glass opacity can be present
Sarcoidosis	Common; seen more often than in UIP; nodular when active; irregular in end-stage
Idiopathic pulmonary fibrosis (IPF) other cause of Usual interstitial pneumonia (UIP)	Sometimes visible but not common; irregular; intralobular thickening and honeycombing usually predominate
Alveolar proteinosis	Common; smooth; ground-glass opacity predominates
Silicosis/Coal worker's pneumoconiosis	Sometimes visible; nodular early; irregular in end-stage disease
Asbestosis	Sometimes visible; irregular; associated with parenchymal bands
Hypersensitivity pneumonitis (chronic)	Uncommon; intralobular thickening and honeycombing usually predominate

bronchiectasis is discussed in greater detail below and in Chapter 7.

Interlobular Septal Thickening

Thickening of the interlobular septa is commonly seen in patients with interstitial lung disease, and can be easily recognized on HRCT (Table 3-2). On HRCT, numerous clearly visible interlobular septa almost always indicates the presence of an interstitial abnormal- ity; only a few septa are visible in normal patients. Septal thickening can be seen in the presence of interstitial fluid, cellular infiltration, or fibrosis.

Within the peripheral lung, thickened septa 1 to 2 cm in length may outline part of, or an entire lobule, and are usually seen extending to the pleural surface, being roughly perpendicular to the pleura (Figs. 3-1,3-8,3-9) (3,4,9,10,24–27). Lobules at the pleural surface may have a variety of appearances, but are often longer than they are wide, resembling a cone or truncated cone. Within the central lung, thickened septa outline

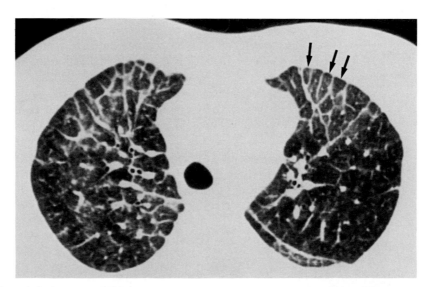

FIG. 3-8. Interlobular septal thickening in a patient with lymphangitic spread of carcinoma. Diffuse interlobular septal thickening outlines numerous pulmonary lobules. Lobules visible in the peripheral lung may appear to be of various sizes and shapes, depending at least partially on the relationship of the lobule to the plane of scan. However, many lobules are conical in shape (*arrows*). In the more central lung, lobules appear more hexagonal or polygonal. The branching or dot-like intralobular vessel is often visible. The septal thickening in this case is primarily smooth in contour, although nodularity is seen in several regions, particularly adjacent to the left major fissure. Long septa that marginate several lobules have been termed "parenchymal bands." The presence of multiple thickened septa form "peripheral" or "polygonal arcades."

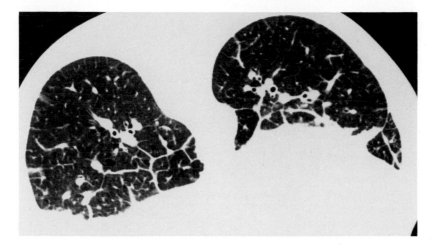

FIG. 3-9. Interlobular septal thickening resulting from pulmonary edema. Prone HRCT shows thickening of numerous interlobular septa in the dependent lung and over the pleural surfaces. Septa within the dependent lung are thickest. Centrilobular arteries appear prominent within most of the lobules surrounded by thickened septa, a finding which reflects thickening of the centrilobular interstitium. Peribronchovascular interstitial thickening is also present.

lobules that are 1 to 2.5 cm in diameter, and appear polygonal, or sometimes hexagonal, in shape (Fig. 3-8). Lobules delineated by thickened septa commonly contain a visible dot-like or branching centrilobular pulmonary artery.

Thickened interlobular septa also have been described using the terms ''septal lines,'' ''peripheral lines,'' ''short lines,'' and ''interlobular lines'' (10,27,28). Thickened septa outlining one or more pulmonary lobules have been described as producing a ''large reticular pattern''(4,6) or ''polygons'' (29), and, if they can be seen contacting the pleural surface, as ''peripheral arcades'' or ''polygonal arcades'' (Figs. 3-8,3-9) (10). Close correlation has been shown between

these HRCT appearances and septal thickening present pathologically, and we consider the terms *interlobular septal thickening, septal thickening*, or *septal lines* to be most appropriate.

Septal thickening can be smooth, nodular, or irregular in contour in different pathologic processes (Table 3-2). Smooth septal thickening is seen in patients with pulmonary edema (Fig. 3-9) (30), lymphangitic spread of carcinoma or lymphoma (Fig. 3-8) (9,10,31), alveolar proteinosis (Fig. 3-10) (32,33), interstitial infiltration associated with amyloidosis (34), in some patients with pneumonia, and in a small percentage of patients with pulmonary fibrosis. Nodular or ''beaded'' septal thickening occurs in lymphangitic spread of carcinoma or

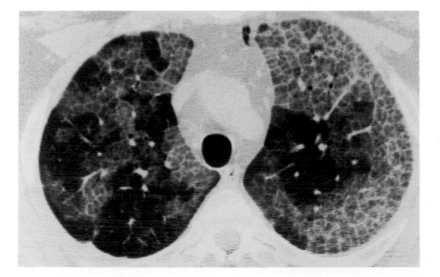

FIG. 3-10. Interlobular septal thickening in alveolar proteinosis. Thickened septa are associated with ground-glass opacity. This appearance is typical of alveolar proteinosis.

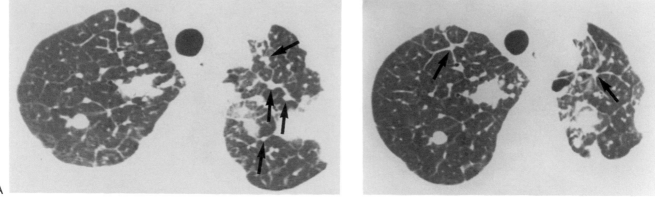

FIG. 3-11. "Beaded" or nodular septal thickening with lymphangitic spread of carcinoma. **A,B:** Generalized septal thickening is associated with some nodularity (*arrows*); this has been termed the beaded septum sign. Septa are well-defined. Several large nodules are also visible in the lung. This is a common appearance in patients with lymphangitic spread of carcinoma.

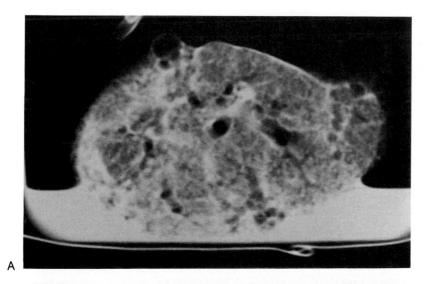

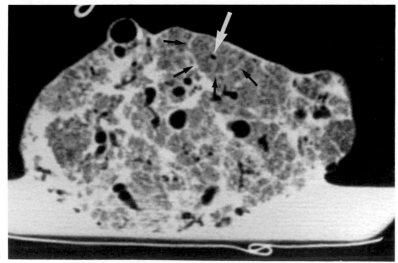

FIG. 3-12. Pulmonary fibrosis in an isolated inflated lung specimen. Scans performed with 1-cm collimation and conventional technique (**A**) and with HRCT technique (**B**). On the HRCT scan, a lobule at the lung surface is well shown. It is marginated with irregularly thickened interlobular septa (*small arrows*). Intralobular interstitial thickening is visible as a fine network of lines. The intralobular bronchiole is also visible (*large white arrow*). The subpleural interstitium is thickened. These findings are not clearly shown with conventional technique. (B from Webb, ref. 3, with permission.)

lymphoma (Fig. 3-11) (9,10,31), sarcoidosis, silicosis or coal worker's pneumoconiosis (14,35-37), and amyloidosis (34). In patients who have interstitial fibrosis, septal thickening visible on HRCT is often irregular in appearance (Figs. 3-12–3-14) (18).

Although interlobular septal thickening can be seen on HRCT in association with fibrosis and honeycombing (28), is not usually a predominant feature (7,25,38). Generally speaking, in the presence of significant fibrosis and honeycombing, distortion of lung architecture make the recognition of thickened septa difficult. Among patients with pulmonary fibrosis and "end-stage" lung disease, the presence of interlobular septal thickening on HRCT is most frequent in patients with sarcoidosis (Fig. 3-14) (present in 56% of patients), and is relatively uncommon in those with usual interstitial pneumonia (UIP) of various causes (Fig. 3-15), asbestosis, and hypersensitivity pneumonitis (38).

The frequency of septal thickening and fibrosis in patients with sarcoidosis reflects the tendency of active sarcoid granulomas to involve the interlobular septa. In patients with idiopathic pulmonary fibrosis or UIP of other cause, the appearance of irregular septal thickening correlates with the presence of fibrosis predominantly affecting the periphery of the secondary lobule (7).

Parenchymal Bands

The term *parenchymal band* has been used to describe non-tapering, reticular opacities, from 2 to 5 cm in length, that can be seen in patients with pulmonary fibrosis or other causes of interstitial thickening (Figs. 3-1,3-14) (27,39); these have also been described as "long lines" (10). They are often peripheral and generally contact the pleural surface.

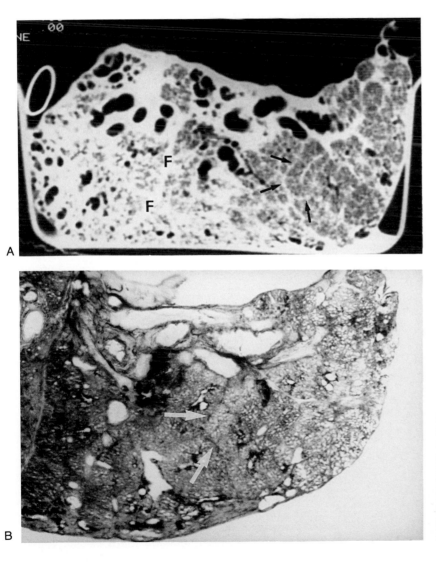

FIG. 3-13. HRCT of pulmonary fibrosis in an isolated inflated lung. The HRCT (**A**) and the corresponding lung section (**B**) are shown for comparison. Typical HRCT findings of fibrosis include interlobular septal thickening that is irregular in contour (*arrows*) and subpleural interstitial thickening shown at the lung surfaces and adjacent to the major fissure (*F*). (From Webb et al., ref. 18, with permission of *Radiology*.)

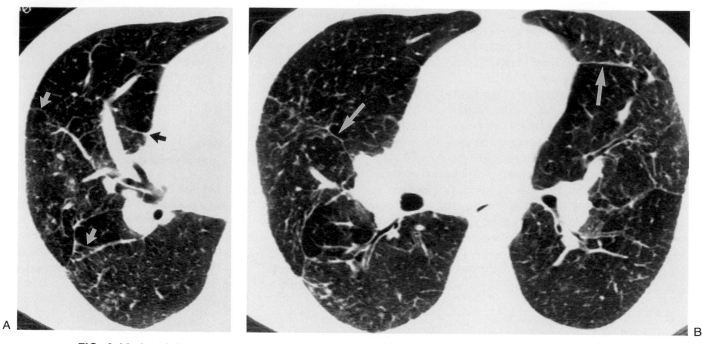

FIG. 3-14. Interlobular septal thickening and parenchymal bands in a patient with end-stage sarcoidosis. **A**: Septa (*arrows*) appear irregular in contour, a finding usually associated with fibrosis. **B**: Longer lines (*arrows*) are "parenchymal bands." As in this patient, these often represent several contiguous thickened septa. Lung distortion is also present, indicative of fibrosis.

In some patients, these bands represent contiguous thickened interlobular septa, and have the same significance and differential diagnosis as septal thickening (28). When parenchymal bands can be identified as thickened septa (Figs. 3-14,3-16), the use of a separate term to describe this finding is unjustified; the term *septal thickening* should suffice.

However, parenchymal bands visible on HRCT can also represent areas of peribronchovascular fibrosis, coarse scars, or atelectasis associated with lung or pleural fibrosis (Fig. 3-17) (28,40). These non-septal bands are often several millimeters thick, irregular in contour, and associated with significant distortion of adjacent lung parenchyma and bronchovascular structures (41).

Parenchymal bands have been reported as most common in patients with asbestos-related lung and pleural disease (Fig. 3-18), sarcoidosis with interstitial fibrosis (Figs. 3-14,3-16), silicosis associated with progressive massive fibrosis and conglomerate masses, and tuberculosis (Table 3-3). In patients with asbestos exposure, multiple parenchymal bands are common;

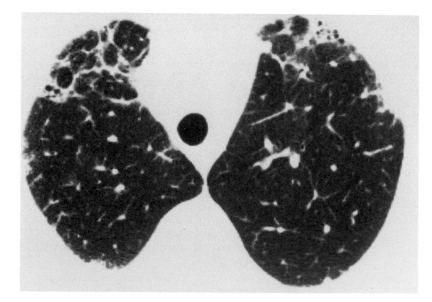

FIG. 3-15. Interlobular septal thickening in a patient with rheumatoid lung disease. Numerous irregularly thickened septa are visible in the anterior right lung.

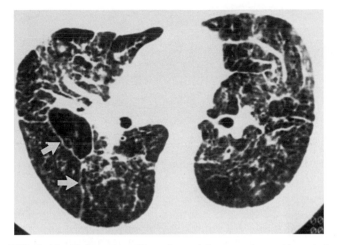

FIG. 3-16. Pulmonary fibrosis and "parenchymal bands" in a patient with sarcoidosis. Irregular septal thickening is present with distortion of lung architecture. Long confluent septa or "parenchymal bands" (*arrows*) are present bilaterally. Peribronchovascular interstitial thickening also results in prominence of the bronchi and pulmonary vessels. The pleural surfaces and the walls of vessels and bronchi appear irregular.

in one study (27) multiple parenchymal bands were seen in 66% of asbestos-exposed patients. In patients with asbestos-related disease, parenchymal bands can reflect thickened interlobular septa, indicating pulmonary fibrosis, or areas of atelectasis and focal scarring occurring in association with pleural plaques. In asbestos-exposed patients, parenchymal bands are frequently associated with areas of thickened pleura and have a basal predominance (27,40).

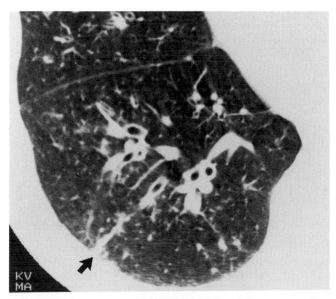

FIG. 3-17. Thick parenchymal band (*arrow*) representing a coarse scar in the peripheral lung. Also note thickening of the bronchial walls because of peribronchovascular fibrosis.

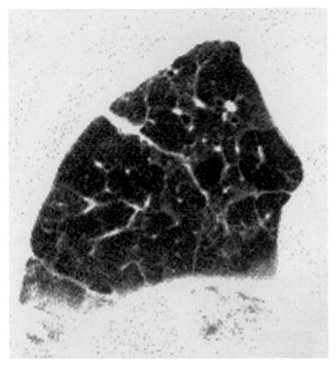

FIG. 3-18. Parenchymal bands in a patient with asbestosis. A prone scan shows both thick and thin bands. Most correspond to thickened septa.

Subpleural Interstitial Thickening

Usually, thickening of the interlobular septa within the peripheral lung is associated with thickening of the "subpleural interstitium" (3,4); both the septa and the subpleural interstitium are part of the "peripheral" interstitial fiber system described by Weibel (Fig. 2-1) (8). Subpleural interstitial thickening can be difficult to recognize in locations where the lung contacts the chest wall or mediastinum, but is easy to see adjacent to the major fissures (Figs. 3-1,3-4,3-8,3-13,3-19). Since two layers of the subpleural interstitium are seen adjacent to each other in this location, any subpleural

TABLE 3-3. *Differential diagnosis of parenchymal bands*

Diagnosis	Comments
Asbestosis	Multiple parenchymal bands common; associated with thickened pleura; septal thickening usually present
Sarcoidosis	Common, associated with septal thickening
Silicosis/Coal worker's pneumoconiosis	In association with PMF and emphysema
Tuberculosis	Associated with scarring

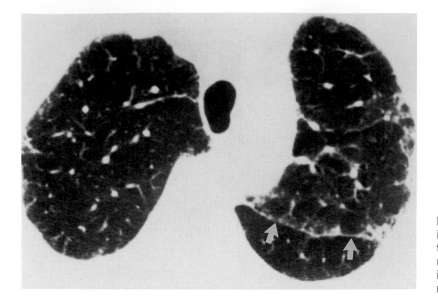

FIG. 3-19. Subpleural interstitial thickening in a patient with pulmonary fibrosis. Apparent thickening of the left major fissure (*arrows*) reflects irregular thickening of the subpleural interstitium. This finding is easiest to recognize adjacent to the fissures.

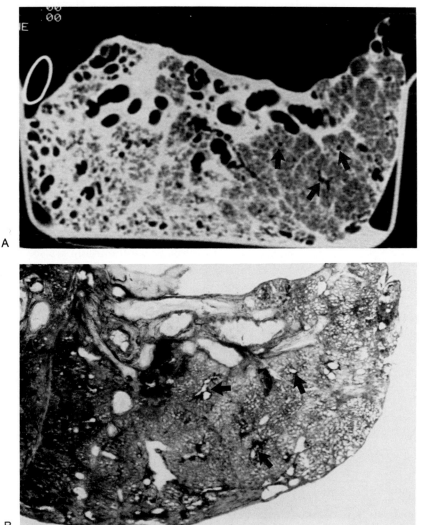

FIG. 3-20. Intralobular interstitial thickening in an isolated lung with pulmonary fibrosis. This is the same specimen as shown in Fig. 3-13. A fine network of lines within visible lobules produces a "spider-web" or "net-like" appearance (**A**). This abnormality contributes to the appearance of irregular interfaces (the "interface sign") at the edges of various structures such as arteries and bronchi. Intralobular bronchioles (*arrows*, A and B) are visible because of a combination of increased attenuation of surrounding lung, thickening of the peribronchiolar interstitium, and dilatation of the bronchiole that occurs as a result of fibrosis. (From Webb et al., ref. 18, with permission of *Radiology*.)

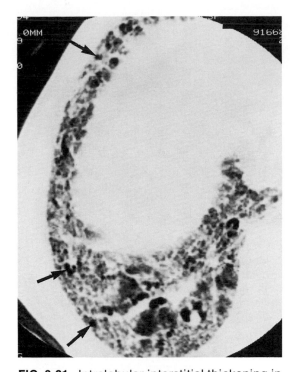

FIG. 3-21. Intralobular interstitial thickening in a patient with idiopathic pulmonary fibrosis. A fine network of lines is visible. Intralobular bronchioles (*arrows*) are visible throughout the peripheral lung as a result of fibrosis and "traction bronchiolectasis."

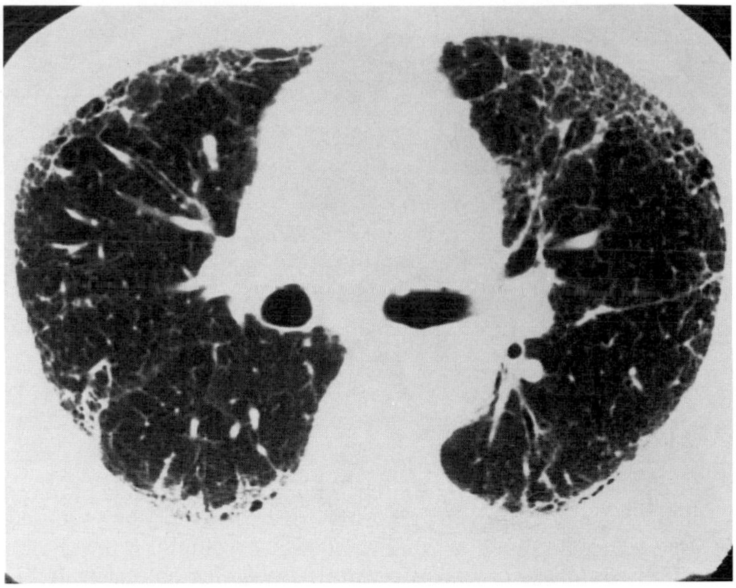

FIG. 3-22. Intralobular interstitial thickening in a patient with idiopathic pulmonary fibrosis. A fine network of lines in the anterior left lung reflects intralobular interstitial thickening.

abnormality appears twice as "abnormal" as it does elsewhere. Thus "thickening of the fissure" can represent subpleural interstitial thickening. If the thickening is smooth, it may be difficult to distinguish from fissural fluid. If the interface sign is present, and the thickening is irregular in appearance (Figs. 3-13,3-19) (4,6), or if the thickening is nodular (Fig. 3-4), an interstitial abnormality is more easily diagnosed.

In general, the differential diagnosis of subpleural interstitial thickening is the same as interlobular septal thickening, although subpleural interstitial thickening is more common than septal thickening in patients with idiopathic pulmonary fibrosis (IPF) or usual interstitial pneumonia of any cause (Table 3-2). The presence of subpleural interstitial fibrosis with irregular or "rugged" pleural surfaces has been reported by Nishimura et al. (7) as a common finding in IPF, correlating with the presence of fibrosis predominantly affecting the lobular periphery; this finding was present in 94% of cases of IPF he studied. A subpleural predominance of fibrosis can also be seen in patients with collagen-vascular diseases and drug reactions (42).

Nodular thickening of the subpleural interstitium can be seen (Fig. 3-4), and has the same differential diagnosis as nodular septal thickening (36). Remy-Jardin et al. (36) have reported the appearance of "subpleural micronodules," defined as less than 7 mm in diameter,

on HRCT in patients with sarcoidosis, coal worker's pneumoconiosis, lymphangitic spread of carcinoma, and in a small percentage of normal subjects. Subpleural nodules are described further below.

Intralobular Interstitial Thickening

Thickening of the intralobular interstitium (Fig. 2-1) results in a fine reticular pattern as seen on HRCT, with the lines of opacity separated by a few millimeters. Lung regions showing this finding characteristically have a fine mesh or net-like appearance that is easy to recognize (Figs. 3-1,3-20). Intralobular bronchioles are often visible on HRCT in patients with intralobular interstitial thickening and fibrosis because of a combination of their dilatation ("traction bronchiolectasis") and thickening of the peribronchiolar interstitium which surrounds them (Figs. 3-20,3-21) (7,18). Interlobular septal thickening may or may not be present in patients with intralobular interstitial thickening; when thickened septa are visible, they appear irregular. The pleural surfaces also appear irregular in the presence of intralobular interstitial thickening. Intralobular interstitial thickening can also be described using the term *intralobular lines* (18). This finding has also been called the *small reticular pattern* (6).

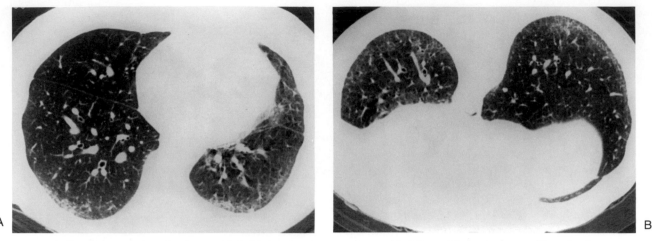

FIG. 3-23. Intralobular interstitial thickening in a patient with idiopathic pulmonary fibrosis. **A:** On a supine scan, an ill-defined increase in opacity is visible posteriorly. This would be difficult to diagnose as abnormal with certainty on this scan alone. **B:** In the prone position, a very fine reticular or web-like pattern is visible posteriorly in the peripheral lung, along with a few thickened septa. This appearance is typical of intralobular interstitial thickening. The peripheral distribution is characteristic of idiopathic pulmonary fibrosis.

Intralobular interstitial thickening as perceived on HRCT reflects thickening of the distal peribronchovascular interstitial tissues, in relation to small arteries and bronchioles, or thickening of the intralobular interstitium. It is most commonly seen in patients with pulmonary fibrosis (Figs. 3-20–3-23) (Table 3-4). In patients with idiopathic pulmonary fibrosis (IPF) or other causes of usual interstitial pneumonia (UIP), such as rheumatoid arthritis, scleroderma, or other collagen-vascular diseases, fibrosis tends to predominantly involve alveoli in the periphery of acini, resulting in a "peripheral acinar distribution" of interstitial fibrosis (7,42); this histologic finding correlates with the presence of intralobular lines on HRCT. In addition, the HRCT pattern of intralobular interstitial thickening can reflect the presence of very small honeycomb cysts or dilated bronchioles associated with surrounding lung fibrosis. Nishimura et al. (7) reviewed 46 cases of idiopathic pulmonary fibrosis with usual interstitial pneumonia (UIP), correlating findings on CT with appearances of lung histology from open biopsy specimens or autopsy. Visibility of centrilobular bronchioles in association with a fine reticulation or increased lung attenuation was visible in 96% of cases, indicating the presence of bronchiolar dilatation, fibrosis, and "microscopic" honeycombing, with dilated bronchioles or

TABLE 3-4. *Differential diagnosis of intralobular interstitial thickening*

Diagnosis	Comments
Idiopathic pulmonary fibrosis (IPF) or other cause of Usual interstitial pneumonia (UIP)	Common; associated with honeycombing
Asbestosis	Common
Hypersensitivity pneumonitis (chronic)	Common
Alveolar proteinosis	Common; associated with septal thickening and ground-glass opacity
Lymphangitic carcinomatosis	Uncommon; septal thickening predominates
Pulmonary edema	Uncommon; septal thickening predominates
Sarcoidosis	Uncommon
Silicosis/Coal worker's pneumoconiosis	Uncommon

TABLE 3-5. *Differential diagnosis of honeycombing*

Diagnosis	Comments
Idiopathic pulmonary fibrosis (IPF) or other cause of Usual interstitial pneumonia (UIP)	Common; peripheral
Asbestosis	Common; peripheral
Hypersensitivity pneumonitis (chronic)	Common; peripheral or diffuse
Sarcoidosis	Sometimes seen
Silicosis/Coal worker's pneumoconiosis	Uncommon
Histiocytosis X	Uncommon; cysts predominate

small cysts measuring approximately 1 mm in diameter (7).

Intralobular interstitial thickening can also be seen in the absence of significant fibrosis, in patients with lymphangitic spread of carcinoma (9), pulmonary edema, and alveolar proteinosis (Fig. 3-10).

Honeycombing

Extensive interstitial and alveolar fibrosis that results in alveolar disruption and bronchiolectasis produces the classic and characteristic appearance of *honeycombing* or *honeycomb lung*. Pathologically, honeycombing is defined by the presence of small air-containing cystic spaces, generally lined by bronchiolar epithelium, and having thickened walls composed of dense fibrous tissue. Honeycombing indicates the presence of "end-stage lung" and can be seen in almost any process leading to end-stage pulmonary fibrosis (Table 3-5) (38,43).

Honeycombing produces a characteristic cystic appearance on HRCT that allows a confident diagnosis of lung fibrosis to be made (18,25). On HRCT, the cystic spaces of honeycombing usually average about 1 cm in diameter, although they can range from several millimeters to several centimeters in size; they are characterized by clearly definable walls 1 to 3 mm in thickness (18,25) (Figs. 3-1,3-2,3-24,3-25). The cysts are air-filled and appear lucent in comparison to normal lung regions or regions of intralobular interstitial thickening. Adjacent honeycomb cysts typically share walls. Honeycombing has been described as producing the "intermediate reticular pattern" by Zerhouni and associates, to distinguish it from the larger pattern seen with interlobular septal thickening, and the smaller pattern visible with intralobular interstitial thickening (6).

Honeycomb cysts often predominate in the peripheral and subpleural lung regions regardless of their cause, and parahilar lung can appear normal despite the presence of extensive peripheral abnormalities

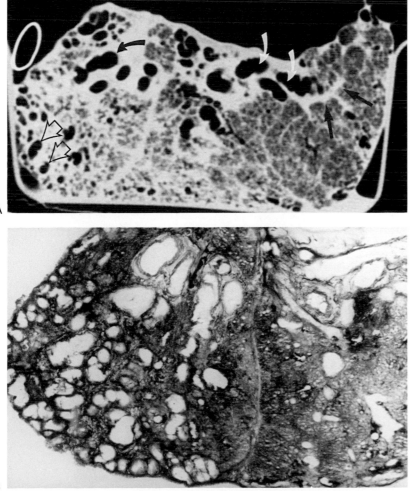

FIG. 3-24. Honeycombing and traction bronchiectasis in the patient with pulmonary fibrosis shown in Figs. 3-13 and 3-20. Large honeycomb cysts present in the posterior lung result in cystic spaces ranging up to several cm in diameter (*large open arrows*). They are characterized by thick, clearly definable, fibrous walls, and are easily identified in the corresponding lung section (**B**). Traction bronchiectasis (*curved arrows*) also reflects extensive fibrosis, and is often seen in patients with honeycombing. The edges of pulmonary vessels (*solid arrows*) appear irregular because of surrounding fibrosis. (From Webb et al., ref. 18, with permission of *Radiology*.)

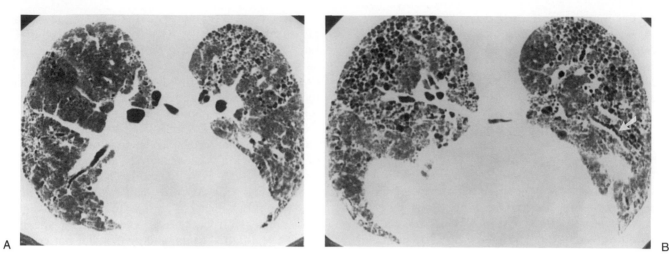

FIG. 3-25. Honeycombing in a patient with idiopathic pulmonary fibrosis (**A,B**; prone HRCT). Honeycombing results in cysts of varying sizes, which have a peripheral predominance. The cysts have thick and clearly definable walls. In areas of honeycombing, lobular anatomy cannot be resolved because of architectural distortion. In less abnormal areas some septal thickening can be seen. Vessels and bronchi have irregular interfaces, and bronchial irregularity (*arrow*) indicates traction bronchiectasis (B). Findings of honeycombing are more severe at the lung bases (B).

(Figs. 3-25,3-26). Subpleural honeycomb cysts typically occur in several contiguous layers (Figs. 3-25,3-26); this finding can allow honeycombing to be distinguished from subpleural emphysema (paraseptal emphysema) since subpleural cysts usually occur in a single layer. In a survey of patients with end-stage lung (38), subpleural honeycombing was present in 96% of patients with UIP associated with IPF or rheumatoid arthritis, 100% of asbestosis patients, 44% of those

with sarcoidosis, and in 75% of those with hypersensitivity pneumonitis (Table 3-5).

Honeycombing is often associated with other findings of lung fibrosis, such as intralobular interstitial thickening, traction bronchiectasis, traction bronchiolectasis, and irregular subpleural interstitial thickening (Fig. 3-24). On the other hand, significant interlobular septal thickening is not commonly visible in association with honeycombing, except in patients

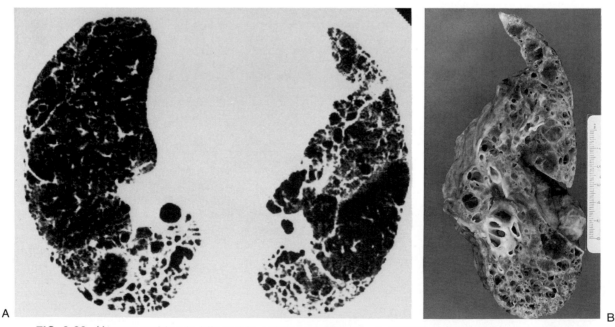

FIG. 3-26. Honeycombing in idiopathic pulmonary fibrosis. **A:** HRCT shows honeycomb cysts to predominate in the peripheral and subpleural regions. Note that the cysts occur in several layers. **B:** The resected left lung in this patient, sectioned at the level of the HRCT shown in A shows the honeycomb cysts, which are most extensive in the posterior and peripheral lung.

with sarcoidosis (38). In patients with HRCT findings of septal thickening, the presence of honeycombing distinguishes fibrosis from other causes of reticulation such as pulmonary edema or lymphangitic spread of carcinoma.

Subpleural Lines

A curvilinear opacity a few millimeters thick, less than 1 cm from the pleural surface, and paralleling the pleura, was first described in patients with asbestosis (44) and was termed the *subpleural curvilinear shadow*. It has been reported that a subpleural curvilinear shadow, or simply *subpleural line*, is much more common in patients with asbestosis than in those with idiopathic pulmonary fibrosis of other causes of UIP (45). Indeed, the presence of a subpleural line in nondependent lung has been reported in as many as 41% of patients with clinical findings of asbestosis (27). However, the presence of this finding is nonspecific and can be seen in a variety of lung diseases (Fig. 3-1). The presence of a subpleural line also has been reported as common in patients with scleroderma who have interstitial disease (46,47).

It was originally suggested that a subpleural line reflects the presence of fibrosis associated with honeycombing (44), and indeed, in some patients, a confluence of honeycomb cysts can result in a somewhat irregular subpleural line (Figs. 3-27,3-28). However, the appearance of a subpleural line has also recently been reported to occur as a result of the confluence of peribronchiolar interstitial abnormalities in patients with asbestosis, representing early fibrosis with associ-

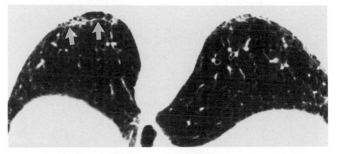

FIG. 3-28. Subpleural line (*arrows*) in a patient with rheumatoid lung disease and fibrosis, shown on a prone scan. Small honeycomb cysts are associated.

ated alveolar flattening and collapse (28). In these patients honeycombing was not present.

A subpleural line can also be seen in normal patients as a result of atelectasis within the dependent lung (Fig. 3-29) (e.g., the posterior lung when the patient is positioned supine); the presence of dependent atelectasis has been confirmed experimentally (48). Also, a thicker, less well-defined subpleural opacity, a so-called dependent density (27), can also be seen in normal subjects as a result of volume loss. Such normal posterior lines or opacities are transient, and disappear in the prone position. In a study by Aberle and associates (27) of patients with asbestos exposure, neither transient subpleural lines nor transient dependent densities correlated with the clinical suspicion of pulmonary fibrosis.

Transient subpleural lines have also been reported in patients with "pulmonary congestion" due to heart failure (49), but the relationship, if any, between the subpleural line and congestion or edema is unclear. Pilate et al. (50) have also suggested that subpleural lines might correspond to the normal subpleural lym-

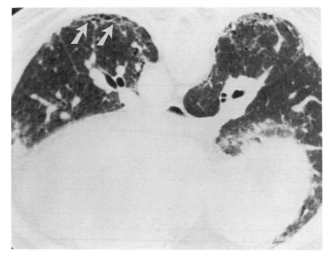

FIG. 3-27. Subpleural line in a patient with asbestosis. An ill-defined subpleural line (*arrows*) on a prone scan, reflects subpleural fibrosis and honeycombing. Other findings of pulmonary fibrosis are also present.

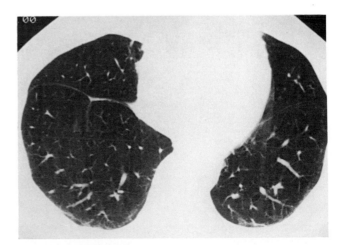

FIG. 3-29. Dependent atelectasis resulting in a posterior subpleural line. An ill-defined subpleural line is present posteriorly. No other findings of fibrosis are present, and this line disappeared in the prone position.

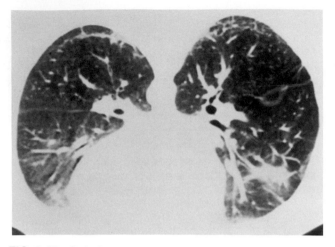

FIG. 3-30. Subpleural line that resolved after treatment in a patient with idiopathic pulmonary fibrosis. In the prone position, bilateral nontransient subpleural lines appear to represent fibrosis. Several small lucencies peripheral to them appear to represent areas of lung destruction or honeycombing. However all these findings cleared following treatment with steroids. This appearance may reflect atelectasis and air trapping within the peripheral lung occurring as a result of an increased closing volume (or in other words, an increased tendency for lung collapse).

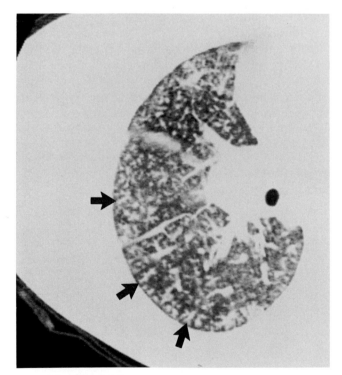

FIG. 3-31. Centrilobular peribronchovascular interstitial thickening. In a patient with lymphangitic spread of carcinoma, the major HRCT abnormality is centrilobular interstitial thickening manifested as increased prominence of the branching arteries (*arrows*) in the lobular core. The absence of associated septal thickening is unusual.

phatic network, but extensive HRCT experience with lymphangitic spread of carcinoma causing lymphatic and perilymphatic abnormalities does not support this contention.

More difficult to explain in some patients with interstitial disease, is a non-transient subpleural line associated with areas of lucency peripheral to it, which can be reversible in a period of weeks or months following treatment (Fig. 3-30). This finding closely mimics the appearance of fibrosis and honeycombing on HRCT, but honeycombing should not be reversible. A reversible subpleural line with peripheral lucency may reflect atelectasis (the line), with small bronchial or bronchiolar obstruction occurring because of the atelectasis, and air trapping within the peripheral lung (the lucency). As such, the presence of this abnormality could reflect an increased closing volume (or in other words, an increased tendency for the lung to collapse) that is known to occur as a result of early interstitial lung disease. In the presence of appropriate treatment, such a finding might disappear. The association of plate-like atelectasis at the junction of "cortical" and "medullary" lung regions, air trapping in the lung peripheral to the atelectasis, and decreased compliance of lung because of interstitial infiltration was first reported by Kubota et al. (51).

Centrilobular (Lobular Core) Abnormalities

Centrilobular linear or reticular abnormalities can reflect interstitial thickening or bronchiolar abnormalities such as bronchiolar dilatation and the finding of "tree-in-bud."

Interstitial Thickening

Diseases that cause interstitial thickening often result in prominence of the centrilobular vessel, which normally appears as a dot, Y-shaped, or X-shaped branching opacity. This finding represents an abnormality of the intralobular component of the peribronchovascular interstitium, termed the *centrilobular interstitium* (Fig. 2-1). It is exactly analogous to the peribronchovascular interstitial thickening described above as visible in the parahilar lung (3,6,10,27). On HRCT, a linear, branching, or dot-like abnormality may be seen (Fig. 3-1).

Thickening of the intralobular bronchovascular interstitium is usually associated with interlobular septal thickening or intralobular interstitial thickening (Figs. 3-1,3-9), but sometimes occurs as an isolated abnormality (Fig. 3-31). Centrilobular interstitial thickening is common in patients with lymphangitic spread of carcinoma or lymphoma (9,10), and interstitial pulmonary edema (Table 3-6) (52). In patients with lung fibrosis, centrilobular interstitial thickening is common but al-

TABLE 3-6. *Differential diagnosis of reticular centrilobular opacities*

Diagnosis	Comments
Idiopathic pulmonary fibrosis (IPF) or other cause of Usual interstitial pneumonia (UIP)	Common in association with other findings of fibrosis; uncommon as a predominant finding
Asbestosis	Common as an isolated finding in early disease; usually appears nodular
Lymphangitic spread of tumor	Common; usually associated with septal thickening
Interstitial pulmonary edema	Common; usually associated with septal thickening
Endobronchial spread of TB; Nontuberculous mycobacteria	Tree-in-bud appearance common
Cystic fibrosis; Bronchiectasis	Tree-in-bud appearance common; associated with bronchiectasis
Bronchopneumonia	Tree-in-bud appearance may be seen; associated with consolidation, ill-defined nodules
Asian panbronchiolitis; Small airways disease	Tree-in-bud appearance common, dilated other air-filled bronchioles, centrilobular nodules

most always associated with honeycombing or intralobular lines. The appearance of centrilobular interstitial thickening is discussed further below (see centrilobular nodules).

Bronchiolar Dilatation and "Tree-in-Bud"

The intralobular bronchiole, which is not seen in normal subjects, is sometimes visible on HRCT in patients with centrilobular interstitial thickening because of a combination of (i) increased attenuation of surrounding lung, (ii) thickening of the peribronchiolar interstitium, and (iii) dilatation of the bronchiole, which occurs as a result of fibrosis (Figs. 3-20,3-21).

Diseases that involve small airways can also result in increased prominence of centrilobular branching structures recognizable as an increase in reticulation on HRCT (53,54). Visibility of the centrilobular bronchiole in the absence of other findings of interstitial thickening should suggest airways disease; this finding can indicate dilatation of the bronchiole and bronchiolar wall thickening, or peribronchiolar fibrosis or inflammation (Figs. 3-1,3-32). In some patients, small airways that are dilated and/or filled with pus, mucus, or inflammatory exudate appear as small, well-defined, centrilobular nodular, linear, or branching structures of soft-tissue opacity (Figs. 3-1,3-33,3-34) (55). This appearance on HRCT has been likened to a *tree-in-bud* (41), a descriptive term which is quite helpful in recognizing this abnormality. The term "budding tree" has also been used to describe small airway filling on bronchography (56). The association of such small airway abnormalities with findings of bronchiectasis, history, or pulmonary function tests can help distinguish small bronchiolar abnormalities from other causes of centrilobular reticulation.

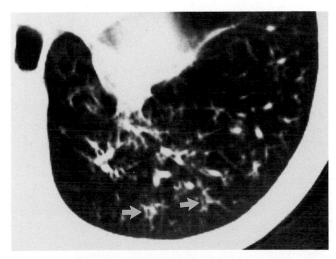

FIG. 3-32. Dilated, air-filled intralobular bronchioles (*arrows*) in the left lower lobe of an 11-year-old patient with hypogammaglobulinemia and bronchiectasis.

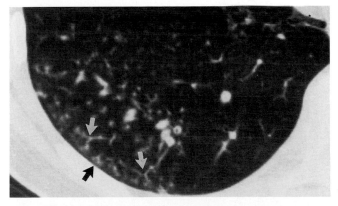

FIG. 3-33. Centrilobular bronchiolar abnormality in a patient with yellow-nails syndrome and chronic bronchial sepsis. Well-defined, fluid-filled centrilobular bronchioles (*arrows*) are visible in the posterior right lower lobe as fine branching structures with nodular tips. These have the appearance of a "tree-in-bud."

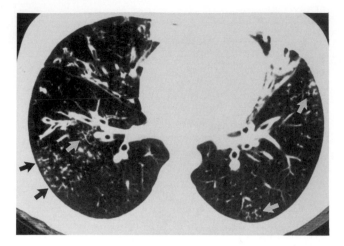

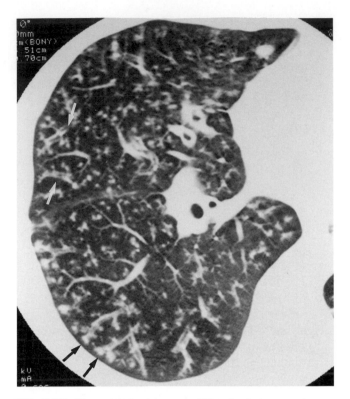

FIG. 3-34. Centrilobular bronchiolar abnormality in a patient with cystic fibrosis. Fluid, mucus, or pus-filled centrilobular bronchioles result in a tree-in-bud appearance in several lung regions (*arrows*). These are associated with findings of bronchiectasis.

Abnormal bronchioles producing a tree-in-bud appearance can usually be distinguished from normal centrilobular vessels by their more irregular appearance, a lack of tapering, or a knobby or bulbous appearance at the tips of small branches. This latter appearance reflects the presence of bronchiolar dilatation or peribronchiolar inflammation. Also, as tree-in-bud is often patchy in distribution even in patients with a diffuse airway abnormality, the appearances of the abnormal airways and normal vessels in other lung regions can be easily contrasted.

Centrilobular bronchiolar abnormalities characterized by dilatation and a tree-in-bud appearance are seen in patients with Asian panbronchiolitis (53,57),

FIG. 3-35. Bronchiolar abnormalities in Asian panbronchiolitis. Dilated and thick-walled bronchioles (*white arrows*) are seen in association with a tree-in-bud appearance (*black arrows*) and multiple centrilobular nodules. These findings correlate pathologically with the presence of dilated bronchioles, inflammatory bronchiolar wall thickening, abundant intraluminal secretions, and peribronchiolar inflammation. (Courtesy of Harumi Itoh, M.D., Chest Disease Research Institute, Kyoto University, Kyoto, Japan.)

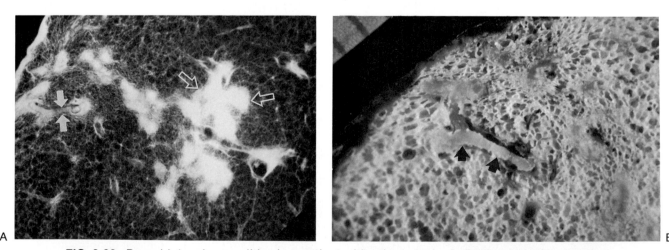

FIG. 3-36. Bronchiolar abnormalities in a patient with tuberculosis. **A:** Radiograph of a resected lung in a patient with endobronchial spread of tuberculosis, shows a branching centrilobular opacity (*solid arrows*), and rosettes of small nodular opacities producing a tree-in-bud appearance (*open arrows*). **B:** On pathologic examination, the branching centrilobular opacity represents caseous material filling bronchioles and alveolar ducts (*arrows*). (Courtesy of Jung-Gi Im, M.D., Seoul National University Hospital, Seoul, Korea.) (From Im et al., ref. 41, with permission.)

endobronchial spread of tuberculosis (41) or nontuberculous mycobacteria, cystic fibrosis (54), bronchopneumonia, bronchiectasis of any cause, and other airway diseases that result in the accumulation of mucus or pus within small bronchi. In patients with Asian panbronchiolitis, prominent, branching centrilobular opacities represent dilated bronchioles with inflammatory bronchiolar wall thickening and abundant intraluminal secretions (Fig. 3-35) (53,58). Similarly, in patients with active tuberculosis, a tree-in-bud appearance was visible in 72% of patients in one study (41), correlating with the presence of solid caseous material within terminal and respiratory bronchioles (Fig. 3-36).

NODULES AND NODULAR OPACITIES

An approach to the assessment and differential diagnosis of multiple nodular opacities is based on a consideration of their size (small or large), distribution, and appearance (well-defined or ill-defined).

Small Nodules

In this book we will use the term *small nodule* to define a rounded opacity less than 1 cm in diameter, whereas *large nodule* will be used to refer to nodules 1 cm or greater in diameter. Some authors have used "micronodule" to describe nodules that are either less than 3 mm (59) or less than 7 mm in diameter (36,60), but it is not clear that this distinction is of value in differential diagnosis (59), and we will not use this term.

Differences in the appearances of nodules that are predominantly "interstitial" or predominantly "air-

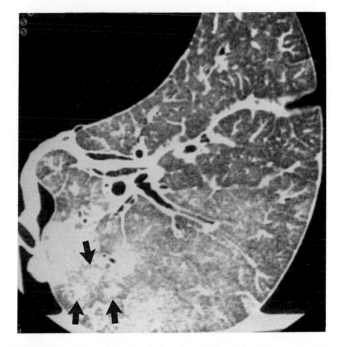

FIG. 3-38. Air-space nodules in an isolated lung. In this patient, centrilobular nodules (*arrows*) representing air-space pulmonary edema are visible in the posterior lung. These are larger and less well-defined than interstitial nodules. (From Webb, ref. 3, with permission.)

space" in origin have been emphasized by several authors. Nodules considered to be interstitial are usually well-defined despite their small size (Fig. 3-37). Nodules as small as 1 to 2 mm in diameter can be detected on HRCT in patients with interstitial diseases such as sarcoidosis (11,14,35,61-63), histiocytosis X (64,65), silicosis and coal worker's pneumoconiosis (36,37,66-68), miliary tuberculosis (26, 70), and metastatic tumor (4,31,69,71). Interstitial nodules usually appear to be

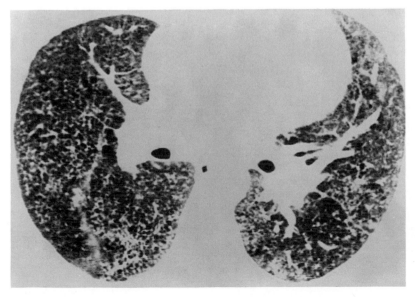

FIG. 3-37. Histiocytosis X with reticular opacities and small nodules. Small nodules best seen in the paravertebral regions are associated with an overall increase in reticular opacities.

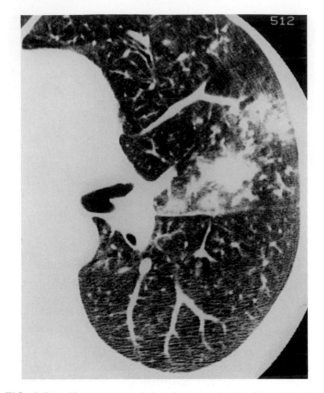

FIG. 3-39. Air-space nodules in a patient with a lobular pneumonia. The nodules are of soft-tissue opacity and obscure vessels. They are centrilobular in location and spare the subpleural lung peripherally and adjacent to the fissures. The small lucency seen within several of the nodules may reflect the centrilobular bronchiole. (From Webb, ref. 3, with permission.)

of soft-tissue attenuation and obscure the edges of vessels or other structures in which they touch (72-77). Air-space nodules, on the other hand, are more likely to be ill-defined (3,26,78-80); they can be of homogeneous soft-tissue attenuation (Figs. 3-38,3-39), thus ob-

scuring vessels, or hazy and less dense than adjacent vessels (so-called ground-glass opacity) (Fig. 3-40). A cluster or rosette of small nodules can also be seen (Fig. 3-36A) (78). Air-space nodules have also been termed "acinar nodules," because they approximate the size of acini, but these nodules are not truly acinar histologically, but tend to be centrilobular and peribronchiolar (79); *ill-defined nodule* or *air-space nodule* are preferable terms.

Despite these differences in appearance, a distinction between interstitial and air-space nodules on the basis of HRCT findings can be quite difficult, and, in fact, is somewhat arbitrary, because many nodular diseases affect both the interstitial and alveolar compartments histologically. The distribution or location of small nodules is generally more valuable in differential diagnosis than their appearance. In different conditions, small nodules can appear randomly distributed, perilymphatic in distribution, or predominantly centrilobular (Fig. 3-41). Although there may be some overlap between these appearances, in most cases, a predominant distribution of nodules is evident on HRCT.

Random Distribution

Small nodules that appear randomly distributed in relation to structures of the secondary lobule (Fig. 3-41) are often seen in patients with miliary tuberculosis (Fig. 3-41) and miliary fungal infections (41,42,70) (Table 3-7). The nodules can be seen in relation to small vessels, interlobular septa, and the pleural surfaces, but do not appear to have a consistent or predominant relationship to any of these. On HRCT, a uniform distribution of nodules without respect for anatomic structures is most typical. In miliary tuberculosis or fungal infections, the nodules tend to be well-defined and up to several millimeters in diameter.

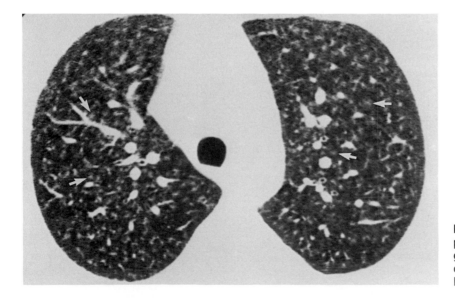

FIG. 3-40. Air-space nodules in organizing pneumonia. Small, ill-defined ground-glass opacity nodules (*arrows*) are visible diffusely. Some can be seen to be centrilobular.

TABLE 3-7. *Differential diagnosis of small nodules—random distribution*

Diagnosis	Comments
Miliary TB, Fungus	Common; nodules may sometimes appear related to vessels
Hematogenous metastases	Common; nodules may sometimes appear related to vessels
Silicosis/Coal worker's pneumoconiosis	When numerous, may appear diffuse and random; centrilobular and subpleural nodules usually predominate; posterior predominance common
Histiocytosis X	When numerous, may appear diffuse and random; otherwise centrilobular

Hematogenous metastases also tend to be randomly distributed in relation to lobular structures (Fig. 5-5), although they have a recognized tendency to predominate in the lung periphery and at the lung bases (71). As with miliary TB, the nodules can be seen in relation

to small vessels in some locations, a fact which likely reflects their mode of dissemination. In a study correlating HRCT and pathologic findings (71), nodules less than 3 mm in diameter had no consistent relationship to lobular structures. Eleven percent of nodules were

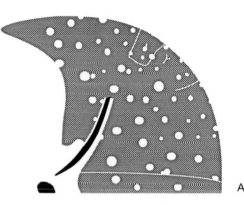

FIG. 3-41. **A:** Appearance of small nodules with a random distribution. Although some nodules can be seen in relation to interlobular septa, vessels, or the pleural surfaces, nodules do not appear to have a consistent or predominant relationship to any of these structures. A uniform distribution is most typical. **B:** Miliary tuberculosis with small nodules. Nodules a few millimeters in diameter have a random distribution, and appear widely and evenly distributed throughout the lung. Some nodules can be seen in relation to small vessels, the pleural surfaces, and the interlobar fissure, but the nodules do not predominate in relation to these structures. (Courtesy of Jung-Gi Im, M.D., Seoul National University Hospital, Seoul, Korea.) (From Im et al., ref. 41, with permission.) **C:** In another patient with miliary tuberculosis, the nodules are smaller than those shown in B. The nodules are widely dispersed. (Courtesy of Shin-Ho Kook, M.D., Koryo General Hospital, Seoul, Korea.)

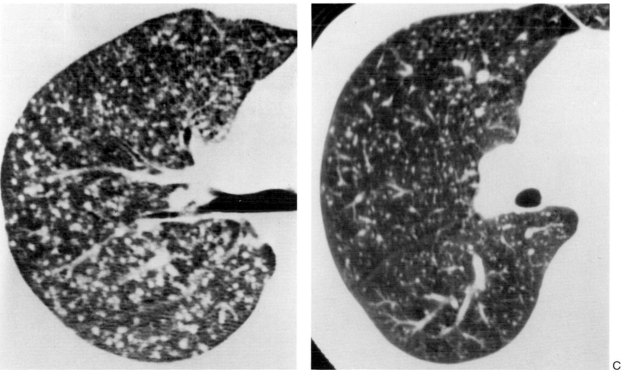

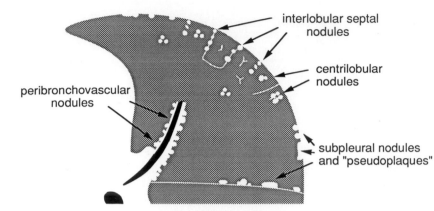

FIG. 3-42. Appearance of small nodules with a perilymphatic distribution. Nodules predominate in relation to the parahilar peribronchovascular interstitium, the centrilobular interstitium, interlobular septa, and the subpleural regions. Conglomerate subpleural nodules can form "pseudoplaques."

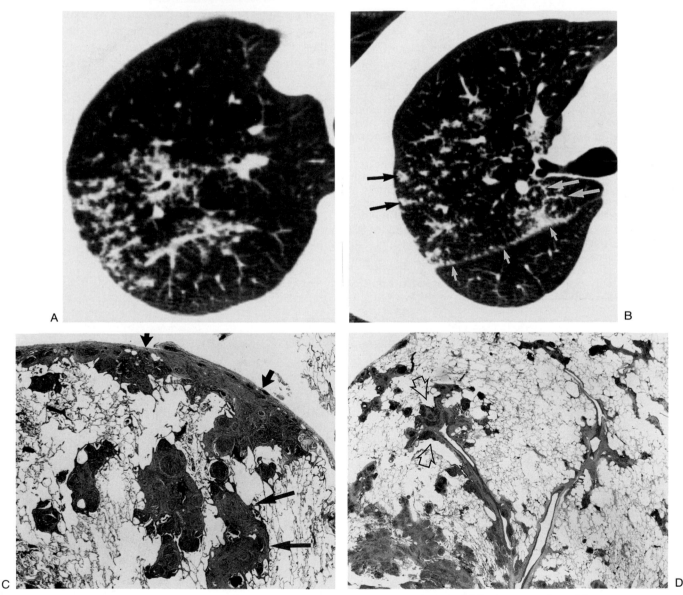

FIG. 3-43. Sarcoidosis showing a "perilymphatic distribution" on HRCT and open lung biopsy. **A:** HRCT through the upper lobe shows small nodules in relation to the peribronchovascular regions and small vessels. Vessels and bronchi show a nodular appearance. **B:** At a lower level, small nodules are seen in the subpleural regions along the fissure (*small white arrows*), in the centrilobular regions (*black arrows*), and interlobular septa (*long white arrows*). **C,D:** Open lung biopsy shows that the small nodules correspond to groups of granulomas which are subpleural (C, *short arrows*), septal (C, *long arrows*), and centrilobular and peribronchiolar (D, *open arrows*).

TABLE 3-8. *Differential diagnosis of small nodules—"perilymphatic" distribution*

Diagnosis	Comments
Sarcoidosis	Common; peribronchovascular and subpleural nodules predominate; septal and centrilobular nodules less common; patchy; upper lobe predominance; rarely cavitate; may calcify
Silicosis/Coal worker's pneumoconiosis	Common; centrilobular and subpleural nodules predominate; peribronchovascular and septal less common; more symmetrical than sarcoid; upper lobe, posterior predominance; may calcify in silicosis
Lymphangitic carcinomatosis, Lymphoma	Nodules not common; peribronchovascular, septal, subpleural nodules predominate
Amyloidosis	Subpleural, septal, centrilobular; may calcify; rare
Lymphocytic interstitial pneumonia (LIP) in AIDS patients	Ill-defined centrilobular nodules; peribronchovascular; septal

seen in relation to the centrilobular pulmonary arteries, 21% were related to interlobular septa , and 68% were located in between. On examination of specimen radiographs and pathology, a similar distribution was noted. Nodules resulting from hematogenous metastasis are characteristically well-defined.

When numerous, nodules in patients with histiocytosis X (Fig. 3-37) or silicosis may appear to be randomly and diffusely distributed (42), and may be difficult to distinguish from the nodules of miliary infection or metastases. However, the more typical appearances of these diseases are described below.

Perilymphatic Distribution

Nodules that predominate in relation to the parahilar peribronchovascular interstitium, the centrilobular interstitium, interlobular septa, and in a subpleural location are typical of patients with sarcoidosis, silicosis and coal worker's pneumoconiosis, and lymphangitic spread of carcinoma (36,42) (Table 3-8) (Fig. 3-42). This

pattern of abnormalities has been termed *lymphatic* or *perilymphatic*, in that it corresponds to the distribution of lymphatics in the lung; also, each of these diseases typically results in histologic abnormalities that occur in relation to lymphatics (36,42). However, these diseases usually show different patterns of involvement of the perilymphatic interstitium that allow their differentiation in most cases.

In nearly all patients with sarcoidosis, HRCT shows nodules, ranging in size from several millimeters to 1 cm or more in diameter (14,35). The nodules often appear sharply defined despite their small size, but can be ill-defined as well. Nodules are most frequently seen in relationship to the parahilar peribronchovascular interstitium (Fig. 3-5), the subpleural interstitium, and small vessels; histologically small clusters of granulomas are visible in these locations (Figs. 3-43,3-44) (14,35,72). Nodules that can be recognized as centrilobular or septal in location are less frequently seen on HRCT in patients with sarcoidosis (Fig. 3-43) (55), but also correlate with typical histologic abnormalities. Large nodules, measuring from 1 to 4 centimeter in

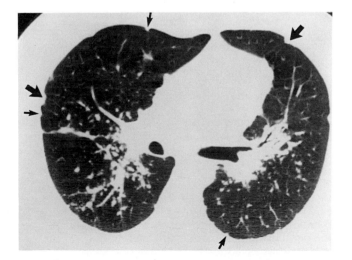

FIG. 3-44. Sarcoidosis with a "perilymphatic" distribution of nodules. Numerous small nodules are seen in relation to the parahilar, bronchovascular interstitium. Bronchial walls appear irregularly thickened. Subpleural nodules (*small arrows*) are also seen bordering the costal pleural surfaces, and right major fissure. This appearance is virtually diagnostic of sarcoidosis. Clusters of subpleural granulomas (*large arrows*) have been termed pseudoplaques.

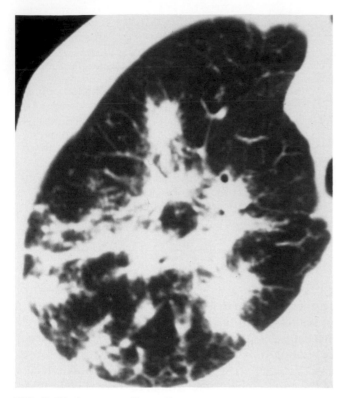

FIG. 3-45. Large peribronchovascular nodules in a patient with sarcoidosis, representing clusters of granulomas. These have irregular margins. Small nodules are also visible.

diameter are seen in 15% to 25% of patients (14,73,74) and represent masses of granulomatous lesions, each granuloma being less than 0.4 millimeters in diameter (72). These large nodules tend to have irregular margins (Fig. 3-45). An upper lobe predominance of nodules is common in sarcoidosis (36). Nodules can cavitate, but this is uncommon; Grenier et al. (59) report this finding in only 3% of cases. Occasionally, nodules visible on HRCT represent nodular areas of fibrosis rather than active granulomas (35).

Silicosis and coal worker's pneumoconiosis are associated with the presence of small nodules, usually measuring from 2 to 5 mm in diameter, which predominantly appear centrilobular and subpleural in location on HRCT (Fig. 3-46) (36,37,66,68,75). These correlate with areas of fibrosis surrounding centrilobular respiratory bronchioles and involving the subpleural interstitium, and are caused by the accumulation of particulate material in these regions (36,68). Parenchymal nodules are visible in 80% of patients with coal worker's pneumoconiosis, while subpleural nodules are seen in 87% (36,37). Nodules occurring in relation to the peribronchovascular interstitium and thickened interlobular septa are less frequent and less conspicuous than in patients with sarcoidosis or lymphangitic spread of tumor. Also, nodules appear more evenly distributed

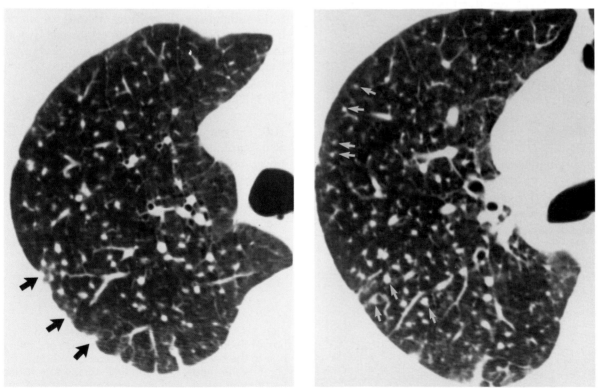

A

B

FIG. 3-46. A,B: Small nodules in a patient with silicosis. Nodules predominate in the subpleural (A, *black arrows*) and centrilobular (B, *white arrows*) regions. Peribronchovascular nodules are less frequent than in patients with sarcoidosis, and the nodules appear more evenly distributed. The nodules often predominate posteriorly and in the upper lobes. (Courtesy of Raymond Glyn Thomas, M.D., The Rand Mutual Hospital, Johannesburg, South Africa.)

than in patients with sarcoidosis; they are present diffusely and bilaterally, but in patients with mild silicosis or coal worker's pneumoconiosis, are usually visible only in the upper lobes. A posterior predominance of nodules is often present (37,66). In patients with silicosis, the nodules can calcify.

In patients with lymphangitic spread of tumor, when nodules are visible, they are most often visible within the thickened peribronchovascular interstitium and interlobular septa (Figs. 3-11,3-47,3-48) (6,9,10,12, 31,67). Peribronchovascular and subpleural nodules are typically not as profuse as in patients with sarcoidosis. Septal thickening results in the appearance of a "beaded" septum (Figs. 3-11,3-47) (11,31,76). In a HRCT study of postmortem lung specimens (31), 19 of 22 cases with interstitial pulmonary metastases showed the appearance of "beaded" or nodular septal thickening on HRCT. The beaded septa corresponded directly to the presence of tumor growing in pulmonary capillaries, lymphatics, and the septal interstitium. In this study (31), beaded septa were not noted in any of the specimens of patients with pulmonary edema, fibrosis, or in normal lungs.

Interstitial thickening with nodularity visible on HRCT in relation to vessels, bronchi, interlobular septa, and the subpleural interstitium has been re-

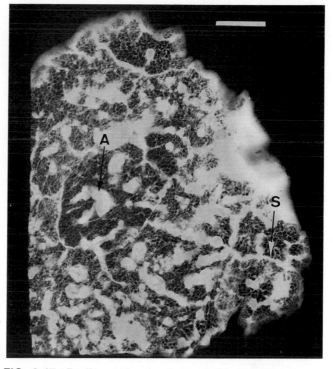

FIG. 3-47. Radiograph of a 1-mm thick lung slice in a patient with lymphangitic spread of tumor. Note the nodular thickening of interlobular septa (S), and the centrilobular interstitium surrounding arteries (A). Bar = 1 cm. (Courtesy of Harumi Itoh, M.D., Chest Disease Research Institute, Kyoto University, Kyoto, Japan.)

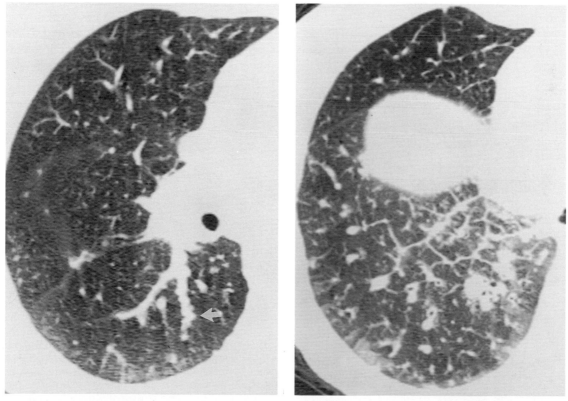

FIG. 3-48. Lymphangitic spread of carcinoma. **A:** Peribronchovascular nodules (*arrow*) give a nodular appearance to a lower lobe pulmonary artery branch. **B:** At a lower level, interlobular septal thickening is also seen, characteristic of lymphangitic spread of carcinoma.

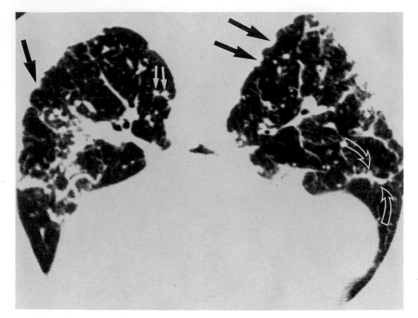

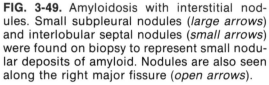

FIG. 3-49. Amyloidosis with interstitial nodules. Small subpleural nodules (*large arrows*) and interlobular septal nodules (*small arrows*) were found on biopsy to represent small nodular deposits of amyloid. Nodules are also seen along the right major fissure (*open arrows*).

ported in a patient with diffuse amyloidosis (Fig. 3-49) (34). The nodules can be calcified. A few small subpleural and centrilobular nodules can also be seen in smokers probably related to the presence of fibrosis and accumulated particulate material in the peribronchial regions and at the bases of interlobular septa, and probably related to pathways of lymphatic drainage. Lymphocytic interstitial pneumonia (LIP) can result in the presence of lymphocytic and plasma cell infiltrates in relation to the peribronchovascular interstitium, interlobular septa, and in the subpleural and centrilobular regions. On HRCT, ill-defined centrilobular opacities can be seen.

A perilymphatic distribution of nodules is most easily diagnosed when nodules are visible in a subpleural location, particularly in relation to the fissures, where they can be easily distinguished from pulmonary vessels. Subpleural nodules have been reported in about 80% of patients with silicosis or coal worker's pneumoconiosis, 50% of patients with sarcoidosis, and are also common with lymphangitic spread of carcinoma (36). In smokers, subpleural nodules can correspond to the presence of fibrosis and accumulated dust at the base of interlobular septa, probably related to pathways of lymphatic drainage, and similar in etiology to the subpleural nodules occurring in coal workers. Confluent

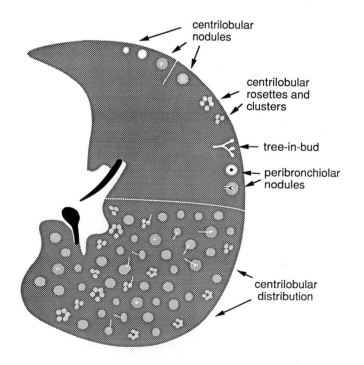

FIG. 3-50. HRCT appearances of centrilobular nodules. Centrilobular nodules are usually separated from the interlobular septa and pleural surfaces by a distance of several millimeters; in the lung periphery the nodules are usually centered 5 to 10 mm from the pleural surface. Also, centrilobular nodules may be associated with small pulmonary artery branches. Because of the similar size of secondary lobules, centrilobular nodules often appear to be evenly spaced. Although they are often ill-defined, this is not always the case. Either a single centrilobular nodule, or a centrilobular rosette of nodules may be seen. In occasional cases, the air-filled centrilobular bronchiole can be recognized as a rounded lucency within a centrilobular nodule.

subpleural nodules can result in the appearance of "pseudoplaques"; linear areas of subpleural opacity several millimeters in thickness that mimic the appearance of asbestos-related parietopleural plaques (Figs. 3-42,3-44). The presence of "pseudoplaques" in these diseases correlates significantly with the profusion of subpleural nodules (36).

Centrilobular Distribution

As indicated above, centrilobular nodules can be seen in association with other abnormalities in patients having a perilymphatic distribution of disease. Nodules limited to the centrilobular regions can also be seen (Fig. 3-50). These nodules may be dense and of homogeneous opacity, or of ground-glass opacity, and range from a few millimeters to a centimeter in size. Either a single centrilobular nodule, or a centrilobular rosette of nodules may be visible (78-80). Although they are often ill-defined, this is not always the case. Because of the similar size of secondary lobules, centrilobular nodules often appear to be evenly spaced.

Centrilobular nodules are usually separated from the interlobular septa and pleural surfaces by a distance of several millimeters; in the lung periphery the nodules are usually centered 5 to 10 mm from the pleural surface (Fig. 3-50). They do not usually occur in relation to interlobular septa or the pleural surfaces, as do random or perilymphatic nodules, and the subpleural lung is typically spared. This difference can be particularly valuable in distinguishing diffuse centrilobular nodules from diffuse, random nodules.

Sometimes, these nodules can be precisely localized as centrilobular by noting their relationship to lobular structures, but this is relatively uncommon. The term *centrilobular nodule* is best thought of as indicating that the nodule is related to *centrilobular structures*, such as small vessels, even if they cannot be precisely localized to the lobular core (Figs. 3-38–3-40,3-50,3-51). Indeed, in most cases, centrilobular nodules can be correctly identified by noting their association with small pulmonary artery branches. It is typical for centrilobular nodules to appear perivascular on HRCT, surrounding or obscuring the smallest pulmonary arteries visible on HRCT (Fig. 3-51). In occasional cases, the air-filled centrilobular bronchiole can be recognized as a rounded lucency within a centrilobular nodule (Fig. 3-39).

Centrilobular nodules can be seen in patients with a variety of diseases that primarily affect centrilobular bronchioles or arteries and result in inflammation or fibrosis of the surrounding interstitium and alveoli (Table 3-9) (42). Bronchiolar diseases most frequently result in this finding, sometimes in association with centrilobular airway dilatation or the appearance of a

tree-in-bud. Well-defined, small peribronchiolar nodules, representing interstitial granulomas, have been described in patients with histiocytosis X (Fig. 3-37) (65). Ill-defined centrilobular opacities can occur in patients with endobronchial spread of tuberculosis or nontuberculous mycobacteria (Fig. 3-36) (26,41,79,81), so-called lobular or bronchopneumonia (Fig. 3-39) (79), Asian panbronchiolitis (Fig. 3-35) (53,57), hypersensitivity pneumonitis (Fig. 3-51) (82-84), bronchiolitis obliterans with organizing pneumonia (BOOP) (Fig. 3-103) (85), respiratory bronchiolitis in smokers (Figs. 6-10,6-11) (86,87), bronchiolitis obliterans (Fig. 3-102) (87), bronchiolectasis with surrounding fibrosis in cigarette smokers (86), asbestosis (Figs. 4-30,4-31) (28,77), pulmonary edema (Figs. 6-41, and 6-42), vasculitis, and talcosis (42,88). Bronchioloalveolar carcinoma (Fig. 5-7) and endobronchial spread of tracheobronchial papillomatosis (Fig. 3-104) can also result in small centrilobular nodules (88).

Centrilobular nodules can reflect the presence of either interstitial or air-space abnormalities, and the histologic correlations reported to occur in association with centrilobular nodules vary with the disease entity

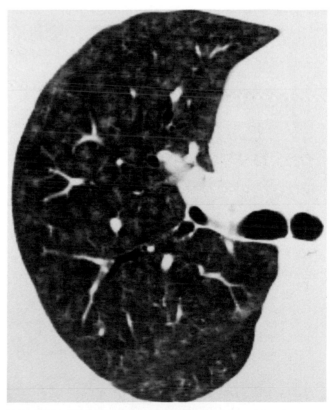

FIG. 3-51. Centrilobular ground-glass opacities in a patient with hypersensitivity pneumonitis. Small ill-defined opacities are visible in relation to small vascular branches throughout the lung. The most peripheral nodules are centered 5 to 10 mm from the pleural surface. The subpleural lung region appears spared.

TABLE 3-9. *Differential diagnosis of small centrilobular nodules*

Diagnosis	Comments
Endobronchial spread of TB, Nontuberculous mycobacteria	Common; associated with bronchiolar abnormalities ("tree-in-bud")
Bronchopneumonia	Common; findings similar to those of bronchogenic spread of TB
Asian panbronchiolitis	Common; associated with bronchiolar abnormalities; bronchiolar dilatation; findings of air trapping
Hypersensitivity pneumonitis	Common; nodules of ground-glass opacity; bronchiolar abnormalities lacking; larger areas of ground-glass opacity may be present
Bronchiolitis obliterans organizing pneumonia/ Cryptogenic organizing pneumonia (BOOP/COP)	Common; areas of ground-glass opacity or consolidation predominate; bronchiolar abnormalities lacking
Respiratory bronchiolitis	Common; nodules of ground-glass opacity; bronchiolar abnormalities lacking; larger areas of ground-glass opacity may be present
Asbestosis	Common in early stages; associated with findings of fibrosis; bronchiolar abnormalities lacking
Edema, Vasculitis, Talcosis	Common with air-space edema; septal thickening may be present; bronchiolar abnormalities lacking
Bronchioloalveolar carcinoma	Bronchiolar abnormalities lacking
Bronchiolitis obliterans	Uncommon; air trapping may predominate; bronchiolar abnormalities lacking

(87). The differential diagnosis of centrilobular opacities, and their histologic correlates is discussed in detail below.

Large Nodules

The term *large nodule* will be used in this book to refer to rounded opacities that are 1 cm or more in diameter. The term *mass* is generally used to describe nodular lesions that are greater than 3 cm in diameter (89). Large nodules can be associated with a variety interstitial or air-space diseases, including those described above. In addition, in patients with diffuse or chronic lung disease, these can represent conglomerate masses of smaller nodules as are common in sarcoidosis, fibrotic masses as are common in sarcoidosis or silicosis, infectious or inflammatory lesions, tumor nodules, infarctions, nodules of Wegener granulomatosis (90), etc.

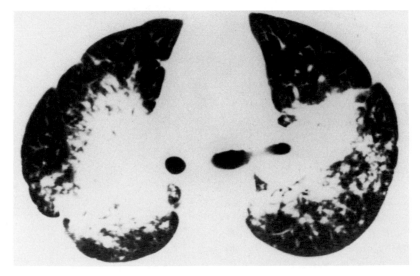

FIG. 3-52. Conglomerate masses of nodules in a patient with sarcoidosis. These masses, which surround central bronchi and vessels, show small discrete nodules at their margins.

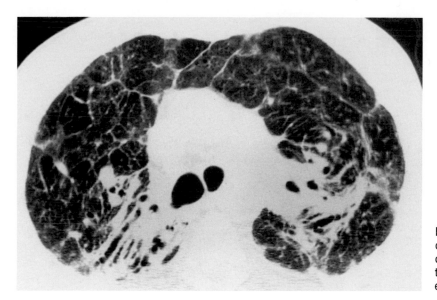

FIG. 3-53. Sarcoidosis with peribronchovascular fibrosis associated with traction bronchiectasis. Volume loss, interlobular septal thickening, and parenchymal bands are also evident.

Conglomerate Nodules or Masses

In patients with disease characterized by small nodules, conglomeration or confluence of nodules can result in large nodular or mass-like opacities (61). Grenier et al. (59) report the presence of confluent nodules greater than 1 cm in 53% of patients with sarcoidosis. In our experience these predominate in the upper lobes and the peribronchovascular regions (Figs. 3-45, 3-52). These nodules or masses are often irregular in shape, surround central bronchi and vessels, and can show small discrete nodules in their periphery (Fig. 3-52). Large nodules were seen in 24% of patients with histiocytosis X, although masses are not generally seen in this disease (59).

Large masses of fibrous tissue may surround and encompass bronchi and vessels within the central or parahilar lung in patients with progressive fibrotic lung disease. The bronchi within these masses may be crowded together, reflecting the volume loss which is present, and are dilated as a result of fibrosis and traction bronchiectasis. In patients with end-stage sarcoidosis, it is not uncommon to see conglomerate masses in the upper lobes, associated with central crowding of vessels and bronchi, presumably as a result of peribronchovascular fibrosis (Figs. 3-6, 3-53). Traction bronchiectasis is often visible within the masses of fibrous tissue. Adjacent areas of emphysema are characteristically absent. Similar upper lobe masses associated with bronchiectasis have been reported in patients with tuberculosis, and are most frequent after treatment (41).

Patients with silicosis and coal workers who have complicated pneumoconiosis or progressive massive

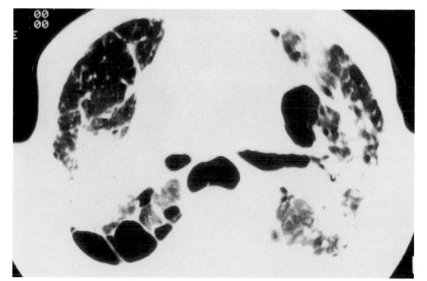

FIG. 3-54. Conglomerate masses of fibrosis in silicosis. Central areas of peribronchovascular fibrosis are associated with peripheral regions of emphysema and bulla formation. (Courtesy of Shin-Ho Kook, M.D., Koryo General Hospital, Seoul, Korea.)

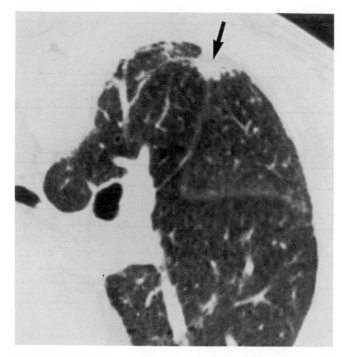

FIG. 3-55. Peripheral fibrotic mass in a patient with pulmonary fibrosis. The focal fibrotic mass (*arrow*) is irregular in shape and is associated with other findings of fibrosis.

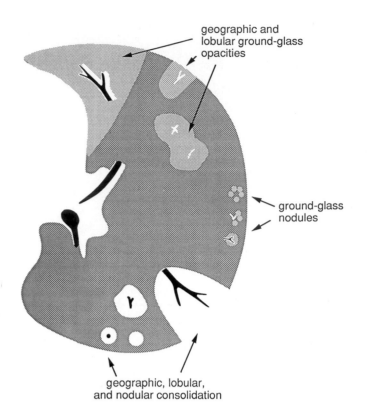

FIG. 3-56. HRCT appearances of increased lung opacity. Ground- glass opacity does not result in obscuration of underlying vessels while consolidation does. Both can be associated with air-bronchograms, and can be nodular, lobular, or patchy and geographic.

fibrosis, also show conglomerate masses in the upper lobes, but these are more typically of homogeneous opacity, and tend to be unassociated with visible traction bronchiectasis as seen in sarcoidosis (Fig. 3-54) (37,66). Also, areas of emphysema peripheral to the conglomerate masses are common. This finding is present in as many as 48% of patients with coal worker's pneumoconiosis (37).

An appearance of progressive massive fibrosis very similar to that occurring in patients with silicosis or sarcoidosis can be seen in intravenous drug users who develop talcosis from injection of talc-containing substances (91). The fibrotic masses can show high attenuation at soft-tissue windows indicating the presence of talc. A parahilar and upper lobe predominance has been seen.

Focal fibrotic masses that are irregular in shape have been described as occurring in the peripheral lung, in relation to pleural abnormalities in patients with asbestos exposure (40). These represent focal areas of scarring or rounded atelectasis (Fig. 3-55). Rounded atelectasis represents a focal, collapsed, and often folded region of lung (40,92–94). It almost always occurs in association with pleural disease, and typically contacts the pleural surface. Rounded atelectasis occurs most commonly in the posterior lung, in the paravertebral regions, and may be bilateral. Bending or bowing of adjacent bronchi and arteries toward the area of atelectasis, because of volume loss or folding of lung is characteristic. This appearance has been likened to a

"comet-tail." Air-bronchograms within the mass can sometimes be seen. In the presence of pleural disease, and these typical findings, the diagnosis can usually be suggested.

INCREASED LUNG OPACITY

Increased lung opacity, or parenchymal opacification, is a common finding on HRCT in patients with

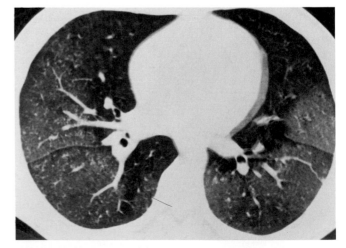

FIG. 3-57. Ground-glass opacity in a 16-year-old boy with Goodpasture's syndrome and pulmonary hemorrhage.

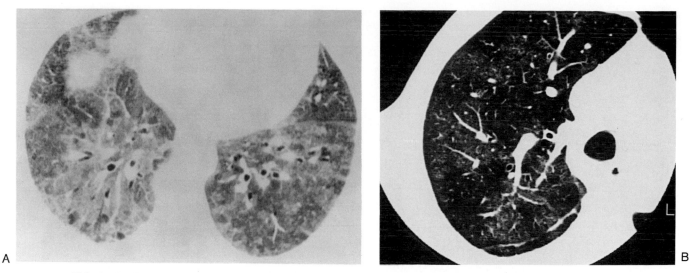

FIG. 3-58. *Pneumocystis carinii* pneumonia with ground-glass opacity. **A:** In one patient, ground-glass opacity is extensive but patchy in distribution. **B:** In another patient, who had a normal chest radiograph, minimal patchy ground-glass opacity is visible.

chronic lung disease. Increased lung opacity is generally described as being *ground-glass opacity* or *consolidation* (5,89) (Fig. 3-56). In some diseases, lung calcification, or other causes of increased attenuation can also be seen.

"Ground-Glass" Opacity

Ground-glass opacity is a nonspecific term referring to the presence on HRCT of a hazy increase in lung opacity that is not associated with obscuration of underlying vessels (Figs. 3-56 and 3-57); if vessels are obscured, the term *consolidation* is generally used (5,89). This finding can reflect the presence of a number of diseases, and can be seen in patients with minimal air-space disease (Fig. 3-58), interstitial thickening (Fig. 3-59), or both (3,88,95–100)

Ground-glass opacity results from the volume averaging of morphologic abnormalities below the resolution of HRCT (97–100). It can reflect the presence of

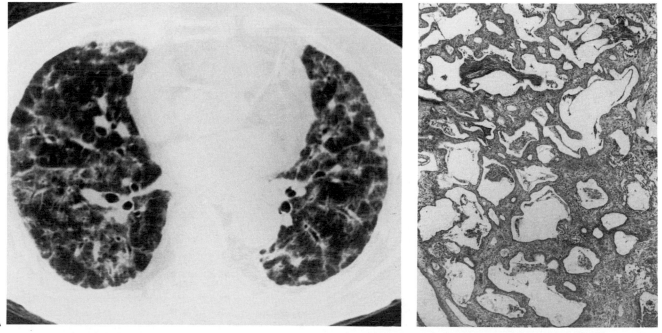

FIG. 3-59. Ground-glass opacity associated with interstitial fibrosis. **A:** HRCT shows patchy areas of ground-glass opacity. **B:** Biopsy specimen shows the abnormality to consist of alveolar wall thickening and fibrosis, with little airspace abnormality. (From Leung et al., ref. 88, with permission of *Radiology*.)

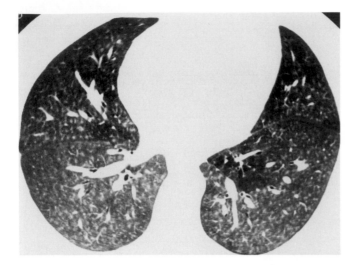

FIG. 3-60. Ground-glass opacity in a patient with idiopathic pulmonary fibrosis and active alveolitis diagnosed on lung biopsy and lavage. Findings of fibrosis are absent.

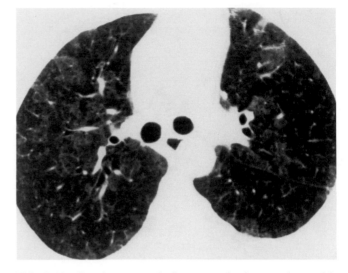

FIG. 3-62. Patchy ground-glass opacity in a patient with hypersensitivity pneumonitis. Some areas of opacity may correspond to secondary lobules.

minimal thickening of the "septal" or alveolar interstitium, thickening of alveolar walls, or the presence of cells or fluid partially filling the alveolar spaces. Ground-glass opacity has been seen in patients with histologic findings of mild or early interstitial inflammation or infiltration (88,101). Also, when a small amount of fluid is present within the alveoli, as can occur in the early stages of an air-space filling disease,

the fluid tends to layer against the alveolar walls, and is indistinguishable on HRCT from alveolar wall thickening (78). In a study comparing the results of lung biopsy with HRCT in 22 patients who showed ground-glass opacity, 14% had diseases primarily affecting airspaces, 32% had a mixed interstitial and air-space abnormality, and 54% had a primarily interstitial abnormality (88).

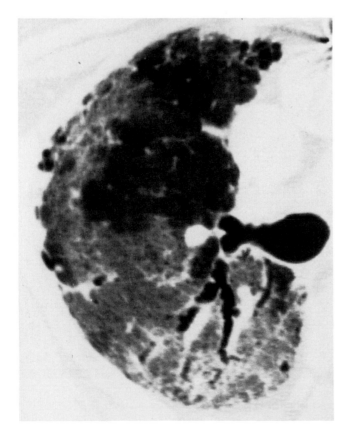

FIG. 3-61. Ground-glass opacity with a peripheral and posterior predominance in a patient with idiopathic pulmonary fibrosis. In addition to the increased lung opacity, there is evidence of increased reticulation, traction bronchiectasis, and some subpleural honeycombing. These findings indicated the presence of fibrosis. End-stage fibrosis was found on biopsy, without evidence of active disease.

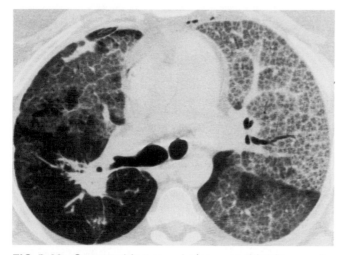

FIG. 3-63. Geographic ground-glass opacities in association with interlobular septal thickening, characteristic of alveolar proteinosis. Note the presence of a "dark bronchus," or air-bronchogram, in the left lung.

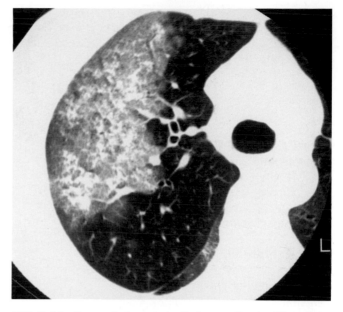

FIG. 3-64. Ground-glass opacity in a patient with pulmonary hemorrhage. Vessels are visible within the area of opacity.

Ground-glass opacity is difficult to recognize if it is of minimal severity and is diffuse in distribution, involving all of the lung to an equal degree. However, this abnormality is usually patchy in distribution, affecting some lung regions while others appear spared; this "geographic" appearance of the lung parenchyma makes it easier to detect and diagnose with confidence (Figs. 3-60–3-64). In some patients, entire lobules may appear abnormally dense, while adjacent lobules appear normal. In others, the abnormal ground-glass opacities are centrilobular and peribronchiolar in location (Fig. 3-51), resulting in the appearance of ill-defined centrilobular nodules (3,26,78,80,82). Ground-glass opacity can also involve individual segments, lobes, or can involve nonsegmental regions of lung. The presence of air-filled bronchi that appear "too black" within an area of lung can also be a clue as to the presence of ground-glass opacity (Figs. 3-60,3-63); this "dark bronchus" appearance is essentially that of an air-bronchogram.

Significance and Differential Diagnosis of Ground-Glass Opacity

Ground-glass opacity is a highly significant finding, as it often indicates the presence of an ongoing, active, and potentially treatable process. Of the 22 patients with ground-glass opacity studied by Leung et al. (88), 18 (82%) were considered to have active or potentially reversible disease on lung biopsy. In a similar study by Remy-Jardin et al. (101) HRCT findings were correlated with histology at 37 biopsy sites in 26 patients. In 24 (65%) of the 37 biopsies, they found that ground-glass opacity corresponded to the presence of inflammation that exceeded or was equal to fibrosis in degree.

In 8 (22%), inflammation was present but fibrosis predominated, while in the remaining 5 (13%), fibrosis was the sole histologic finding. Because of its association with active lung disease, the presence of ground-glass opacity often leads to further diagnostic evaluation, including lung biopsy, depending on the clinical status of the patient. Also, when a lung biopsy is performed, areas of ground-glass opacity can be targeted by the surgeon or bronchoscopist. Since such areas are most likely to be active, they are most likely to yield diagnostic material.

Because ground-glass opacity can reflect the presence of either fibrosis or inflammation, one should be careful to diagnose an active process only when ground-glass opacity is unassociated with HRCT findings of fibrosis, or is the predominant finding (Figs. 3-60,3-62). If ground-glass opacity is only seen in lung regions also showing significant HRCT findings of fibrosis, such as traction bronchiectasis or honeycombing, it is most likely that fibrosis will be the predominant histologic abnormality (Fig. 3-61). For example, in a study by Remy-Jardin et al. (101), patients showing traction bronchiectasis or bronchiolectasis on HRCT in regions of ground-glass opacity all had fibrosis on lung biopsy. On the other hand, in patients without traction bronchiectasis in areas of ground-glass opacity, 92% were found to have active inflammatory disease on lung biopsy.

A large number of diseases can be associated with ground-glass opacity on HRCT (Table 3-10). In many, this reflects the presence of similar histologic reactions in the early or active stages of disease, with inflamma-

TABLE 3-10. *Differential diagnosis of ground-glass opacity*

Diagnosis	Comments
Usual interstitial pneumonia (UIP)	Often present; patchy; usually dominant in peripheral, posterior, and basal regions; findings of fibrosis often present; consolidation much less common
Desquamative interstitial pneumonia (DIP)	Always present; diffuse or patchy; usually dominant in basal, peripheral regions; findings of fibrosis less common than in UIP; consolidation much less common
Lymphocytic interstitial pneumonia (LIP)	Diffuse, patchy, or centrilobular
Bronchiolitis obliterans organizing pneumonia/ Cryptogenic organizing pneumonia (BOOP/COP)	Common, consolidation may also be present; can be dominant in peripheral regions; can be nodular
Sarcoidosis	Present in about 25%; patchy; nodules usually predominate; consolidation less common
Hypersensitivity pneumonitis	Very common; patchy or nodular; can be centrilobular; consolidation less common
Alveolar proteinosis	Very common; patchy or diffuse; septal thickening common; fibrosis rare; consolidation much less common
Acute interstitial pneumonia	Always present; consolidation common; patchy or diffuse
Pneumocystis carinii pneumonia, CMV pneumonia	Common; diffuse or patchy; consolidation can be present; septal thickening in subacute stage
Eosinophilic pneumonia	Sometimes seen; consolidation more common
Respiratory bronchiolitis	Common; patchy or nodular; can be centrilobular; consolidation not reported
Pulmonary edema	Diffuse or centrilobular; septal thickening also present
Pulmonary hemorrhage	Patchy or focal

tory exudates involving the alveolar septa and alveolar spaces, although this pattern can be the result of a variety of pathologic processes. The most common causes of ground-glass opacity include usual interstitial pneumonia (UIP) or desquamative interstitial pneumonia (DIP) associated with idiopathic pulmonary fibrosis (Figs. 3-59–3-61) or scleroderma (88,101–103), bronchiolitis obliterans organizing pneumonia (Fig. 3-65) (88,101), sarcoidosis (Figs. 5-16 and 5-17) (35,61,88,

101,104), and hypersensitivity pneumonitis (Figs. 3-51,3-62) (82–84,101). Other diseases associated with this finding include pneumonia (particularly *Pneumocystis carinii* pneumonia (15,105–107)) (Fig. 3-58), alveolar proteinosis (Fig. 3-63) (32,33,108), acute interstitial pneumonia (Figs. 6-39,6-40,6-43) (109) or other causes of diffuse alveolar damage or the adult respiratory distress syndrome (ARDS), pulmonary edema of various causes (Figs. 6-41,6-42) (15), pulmonary hem-

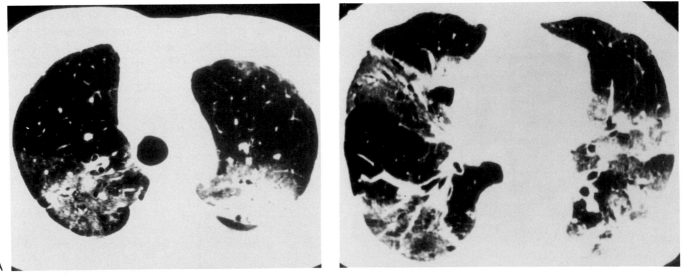

A

B

FIG. 3-65. A,B: Bronchiolitis obliterans organizing pneumonia (BOOP) with patchy areas of consolidation and ground-glass opacity. A peripheral distribution is typical.

orrhage (Figs. 3-57,3-64), respiratory bronchiolitis (Figs. 6-10,6-11) (86,87,110), and early radiation pneumonitis (111,112).

In patients with ground-glass opacity, the nature of the histologic abnormalities associated with this finding vary according to the typical histologic features of the disease (72,82,86–88,113,114) (Table 3-11). In patients with UIP or DIP associated with idiopathic pulmonary fibrosis, scleroderma, or other collagen-vascular diseases, a number of studies have correlated the presence of ground-glass opacity on HRCT with biopsy results, response to treatment, and patient survival (7,95,98–100,102,103,115–117). In histologic studies of patients with interstitial pneumonia, ground-glass opacity has been shown to be associated with the presence of alveolar wall or intra-alveolar inflammation in most. For example, in a study of scleroderma patients by Wells et al. (98), increased opacity on HRCT correlated with predominant inflammation on biopsy in 4 of 7 cases, while reticulation on HRCT indicated fibrosis in 12 of 13 (98). In another study, of 14 patients with idiopathic pulmonary fibrosis and ground-glass opacity on HRCT, 12 had inflammation on biopsy (88). In patients with UIP, ground-glass opacity is associated with alveolar septal inflammation, varying numbers of intra-alveolar histiocytes, and varying degrees of fibrosis; ground-glass opacity in patients with DIP largely reflects the presence of macrophages within alveoli (7,88,98,103).

Technical Considerations and Pitfalls in the Diagnosis of Ground-Glass Opacity

There are several potential pitfalls in the recognition and diagnosis of ground-glass opacity. First, it is important to recognize that since ground-glass opacity reflects the volume averaging of morphologic abnormalities below the resolution of this technique, the thicker the collimation used for scanning, the more likely volume averaging will occur, regardless of the nature of the anatomic abnormality. Thus, ground-glass opacity should be diagnosed only on scans obtained with thin collimation.

The diagnosis of ground-glass opacity is largely subjective and based on a qualitative assessment of lung attenuation (97). The use of lung attenuation measurements to determine the presence of increased lung density in patients with ground-glass opacity is difficult because of the variations in attenuation measurements that are known to be associated with gravitational density gradients in the lung, the level of inspiration, and fluctuations that occur as a result of patient size, position, chest wall thickness, and kVp. Using consistent window settings for the interpretation of HRCT is very important. Using too low a window mean in conjunction with a relatively narrow window width can give the appearance of a diffuse ground-glass abnormality (97). In addition, using a wider window width than one is accustomed to, without changing window mean can give the impression of increased lung attenuation. In assessing the attenuation of lung parenchyma, it is often helpful to compare its appearance to that of air in the trachea or bronchi; if tracheal air appears gray instead of black, then increased attenuation or "grayness" of the lung parenchyma may not be significant.

Also, as previously indicated, increased lung opacity is commonly seen in dependent lung on HRCT, largely as a result of volume loss in the dependent lung parenchyma; so-called dependent density (27). This can result in a stripe of ground-glass opacity several centime-

TABLE 3-11. *Histologic abnormalities associated with ground-glass opacity*

Diagnosis	Histologic findings
Usual interstitial pneumonia (UIP)	Alveolar septal inflammation; intra-alveolar histiocytes; fibrosis
Desquamative interstitial pneumonia (DIP)	Alveolar macrophages; interstitial inflammatory infiltrate
Lymphocytic interstitial pneumonia (LIP)	Mature lymphocytic and plasma cell infiltrates in relation to lymphatics
Bronchiolitis obliterans organizing pneumonia/ Cryptogenic organizing pneumonia (BOOP/COP)	Alveolar septal inflammation; alveolar cellular desquamation
Sarcoidosis	Largely due to numerous small granulomas; alveolitis less important
Hypersensitivity pneumonitis	Alveolitis, interstitial infiltrates, poorly defined granulomas, cellular bronchiolitis
Alveolar proteinosis	Intra-alveolar lipo-proteinaceous material
Acute interstitial pneumonia	Interstitial inflammatory exudate; edema; diffuse alveolar damage with hyaline membranes
Pneumocystis carinii pneumonia	Alveolar inflammatory exudate, alveolar septal thickening
Eosinophilic pneumonia	Eosinophilic interstitial infiltrate; alveolar eosinophils and histiocytes
Respiratory bronchiolitis	Pigment-containing alveolar macrophages

ters thick in the posterior lung of supine patients; prone scans allow this transient finding to be distinguished from a true abnormality. Similarly, on expiration, because of a reduction of the amount of air within alveoli, lung regions increase in attenuation and can mimic the appearance of ground-glass opacity resulting from lung disease.

Furthermore, in patients who have emphysema or other causes of lung hyperlucency such as airways obstruction and air trapping, normal lung regions can appear relatively dense, thus mimicking the appearance of ground-glass opacity. This pitfall can usually be avoided if consistent window settings are used for interpretation of scans, and the interpreter is accustomed to the appearances of normal lung, lung of increased attenuation, and lung of decreased attenuation. Also, "dark bronchi" will not be seen within the relatively dense, normal lung regions, as they are in patients with true ground-glass opacity. The use of expiratory HRCT can also be of value in distinguishing the presence of heterogeneous lung attenuation resulting from emphysema or air trapping from that representing ground-glass opacity. This is described further below.

Consolidation

Increased lung attenuation with obscuration of underlying pulmonary vessels is referred to as consolidation (Figs. 3-56,3-65,3-66)(5,89); air-bronchograms may be present. HRCT has little to add to the diagnosis of patients with clear-cut evidence of consolidation visible on chest radiographs. However, HRCT can allow the detection of consolidation before it becomes diagnosable radiographically. Some evidence of consolidation can be seen in patients with a variety of diffuse lung diseases.

By definition, diseases that produce consolidation, are characterized by a replacement of alveolar air by fluid, cells, tissue, or other material (78,89,108). Most are associated with air-space filling, but diseases that produce an extensive, confluent interstitial abnormality, such as UIP or sarcoidosis, can also result in this finding (88). Air-space nodules or focal areas of ground-glass opacity are often seen in association with areas of frank consolidation.

The differential diagnosis of consolidation overlaps that listed above for ground-glass opacity, and, in fact, many of the diseases listed in Table 3-10 can show a mixture of both findings. The differential diagnosis of consolidation includes pneumonia of different causes including *Pneumocystis carinii* pneumonia (78,106), bronchiolitis obliterans organizing pneumonia (Fig. 3-65) (85), hypersensitivity pneumonitis (84), eosinophilic pneumonia (Fig. 3-66) (118), radiation pneumonitis (111,112,119,120), bronchioloalveolar carcinoma and lymphoma (78,88), UIP (88,95), alveolar pro-

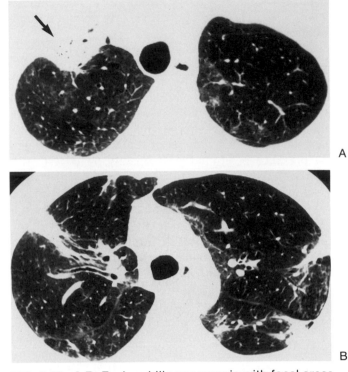

FIG. 3-66. A,B: Eosinophilic pneumonia with focal areas of consolidation and ground-glass opacity. As in patients with BOOP, a peripheral distribution is typical. Note the presence of air bronchograms and obscuration of vessels in the apical opacity (*arrow*).

teinosis (33), acute interstitial pneumonia (109), sarcoidosis (73), drug reactions (121), pulmonary edema, and ARDS (78).

Lung diseases causing consolidation can have widely differing appearances and distributions depending on the nature of the pathologic process responsible. Lobar consolidation is often due to infection, although consolidation due to alveolar proteinosis can also have a lobar predominance. Chronic lung diseases that result in consolidation often involve the lung in a patchy fashion. Patchy consolidation can show a nonanatomic and nonsegmental distribution, but can also be "panlobular," involving individual lobules, or can appear nodular and centrilobular on HRCT (3,62,78).

Lung Calcification and Increased Lung Opacity

Multifocal lung calcification, often associated with lung nodules, has been reported in association with infectious granulomatous diseases such as tuberculosis (41), sarcoidosis (Fig. 3-67) (36), silicosis (36,37), talcosis (91), amyloidosis (34), and fat embolism associated with ARDS (122). Diffuse and dense lung calcification can be seen in the presence of metastatic calcification, disseminated pulmonary ossification, or alveolar microlithiasis. Diffuse, increased lung attenu-

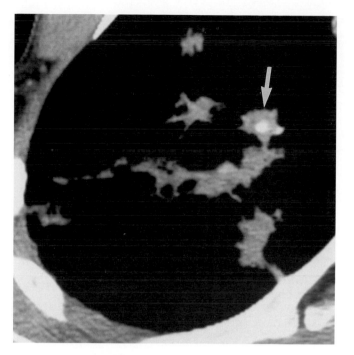

FIG. 3-67. Calcification (*arrow*) within nodular lung disease in a patient with sarcoidosis.

ation in the absence of calcification can be seen as a result of amiodarone lung toxicity.

Disseminated pulmonary ossification is a rare condition in which very small deposits of mature bone form within the lung parenchyma (123). It can be associated with chronic heart disease, such as mitral stenosis, or chronic interstitial fibrosis, such as IPF, asbestosis, or related to drugs. Such calcification is usually invisible on chest radiographs and on HRCT.

Metastatic Calcification

Deposition of calcium within the lung parenchyma (metastatic calcification) can occur due to hypercalcemia in patients with abnormal calcium and phosphate metabolism, and is most common in patients with chronic renal failure and secondary hyperparathyroidism (Fig. 3-68) (124–126). Metastatic calcification is typically interstitial, involving the alveolar septa, bronchioles, and arteries, and can be associated with secondary lung fibrosis. Plain radiographs are relatively insensitive in detecting this calcification; HRCT can show calcification in the absence of radiographic findings. Calcifications can be focal, centrilobular, or diffuse (Fig. 3-68). Ground-glass opacities with a centrilobular distribution have been reported in association with metastatic calcification (126).

Hartman et al. (126) reviewed the chest radiographs and CT and HRCT scans of 7 patients with hypercalcemia and biopsy-proven metastatic calcification. In 5 patients, the radiographic findings were nonspecific, consisting of poorly defined nodular opacities and patchy areas of parenchymal consolidation, while in 2 patients calcified nodules were visible. CT and HRCT findings consisted of numerous fluffy and poorly defined nodules measuring 3 to 10 mm in diameter. The nodules primarily involved the upper lobes in 3 patients, were diffuse in 3, and were predominant in the lower lung zones in 1. Areas of ground-glass opacity were present in 3 of the 7 patients, and patchy areas of consolidation were present in 2. Calcification of some or all of the nodules was seen on CT in 4 of the 7 patients. Six of the 7 patients also had evidence of calcification in the vessels of the chest wall, and 1 had calcification of the left atrial wall.

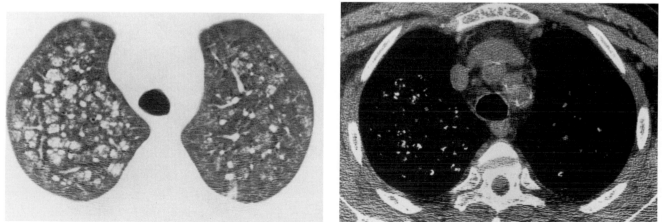

A

B

FIG. 3-68. A 42-year-old man with chronic renal failure and metastatic calcification. **A:** HRCT shows nodular areas of opacity that appear centrilobular, as well as some ground-glass opacities. **B:** Soft-tissue window scan shows multiple areas of calcification within these opacities.

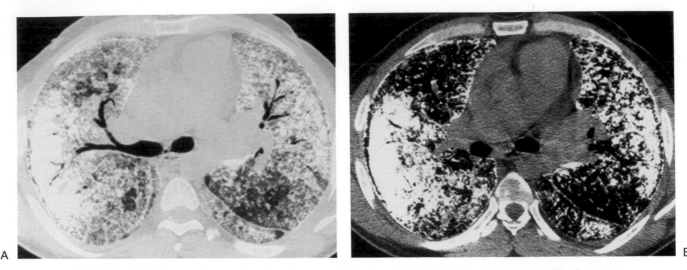

FIG. 3-69. HRCT in a patient with alveolar microlithiasis, with lung **(A)** and soft-tissue **(B)** windows. Calcifications that are very small and diffuse show a subpleural predominance. (Courtesy of Joseph Cherian, M.D., Al-Sabah Hospital, Kuwait.)

Alveolar Microlithiasis

The high-resolution CT appearances of several patients with pulmonary alveolar microlithiasis have been reported, corresponding closely to pathologic findings in this disease (127,128). Alveolar microlithiasis is characterized by widespread intra-alveolar calcifications, representing so-called microliths or cal-

cospheres. HRCT shows a posterior and lower lobe predominance of the calcifications with an high concentration in the subpleural parenchyma and in association with bronchi and vessels (Fig. 3-69). A perilobular and centrilobular distribution of the calcifications may be seen, or calcifications may be associated with interlobular septa. Intraparenchymal cysts or paraseptal emphysema may be associated (127,128).

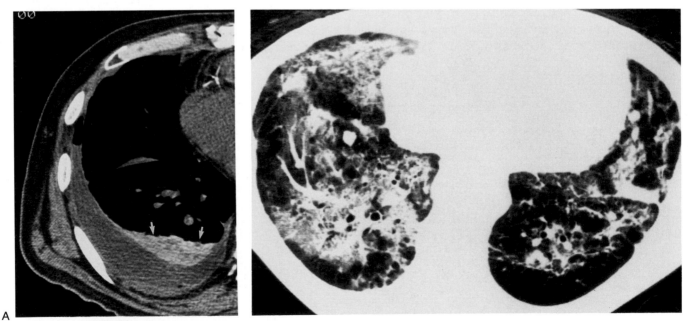

FIG. 3-70. HRCT in pulmonary amiodarone toxicity. **A:** On an unenhanced HRCT, a focal area of dense lung consolidation is present in the posterior lung. A pleural effusion is also visible, due to cardiac decompensation. **B:** In another patient with amiodarone toxicity, a lung window scan shows areas of ground-glass opacity, consolidation, nodular opacities, and abnormal reticulation. The high attenuation cannot be appreciated with this window setting.

Amiodarone Pulmonary Toxicity

Amiodarone is a triiodinated drug used to treat refractory tachyarrhythmias. It accumulates in lung, largely within macrophages and type-2 pneumocytes, where it forms lamellar inclusion bodies and has a very long half-life. In some patients, accumulation of the drug results in pulmonary toxicity with interstitial pneumonia and fibrosis, although the mechanisms of disease are unclear. CT in patients with amiodarone can show high-attenuation areas of consolidation or high attenuation nodules or masses, sometimes in association with an abnormal reticulation or ground-glass opacity (Fig. 3-70) (121,129). High attenuation consolidation or masses were seen in 8 of 11 patients in one series (129), correlating with the presence of numerous foamy macrophages in the interstitium and alveolar spaces. Unconsolidated lung parenchyma does not appear abnormally dense. Because the drug also accumulates in the liver and spleen, these also appear dense.

DECREASED LUNG OPACITY AND CYSTIC ABNORMALITIES

A variety of abnormalities result in decreased lung attenuation or air-filled cystic lesions on HRCT. These include honeycombing, bronchiectasis, emphysema, lung cysts, cavitary nodules, mosaic perfusion, and air-trapping due to airways disease (Fig. 3-71). In most cases these can be readily distinguished on the basis of HRCT findings (130).

Honeycombing

In patients with interstitial fibrosis, alveolar disruption, dilatation of alveolar ducts, and bronchiolar dilatation can result in the formation of honeycomb cysts (7,131). These cysts have fibrous walls and are lined by bronchiolar epithelium. On HRCT, honeycombing is characterized by the presence of air-filled, cystic spaces several millimeters to several centimeters in diameter, which often predominate in a peripheral and subpleural location, occur in several layers, and are characterized by clearly definable walls, 1 to 3 mm in thickness (18,25) (Figs. 3-24,3-26,3-72,3-73). In contradistinction to the lung cysts seen in patients with lymphangiomyomatosis and histiocytosis X, and the lucencies seen in patients with centrilobular emphysema, honeycomb cysts tend to share walls. The presence of honeycombing on HRCT indicates the presence of severe fibrosis.

Large subpleural cystic spaces, several centimeters in diameter, can be associated with honeycombing, mimicking the appearance of bullae (Fig. 3-73). These large cysts tend to predominate in the upper lobes. These large honeycomb cysts decrease in size on expi-

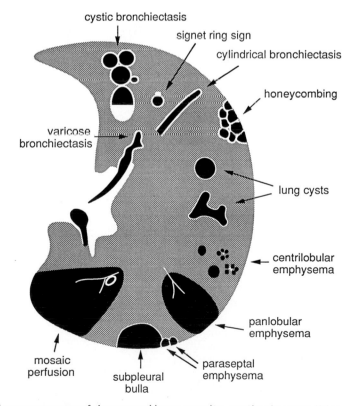

FIG. 3-71. HRCT appearances of decreased lung opacity, cystic abnormalities, emphysema, bronchiectasis, and mosaic perfusion.

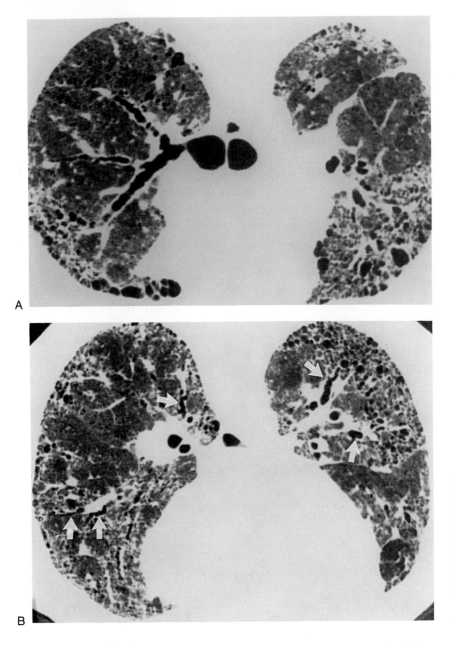

FIG. 3-72. Honeycombing in a patient with idiopathic pulmonary fibrosis. A,B: On HRCT, honeycombing cysts have clearly definable walls a few millimeters in thickness. In areas of honeycombing, lobular anatomy cannot be resolved because of architectural distortion. Bronchial irregularity and traction bronchiectasis (arrows, B) are often present in patients with severe fibrosis and may be difficult to distinguish from honeycombing.

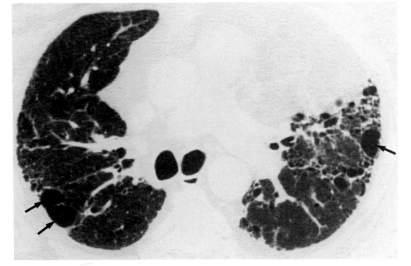

FIG. 3-73. Honeycombing with large lung cysts. In a patient with idiopathic pulmonary fibrosis, peripheral honeycombing, traction bronchiectasis, and several large lung cysts (arrows) are visible.

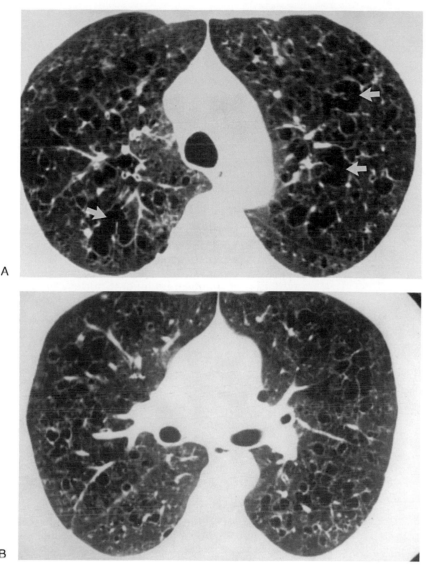

A

B

FIG. 3-74. Histiocytosis X with lung cysts. High-resolution CT at two levels show numerous thin-walled lung cysts. The cysts are larger and most numerous in the upper lobes **(A)** than in the lower **(B)**, as is characteristic of this disease. Some cysts (*arrows*) are confluent, branching, or irregular in shape. Note that the intervening lung appears normal. The peripheral predominance commonly seen with honeycombing is absent.

ratory scans (132); this change would not be expected of bullae.

Lung Cysts

On HRCT, the term *lung cyst* is used to refer to a thin-walled (usually > 3 mm), well-defined and circumscribed, air-containing lesion (Figs. 3-71,3-74–3-77) (130). Lung cysts are also defined as having a wall composed of one of a variety of cellular elements, usually fibrous or epithelial in nature (89). For example, in patients with end-stage pulmonary fibrosis, honeycomb cysts are lined by bronchiolar epithelium; on the other hand, in patients with lymphangiomyomatosis the cysts are lined by abnormal spindle cells resembling smooth muscle.

Lymphangiomyomatosis (LAM) and histiocytosis X often produce multiple lung cysts, whose appearance

on HRCT is usually quite distinct from that of honeycombing (64,65,133–137). The cysts have a thin but easily discernible wall in most instances, ranging up to a few millimeters in thickness (Figs. 3-74–3-77). Associated findings of fibrosis are usually absent or much less conspicuous than they are in patients with honeycombing and end-stage lung disease. In LAM and histiocytosis X, the cysts are usually interspersed within areas of normal-appearing lung.

In patients with histiocytosis X, the cysts can have bizarre shapes because of the fusion of several cysts or perhaps because they represent ectatic and thick-walled bronchi (Figs. 3-74–3-75). Although confluent cysts can also be seen with lymphangiomyomatosis, they are less common; in patients with LAM, cysts generally appear rounder, and more uniform in size, than those seen with histiocytosis X (Figs. 3-76–3-77).

As described above, the term *lung cyst* refers to a specific type of cystic space within the lung paren-

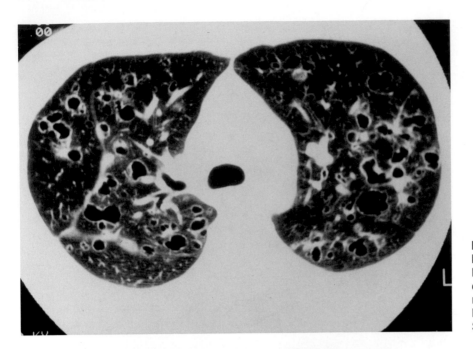

FIG. 3-75. HRCT in a patient with cystic lung disease typical of histiocytosis X. Multiple lung cysts, many bifurcating or complex, are interspersed within normal-appearing lung. (Courtesy of Shin-Ho Kook, M.D., Koryo General Hospital, Seoul, Korea.)

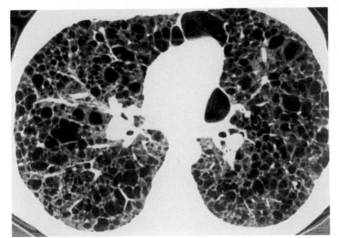

FIG. 3-76. HRCT in a patient with tuberous sclerosis and lymphangiomyomatosis. Cystic airspaces have clearly defined walls measuring up to 2 mm in thickness.

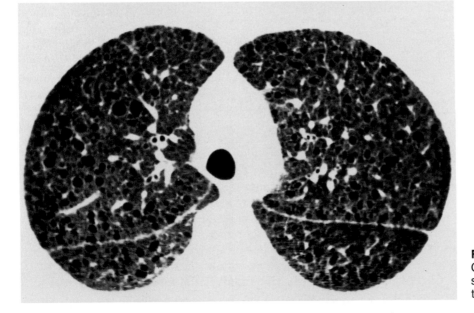

FIG. 3-77. HRCT in a woman with LAM. Cysts are rounder and more regular in size than those seen in patients with histiocytosis X.

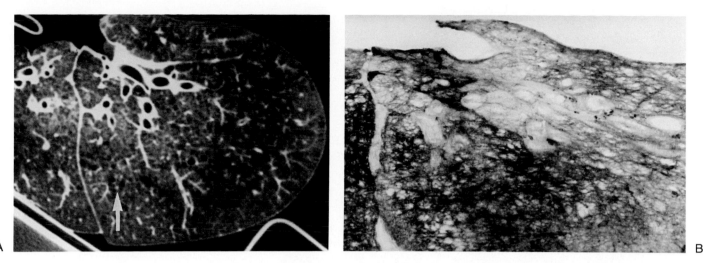

A

B

FIG. 3-78. Isolated inflated lung from a patient with centrilobular emphysema. **A:** Small lucencies without identifiable walls are present. Some lucencies are seen to cluster around a centrilobular artery (*arrow*). This appearance is typical of centrilobular emphysema. **B:** On the corresponding lung section, the small centrilobular foci of destruction are clearly seen. (From Webb et al., ref. 18, with permission of *Radiology*.)

chyma. Lung cysts should be distinguished from other air-containing spaces such as emphysematous bullae, blebs, and pneumatoceles (for example, those associated with *Pneumocystis carinii* pneumonia), which are described below; none of these are true "lung cysts."

Emphysema

Emphysema is defined as a permanent, abnormal enlargement of airspaces distal to the terminal bronchiole, accompanied by the destruction of the walls of the involved airspaces (130). Emphysema can be accurately diagnosed using HRCT (18,26,69,138–140), and results in focal areas of very low attenuation that can be easily contrasted with surrounding, higher attenuation, normal lung parenchyma if sufficiently low-window means (−600 HU to −800 HU) are used (Figs. 3-71–3-78). Although some types of emphysema can have walls visible on HRCT, these are usually inconspicuous.

In many patients it is possible to classify the type of emphysema on the basis of its HRCT appearance (18,26). *Centrilobular (proximal or centriacinar) emphysema*, is characterized on HRCT by the presence of multiple small lucencies that predominate in the upper lobes, and in some subjects, or in some regions, may appear centrilobular (Figs. 3-71,3-78,3-79). Even if the centrilobular location of these lucencies is not visible, a spotty distribution is typical of centrilobular emphysema (Fig. 3-80). In most cases, the areas of low attenuation seen on HRCT in patients with centrilobular emphysema lack a visible wall, although very thin walls are occasionally visible, and are related to areas of fi-

brosis (Fig. 3-80). In severe cases, the areas of centrilobular emphysema become confluent. *Panlobular (panacinar) emphysema* typically results in an overall decrease in lung attenuation, and a reduction in size of pulmonary vessels, without the focal areas of lucency typically seen in patients with centrilobular emphysema (Fig. 3-81). Areas of panlobular emphysema typically lack visible walls. This form of emphysema has been aptly described as a diffuse simplification of lung architecture. Severe or confluent centrilobular emphysema can mimic this appearance (Fig. 3-82). *Paraseptal (distal acinar) emphysema* results in the presence of subpleural lucencies, which often share very thin walls that are visible on HRCT; paraseptal emphysema can be seen as an isolated abnormality, but is often associated with centrilobular emphysema (Figs. 3-83,3-84). *Irregular air-space enlargement*, previously known as irregular or cicatricial emphysema, can be seen in association with fibrosis, as in patients with silicosis and progressive massive fibrosis (Fig. 3-54) (68,141). These types of emphysema and their HRCT appearances are further described in detail in Chapter 7.

Panlobular emphysema usually results in a distinct appearance on HRCT, and it is not typically confused with other entities. However, the appearance of panlobular and centrilobular emphysema can mimic the presence of honeycombing or lung cysts in some patients.

Paraseptal Emphysema vs. Honeycombing

In patients with paraseptal emphysema, areas of lung destruction are typically marginated by thin linear

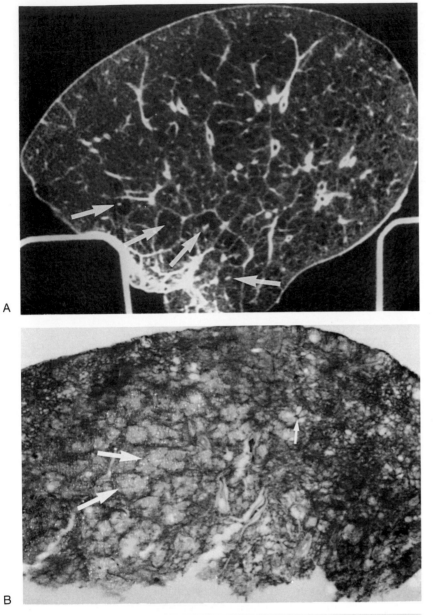

A

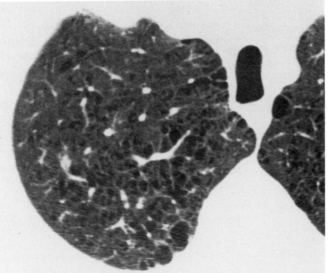

B

FIG. 3-79. Centrilobular emphysema in an isolated lung. **A:** More severe, but patchy, emphysema is visible on the HRCT. As in Fig. 3-89, the areas of destruction cluster about the centrilobular arteries (*arrows*). (From Webb et al., ref. 18, with permission of *Radiology*.) **B:** On the pathologic specimen, some lobules (*large arrows*) show extensive destruction. In some, the centrilobular artery remains visible (*small arrow*) within the area of emphysema.

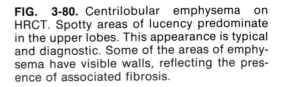

FIG. 3-80. Centrilobular emphysema on HRCT. Spotty areas of lucency predominate in the upper lobes. This appearance is typical and diagnostic. Some of the areas of emphysema have visible walls, reflecting the presence of associated fibrosis.

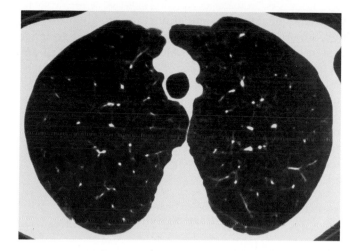

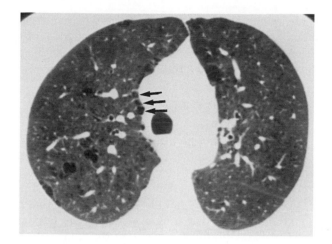

FIG. 3-81. Panlobular emphysema. On HRCT, lung volumes are increased, the lungs appear lucent, and size of pulmonary vessels are diminished in size. Focal lucencies, as seen in patients with centrilobular emphysema are not visible.

FIG. 3-83. Centrilobular and paraseptal emphysema. Small isolated areas of destruction are present within the central upper lobes and adjacent to the mediastinal pleura. Some of the paramediastinal cysts (*arrows*) have visible walls, as is characteristic of paraseptal emphysema.

opacities, visible on HRCT, that extend to the pleural surface. These linear opacities often correspond to interlobular septa and sometimes are associated with minimal fibrosis (Figs. 3-71,3-82–3-84). Because they are subpleural and marginated by visible walls, areas of paraseptal emphysema can resemble the appearance of honeycombing. However, several features allow these two entities to be distinguished in the large majority of cases. Honeycomb cysts are usually smaller, usually occur in several layers, tend to predominate at

the lung bases, and are associated with disruption of lobular architecture and other findings of fibrosis. On the other hand, areas of paraseptal emphysema are often larger and associated with bullae, usually occur in a single layer, predominate in the upper lobes, and may be associated with other findings of emphysema, but are typically unassociated with significant fibrosis.

Centrilobular Emphysema vs. Lung Cysts

In some patients, areas of centrilobular emphysema can show very thin walls on HRCT, corresponding to minimal lung fibrosis or compressed adjacent lung parenchyma. However, these walls are usually less well-defined than walls seen in patients with cystic lung disease. Also, lung cysts often appear larger than do areas

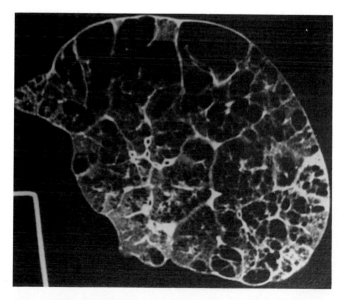

FIG. 3-82. Confluent centrilobular emphysema. On HRCT, areas of centrilobular emphysema have coalesced to form peripheral bulla. These are marginated by residual normal septa. Because of its peripheral location, this may be termed paraseptal emphysema.

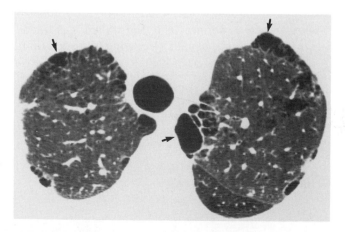

FIG. 3-84. HRCT in a patient with paraseptal and centrilobular emphysema. The larger areas of subpleural emphysema (*arrows*) are most appropriately termed bullae.

of centrilobular emphysema. In patients with centrilobular emphysema, lucencies can often be seen to involve only one part of an otherwise normal-appearing secondary lobule (Fig. 3-71); this appearance is diagnostic.

Bullae and Blebs

Emphysematous bullae are well seen using HRCT. A *bulla* has been defined as a sharply demarcated area of emphysema measuring 1 cm or more in diameter, and possessing a wall less than 1 mm in thickness (Fig. 3-84) (89). Although it is not always possible to distinguish a bulla from a true lung cyst, bullae are uncommon as isolated findings, except in the lung apices, but are usually associated with evidence of extensive centrilobular or paraseptal emphysema. Subpleural bullae often reflect the presence of areas of paraseptal emphysema. When emphysema is associated with predominant bullae, it may be termed *bullous emphysema* (142).

On HRCT, bullae show a distinct wall, which usually appears about 1 mm in thickness. Bullae can range up to 20 cm in diameter, but are usually between 2 and 8 cm in diameter. Bullae can be seen in both a subpleural location and within the lung parenchyma, but subpleural bullae are more frequent. In patients with bullous emphysema, bullae are often asymmetric, with one lung being involved to a greater degree (142).

The term bleb is used pathologically to refer to a gas-containing space within the visceral pleura (89). Radiographically, this term is sometimes used to describe a focal thin-walled lucency, contiguous with the pleura, usually at the lung apex. However, the distinction between bleb and bulla is of little practical significance and is seldom justified. The term *bulla* is preferred (89).

Pneumatocele

Pneumatocele is defined as a thin-walled, gas-filled space within the lung, usually occurring in association with acute pneumonia, and almost invariably transient (89). Pneumatocele has an appearance similar to lung cyst or bulla on HRCT and cannot be distinguished on the basis of HRCT findings. The association of such an abnormality with acute pneumonia, particularly resulting from *Pneumocystis carinii* or *Staphylococcus*, would suggest the presence of a pneumatocele, but a spectrum of cystic abnormalities can be seen in such patients (Fig. 3-85) (143–145). The association of lung cysts or bullae with *P. carinii* pneumonia is discussed in Chapter 7.

Cavitary Nodules

Cavitary nodules have thicker and more irregular walls than do lung cysts, but there is some overlap between these appearances (Fig. 3-86). Such nodules have been reported in histiocytosis X (64,65), tuberculosis (41), fungal infections, and sarcoidosis (72), but could also be seen in patients with rheumatoid lung disease, septic embolism, pneumonia, metastatic tumor, Wegener granulomatosis, etc. Also, some nodular opacities having central lucencies, may represent dilated bronchioles surrounded by areas of consolidation or interstitial thickening (64).

Bronchiectasis

Bronchiectasis is generally defined as localized, irreversible bronchial dilatation (146). While bronchiectasis usually results from chronic infection, airway obstruction by tumor, stricture, impacted material, or inherited abnormalities can also play a significant role. Bronchiectasis has been classified into three types, depending on the morphology of the abnormal bronchi, although these distinctions are of little clinical value (130). The HRCT diagnosis of bronchiectasis is described in detail in Chapter 7.

Cylindrical bronchiectasis, the mildest form of this disease, is characterized on HRCT by the presence of thick-walled bronchi, which extend into the lung pe-

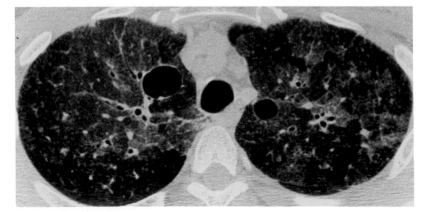

FIG. 3-85. HRCT in a patient with *Pneumocystis carinii* pneumonia shows ground-glass opacity and focal lung cysts representing pneumatoceles.

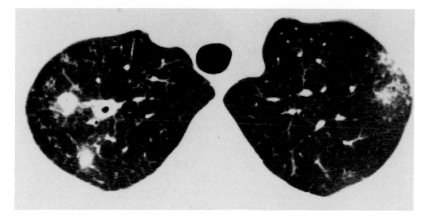

FIG. 3-86. Cavitary nodules in an AIDS patient with a fungal pneumonia. Nodules appear both solid and cavitary. The cavitated nodule in the right upper lobe is thick walled.

riphery and fail to show normal tapering. On HRCT, bronchi are not normally visible in the peripheral 2 cm of lung, but in patients with bronchiectasis, bronchial wall thickening, peribronchial fibrosis, and dilatation of the bronchial lumen, allow them to be seen in the lung periphery. Depending on their orientation relative to the scan plane they can simulate ''tram tracks'' or can show the ''signet-ring sign,'' in which the dilated, thick-walled bronchus and its accompanying pulmonary artery branch are seen adjacent to each other (19). Ectatic bronchi containing fluid or mucus appear as tubular opacities (Fig. 3-7).

Varicose bronchiectasis is similar in appearance to cylindrical bronchiectasis; however, with varicose bronchiectasis the bronchial walls are more irregular,

and can assume a beaded appearance (Fig. 3-87). The term *string of pearls* has been used to describe varicose bronchiectasis. Traction bronchiectasis often appears varicose.

Cystic bronchiectasis most often appears as a group or cluster of air-filled cysts, but cysts can also be fluid-filled, giving the appearance of a ''cluster of grapes.'' Cystic bronchiectasis is often patchy in distribution, allowing it to be distinguished from a cystic lung disease such as LAM (Fig. 3-88). Also, air-fluid levels, which may be present in the dependent portions of the cystic dilated bronchi, are a very specific sign of bronchiectasis, and are not usually seen in patients with lung cysts.

Traction Bronchiectasis

In patients with lung fibrosis and distortion of lung architecture, traction bronchiectasis is commonly

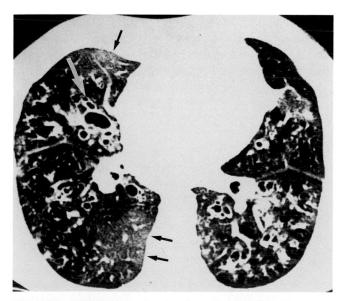

FIG. 3-87. HRCT in a patient with varicose bronchiectasis resulting from allergic bronchopulmonary aspergillosis. A string of pearls (*white arrow*) is visible in the anterior right lung. Dilatation of small bronchioles in the peripheral lung is also visible. Patchy lung opacity, with focal regions of decreased and increased attenuation (*black arrows*), reflect mosaic perfusion.

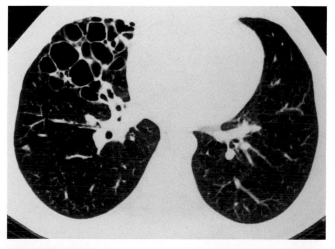

FIG. 3-88. Cystic bronchiectasis involving the right middle lobe. The focal distribution allows distinction of this entity from cystic lung disease, such as seen in LAM.

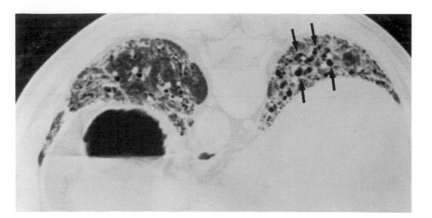

FIG. 3-89. Traction bronchiectasis in a patient with idiopathic pulmonary fibrosis. Dilated bronchi (*arrows*) are visible in the posterior lung base.

present (Figs. 3-24, 3-53,3-61,3-89). In this condition, traction by fibrous tissue on the walls of bronchi results in irregular bronchial dilatation, or bronchiectasis, which is typically "varicose" in appearance (17,18). Traction bronchiectasis usually involves the segmental and subsegmental bronchi, can also affect small peripheral bronchi or bronchioles. Dilatation of intralobular bronchioles because of surrounding fibrosis is termed *traction bronchiolectasis*. In patients with honeycombing, bronchiolar dilatation contributes to the cystic appearance seen on HRCT (7).

The increased transpulmonary pressure and elastic recoil associated with advanced pulmonary fibrosis, along with local distortion of airways by fibrotic tissue, all contribute to the varicose dilatation of airways seen in these conditions. Because of peribronchial interstitial thickening, bronchial walls can appear to measure up to several millimeters in thickness. Traction bronchiectasis is usually most marked in areas of lung that show the most severe fibrosis. It is commonly seen in association with honeycombing, as is bronchiolectasis.

"Mosaic Perfusion"

Lung density and attenuation are partially determined by the amount of blood present in lung tissue. On HRCT, inhomogeneous lung opacity can result from regional differences in lung perfusion in patients with airways disease or pulmonary vascular disease (147–149). Because this phenomenon is often patchy or mosaic in distribution, with adjacent areas of lung having relatively decreased and increased opacity, it has been termed *mosaic perfusion* (5) or *mosaic oligemia* (149), although the former term is most appropriate. Areas of relatively decreased lung opacity seen on HRCT can be of varying sizes, and sometimes appear to correspond to lobules, segments, lobes, or an entire lung (Figs. 3-87,3-90–3-92).

In almost all cases, mosaic perfusion is seen in association with diseases causing regional decreases in lung perfusion. However, differences in attenuation between normal and abnormal lung regions, recognizable on HRCT, are accentuated by compensatory increased perfusion of normal or relatively normal lung areas.

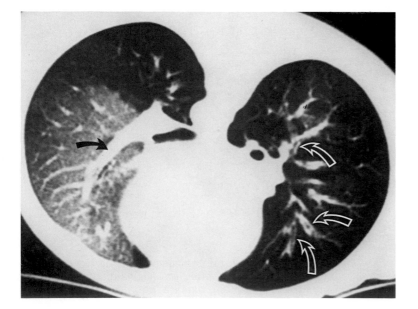

FIG. 3-90. Decreased lung attenuation and "mosaic perfusion" in a patient with bronchiolitis obliterans. On this prone scan, abnormal lucency of the right lung and left lower lobe are associated with bronchial wall thickening (*open arrows*). The lucency reflects air trapping and/or poor perfusion of these areas. The relatively dense left upper lobe is normally perfused or overperfused because of shunting of blood away from the abnormal areas. Note the large size of the vessels (*solid arrow*) in the area of relatively increased attenuation.

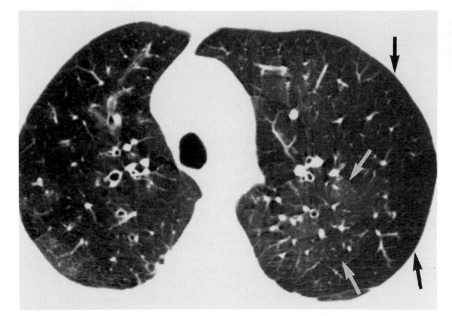

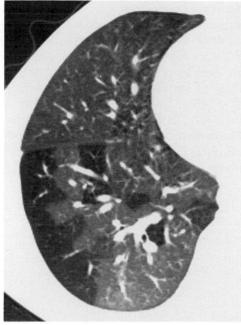

FIG. 3-91. HRCT in a patient with bronchiolitis obliterans related to rheumatoid arthritis. Bronchiectasis is visible, along with patchy lung attenuation, a finding that reflects mosaic perfusion. Note that the pulmonary vessels in the lucent-appearing peripheral left lung (*black arrows*) are smaller than vessels in the denser medial left lung (*white arrows*).

FIG. 3-92. HRCT in a 9-year-old boy with post-infectious bronchiolitis obliterans. Patchy areas of mosaic perfusion are visible, with decreased vascular size within the lucent regions.

Mosaic perfusion is most frequent in patients with airway diseases that result in focal air-trapping or poor ventilation of lung parenchyma (54,147,148); in these patients, areas of poorly ventilated lung are poorly perfused because of reflex vasoconstriction or because of a permanent reduction in the pulmonary capillary bed. In our experience, this finding has been most common in patients with bronchiolitis obliterans, or other diseases associated with small airways obstruction such as cystic fibrosis or bronchiectasis of any cause (Fig. 3-87), but can also be seen as a result of large bronchial obstruction.

Mosaic perfusion has also been reported in association with pulmonary vascular obstruction such as that caused by pulmonary embolism (Fig. 3-93) (149–151). In one study of patients with chronic pulmonary embolism (151), 58 (77%) of 75 of patients showed a mosaic pattern on CT with areas of both increased and decreased attenuation; areas of increased attenuation averaged −727 HU, while areas of decreased attenuation averaged −868 HU.

Regardless of its cause, when mosaic perfusion is present, pulmonary vessels in the areas of decreased opacity often appear smaller than vessels in relative dense areas of lung (54,148,151) (Figs. 3-90–3-93). This difference reflects differences in regional blood flow, and can be quite helpful in distinguishing mosaic perfusion from ground-glass opacity, which can otherwise have a similar patchy appearance. In patients with

ground-glass opacity, vessels usually appear equal in size throughout the lung. Furthermore, in patients with mosaic perfusion due to bronchiolitis obliterans, cystic fibrosis, or other airway diseases, gross abnormalities of large bronchi (i.e., bronchiectasis) can often be seen in the relatively lucent areas of lung (54,147,148). In patients with mosaic perfusion occurring in association with chronic pulmonary embolism, enlargement of the main pulmonary arteries may be visible, because of pulmonary hypertension.

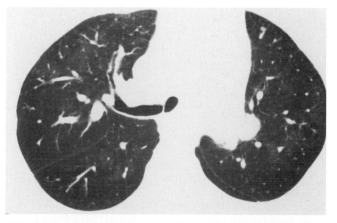

FIG. 3-93. Mosaic perfusion with patchy lung attenuation in a patient with chronic pulmonary embolism and pulmonary hypertension. Peripheral pulmonary vessels are largest in the relatively dense anterior right upper lobe.

In some cases, however, it can be very difficult to distinguish mosaic perfusion from patchy ground-glass opacity on HRCT; this distinction is important to make for the purposes of differential diagnosis. Obtaining post-expiratory HRCT can be very helpful in differentiating patients with mosaic perfusion related to airways obstruction from patients with ground-glass opacity. Differences in lung attenuation resulting from airways obstruction and mosaic perfusion are accentuated on expiratory HRCT scans; this is not the case with ground-glass opacity.

Expiratory HRCT and the Diagnosis of Air-trapping

Obtaining HRCT scans at selected levels following expiration may be useful (i) in the diagnosis of obstructive or airways disease unassociated with distinct mor-

phologic abnormalities, and (ii) in distinguishing mosaic perfusion from ground-glass opacity (148).

Use of Expiratory CT To Diagnose Airways Disease

Recently, CT scans performed at suspended full expiration have been used to demonstrate air trapping in patients with emphysema (152), asthma (148), the Swyer-James syndrome (147,153), and in patients with a variety of airway abnormalities. Dynamic expiratory CT (154–156) has also been used to detect air trapping. Expiratory CT techniques are described in Chapter 1.

In normal subjects, lung increases significantly in attenuation during expiration (see Chapter 2, Figs. 2-19–2-21). In the presence of airways obstruction and air trapping, lung remains lucent on expiration, and shows little change in cross-sectional area. In some patients with airways obstruction, expiratory CT shows evidence of air trapping in the absence of morphologic or lung attenuation abnormalities recognizable on inspiratory HRCT (148).

The diagnosis of air trapping on expiratory HRCT is easiest when the abnormality is patchy in distribution, and normal lung regions can be contrasted with abnormal, lucent, lung regions on the expiratory scans (Figs. 3-94–3-96,3-98) (148). Areas of air trapping, which remain lucent on expiration, can be patchy and nonanatomic, or can correspond to individual secondary pulmonary lobules, segments, lobes, or an entire lung. In patients with airways disease or emphysema who have a diffuse abnormality, expiratory inhomogeneities in lung attenuation may not be visible, but air trapping can be detected by measuring the lung attenuation increase occurring with expiration (155,156).

In patients with airways obstruction and patchy air-trapping, areas of lung that appear relatively lucent on expiration usually show an increase in attenuation

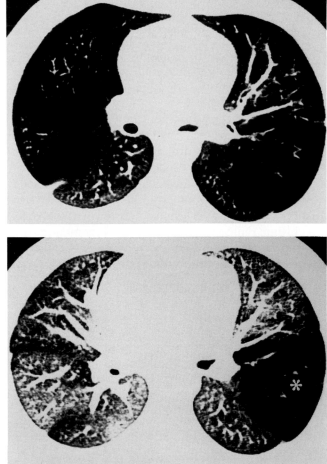

A

B

FIG. 3-94. Dynamic inspiratory **(A)** and expiratory **(B)** HRCT in a patient with post-infectious bronchiolitis obliterans. On expiration, marked inhomogeneity in lung attenuation is noted, with focal air-trapping in the left upper lobe (*asterisk*). Note the relatively small size of pulmonary vessels in the region of air trapping. A region of interest placed in the area of air-trapping shows a paradoxical decrease in lung attenuation of 30 HU during expiration.

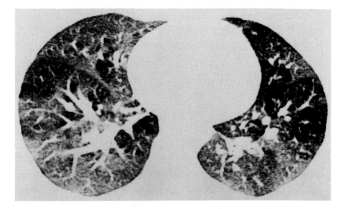

FIG. 3-95. Dynamic expiratory HRCT in a patient with asthma. On expiration, marked inhomogeneity in lung attenuation is noted, with multifocal regions of air trapping. (From Webb, ref. 148, with permission.)

measuring less than 50 HU, or sometimes show a paradoxical decrease in attenuation (Figs. 3-94–3-96); normal-appearing areas of lung usually increase in attenuation by 150 HU or more (156,157). Although a specific value of post-expiratory increase in lung attenuation, useful in distinguishing normals from abnormals, has not been established, in recent studies of dynamic expiratory HRCT obtained during forced expiration (156), all patients with obstructive disease showed areas of lung parenchyma that increased in attenuation by less than 100 HU on expiration; this finding was rarely seen in normals (158).

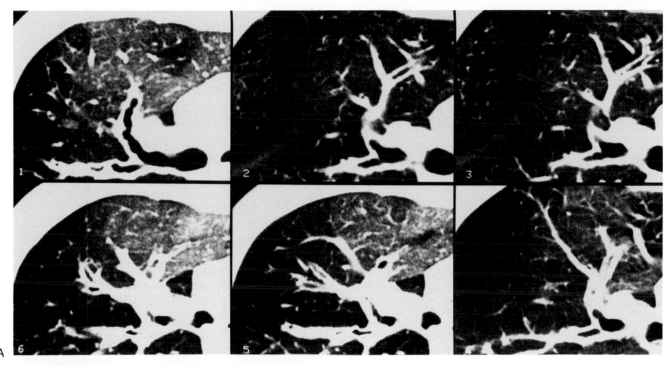

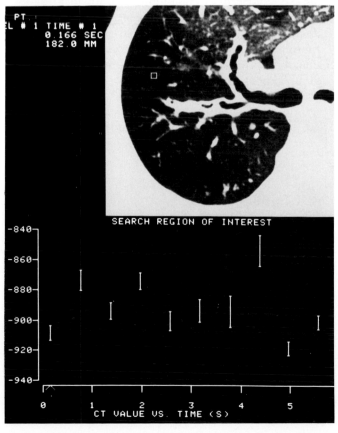

FIG. 3-96. Dynamic expiratory HRCT in a patient with cystic fibrosis. **A:** Six dynamic images from a sequence of 10, through the right upper lobe region, shown sequentially in a clockwise fashion from the upper left to lower left. On inspiration (*top middle*), lung opacity appears homogeneous. On expiration (*lower left corner*), a part of the anterior segment shows a normal increase in opacity, while the remainder of the upper lobe remains lucent. **B:** Time-attenuation curve measured in a lucent region of the upper lobe shows little change in attenuation during expiration.

In a series of patients with obstructive disease evaluated using expiratory CT, the extent of air-trapping measured on the scans series correlated closely with pulmonary function test measures of obstruction; correlation of FEV1, percent predicted, with the extent of air trapping measured using DUHRCT was highly significant ($r = -0.92$; $p = 0.0004$) (156). Percent predicted values of peak flow rate, FVC, and the mean forced expiratory flow rate during the middle of the FVC also correlated closely with the dynamic CT extent of air trapping. Respectively, these r values measured -0.91 ($p = 0.004$), -0.92 ($p = 0.0005$), and -0.90 ($p = 0.003$). In some patients, significant air trapping can be detected using expiratory HRCT in the absence of definite pulmonary function abnormalities (155).

In patients with air trapping, collapse or obstruction of large or small bronchi can sometimes be seen, although this is uncommon. A lung region trapping area may show little change in area on the scan as compared to surrounding lung regions, although this observation can be quite subjective.

Areas of inhomogeneous lung attenuation visible on expiratory scans, and mimicking the appearance of air trapping, can sometimes be seen in patients with fibrotic lung disease and restrictive lung physiology. Although this finding could reflect the presence of airways obstruction resulting from peribronchial fibrosis, it is more likely the result of regional differences in lung compliance due to patchy lung fibrosis. It is important to keep in mind that the function of adjacent lung units, be they alveoli, lobules, or segments, are interdependent, with the movement and ventilation of one area of lung being affected by the movement and ventilation of surrounding lung (159). In patients with patchy lung fibrosis, the rapid decrease in local lung volume that occurs during exhalation in the areas of fibrosis could have the effect of maintaining the volume of adjacent areas of relatively normal and more compliant lung. These areas of relatively normal lung would appear lucent during exhalation.

Use of Expiratory CT to Differentiate Mosaic Perfusion From Ground-Glass Opacity

Inhomogeneous lung attenuation visible on inspiratory scans can be the result of (i) ground-glass opacity, (ii) mosaic perfusion resulting from airways obstruction and reflex vasoconstriction, or (iii) mosaic perfusion resulting from vascular obstruction. In many patients with mosaic perfusion, HRCT findings of decreased vascular caliber in lucent lung regions, or airway abnormalities can be diagnostic; however, in others, HRCT findings are nonspecific.

Expiratory scans can usually allow the differentiation of patients with ground-glass opacity from those with mosaic perfusion resulting from airways obstruction. In patients with ground-glass opacity, expiratory HRCT typically shows a proportional increase in attenuation in areas of both increased and decreased opacity (Fig. 3-97). In patients with mosaic perfusion resulting from airways disease, attenuation differences are accentuated on expiration (Fig. 3-98); relatively dense areas increase in attenuation, while lower attenuation regions remain lucent. In patients with mosaic perfusion resulting from vascular disease, expiratory HRCT findings mimic those seen in patients with ground-glass opacity; both low-attenuation and high-attenuation regions increase in opacity.

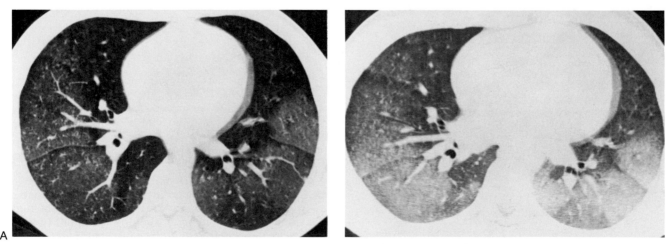

FIG. 3-97. Inspiratory and post-expiratory HRCT in a patient with pulmonary hemorrhage and ground-glass opacity. **A:** Patchy differences in lung opacity are visible on the inspiratory scan. This appearance mimics mosaic perfusion. **B:** On post-expiration scan, proportional increases in lung opacity are seen throughout the lungs. Lung attenuation increased by 150 to 200 HU on the expiratory scan in all lung regions.

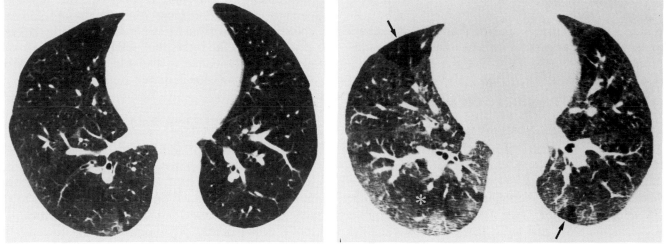

FIG. 3-98. Inspiratory and post-expiratory HRCT in a patient with bronchiolitis obliterans. **A:** Inspiratory scan shows subtle differences in opacity in different lung regions, representing mosaic perfusion. **B:** Post-expiratory HRCT shows a marked accentuation in attenuation inhomogeneities due to air trapping. Regions of lucency increased in attenuation by approximately 50 HU on expiration. While some areas of air-trapping appear patchy and nonanatomic (*asterisk*), others appear subsegmental or lobular (*arrows*).

THE DISTRIBUTION OF PARENCHYMAL ABNORMALITIES IN THE DIAGNOSIS OF LUNG DISEASE

When attempting to reach a diagnosis or differential diagnosis of lung disease using HRCT, the distribution of pulmonary abnormalities should be considered along with their morphology and HRCT appearance (24,62,67,76). Many lung diseases show specific regional distributions or preferences, a fact which is likely related to their underlying pathogenesis and pathophysiology (160).

Preferential or predominant involvement of one or more lung regions is commonly seen on HRCT, even in patients with chest radiographs showing a "diffuse" abnormality. For the purposes of interpreting HRCT, the regional distribution of lung abnormalities can be categorized in several ways—central lung vs. peripheral lung, upper lung vs. lower lung, anterior lung vs. posterior lung, or unilateral vs. bilateral. Also, as indicated above, HRCT abnormalities can often be localized to specific regions or parts of the secondary pulmonary lobule.

An important caveat to keep in mind when reading

TABLE 3-12. *Predominance of lung disease on HRCT—central lung vs. peripheral lung*

Lung diseases	Findings
Central Lung	
Sarcoidosis	Peribronchovascular nodules, conglomerate fibrosis with traction bronchiectasis
Silicosis	Conglomerate masses of fibrosis
Talcosis	Conglomerate masses of fibrosis
Lymphangitic spread of carcinoma	Peribronchovascular interstitial thickening or nodules
Large airways diseases (e.g., cystic fibrosis)	Bronchiectasis
Peripheral Lung	
Idiopathic pulmonary fibrosis, Scleroderma, Rheumatoid lung disease	Subpleural fibrosis, honeycombing, ground-glass opacity
Asbestosis	Subpleural fibrosis, honeycombing
Hematogenous metastases	Nodules
Eosinophilic pneumonia	Consolidation, ground-glass opacity
BOOP/COP	Consolidation, ground-glass opacity
Hypersensitivity pneumonitis	Ground-glass opacity, centrilobular nodules
Desquamative interstitial pneumonia	Consolidation, ground-glass opacity, fibrosis
Sarcoidosis	Nodules—subpleural, septal, centrilobular
Acute interstitial pneumonia	Consolidation, ground-glass opacity

the following section, is that significant variations in "classical" patterns of lung involvement can be seen in individual patients. A specific diagnosis should not be excluded because of an atypical distribution of abnormalities.

Central Lung vs. Peripheral Lung

Some diseases have a central, parahilar, "bronchocentric," or "bronchovascular" distribution (62), while others favor the peripheral or subpleural parenchyma, or lung "cortex" (Table 3-12). Diseases that can have a central or parahilar predominance include sarcoidosis (Fig. 3-52), silicosis, lymphangitic spread of carcinoma (163), and large airway diseases such as bronchiectasis, cystic fibrosis, and allergic bronchopulmonary aspergillosis (Fig. 3-87) (9,10,24,35,61, 67,76). In a recent study by Grenier et al. (161), a predominantly central distribution of abnormalities was visible in 16% of patients with sarcoidosis, 31% of patients with silicosis, and 8% of those with lymphangitic spread of carcinoma. In another study (67), a central or peribronchovascular predominance was seen in 70% of patients with sarcoidosis and in 60% of patients with lymphangitic spread of carcinoma.

A peripheral, cortical, or subpleural predominance of abnormalities has been reported in nearly all patients with eosinophilic pneumonia (Fig. 3-66) (118) and asbestosis (38), in from 81% to 94% of patients with idiopathic pulmonary fibrosis (Figs. 3-22,3-61) (38,59,67), and in a similar high percentage of patients with scleroderma, rheumatoid lung disease (Figs. 3-15,3-28), or interstitial pneumonia of other causes (102,161). Peripheral predominance of abnormalities is somewhat less common, visible in approximately half of patients, in BOOP/COP (Fig. 3-65) and desquamative interstitial

pneumonia (38,67,85,103). It is occasionally present in patients with hypersensitivity pneumonitis and sarcoidosis, ranging from a few percent to 18% in different studies, and acute interstitial pneumonia (109). A subpleural predominance is also typical of amyloidosis, although this disease is quite rare.

Upper Lung vs. Lower Lung

The relative extent and severity of abnormalities in the upper lungs, midlungs, and at the lung bases can be determined on HRCT if scans have been obtained at several levels, and if one level is compared to the others. Some diseases tend to predominate in the upper lobes, while others predominate in the lower lobes (Table 3-13) (162).

Diseases that have been recognized to have an upper lobe predominance on HRCT include sarcoidosis (Figs. 3-5,3-6,3-52), histiocytosis X (Figs. 3-74,3-75), coal worker's pneumoconiosis and silicosis (Figs. 3-46,3-54), and centrilobular emphysema (Fig. 3-80) (14,37,59,61,64,65,67,76,161). An upper lobe predominance of abnormalities is present in nearly equal percentages of patients with sarcoidosis (47% to 50%), histiocytosis X (57% to 62%), and silicosis (55% to 69%), while a lower lobe preponderance is present in less than 10% of patients with these diseases (59,161). An upper lobe predominance may be present in patients with respiratory bronchiolitis (86).

A basal distribution is most typical of lymphangitic metastasis (46%), hematogenous metastases, idiopathic pulmonary fibrosis (68%) (Fig. 3-25), collagen-vascular diseases such as rheumatoid lung disease and scleroderma (80%), and asbestosis (24,25,27,38,39,59, 67,102,161). Pulmonary fibrosis of any cause has a basal predominance in about 60% of cases (59,67). Al-

TABLE 3-13. *Predominance of lung disease on HRCT—upper lung vs. lower lung*

Lung disease	Findings
Upper Lung	
Sarcoidosis	Nodules, fibrosis, conglomerate masses
Histiocytosis X	Nodules, cysts
Silicosis	Nodules, conglomerate masses, emphysema
Talcosis	Conglomerate masses
TB	Consolidation, nodules, cavities, scarring
Centrilobular emphysema	Patchy lucencies
Respiratory bronchiolitis	Ground-glass opacity
Lower Lung	
Hypersensitivity pneumonitis	Ground-glass opacity, nodules, fibrosis
Hematogenous or Lymphangitic metastases	Nodules, septal thickening
Idiopathic pulmonary fibrosis, Scleroderma, Rheumatoid lung disease	Subpleural fibrosis, honeycombing, ground-glass opacity
Asbestosis	Subpleural fibrosis, honeycombing
Lipoid pneumonia	Consolidation, ground-glass opacity

TABLE 3-14. *Predominance of lung disease on HRCT—posterior lung*

Lung disease	Findings
Posterior Lung	
Asbestosis	Fibrosis
Scleroderma	Fibrosis, ground-glass opacity
Silicosis	Nodules
Sarcoidosis	Peribronchovascular, subpleural, and septal nodules
Hypersensitivity pneumonitis	Ground-glass opacity, nodules, fibrosis
Pulmonary edema	Septal thickening, ground-glass opacity

though hypersensitivity pneumonitis has been thought of as having an upper lobe predominance, it more often appears to be diffuse or preponderant in the midlung zones (13,38), or lower lung zones (30%) (161).

Posterior Lung Predominance

Some diseases produce their initial or most extensive abnormalities in the posterior lung (Table 3-14). The distinction between anterior and posterior, of course, is easily made on HRCT. However, it is important to recognize the value of using both prone and supine scans in this regard. Areas of increased attenuation that are limited to the posterior lung on scans obtained in the supine position can reflect normal dependent volume loss; prone scans are essential in making a confident diagnosis of early posterior lung disease. Although the percentages vary in different series, a posterior preponderance of disease is particularly common in scleroderma (60%), sarcoidosis (32% to 36%) (Fig. 3-53), silicosis (31% to 38%) (Fig. 3-46), hypersensitivity pneumonitis (23%), idiopathic pulmonary fibrosis (9% to 21%), and other causes of UIP (Figs. 3-26,3-28) (37,59,61,67,161). A posterior predominance of abnormalities is also common in patients with asbestosis, lymphangitic carcinomatosis, and pulmonary edema (24,27,39,59,61,67,102,161). In patients with pulmonary edema, the predominant abnormality is more appropriately referred to as dependent (Fig. 3-9) rather than posterior.

TABLE 3-15. *Predominance of lung disease on HRCT—unilateral or markedly asymmetric disease*

Lung disease	Findings
Pneumonia	Variable
Lymphangitic spread of carcinoma	Peribronchovascular interstitial thickening, nodules, septal thickening
Sarcoidosis	Peribronchovascular, subpleural, septal nodules
Bronchiectasis	Findings of bronchiectasis

Unilateral vs. Bilateral

A unilateral predominance of abnormalities is most typical of lymphangitic spread of carcinoma, which is often asymmetric in distribution (Table 3-15); this was seen in nearly 40% of patients with lymphangitic spread of carcinoma in one series (Fig. 3-4) (67). Asymmetry or unilateral predominance of findings is also common in patients with sarcoidosis, ranging from 9% to 21%. It is somewhat less frequent in association with silicosis (2% to 21%), pulmonary fibrosis (3% to 14%), histiocytosis X (12%), and hypersensitivity pneumonitis (5%) (59,67).

Diffuse Lung Involvement

Some diseases that appear "diffuse" on chest films, are in fact diffuse, and involve the lung uniformly from apex to base, from anterior to posterior, and from central to peripheral (Table 3-16) (67,76). This is not to say that the disease may not be patchy in distribution, with some areas much more abnormal than others, but that there is no consistent pattern to the disease. Many of the diseases that are described above as showing a particular distribution can also be diffuse; these include lymphangitic spread of carcinoma, sarcoidosis, and silicosis. One disease that typically shows this uniform distribution is hypersensitivity pneumonitis (67,76,82). Lymphangiomyomatosis tends to be diffuse while histiocytosis X does not (137).

DISTRIBUTION OF DISEASE RELATIVE TO THE SECONDARY LOBULE

Some lung diseases can show predominant involvement of different parts of the secondary pulmonary lobule, specifically, the perilobular or septal regions or the centrilobular regions (42,62,160).

TABLE 3-16. *Diffuse lung disease*

Lung disease	Findings
Diffuse pneumonia	Ground-glass opacity, consolidation
Lymphangitic spread of carcinoma	Peribronchovascular interstitial thickening, nodules, septal thickening
Hematogenous metastases	Nodules
Sarcoidosis	Nodules
Silicosis	Nodules
Bronchiectasis	Findings of bronchiectasis
Hypersensitivity pneumonitis	Ground-glass opacity, nodules, fibrosis
Lymphangiomyomatosis	Lung cysts

Perilobular or Septal Opacities

Diseases that are primarily "perilobular" (62) with predominant involvement of the interlobular septa include lymphangitic spread of carcinoma (Fig. 3-8) (9,10,62), lymphoma (62), sarcoidosis (Fig. 3-14) (35,61,62), asbestosis (Fig. 3-18) (27,62), idiopathic pulmonary fibrosis or UIP (Fig. 3-15) (7,18), pulmonary edema (Fig. 3-9), and some drug reactions (42).

Perilobular or septal opacities can appear smooth, nodular, or irregular in different diseases. Smooth septal thickening is seen most frequently in patients with pulmonary edema (Fig. 3-9), lymphangitic spread of carcinoma (Fig. 3-8) or lymphoma (9,10,31), and in a small percentage of patients with pulmonary fibrosis. Nodular or "beaded" septal thickening occurs primarily in patients with lymphangitic spread of carcinoma or lymphoma (Figs. 3-11,3-43) (9,10,31), sarcoidosis, and silicosis (35,36). In patients who have interstitial fibrosis, septal thickening visible on HRCT is often irregular in appearance and associated with distortion of lung architecture (18).

Among patients with pulmonary fibrosis and "end-stage" lung disease, the presence of perilobular opacities or interlobular septal thickening on HRCT is most frequent in those with sarcoidosis (Fig. 3-14) (56% of patients) and asbestosis (Fig. 3-18) (27,38,163). Septal thickening is relatively uncommon in patients with IPF and other causes of usual interstitial pneumonia (UIP), and hypersensitivity pneumonitis (38). The differential diagnosis of interlobular septal thickening is reviewed in Table 3-2.

Centrilobular Opacities

A number of diseases can result in the presence of opacities that appear predominantly centrilobular on HRCT (55). An increase in the prominence of centrilobular branching structures can reflect the presence of interstitial thickening surrounding the centrilobular arteries, or dilatation and filling of the centrilobular bronchiole, resulting in a tree-in-bud appearance (Figs. 3-33–3-36). Centrilobular nodular opacities can be well-defined or ill-defined, and can appear as a single opacity or as a rosette of small opacities (Figs. 3-36,3-50,3-51). In general, nodules can be diagnosed on HRCT as centrilobular if they (i) are adjacent to, surround, or obscure centrilobular arteries, (ii) occur in relation to small (centrilobular) vascular branches, or (iii) are centered 5 to 10 mm from the lobular periphery or pleural surface, but do not reach the pleura.

A centrilobular distribution of abnormalities recognizable on HRCT has been reported in a variety of diseases that predominantly affect the centrilobular bronchioles, pulmonary arteries, and lymphatics, often associated with secondary involvement of the peribronchovascular interstitium or alveoli. The recognition of a centrilobular abnormality on HRCT can thus suggest the presence of a bronchiolar, vascular, or lymphatic disease, and a relatively short list of possible diagnoses (Table 3-17) (26,62,160). In addition, a centrilobular predominance of abnormalities is strong evidence that a transbronchial biopsy would provide abnormal material, although it may not always be diagnostic of a specific disease.

It is most helpful to categorize diseases presenting with centrilobular abnormalities relative to their predominant cause (55).

Bronchiolar and Peribronchiolar Diseases

Bronchiolar diseases that secondarily involve the peribronchiolar interstitium and/or alveoli are the most frequent cause of centrilobular opacities seen on HRCT. Their histologic correlates and HRCT appearances vary with the nature of the disease.

Increased prominence, and often irregularity, of centrilobular branching structures commonly reflects the presence of bronchiolar dilatation and filling of the bronchiolar lumen with mucus, fluid, or pus (Figs. 3-33–3-36). This finding has been aptly described as tree-in-bud by Im et al. (41), and is usually seen in patients with small airway diseases associated with mucus retention or infection. Bronchiolar dilatation and wall thickening can sometimes be seen if the dilated bronchioles are air filled (Fig. 3-32). Either of these findings is diagnostic of a small airway abnormality.

Ill-defined centrilobular opacities or nodules, surrounding the centrilobular artery or sometimes seen in association with a tree- in-bud appearance, can also reflect bronchiolar abnormalities and peribronchiolar interstitial or alveolar inflammation or fibrosis. Centrilobular nodules, in the absence of a tree-in-bud appearance, are most typical of bronchiolar diseases not associated with infection.

Bronchiolar diseases with centrilobular opacities are also often associated with large airway abnormalities and bronchiectasis, which can be a clue to their diagnosis (55). The differential diagnosis of airway diseases associated with centrilobular abnormalities includes the following entities:

Cystic Fibrosis

In patients with cystic fibrosis, thick-walled, mucus or pus-filled bronchioles are seen as rounded or branching centrilobular opacities, usually in association with central bronchiectasis (Fig. 3-34) (54,62,148). The centrilobular bronchiolar abnormalities can be an early finding, and can be patchy in distribution.

TABLE 3-17. *Differential diagnosis of centrilobular opacities*

Diagnosis	Comments
Peribronchiolar Diseases	
Cystic fibrosis, Bronchiectasis	Bronchiolar dilatation; large bronchi abnormal
Panbronchiolitis	Bronchiolar dilatation; centrilobular nodules; air trapping
Bronchogenic spread of TB	Bronchiolar dilatation; centrilobular nodules
Bronchopneumonia	Bronchiolar dilatation; centrilobular nodules
Bronchiolitis obliterans	Centrilobular nodules; air trapping predominant
Bronchiolitis obliterans organizing pneumonia	Centrilobular nodules; ground-glass opacity or consolidation predominant
Respiratory bronchiolitis	Centrilobular nodules of ground-glass opacity
Asbestosis	Centrilobular nodules in early stages
Silicosis	Centrilobular nodules; subpleural nodules
Histiocytosis X	Well-defined centrilobular nodules in early stages
Hypersensitivity pneumonitis	Centrilobular ground-glass opacities
Bronciolalveolar carcinoma, Tracheobronchial papillomatosis	Centrilobular nodules
Perilymphatic Diseases	
Lymphangitic spread of carcinoma	Prominent centrilobular branching structures; septal thickening almost always present
Sarcoidosis	Centrilobular, peribronchovascular, subpleural nodules
Silicosis	Centrilobular nodules; subpleural nodules
Lymphocytic interstitial pneumonitis (LIP) in AIDS patients	Centrilobular nodules
Perivascular Diseases	
Edema	Centrilobular nodules; septal thickening
Talcosis	Centrilobular nodules
Vasculitis	Centrilobular nodules

Bronchiectasis

Findings similar to those of cystic fibrosis can be seen in patients with chronic bronchiectasis of any cause, including congenital immunodeficiency states, ciliary dysmotility syndrome, and the syndrome of yellow nails and lymphedema (Figs. 3-33–3-99). Typically, both large airway abnormalities and a tree-in-bud appearance are visible.

Panbronchiolitis

In patients with Asian panbronchiolitis, aggregates of histiocytes, lymphocytes, and plasma cells infiltrate the walls of respiratory bronchioles and extend into the peribronchiolar tissues. HRCT (Fig. 3-35) can show:

1. Prominent branching centrilobular opacities representing dilated bronchioles with inflammatory bronchiolar wall thickening and abundant intraluminal secretions,

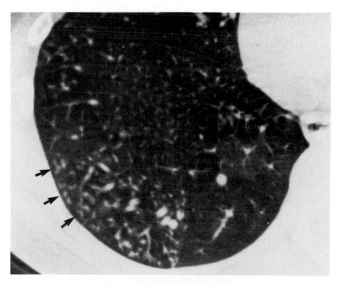

FIG. 3-99. Centrilobular nodules and a "tree-in-bud" appearance (*arrows*) are visible in the posterior lower lobe of a patient with yellow-nails syndrome, bronchiectasis, and chronic airway infection.

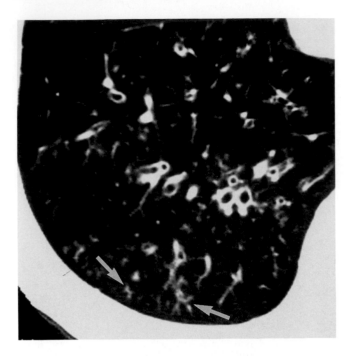

FIG. 3-100. Nontuberculous mycobacterial infection with endobronchial spread. Coned view of the right lower lobe in a patient with chronic obstructive lung disease and *Mycobacterium avium-intracellulare complex* (MAC) infection on sputum cultures. Central bronchi are dilated and thick walled; centrilobular bronchioles are also dilated, with a "tree-in-bud" appearance (*arrows*). (From Gruden et al., ref. 55, with permission.)

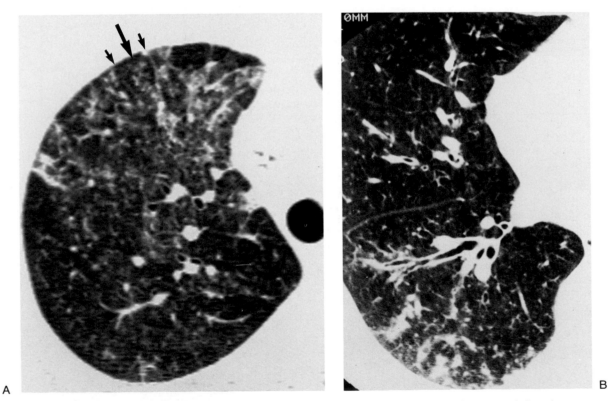

FIG. 3-101. A,B: Bronchopneumonia in two patients. **A:** HRCT of the right upper lobe shows ill-defined areas of centrilobular opacity predominating in the anterior segment. Centrilobular branching opacities are present with a "tree-in-bud" appearance (*large arrow*) typical of bronchiolar impaction with mucus or pus. *Small arrows* indicate the location of interlobular septa. Sputum cultures grew *Staphylococcus aureus*. (From Gruden et al., ref. 55, with permission.) **B:** In another patient, HRCT shows a left lower lobe bronchopneumonia with ill-defined centrilobular nodules and bronchiolar dilatation. Lower lobe bronchi also appear thick walled.

2. Bronchiolar dilatation that tends to occur late in the disease process (53,57,58) and is typically proximal to the nodular peribronchiolar opacities, and

3. Centrilobular nodules that reflect bronchiolar and peribronchiolar inflammation and fibrosis (57).

Endobronchial Spread of Tuberculosis, Nontuberculous Mycobacteria, and Other Granulomatous Infections

Bronchogenic dissemination of infection can occur in patients with active tuberculosis and nontuberculous mycobacterial disease (Figs. 3-36,3-100). Nodules, or clusters of nodules, that reflect peribronchiolar consolidation or granuloma formation are common, visible on HRCT in as many as 97% of patients with active tuberculosis, and are also common in patients with nontuberculous mycobacterial infection (26,41,62,79,81,164). Bronchioles filled with infected material can also result in the appearance of tree-in-bud (41).

Bronchopneumonia

Bronchopneumonia resulting from other organisms, most commonly bacteria, is associated with bronchial and peribronchiolar inflammatory exudates, which also involve surrounding alveoli. HRCT findings are quite similar to those of endobronchial spread of tuberculosis (Fig. 3-101) (3,55,62,78). Viral infections and PCP can also result in the appearance of centrilobular nodules.

Bronchiolitis and Bronchiolitis Obliterans

Acute bronchiolitis is characterized by epithelial injury, intraluminal exudation, and peribronchiolar inflammation. Bronchiolitis obliterans is characterized by the presence of inflammatory cells lining the walls of the terminal and respiratory bronchioles with plugs of granulation tissue filling and obstructing the airway lumen; it can represent the organizational phase of acute bronchiolitis. In patients with bronchiolitis and bronchiolitis obliterans, centrilobular opacities can be seen on HRCT, largely reflecting peribronchiolar inflammation (Fig. 3-102) (55). However, this is not a

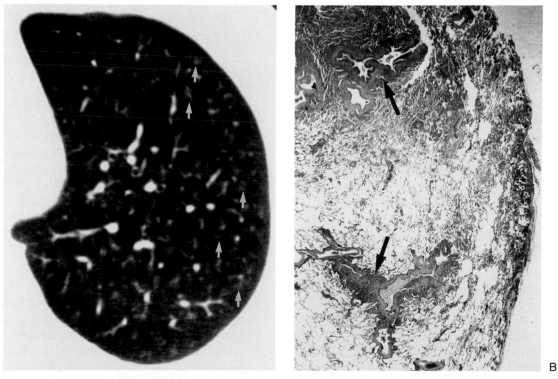

FIG. 3-102. Bronchiolitis obliterans with centrilobular opacities. **A:** Ill-defined nodular opacities (*arrows*) are scattered throughout the left upper lobe in this patient who had received an allogeneic bone marrow transplant several years previously. Their centrilobular location can be inferred in that they surround small artery branches. **B:** Open lung biopsy shows bronchioles (*arrows*) partially occluded by plugs of granulation tissue, features diagnostic of bronchiolitis obliterans. Inflammation surrounding the bronchioles probably accounts for the opacities seen on HRCT. (From Gruden et al., ref. 55, with permission.)

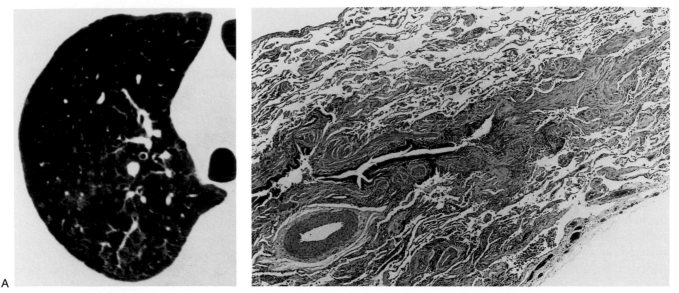

A   B

FIG. 3-103. BOOP with centrilobular nodules. **A:** Multifocal areas of ill-defined opacity are present in the right upper lobe. Note that small pulmonary artery branches are partially obscured by the centrilobular opacities. **B:** Open lung biopsy showed features of bronchiolitis obliterans organizing pneumonia (BOOP). Bronchioles are compressed and occluded by granulation tissue; organizing pneumonia and loose connective tissue are also present, surrounding the bronchioles. (From Gruden et al., ref. 55, with permission.)

common finding (62). The appearance of tree-in-bud is absent.

Bronchiolitis Obliterans Organizing Pneumonia/ Cryptogenic Organizing Pneumonia (BOOP/COP)

If a significant organizing pneumonia is associated with histologic findings of bronchiolitis, the terms *BOOP* or *COP* are generally used to describe the abnormality. Because the organizing pneumonia is distributed in the peribronchiolar airspaces, centrilobular opacities can be present in patients with BOOP/COP (Fig. 3-103). Frank consolidation or larger areas of ground-glass opacity, however, are more common (Fig. 3-65) (85,88). The appearance of tree-in-bud is absent.

Respiratory Bronchiolitis

Respiratory bronchiolitis is thought to represent a nonspecific reaction to inhaled irritants; it is almost always seen in smokers. Inflammation of the respiratory bronchioles with filling of the bronchioles by brown-pigmented macrophages, plasma cells, and lymphocytes are present histologically. In symptomatic patients, macrophages and inflammatory cells extend into the peribronchiolar airspaces and alveolar walls. HRCT findings in symptomatic patients include multifocal ground-glass opacities with a centrilobular distribution that reflects the peribronchiolar nature of this

disease (Figs. 6-10,6-11) (86,87,110). Patchy opacities can also be seen. The appearance of tree-in-bud is absent.

Cigarette Smoking

A few small subpleural and centrilobular nodules can be seen in subjects who smoke or have a history of smoking. Ill-defined centrilobular nodules have been reported in as many as 12% to 27% of smokers studied using HRCT, reflecting the presence of bronchiolectasis and peribronchiolar fibrosis (86,165), although in our experience, this is not a common finding. The appearance of tree-in-bud is absent.

Asbestosis

In patients with early asbestosis, the histologic abnormality is nearly identical to that seen in patients with respiratory bronchiolitis, but asbestos fibers can be identified in the peribronchiolar tissues. Fiber deposition in the respiratory bronchioles results in a peribronchiolar cellular response and fibrosis that eventually extends to involve the contiguous airspaces and alveolar interstitium. Ill-defined centrilobular opacities have been reported on HRCT in as many as half of patients with early asbestosis (Figs. 4-30,4-31) (77). Nodules predominate posteriorly and at the lung bases, probably due to the gravitational effects of fiber deposition (28,77). Other inhaled inorganic materials can result in similar histologic and imaging abnormalities. Tree-in-bud is absent.

Silicosis

In patients with silicosis, early lesions are centrilobular, and peribronchiolar and perilymphatic nodules are a few millimeters in diameter and consist of layers of laminated connective tissue (Fig. 3-46). The characteristic lesion of coal worker's pneumoconiosis (CWP) is the so-called coal macule, which consists of a focal accumulation of coal dust surrounded by a small amount of fibrous tissue. Small centrilobular or subpleural nodules are characteristic of both silicosis and CWP on HRCT (37,68). The appearance of tree-in-bud is absent.

Histiocytosis X

Initially, granulomas form in the peribronchiolar tissues and adjacent alveolar interstitium. Mononuclear Langerhans cells are present in the early stages of the disease; later, the cellular response diminishes and fibrosis dominates. Centrilobular nodules on HRCT reflect the peribronchiolar abnormality (Fig. 7-3) (65). Later in the course of the disease, cavitation of nodules, cyst formation, and centrilobular bronchiolectasis can be seen.

Hypersensitivity Pneumonitis

An immunologic response to a variety of inhaled allergens in sensitized persons, subacute hypersensitivity pneumonitis (extrinsic allergic alveolitis) is characterized by a peribronchiolar and perivascular lymphocytic and plasma cell infiltrate, with formation of poorly defined granulomas (82). There may be associated plugs of granulation tissue within bronchiolar lumens (bronchiolitis obliterans). Centrilobular nodules of ground-glass opacity seen on HRCT are typical (Fig. 3-51), reflecting the histologic abnormality (83). Tree-in-bud is absent.

Endobronchial Spread of Neoplasm

Centrilobular nodules can be seen in bronchioloalveolar carcinoma (Fig. 5-7) or tracheobronchial papillomatosis (Fig. 3-104) when endobronchial spread of tumor occurs (166). These can be well-defined or ill-defined. Large airway papillomas or cystic lesions may also be visible in patients with tracheobronchial papillomatosis.

Lymphatic and Perilymphatic Diseases

Pulmonary lymphatics are located in the peribronchovascular interstitial compartment and in the peripheral interstitial compartment (within the interlobular septa and in the subpleural regions). Diseases that involve the lymphatics commonly result in both centrilobular and septal abnormalities, along with other manifestations of "perilymphatic" disease. Although it is unusual for a centrilobular abnormality to predominate, this can occur.

Lymphangitic Spread of Carcinoma

Tumor, edema, and fibrosis involving the lymphatics in the peribronchovascular interstitium and interlobular septa are typically present histologically. Although interlobular septal thickening is usually a predominant feature, in some subjects, centrilobular peribronchovascular interstitial thickening, with accentuation of normal centrilobular branching structures is the primary HRCT finding, at least in some lung regions (Fig. 3-47) (55). Other findings include thickening of the peribronchovascular interstitium surrounding vessels and bronchi in the parahilar lung, small nodules, and a preservation of normal lung architecture at the lobular level.

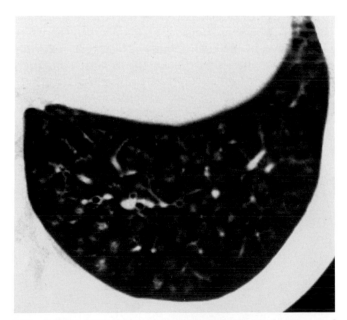

FIG. 3-104. Endobronchial spread of tracheobronchial papillomatosis. Multiple small, ill-defined, centrilobular nodules are present in the posterior left lower lobe. Many appear to be about 1 cm from the pleural surface or are related to small vessels.

Sarcoidosis

Sarcoid granulomas, the hallmark of this disease, are typically distributed along lymphatics in the peribronchovascular interstitial space (both in the parahilar regions and lobular core), and, to a lesser extent, in the interlobular septa and subpleural interstitial space (Fig. 3-43) (35,62). This characteristic "perilymphatic" distribution is helpful in making a histologic and radiographic diagnosis (36).

Lymphocytic Interstitial Pneumonia

Lymphocytic interstitial pneumonia (LIP) in AIDS patients can result in the presence of ill-defined centrilobular opacities (Fig. 3-105). LIP is associated with a lymphocytic and plasma cell infiltrate in relation to lymphatics; it may predominate in the centrilobular regions.

Vascular and Perivascular Diseases

Vascular pathology, either localized to the walls of arteries or to perivascular tissues, can cause centrilobular abnormality. Since airways are not involved, bronchiolectasis is absent, although if the cellular response extends into the peribronchiolovascular interstitium, apparent bronchiolar wall thickening may result.

Pulmonary Edema

Mild cases of edema may show hazy, ill-defined centrilobular opacities (Figs. 6-41,6-42) (79). Increased prominence of the centrilobular artery resulting from perivascular interstitial thickening is also commonly

visible (Fig. 3-9). Septal thickening is variably associated. Pleural effusion may also be present.

Vasculitis

Processes resulting in an vascular and perivascular inflammatory response, including vasculitis and reaction to injected substances, such as talc (55,68,91), can result in ill-defined centrilobular opacities on HRCT.

Centrilobular Lucencies

Centrilobular lucencies can reflect dilation of air-containing centrilobular bronchioles, or centrilobular emphysema.

Centrilobular Bronchiolectasis

This can result from some of the small airways abnormalities described above, particularly panbronchiolitis, cystic fibrosis, bronchiectasis, and histiocytosis X (Fig. 3-75). Centrilobular bronchiolectasis can also be seen in the presence of pulmonary fibrosis (traction bronchiolectasis).

Centrilobular Emphysema

The respiratory bronchioles, predominantly in the upper lobes, are primarily affected in this entity. Focal areas of low attenuation are present in a centrilobular location or clustered around the centrilobular structures (Figs. 3-78,3-79). On HRCT, centrilobular emphysema appears as multiple, scattered foci of lucency, without visible walls, interspersed with areas of normal

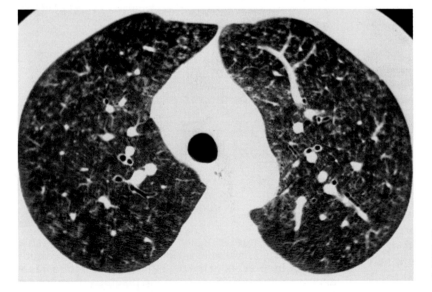

FIG. 3-105. Lymphocytic interstitial pneumonia (LIP) in a 38- year-old woman with AIDS. Ill-defined centrilobular nodules are visible diffusely.

lung. The centrilobular distribution of the emphysematous areas is sometimes visible on clinical scans (18,26,62).

Panlobular Abnormalities

A "panlobular" distribution, that is, uniform involvement of secondary pulmonary lobules by the pathologic process (62), is typical of diseases that produce air-space consolidation, such as bronchopneumonia or lobular pneumonia (41), but can be seen in a variety of diffuse interstitial diseases characterized by ground-glass opacity (Fig. 3-62), and is nonspecific.

Patchy areas of panlobular lucency can represent paraseptal emphysema (Fig. 3-84), severe centrilobular emphysema (Fig. 3-82), or mosaic perfusion in patients with airways obstruction (Fig. 3-92). A diffuse distribution of panlobular lucencies can represent panlobular emphysema, or severe confluent centrilobular emphysema.

REFERENCES

1. Müller NL, Miller RR. Computed tomography of chronic diffuse infiltrative lung disease: part 1. *Am Rev Respir Dis* 1990; 142:1206–1215.
2. Müller NL, Miller RR. Computed tomography of chronic diffuse infiltrative lung disease: part 2. *Am Rev Respir Dis* 1990; 142:1440–1448.
3. Webb WR. High-resolution CT of the lung parenchyma. *Radiol Clin North Am* 1989;27:1085–1097.
4. Zerhouni E. Computed tomography of the pulmonary parenchyma: an overview. *Chest* 1989;95:901–907.
5. Webb WR, Müller NL, Naidich DP. Standardized terms for high-resolution computed tomography of the lung: a proposed glossary. *J Thorac Imaging* 1993;8:167–185.
6. Zerhouni EA, Naidich DP, Stitik FP, Khouri NF, Siegelman SS. Computed tomography of the pulmonary parenchyma. Part 2: interstitial disease. *J Thorac Imaging* 1985;1:54–64.
7. Nishimura K, Kitaichi M, Izumi T, Nagai S, Itoh H. Usual interstitial pneumonia: histologic correlation with high-resolution CT. *Radiology* 1992;182:337–342.
8. Weibel ER. Looking into the lung: what can it tell us? *AJR* 1979;133:1021–1031.
9. Munk PL, Müller NL, Miller RR, Ostrow DN. Pulmonary lymphangitic carcinomatosis: CT and pathologic findings. *Radiology* 1988;166:705–709.
10. Stein MG, Mayo J, Müller N, Aberle DR, Webb WR, Gamsu G. Pulmonary lymphangitic spread of carcinoma: appearance on CT scans. *Radiology* 1987;162:371–375.
11. Bergin CJ, Müller NL. CT in the diagnosis of interstitial lung disease. *AJR* 1985;145:505–510.
12. Johkoh T, Ikezoe J, Tomiyama N, et al. CT findings in lymphangitic carcinomatosis of the lung: correlation with histologic findings and pulmonary function tests. *AJR* 1992;158: 1217–1222.
13. Adler BD, Padley SP, Müller NL, Remy-Jardin M, Remy J. Chronic hypersensitivity pneumonitis: high-resolution CT and radiographic features in 16 patients. *Radiology* 1992;185:91–95.
14. Müller NL, Kullnig P, Miller RR. The CT findings of pulmonary sarcoidosis: analysis of 25 patients. *AJR* 1989;152:1179–1182.
15. Bessis L, Callard P, Gotheil C, Biaggi A, Grenier P. High-resolution CT of parenchymal lung disease: precise correlation with histologic findings. *Radiographics* 1992;12:45–58.
16. Weibel ER, Taylor CR. Design and structure of the human lung. In: *Pulmonary Diseases and Disorders*. Weibel ER, Taylor CR. New York: McGraw-Hill; 1988:11–60.
17. Westcott JL, Cole SR. Traction bronchiectasis in end-stage pulmonary fibrosis. *Radiology* 1986;161:665–669.
18. Webb WR, Stein MG, Finkbeiner WE, Im JG, Lynch D, Gamsu G. Normal and diseased isolated lungs: high-resolution CT. *Radiology* 1988;166:81–87.
19. Naidich DP, McCauley DI, Khouri NF, Stitik FP, Siegelman SS. Computed tomography of bronchiectasis. *J Comput Assist Tomogr* 1982;6:437–444.
20. Grenier P, Maurice F, Musset D, Menu Y, Nahum H. Bronchiectasis: assessment by thin-section CT. *Radiology* 1986;161: 95–99.
21. Munro NC, Cooke JC, Currie DC, Strickland B, Cole PJ. Comparison of thin section computed tomography with bronchography for identifying bronchiectatic segments in patients with chronic sputum production. *Thorax* 1990;45:135–139.
22. Grenier P, Lenoir S, Brauner M. Computed tomographic assessment of bronchiectasis. *Semin Ultrasound CT MR* 1990; 11:430–441.
23. Neeld DA, Goodman LR, Gurney JW, Greenberger PA, Fink JN. Computerized tomography in the evaluation of allergic bronchopulmonary aspergillosis. *Am Rev Respir Dis* 1990;142: 1200–1206.
24. Swensen SJ, Aughenbaugh GL, Brown LR. High-resolution computed tomography of the lung. *Mayo Clin Proc* 1989;64: 1284– 1294.
25. Müller NL, Miller RR, Webb WR, Evans KG, Ostrow DN. Fibrosing alveolitis: CT-pathologic correlation. *Radiology* 1986;160:585–588.
26. Murata K, Itoh H, Todo G, et al. Centrilobular lesions of the lung: demonstration by high-resolution CT and pathologic correlation. *Radiology* 1986;161:641–645.
27. Aberle DR, Gamsu G, Ray CS, Feuerstein IM. Asbestos-related pleural and parenchymal fibrosis: detection with high-resolution CT. *Radiology* 1988;166:729–734.
28. Akira M, Yamamoto S, Yokoyama K, et al. Asbestosis: high-resolution CT-pathologic correlation. *Radiology* 1990;176: 389–394.
29. Bergin CJ, Coblentz CL, Chiles C, Bell DY, Castellino RA. Chronic lung diseases: specific diagnosis using CT. *AJR* 1989; 152:1183–1188.
30. Cassart M, Genevois PA, Kramer M, et al. Pulmonary venoocclusive disease: CT findings before and after single-lung transplantation. *AJR* 1993;160:759–760.
31. Ren H, Hruban RH, Kuhlman JE, et al. Computed tomography of inflation-fixed lungs: the beaded septum sign of pulmonary metastases. *J Comput Assist Tomogr* 1989;13:411–416.
32. Murch CR, Carr DH. Computed tomography appearances of pulmonary alveolar proteinosis. *Clin Radiol* 1989;40:240–243.
33. Godwin JD, Müller NL, Takasugi JE. Pulmonary alveolar proteinosis: CT findings. *Radiology* 1988;169:609–613.
34. Graham CM, Stern EJ, Finkbeiner WE, Webb WR. High-resolution CT appearance of diffuse alveolar septal amyloidosis. *AJR* 1992;158:265–267.
35. Lynch DA, Webb WR, Gamsu G, Stulbarg M, Golden J. Computed tomography in pulmonary sarcoidosis. *J Comput Assist Tomogr* 1989;13:405–410.
36. Remy-Jardin M, Beuscart R, Sault MC, Marquette CH, Remy J. Subpleural micronodules in diffuse infiltrative lung diseases: evaluation with thin-section CT scans. *Radiology* 1990;177: 133–139.
37. Remy-Jardin M, Degreef JM, Beuscart R, Voisin C, Remy J. Coal worker's pneumoconiosis: CT assessment in exposed workers and correlation with radiographic findings. *Radiology* 1990;177:363–371.
38. Primack SL, Hartman TE, Hansell DM, Müller NL. End-stage lung disease: CT findings in 61 patients. *Radiology* 1993;189: 681–686.
39. Aberle DR, Gamsu G, Ray CS. High-resolution CT of benign asbestos-related diseases: clinical and radiographic correlation. *AJR* 1988;151:883–891.

40. Lynch DA, Gamsu G, Ray CS, Aberle DR. Asbestos-related focal lung masses: manifestations on conventional and high-resolution CT scans. *Radiology* 1988;169:603–607.

41. Im JG, Itoh H, Shim YS, et al. Pulmonary tuberculosis: CT findings—early active disease and sequential change with antituberculous therapy. *Radiology* 1993;186:653–660.

42. Colby TV. Anatomic distribution and histopathologic patterns in interstitial lung disease. In: Schwarz MI, King TE Jr, eds. *Interstitial Lung Disease*. St. Louis: Mosby Year Book; 1993: 59–77.

43. Genereux GP. The end-stage lung: pathogenesis, pathology, and radiology. *Radiology* 1975;116:279–289.

44. Yoshimura H, Hatakeyama M, Otsuji H, et al. Pulmonary asbestosis: CT study of subpleural curvilinear shadow. Work in progress. *Radiology* 1986;158:653–658.

45. Al Jarad N, Strickland B, Pearson MC, Rubens MB, Rudd RM. High-resolution computed tomographic assessment of asbestosis and cryptogenic fibrosing alveolitis: a comparative study. *Thorax* 1992;47:645–650.

46. Schurawitzki H, Stiglbauer R, Graninger W, et al. Interstitial lung disease in progressive systemic sclerosis: high-resolution CT versus radiography. *Radiology* 1990;176:755–759.

47. Swensen SJ, Aughenbaugh GL, Douglas WW, Myers JL. High-resolution CT of the lungs: findings in various pulmonary diseases. *AJR* 1992;158:971–979.

48. Morimoto S, Takeuchi N, Imanaka H, et al. Gravity dependent atelectasis: radiologic, physiologic and pathologic correlation in rabbits on high-frequency ventilation. *Invest Radiol* 1989; 24:522–530.

49. Arai K, Takashima T, Matsui O, Kadoya M, Kamimura R. Transient subpleural curvilinear shadow caused by pulmonary congestion. *J Comput Assist Tomogr* 1990;14:87–88.

50. Pilate I, Marcelis S, Timmerman H, Beeckman P, Osteaux MJC. Pulmonary asbestosis: CT study of subpleural curvilinear shadow [Letter]. *Radiology* 1987;164:584.

51. Kubota H, Hosoya T, Kato M, Uchimura F, Itagaki T, Yamaguchi K. Plate-like atelectasis at the corticomedullary junction of the lung: CT observation and hypothesis. *Radiat Med* 1983; 1:305–310.

52. Todo G, Herman PG. High-resolution computed tomography of the pig lung. *Invest Radiol* 1986;21:689–696.

53. Akira M, Kitatani F, Lee Y-S, et al. Diffuse panbronchiolitis: evaluation with high-resolution CT. *Radiology* 1988;168: 433–438.

54. Lynch DA, Brasch RC, Hardy KA, Webb WR. Pediatric pulmonary disease: assessment with high-resolution ultrafast CT. *Radiology* 1990;176:243–248.

55. Gruden JF, Webb WR, Warnock M. Centrilobular opacities in the lung on high-resolution CT: diagnostic considerations and pathologic correlation. *AJR* 1994;162:569–574.

56. Reid L, Simon G. The peripheral pattern in the normal bronchogram and its relation to peripheral pulmonary anatomy. *Thorax* 1958;13:103–109.

57. Nishimura K, Kitaichi M, Izumi T, Itoh H. Diffuse panbronchiolitis: correlation of high-resolution CT and pathologic findings. *Radiology* 1992;184:779–785.

58. Akira M, Higashihara T, Sakatani M, Hara H. Diffuse panbronchiolitis: follow-up CT examination. *Radiology* 1993;189: 559–562.

59. Grenier P, Valeyre D, Cluzel P, Brauner MW, Lenoir S, Chastang C. Chronic diffuse interstitial lung disease: diagnostic value of chest radiography and high-resolution CT. *Radiology* 1991;179:123–132.

60. Remy-Jardin M, Remy J, Deffontaines C, Duhamel A. Assessment of diffuse infiltrative lung disease: comparison of conventional CT and high-resolution CT. *Radiology* 1991;181: 157–162.

61. Brauner MW, Grenier P, Mompoint D, Lenoir S, de Cremoux H. Pulmonary sarcoidosis: evaluation with high-resolution CT. *Radiology* 1989;172:467–471.

62. Murata K, Khan A, Herman PG. Pulmonary parenchymal disease: evaluation with high-resolution CT. *Radiology* 1989;170: 629–635.

63. Nakata H, Kimoto T, Nakayama T, Kido M, Miyazaki N, Harada S. Diffuse peripheral lung disease: evaluation by high-resolution computed tomography. *Radiology* 1985;157:181–185.

64. Brauner MW, Grenier P, Mouelhi MM, Mompoint D, Lenoir S. Pulmonary histiocytosis X: evaluation with high resolution CT. *Radiology* 1989;172:255–258.

65. Moore AD, Godwin JD, Müller NL, et al. Pulmonary histiocytosis X: comparison of radiographic and CT findings. *Radiology* 1989;172:249–254.

66. Bergin CJ, Müller NL, Vedal S, Chan Yeung M. CT in silicosis: correlation with plain films and pulmonary function tests. *AJR* 1986;146:477–483.

67. Mathieson JR, Mayo JR, Staples CA, Müller NL. Chronic diffuse infiltrative lung disease: comparison of diagnostic accuracy of CT and chest radiography. *Radiology* 1989;171: 111–116.

68. Akira M, Higashihara T, Yokoyama K, et al. Radiographic type p pneumoconiosis: high-resolution CT. *Radiology* 1989;171: 117–123.

69. Hruban RH, Meziane MA, Zerhouni EA, et al. High resolution computed tomography of Inflation fixed lungs: pathologic-radiologic correlation of centrilobular emphysema. *Am Rev Respir Dis* 1987;136:935–940.

70. Lee KS, Song KS, Lim TH, Kim PN, Kim IY, Lee BH. Adult-onset pulmonary tuberculosis: findings on chest radiographs and CT scans. *AJR* 1993;160:753–758.

71. Murata K, Takahashi M, Mori M, et al. Pulmonary metastatic nodules: CT-pathologic correlation. *Radiology* 1992;182: 331–335.

72. Nishimura K, Itoh H, Kitaichi M, Nagai S, Izumi T. Pulmonary sarcoidosis: correlation of CT and histopathologic findings. *Radiology* 1993;189:105–109.

73. Brauner MW, Lenoir S, Grenier P, Cluzel P, Battesti JP, Valeyre D. Pulmonary sarcoidosis: CT assessment of lesion reversibility. *Radiology* 1992;182:349–354.

74. Bergin CJ, Bell DY, Coblentz CL, et al. Sarcoidosis: correlation of pulmonary parenchymal pattern at CT with results of pulmonary function tests. *Radiology* 1989;171:619–624.

75. Bégin R, Bergeron D, Samson L, Boctor M, Cantin A. CT assessment of silicosis in exposed workers. *AJR* 1987;148: 509–514.

76. Bergin CJ, Müller NL. CT of interstitial lung disease: a diagnostic approach. *AJR* 1987;148:9–15.

77. Akira M, Yokoyama K, Yamamoto S, et al. Early asbestosis: evaluation with high-resolution CT. *Radiology* 1991;178: 409–416.

78. Naidich DP, Zerhouni EA, Hutchins GM, Genieser NB, McCauley DI, Siegelman SS. Computed tomography of the pulmonary parenchyma. Part 1: distal air-space disease. *J Thorac Imaging* 1985;1:39–53.

79. Itoh H, Tokunaga S, Asamoto H, et al. Radiologic-pathologic correlations of small lung nodules with special reference to peribronchiolar nodules. *AJR* 1978;130:223–231.

80. Murata K, Herman PG, Khan A, Todo G, Pipman Y, Luber JM. Intralobular distribution of oleic acid-induced pulmonary edema in the pig: evaluation by high-resolution CT. *Invest Radiol* 1989;24:647–653.

81. Lee KS, Kim YH, Kim WS, Hwang SH, Kim PN, Lee BH. Endobronchial tuberculosis: CT features. *J Comput Assist Tomogr* 1991;15:424–428.

82. Silver SF, Müller NL, Miller RR, Lefcoe MS. Hypersensitivity pneumonitis: evaluation with CT. *Radiology* 1989;173:441–445.

83. Lynch DA, Rose CS, Way D, King TE. Hypersensitivity pneumonitis: sensitivity of high-resolution CT in a population-based study. *AJR* 1992;159:469–472.

84. Akira M, Kita N, Higashihara T, Sakatani M, Kozuka T. Summer-type hypersensitivity pneumonitis: comparison of high-resolution CT and plain radiographic findings. *AJR* 1992;158: 1223–1228.

85. Müller NL, Staples CA, Miller RR. Bronchiolitis obliterans organizing pneumonia: CT features in 14 patients. *AJR* 1990; 154:983–987.

86. Remy-Jardin M, Remy J, Gosselin B, Becette V, Edme JL. Lung parenchymal changes secondary to cigarette smoking: pathologic-CT correlations. *Radiology* 1993;186:643–651.

87. Gruden JF, Webb WR. CT findings in a proved case of respiratory bronchiolitis. *AJR* 1993;161:44–46.

88. Leung AN, Miller RR, Müller NL. Parenchymal opacification in chronic infiltrative lung diseases: CT-pathologic correlation. *Radiology* 1993;188:209–214.

89. Tuddenham WJ. Glossary of terms for thoracic radiology: recommendations of the Nomenclature Committee of the Fleischner Society. *AJR* 1984;143:509–517.

90. Weir IH, Müller NL, Chiles C, Godwin JD, Lee SH, Kullnig P. Wegener's granulomatosis: findings from computed tomography of the chest in 10 patients. *Can Assoc Radiol J* 1992;43:31–34.

91. Padley SPG, Adler BD, Staples CA, Miller RR, Müller NL. Pulmonary talcosis: CT findings in three cases. *Radiology* 1993;186:125–127.

92. Doyle TC, Lawler GA. CT features of rounded atelectasis of the lung. *AJR* 1984;143:225–228.

93. Ren H, Hruban RH, Kuhlman JE, et al. Computed tomography of rounded atelectasis. *J Comput Assist Tomogr* 1988;12:1031–1034.

94. McHugh K, Blaquiere RM. CT features of rounded atelectasis. *AJR* 1989;153:257–260.

95. Müller NL, Staples CA, Miller RR, Vedal S, Thurlbeck WM, Ostrow DN. Disease activity in idiopathic pulmonary fibrosis: CT and pathologic correlation. *Radiology* 1987;165:731–734.

96. Engeler CE, Tashjian JH, Trenkner SW, Walsh JW. Ground-glass opacity of the lung parenchyma: a guide to analysis with high-resolution CT. *AJR* 1993;160:249–251.

97. Remy-Jardin M, Remy J, Giraud F, Wattinne L, Gosselin B. Computed tomography assessment of ground-glass opacity: semiology and significance. *J Thorac Imaging* 1993;8:249–264.

98. Wells AU, Hansell DM, Corrin B, et al. High resolution computed tomography as a predictor of lung histology in systemic sclerosis. *Thorax* 1992;47:508–512.

99. Wells AU, Hansell DM, Rubens MB, Cullinan P, Black CM, du Bois RM. The predictive value of appearances of thin-section computed tomography in fibrosing alveolitis. *Am Rev Respir Dis* 1993;148:1076–1082.

100. Wells AU, Rubens MB, du Bois RM, Hansell DM. Serial CT in fibrosing alveolitis: prognostic significance of the initial pattern. *AJR* 1993;161:1159–1165.

101. Remy-Jardin M, Giraud F, Remy J, Copin MC, Gosselin B, Duhamel A. Importance of ground-glass attenuation in chronic diffuse infiltrative lung disease: pathologic-CT correlation. *Radiology* 1993;189:693–698.

102. Remy-Jardin M, Remy J, Wallaert B, Bataille D, Hatron PY. Pulmonary involvement in progressive systemic sclerosis: sequential evaluation with CT, pulmonary function tests, and bronchoalveolar lavage. *Radiology* 1993;188:499–506.

103. Hartman TE, Primack SL, Swensen SJ, Hansell D, McGuinness G, Müller NL. Desquamative interstitial pneumonia: thin-section CT findings in 22 patients. *Radiology* 1993;187:787–790.

104. Murdoch J, Müller NL. Pulmonary sarcoidosis: changes on follow-up CT examinations. *AJR* 1992;159:473–477.

105. Bergin CJ, Wirth RL, Berry GJ, Castellino RA. Pneumocystis carinii pneumonia: CT and HRCT observations. *J Comput Assist Tomogr* 1990;14:756–759.

106. Moskovic E, Miller R, Pearson M. High resolution computed tomography of Pneumocystis carinii pneumonia in AIDS. *Clin Radiol* 1990;42:239–243.

107. Graham NJ, Müller NL, Miller RR, Shepherd JD. Intrathoracic complications following allogeneic bone marrow transplantation: CT findings. *Radiology* 1991;181:153–156.

108. Hommeyer SH, Godwin JD, Takasugi JE. Computed tomography of air-space disease. *Radiol Clin North Am* 1991;29:1065–1084.

109. Primack SL, Hartman TE, Ikezoe J, Akira M, Sakatani M, Müller NL. Acute interstitial pneumonia: radiographic and CT findings in nine patients. *Radiology* 1993;188:817–820.

110. Holt RM, Schmidt RA, Godwin JD, Raghu G. High resolution CT in respiratory bronchiolitis-associated interstitial lung disease. *J Comput Assist Tomogr* 1993;17:46–50.

111. Ikezoe J, Takashima S, Morimoto S, et al. CT appearance of acute radiation-induced injury in the lung. *AJR* 1988;150:765–770.

112. Ikezoe J, Morimoto S, Takashima S, Takeuchi N, Arisawa J, Kozuka T. Acute radiation-induced pulmonary injury: computed tomographic evaluation. *Semin Ultrasound CT MR* 1990;11:409–416.

113. Nishimura K, Itoh H. High-resolution computed tomographic features of bronchiolitis obliterans organizing pneumonia. *Chest* 1992;102:26S-31S.

114. Müller NL, Miller RR. Ground-glass attenuation, nodules, alveolitis, and sarcoid granulomas. *Radiology* 1993;189:31–32.

115. Lee JS, Im JG, Ahn JM, Kim YM, Han MC. Fibrosing alveolitis: prognostic implication of ground-glass attenuation at high-resolution CT. *Radiology* 1992;184:415–454.

116. Akira M, Sakatani M, Ueda E. Idiopathic pulmonary fibrosis: progression of honeycombing at thin-section CT. *Radiology* 1993;189:687–691.

117. Terriff BA, Kwan SY, Chan-Yeung MM, Müller NL. Fibrosing alveolitis: chest radiography and CT as predictors of clinical and functional impairment at follow-up in 26 patients. *Radiology* 1992;184:445–449.

118. Mayo JR, Müller NL, Road J, Sisler J, Lillington G. Chronic eosinophilic pneumonia: CT findings in six cases. *AJR* 1989;153:727–730.

119. Bourgouin P, Cousineau G, Lemire P, Delvecchio P, Hebert G. Differentiation of radiation-induced fibrosis from recurrent pulmonary neoplasm by CT. *Can Assoc Radiol J* 1987;38:23–26.

120. Libshitz HI, Shuman LS. Radiation-induced pulmonary change: CT findings. *J Comput Assist Tomogr* 1984;8:15–19.

121. Kuhlman JE. The role of chest computed tomography in the diagnosis of drug-related reactions. *J Thorac Imaging* 1991;6(1):52–61.

122. Hamrick-Turner J, Abbitt PL, Harrison RB, Cranston PE. Diffuse lung calcification following fat emboli and adult respiratory distress syndromes: CT findings. *J Thorac Imaging* 1994;9:47–50.

123. Gevenois PA, Abehsera M, Knoop C, Jacobovitz D, Estenne M. Disseminated pulmonary ossification in end-stage pulmonary fibrosis: CT demonstration. *AJR* 1994;162:1303–1304.

124. Kuhlman JE, Ren H, Hutchins GM, Fishman EK. Fulminant pulmonary calcification complicating renal transplantation: CT demonstration. *Radiology* 1989;173:459–460.

125. Johkoh T, Ikezoe J, Nagareda T, Kohno N, Takeuchi N, Kozuka T. Metastatic pulmonary calcification: early detection by high-resolution CT. *J Comput Assist Tomogr* 1993;17:471–473.

126. Hartman TE, Müller NL, Primack SL, Johkoh T, Takeuchi N, Ikezoe J, Swensen SJ. Metastatic pulmonary calcification in patients with hypercalcemia: findings on chest radiographs and CT scans. *AJR* 1994;162:799–802.

127. Cluzel P, Grenier P, Bernadac P, Laurent F, Picard JD. Pulmonary alveolar microlithiasis: CT findings. *J Comput Assist Tomogr* 1991;15:938–942.

128. Korn MA, Schurawitzki H, Klepetko W, Burghuber OC. Pulmonary alveolar microlithiasis: findings on high-resolution CT. *AJR* 1992;158:981–982.

129. Kuhlman JE, Teigen C, Ren H, Hurban RH, Hutchins GM, Fishman EK. Amiodarone pulmonary toxicity: CT findings in symptomatic patients. *Radiology* 1990;177:121–125.

130. Naidich DP. High-resolution computed tomography of cystic lung disease. *Semin Roentgenol* 1991;26:151–174.

131. Hogg JC. Benjamin Felson lecture. Chronic interstitial lung disease of unknown cause: a new classification based on pathogenesis. *AJR* 1991;156:225–233.

132. Aquino SL, Webb WR, Zaloudek CJ, Stern EJ. Lung cysts associated with honeycombing: change in size on expiratory CT scans. *AJR* 1994;162:583–584.

133. Lenoir S, Grenier P, Brauner MW, et al. Pulmonary lymphangiomyomatosis and tuberous sclerosis: comparison of radiographic and thin-section CT findings. *Radiology* 1990;175:329–334.

134. Templeton PA, McLoud TC, Müller NL, Shepard JA, Moore EH. Pulmonary lymphangioleiomyomatosis: CT and pathologic findings. *J Comput Assist Tomogr* 1989;13:54–57.

135. Sherrier RH, Chiles C, Roggli V. Pulmonary lymphangioleiomyomatosis: CT findings. *AJR* 1989;153:937–940.
136. Rappaport DC, Weisbrod GL, Herman SJ, Chamberlain DW. Pulmonary lymphangioleiomyomatosis: high-resolution CT findings in four cases. *AJR* 1989;152:961–964.
137. Müller NL, Chiles C, Kullnig P. Pulmonary lymphangiomyomatosis: correlation of CT with radiographic and functional findings. *Radiology* 1990;175:335–339.
138. Sanders C, Nath PH, Bailey WC. Detection of emphysema with computed tomography: correlation with pulmonary function tests and chest radiography. *Invest Radiol* 1988;23:262–266.
139. Müller NL, Staples CA, Miller RR, Abboud RT. "Density mask": an objective method to quantitate emphysema using computed tomography. *Chest* 1988;94:782–787.
140. Miller RR, Müller NL, Vedal S, Morrison NJ, Staples CA. Limitations of computed tomography in the assessment of emphysema. *Am Rev Respir Dis* 1989;139:980–983.
141. Kinsella N, Müller NL, Vedal S, Staples C, Abboud RT, Chan-Yeung M. Emphysema in silicosis: a comparison of smokers with nonsmokers using pulmonary function testing and computed tomography. *Am Rev Respir Dis* 1990;141:1497–1500.
142. Stern EJ, Webb WR, Weinacker A, Müller NL. Idiopathic giant bullous emphysema (vanishing lung syndrome): imaging findings in nine patients. *AJR* 1994;162:279–282.
143. Feuerstein I, Archer A, Pluda JM, et al. Thin-walled cavities, cysts, and pneumothorax in Pneumocystis carinii pneumonia: further observations with histopathologic correlation. *Radiology* 1990;174:697–702.
144. Panicek DM. Editorial. Cystic pulmonary lesions in patients with AIDS. *Radiology* 1989;173:12–14.
145. Gurney JW, Bates FT. Pulmonary cystic disease: comparison of Pneumocystis carinii pneumatoceles and bullous emphysema due to intravenous drug abuse. *Radiology* 1989;173:27–31.
146. Grenier P, Cordeau MP, Beigelman C. High-resolution computed tomography of the airways. *J Thorac Imaging* 1993;8:213–229.
147. Marti-Bonmati L, Ruiz PF, Catala F, Mata JM, Calonge E. CT findings in Swyer-James syndrome. *Radiology* 1989;172:477–480.
148. Webb WR. High-resolution computed tomography of obstructive lung disease. *Radiol Clin North Am* 1994;32:745–757.
149. Martin KW, Sagel SS, Siegel BA. Mosaic oligemia simulating pulmonary infiltrates on CT. *AJR* 1986;147:670–673.
150. King MA, Bergin CJ, Yeung DWC, et al. Chronic pulmonary thromboembolism: detection of regional hypoperfusion with CT. *Radiology* 1994;191:359–363.
151. Schwickert HC, Schweden F, Schild HH, et al. Pulmonary arteries and lung parenchyma in chronic pulmonary embolism: preoperative and postoperative CT findings. *Radiology* 1994;191:351–357.
152. Knudson RJ, Standen JR, Kaltenborn WT, et al. Expiratory computed tomography for assessment of suspected pulmonary emphysema. *Chest* 1991;99:1357–1366.
153. Moore ADA, Godwin JD, Dietrich PA, Verschakelen JA, Henderson WR. Swyer-James syndrome: CT findings in eight patients. *AJR* 1992;158:1211–1215.
154. Stern EJ, Webb WR, Warnock ML, Salmon CJ. Bronchopulmonary sequestration: dynamic, ultrafast, high-resolution CT evidence of air trapping. *AJR* 1991;157:947–949.
155. Stern EJ, Webb WR, Golden JA, Gamsu G. Cystic lung disease associated with eosinophilic granuloma and tuberous sclerosis: air trapping at dynamic ultrafast high-resolution CT. *Radiology* 1992;182:325–329.
156. Stern EJ, Webb WR, Gamsu G. Dynamic quantitative computed tomography: a predictor of pulmonary function in obstructive lung diseases. *Invest Radiol* 1994;29:564–569.
157. Stern EJ, Webb WR. Dynamic imaging of lung morphology with ultrafast high-resolution computed tomography. *J Thorac Imaging* 1993;8:273–282.
158. Webb WR, Stern EJ, Kanth N, Gamsu G. Dynamic pulmonary CT: findings in normal adult men. *Radiology* 1993;186:117–124.
159. Menkes HA, Traystman RJ. State of the art: collateral ventilation. *Am Rev Respir Dis* 1977;116:287–309.
160. Gurney JW. Cross-sectional physiology of the lung. *Radiology* 1991;178:1–10.
161. Grenier P, Chevret S, Beigelman C, Brauner MW, Chastang C, Valeyre D. Chronic diffuse infiltrative lung disease: determination of the diagnostic value of clinical data, chest radiography, and CT with Bayesian analysis. *Radiology* 1994;1994:383–390.
162. Gurney JW, Schroeder BA. Upper lobe disease: physiological correlates. *Radiology* 1988;167:359–366.
163. Staples CA. Computed tomography in the evaluation of benign asbestos-related disorders. *Radiol Clin North Am* 1992;30:1191–1207.
164. Hartman TE, Swensen SJ, Williams DE. Mycobacterium avium-intracellulare complex: evaluation with CT. *Radiology* 1993;187:23–26.
165. Remy-Jardin M, Remy J, Boulenguez C, Sobaszek A, Edme JL, Furon D. Morphologic effects of cigarette smoking on airways and pulmonary parenchyma in healthy adult volunteers: CT evaluation and correlation with pulmonary function tests. *Radiology* 1993;186:107–115.
166. Gruden JF, Webb WR, Sides DM. Adult-onset disseminated tracheobronchial papillomatosis: CT features. *J Comput Assist Tomogr* 1994;18:640–642.

FOUR

Diseases Characterized Primarily by Linear and Reticular Opacities

The first group of diseases we will discuss are those primarily characterized by the presence of fibrosis and linear or reticular abnormalities on HRCT. These notably include the chronic interstitial pneumonias (UIP and DIP), idiopathic pulmonary fibrosis (IPF), collagen-vascular diseases, and asbestosis. Also reviewed in this chapter are drug-induced lung diseases, and radiation fibrosis. It should be recognized, however, that many of the other lung diseases discussed in this book result in pulmonary fibrosis and may produce similar HRCT abnormalities; the differential diagnosis of reticular abnormalities should not be limited to the diseases reviewed in this chapter.

Although the diseases discussed in this chapter are primarily reticular, they commonly show other HRCT findings as well. In this, and in the following three chapters, lung diseases have been classified according to their most common and most diagnostic appearances. In the discussion of individual diseases, however, the entire spectrum of abnormalities seen with each will be reviewed.

CHRONIC INTERSTITIAL PNEUMONIAS AND IDIOPATHIC PULMONARY FIBROSIS

During the 1960s, Liebow classified the chronic interstitial pneumonias into five types, based on their differences in histologic appearance. These five were usual interstitial pneumonia (UIP), desquamative interstitial pneumonia (DIP), lymphocytic interstitial pneumonia (LIP), giant-cell interstitial pneumonia (GIP), and bronchiolitis with interstitial pneumonia (BIP) (1). With the exception of BIP, these terms have become widely accepted.

It should be clearly understood that the interstitial pneumonias do not represent "diseases" per se; rather, they represent fundamental responses of the lung to injury or the presence of a pathologic condition. Each of the interstitial pneumonias can be produced by a number of different disease entities, and conversely, more than one type of interstitial pneumonia can be seen in a single patient, or a single lung.

Although we do not plan to discuss Liebow's interstitial pneumonias in great detail, but prefer to describe the appearances of specific diseases, we will briefly review the two that are most common—UIP and DIP. These two terms are commonly used by lung pathologists in the interpretation of lung biopsy specimens, and thus, a basic understanding of their HRCT characteristics is desirable.

The remaining three types of interstitial pneumonia will be reviewed only briefly. Lymphocytic interstitial pneumonia is uncommon, being seen mainly in patients with dysproteinemia, autoimmune disease, particularly Sjögren's syndrome, and more recently, in patients with AIDS (2–5). Many cases initially classified as LIP are now considered to be lymphomas (6) and Spencer considers LIP a "pre-lymphomatous" condition (7), except in patients with AIDS. LIP results in the presence of mature lymphocytic and plasma cell infiltrates in relation to lymphatics, and in particular, in association with the peribronchovascular interstitium, interlobular septa, subpleural interstitium, and in the centrilobular regions. Fibrosis is uncommon. Symptoms are nonspecific and often those of the patient's underlying disease; cough and dyspnea are the most frequent respiratory complaints. Chest radiographs are nonspecific, showing reticular or nodular opacities, or consolidation, often with a lower lobe predominance.

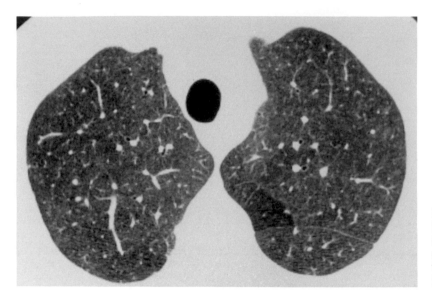

FIG. 4-1. Lymphocytic interstitial pneumonia (LIP) in a 75-year-old man with AIDS. HRCT demonstrates extensive bilateral areas of ground-glass opacity and small, poorly defined nodules, some of which appear centrilobular.

On HRCT, patchy ground-glass attenuation or ill-defined centrilobular nodules can be seen (Figs. 3-57, 4-1).

Giant-cell interstitial pneumonia is very rare and found almost exclusively in workers exposed to hard-metal, an alloy of tungsten carbide and cobalt (8). It therefore should be considered a form of pneumoconiosis. The term BIP has been replaced by the expressions *bronchiolitis obliterans organizing pneumonia (BOOP) or cryptogenic organizing pneumonia (COP)*, as the abnormality is not purely interstitial but mainly air-space (6). BOOP/COP has often been confused with UIP, but has distinct radiologic and pathologic features (9–12); BOOP/COP will be discussed in a subsequent chapter.

Usual Interstitial Pneumonia (UIP) and Desquamative Interstitial Pneumonia (DIP)

It should be emphasized that although UIP and DIP have distinct pathologic and histologic appearances (Figs. 4-2, 4-3), they are not distinct disease processes, but probably represent different phases, stages, or degrees of abnormality caused by the same lung injury or disease state (6,13,14). UIP and DIP can be seen simultaneously in the same patient with lung disease.

Usual interstitial pneumonia, as the name implies, is the most common type of chronic interstitial pneumonia (1,6). In its early stages, UIP is characterized histologically by alveolitis and increased cellularity of the alveolar wall. As this process progresses, fibrosis and honeycombing develop (Fig. 4-2). Clinically, the term UIP is often used synonymously with idiopathic pulmonary fibrosis (or cryptogenic fibrosing alveolitis as it is called in the United Kingdom), but identical

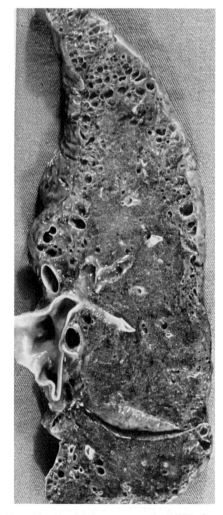

FIG. 4-2. Usual interstitial pneumonia (UIP). Gross pathologic specimen of a patient with IPF and UIP, which has been cut in the transverse plane. Fibrosis and honeycombing, which almost exclusively involve the lung periphery, are typical.

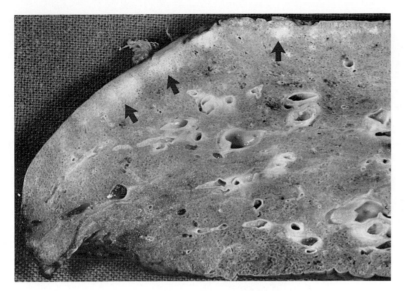

FIG. 4-3. Desquamative interstitial pneumonia (DIP). A gross pathologic specimen of a patient with DIP cut in the transverse plane, shows foci of air-space consolidation in the subpleural lung regions (*arrows*). The remaining lung is normal. Such a peripheral distribution of abnormalities is present in some but not all patients with DIP.

findings of UIP can be seen in patients with other diseases, particularly those with collagen-vascular diseases such as rheumatoid arthritis and scleroderma or certain drug reactions. In this book, we will use the term UIP only to refer to the histologic abnormality described by Liebow; we will use the term idiopathic pulmonary fibrosis (IPF) to describe the syndrome or disease that so commonly results in this histological finding.

Desquamative interstitial pneumonia was initially described as being characteristically associated with mild symptoms, mild fibrosis, and a large number of cells in the alveolar airspaces (Fig. 4-3) (15). These cells were originally thought to be type II pneumocytes, desquamated into the alveolar spaces from the alveolar walls, but this has since been shown to be incorrect. Most of the intra-alveolar cells present in DIP represent macrophages rather than type II alveolar cells (16).

The differences between the clinical and pathologic features of UIP and DIP have been emphasized by Carrington et al. (17) and others (16). Most significant is the fact that DIP has a much better prognosis than UIP. When corrected for normal life expectancy, the 5-year mortality for DIP in the study by Carrington et al. (17), was 4.8% compared to 44.6% for UIP, and 61% of patients with DIP responded to treatment as compared to only 11% of patients with UIP.

In one report (15), it was concluded that patients with DIP were more likely to show ground-glass opacities on chest radiographs, particularly at the lung bases and costophrenic angles, than were patients with UIP. However, in the study by Carrington et al. (17), there was no qualitative difference between the radiographic findings in patients with DIP and UIP, but the radiographic abnormalities associated with DIP were considered to be of a milder degree (17). In 3% to 22% of patients with DIP, chest radiographs are normal despite the presence of extensive parenchymal disease (16–18).

HRCT Findings

The HRCT appearances of UIP have been described in a number of studies of patients with biopsy proven UIP, IPF, or collagen-vascular disease (19–23); the HRCT appearances of UIP associated with these diseases are described in detail below. On HRCT, UIP is characterized by a predominance of reticular opacities, which correspond to areas of irregular fibrosis, lung destruction, honeycombing, and traction bronchiectasis; these findings are visible in virtually all patients with UIP, and frequently show a peripheral, subpleural, and basal predominance (Figs. 4-4–4-10) (19–23). Ground-glass attenuation is seen in less than half of patients with UIP, usually related to the presence of alveolitis, alveolar wall thickening, or early fibrosis (Figs. 4-11–4-13).

Descriptions of the HRCT abnormalities associated with DIP have been limited to a few reports (16,24–26). Although the spectrum of abnormalities visible in DIP is similar to that seen in UIP, ground-glass opacities rather than reticular opacities predominate; areas of ground-glass opacity are seen in nearly all patients with DIP, and reflect the presence of intra-alveolar macrophages and interstitial inflammation (Figs. 4-14–4-16) (16). Irregular reticulation suggestive of fibrosis has been described in 50% of cases of DIP, with honeycombing present in 30% (16). However, in comparison to patients with UIP, findings of fibrosis are limited in extent and relatively mild (16).

Text continues on page 118.

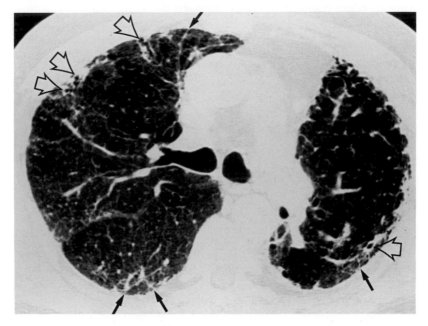

FIG. 4-4. Reticular opacities in a 69-year-old man with mild idiopathic pulmonary fibrosis. HRCT at the level of the right upper-lobe bronchus demonstrates irregular reticular opacities bilaterally in the subpleural lung regions. In several areas, irregular septal thickening (*small arrows*) and traction bronchiolectasis (*open arrows*) are visible. Irregular interfaces are present along the mediastinal and costal lung surfaces.

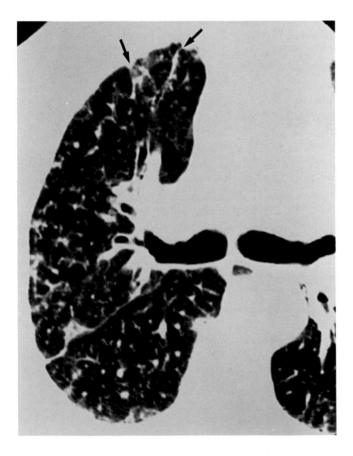

FIG. 4-5. Reticular opacities in a 58-year-old woman with IPF. HRCT targeted to right upper lobe. Reticular opacities are slightly more prominent in the subpleural regions. Irregular septal thickening (*small arrows*) is visible in several locations.

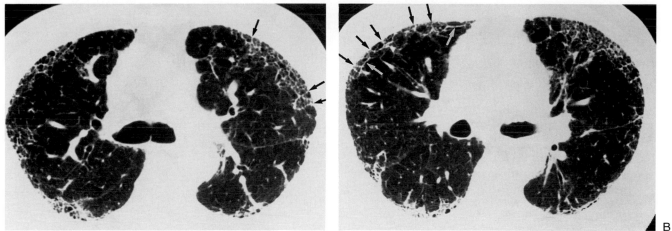

FIG. 4-6. Reticular opacities in a patient with IPF. Scans at two levels (**A,B**), show a peripheral predominance of abnormalities indicative of fibrosis, including irregular interlobular septal thickening (*black arrows*) and subpleural lines (*white arrows*). However, the predominant pattern is that of intralobular interstitial thickening with areas of honeycombing.

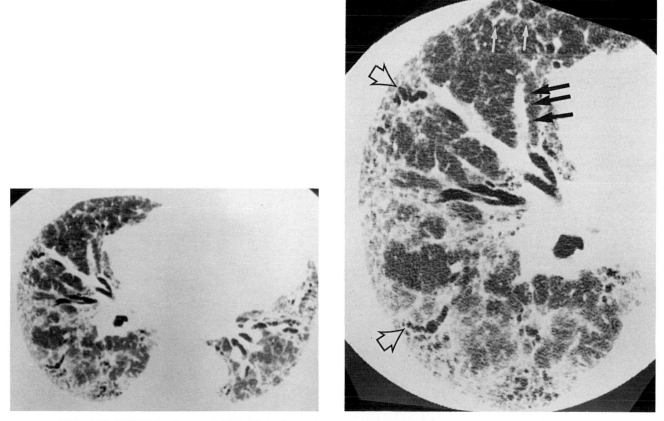

FIG. 4-7. HRCT findings of IPF; fibrosis and a peripheral, subpleural predominance. **A:** A 1.5-mm collimation scan using the standard reconstruction algorithm demonstrates a patchy distribution of reticular opacities in the peripheral aspects of both lungs. **B:** The distinction between normal and abnormal lung parenchyma is more readily made on this image targeted to the right lung and reconstructed using the bone algorithm; the patchy distribution of abnormalities is clearly seen. The fine reticular pattern visible largely reflects intralobular interstitial thickening, but irregular septal thickening (*white arrows*) is visible anteriorly, in areas that are less abnormal. Irregular interfaces (*black arrows*) are visible throughout the lung, at the margins of vessels and bronchi. Traction bronchiectasis and bronchiolectasis are seen within the peripheral lung regions (*open arrows*). Ground-glass opacities are visible in the right lower lobe. (From Müller, ref. 27, with permission.)

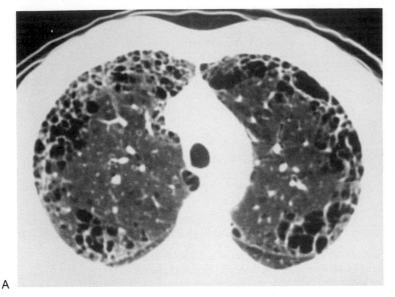

A

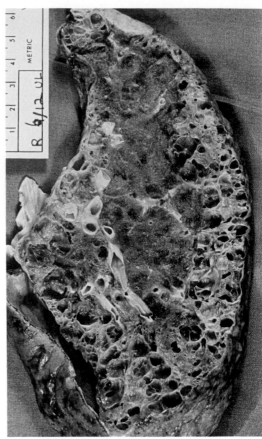

B

FIG. 4-8. Peripheral honeycombing in a 60-year-old patient with IPF. **A:** A 1.5-mm collimation scan (reconstructed with the standard algorithm) at the level of the aortic arch shows honeycombing, which is almost exclusively in the subpleural lung regions. **B:** The macroscopic pathologic specimen of the right upper lobe, cut in the same plane and at the same level as the HRCT, mirrors the appearance of the HRCT image. Honeycomb cysts measuring 2 to 10 mm in diameter are present in the subpleural lung regions; the remaining parenchyma is normal. (From Müller, ref. 21, with permission.)

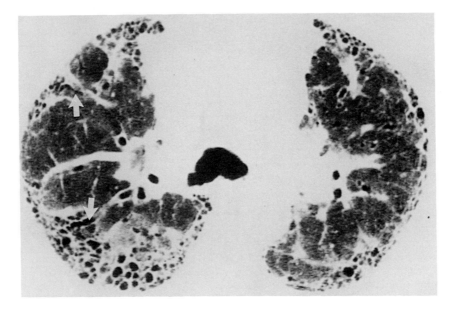

FIG. 4-9. End-stage idiopathic pulmonary fibrosis. Typical honeycomb cysts are present mainly in the subpleural lung regions. Also noted is traction bronchiectasis (*arrows*).

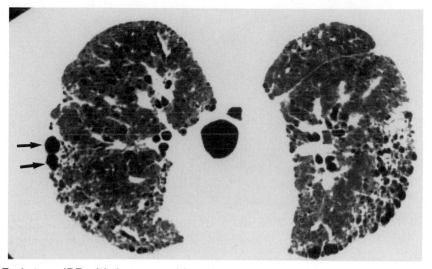

FIG. 4-10. End-stage IPF with honeycombing. A prone scan shows subpleural cysts typical of honeycombing. Some cysts (*arrows*) can be large. Honeycomb cysts typically share walls on HRCT and usually occur in several layers in the subpleural lung.

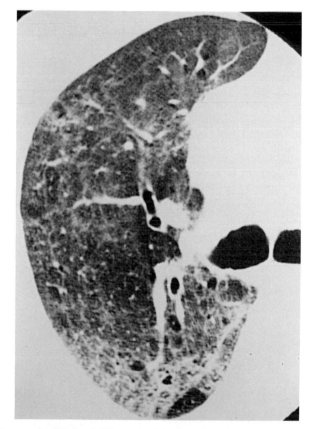

FIG. 4-11. Ground-glass opacity in a 65-year-old man with IPF. HRCT at the level of the right upper lobe shows a ground-glass increase in lung opacity involving most of the right lung. This ground-glass pattern reflects the presence of active disease. Reticular abnormalities indicating fibrosis are few, but some septal thickening is visible.

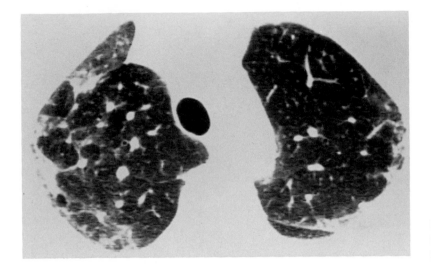

FIG. 4-12. Active IPF in a 63-year-old woman. HRCT shows ground-glass opacities in the sub-pleural lung regions, particularly on the right.

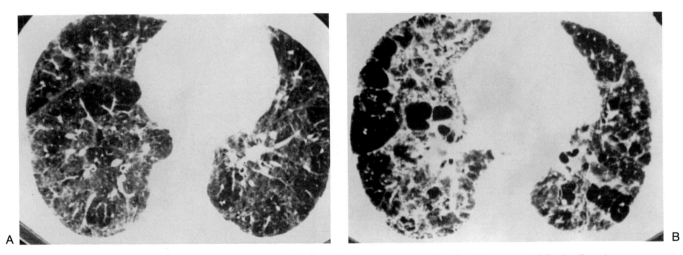

A   B

FIG. 4-13. Ground-glass opacity progressing to fibrosis in patient with active IPF. **A:** Patchy ground-glass opacity is present bilaterally. There is a mild increase in interstitial opacities. The patient refused treatment. **B:** A repeat HRCT, near the same level, 1 year later shows findings of fibrosis.

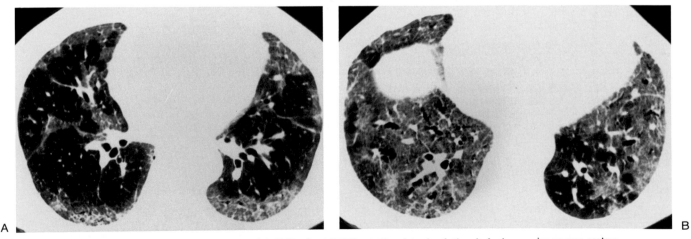

A   B

FIG. 4-14. A 71-year-old man with DIP. **A:** HRCT at the level of the inferior pulmonary veins demonstrates bilateral areas of ground-glass opacity involving mainly the subpleural lung regions. **B:** HRCT through the lung bases demonstrates more extensive bilateral involvement. There is a mild increase in reticulation.

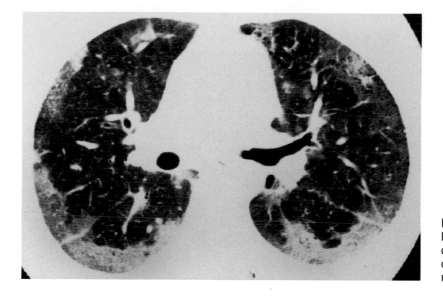

FIG. 4-15. A 45-year-old woman with DIP. HRCT at the level of the bronchus intermedius demonstrates bilateral areas of ground-glass opacity predominantly involving the subpleural lung regions.

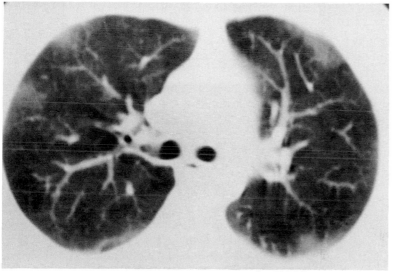

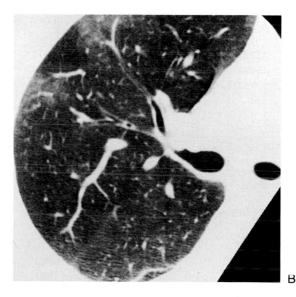

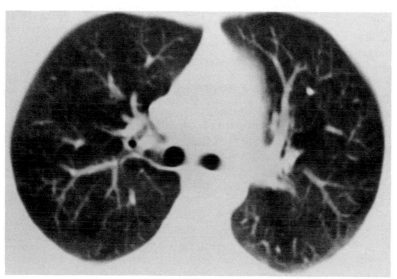

FIG. 4-16. Ground-glass opacities in a 36-year-old man with DIP. **A:** A 10-mm collimation scan shows patchy areas of ground-glass opacity in the subpleural lung regions. **B:** HRCT scan shows sharp demarcation between normal and abnormal areas of lung parenchyma. **C:** A 10-mm collimation CT scan obtained 3 months after initiation of steroid therapy. Areas represented by ground-glass opacity have resolved. (From Müller, ref. 27, with permission.)

The distribution of abnormalities seen on HRCT in patients with DIP is quite similar to that seen with UIP, being predominantly peripheral, subpleural, and lower lobe (Figs. 4-14–4-16) (16). This is not surprising, considering the hypothesis that DIP and UIP represent different stages or manifestations of the same disease process. The ground-glass opacity may be patchy or diffuse in distribution, but tends to predominantly involve the lower lung zones. In the study by Hartman et al. (16), all patients with DIP had ground-glass opacity involving mid and lower-lung zones, while 82% also had upper lobe opacities; 73% of these patients were felt to have a lower lobe predominance of abnormalities. In approximately 60% of patients with DIP, the areas of ground-glass opacity mainly involve the subpleural lung regions. In cases of DIP, areas of ground-glass opacity may improve or resolve completely following treatment with corticosteroids (27). The appearance of DIP is discussed further in Chapter 6.

Idiopathic Pulmonary Fibrosis

Idiopathic pulmonary fibrosis (IPF), or cryptogenic fibrosing alveolitis, occurs most commonly in patients between 40 and 60 years of age, although it has also been described in children and in the elderly (13,14,17,28). Patients with IPF typically present with progressive shortness of breath and a dry cough. On physical examination finger clubbing is seen in 25% to 50% of cases, and on auscultation, late inspiratory crackles (so-called Velcro rales) are characteristic. Pulmonary function tests show a restrictive pattern with reduced lung volumes and impairment in gas exchange (17,28). Idiopathic pulmonary fibrosis has a poor prognosis, with a mean survival of 4 years from the onset of symptoms (range 0.4 to 20 years) (29).

Pathologically, the vast majority of patients with IPF show typical histologic findings of usual interstitial pneumonia (UIP) and/or desquamative interstitial pneumonia (DIP). The earliest histologic abnormality in IPF is alveolitis with increased cellularity of the alveolar walls (6,13). This inflammatory process can lead to progressive fibrosis (14). Alveolar wall inflammation and intra-alveolar macrophages in IPF indicate disease activity and are potentially reversible (30,31). Fibrosis and honeycombing are considered to be irreversible.

A wide spectrum of histologic abnormalities can be seen in different patients with IPF (14). Thus the findings shown in individual cases range from those typical of alveolitis, with many intra-alveolar mononuclear cells and little fibrosis (which would be called DIP), to those of extensive fibrosis with relatively few intra-alveolar cells (which would be called UIP) (14). All patients with IPF have mononuclear cells in their alveoli, but the relative number of these cells varies con-

siderably among different patients and often varies considerably in different areas of the same open lung biopsy specimen. Since findings of both UIP and DIP are often seen in the same patient, it is probable that DIP represents the early stage of the disease process, whereas UIP represents the late stage (6,13,14).

One of the most characteristic features of IPF is its patchy distribution within the lung parenchyma. Areas of normal lung, active inflammation or alveolitis, and end-stage fibrosis are often present within the same open lung biopsy specimen (6,13).

The plain chest radiographic findings of IPF consist initially of ill-defined or ground-glass opacity, presumably due to alveolitis (6,32). As fibrosis develops, a fine reticular pattern appears, which may be diffuse, but is often first seen and is more severe in the lower-lung zones. As fibrosis progresses, the reticular pattern becomes coarser, and there is progressive loss of lung volume. In the end stage there is diffuse honeycombing. It is well known, however, that the plain radiographic pattern of IPF is nonspecific, being similar to that seen in many other interstitial diseases. Further, it has been repeatedly demonstrated that the severity of interstitial disease assessed on the chest radiograph correlates poorly with the clinical and functional impairment (13,22,33). Patients may have severe dyspnea and a normal chest radiograph, or they may have extensive changes on the radiograph and minimal symptomatology.

CT and HRCT Findings

On HRCT, IPF is characterized by the presence of reticular opacities, which correspond to areas of irregular fibrosis (Figs. 4-4,4-5) and reflect the typical pathologic features of UIP (Table 4-1) (13,21,22,27, 34,35). The predominant HRCT features of IPF include intralobular interstitial thickening and honeycombing; irregular interlobular septal thickening and ground-glass opacity may also be present but are usually less conspicuous findings.

TABLE 4-1. *HRCT findings in idiopathic pulmonary fibrosis*[a,b]

1. **Findings of Fibrosis**
   Intralobular Interstitial Thickening, Irregular Interfaces, Visible Intralobular Bronchioles, Honeycombing, Traction Bronchiectasis
2. Irregular Interlobular Septal Thickening
3. **Ground-glass Opacity**
4. *Peripheral and Subpleural Predominance of Abnormalities*
5. *Lower Lung Zone and Posterior Predominance*

[a] Most common findings in boldface.
[b] Findings most helpful in differential diagnosis in boldface italics.

Intralobular interstitial thickening is often visible on HRCT in patients with IPF (Figs. 4-6,4-7), resulting in a fine reticular pattern which frequently predominates in patients with this disease (36). Nishimura et al. (23) reported the presence of a fine reticulation or ill-defined increased lung attenuation in 96% of cases, associated with visibility of centrilobular bronchioles. Thickening of the intralobular interstitium also results in the presence of irregular interfaces between the lung and pulmonary vessels, bronchi, and pleural surfaces (Fig. 4-7) (37,38). In areas of severe fibrosis, the segmental and subsegmental bronchi become dilated and tortuous, a finding referred to as traction bronchiectasis (Fig. 4-7) (39). Subpleural lines can also be seen, usually indicating fibrosis (Fig. 4-6).

In many cases of IPF, findings of honeycombing predominate (21,36). In such cases, there is gross distortion of lung architecture, and individual lobules are no longer visible (Figs. 4-8–4-10). Honeycomb cysts usually range from 2 to 20 mm in diameter, but can be larger (Figs. 4-8–4-10) (21,36,40). They typically appear to share walls on HRCT and usually occur in several layers in the subpleural lung. Honeycomb cysts have been reported on HRCT in 24% to 90% of patients with IPF (22,23), and the frequency of this finding varies with the severity or stage of the disease.

Interlobular septal thickening is sometimes seen on HRCT in patients with IPF, but is a less conspicuous finding than intralobular interstitial thickening or honeycombing (Figs. 4-4–4-6). Usually, in patients who have honeycombing, findings of septal thickening are visible only in less abnormal lung regions. When visible, septal thickening is characteristically irregular in contour (Figs. 4-4–4-6) (36), and septa marginate

pulmonary lobules that can appear irregular in shape or distorted. Abnormal prominence of the centrilobular vessel, which normally appears as a dot- or Y-shaped branching opacity in the lobular core, is often present in patients who show septal thickening, but is not a conspicuous finding in most patients (36). In addition, the centrilobular bronchiole, which is not normally seen, is sometimes visible because of a combination of dilatation, thickening of the peribronchiolar interstitium, and increased opacity of surrounding lung (Figs. 4-4,4-7) (36).

Ground-glass attenuation is often visible on HRCT in patients with IPF. It usually indicates the presence of disease activity and potentially treatable disease (Figs. 4-11–4-13) (25), but can also be seen in the presence of fibrosis or honeycombing below the resolution of HRCT. Ground-glass attenuation should be considered to represent an active process only when there are no associated HRCT findings of fibrosis. Findings of fibrosis in association with ground-glass attenuation, thus suggesting an inactive process, include intralobular interstitial thickening, honeycombing, and traction bronchiectasis and bronchiolectasis (24).

In patients with IPF, ground-glass attenuation may be seen either as a result of the active alveolitis associated with UIP (Figs. 4-11–4-13) or DIP (Figs. 4-14–4-16) (20,25,27,41,42). It should be realized, however, that while patients with DIP typically respond to treatment (Fig. 4-16) and have a good long-term prognosis, patients with UIP have a relatively poor prognosis. The majority of patients with UIP have evidence of extensive fibrosis at presentation and do not respond well to treatment (17,19,43). In untreated patients with IPF, areas of ground-glass opacity frequently can be seen to progress to fibrosis and honeycombing (Fig. 4-13) (20).

Another hallmark of IPF on HRCT is its patchy distribution (Figs. 4-7,4-17). Areas of mild and severe fibrosis, mild and marked inflammatory activity, and normal lung are often present in the same patient, in the same lung, and in the same lobe. Also, and most important diagnostically, is that findings of IPF often predominate in the peripheral, subpleural regions (Figs. 4-2,4-4,4-6–4-8) and in the lung bases (21). Concentric subpleural honeycombing is characteristic of IPF (Figs. 4-2,4-8–4-10). Like the reticular opacities seen in patients with IPF, areas of ground-glass attenuation usually predominate in the subpleural regions.

Clinical Utility of HRCT

Several studies have shown that CT and HRCT are superior to plain chest radiographs in the assessment of patients with IPF. For example, honeycombing is seen in up to 90% of CT studies as compared to 30%

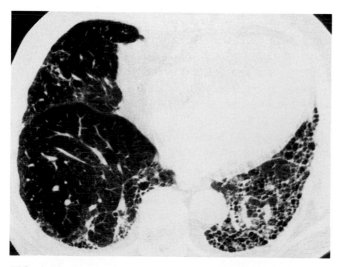

FIG. 4-17. A 73-year-old man with idiopathic pulmonary fibrosis. HRCT through the lung bases shows a patchy distribution of abnormalities, with mild honeycombing in the right lower lobe and extensive honeycombing and marked loss of lung volume in the left lower lobe.

of cases on plain radiographs (22). HRCT findings have been shown to correlate with symptoms and pulmonary function abnormalities in patients with IPF. Staples et al. (22) compared CT with clinical, functional, and radiologic findings in 23 patients with IPF. The CT scans provided a better estimate of the pattern, distribution, and extent of pulmonary fibrosis and showed more extensive honeycombing than did radiographs. In this study, there was also good correlation between the extent of disease, assessed by the percentage of lung showing evidence of fibrosis on CT, and the severity of dyspnea ($r = 0.64$, $p < 0.001$). A significant correlation between the extent of ground-glass opacities seen on CT or HRCT and the severity of dyspnea, and reduction in total lung capacity and carbon monoxide diffusing capacity ($p < 0.01$) has also been found (19).

Both the long-term survival in IPF and its response to treatment with corticosteroids correlate with the histologic findings at biopsy. The best response to steroids is observed in patients with marked disease activity and little fibrosis (30–33). Although open lung biopsy provides the "gold standard" for evaluating patients with IPF, it has limitations. Most importantly, it is invasive and usually assesses only a small part of the lung. Thus, the region sampled may not be representative of the lung as a whole, and the presence of alveolitis or DIP (active disease) may be missed.

Recent studies have demonstrated that HRCT allows a distinction of active, potentially reversible alveolitis from irreversible fibrosis in the majority of patients with IPF, without the need for lung biopsy (20,25,27,41,42). Several investigators now routinely use HRCT to assess disease activity in patients with IPF, with HRCT findings governing treatment. In some patients with IPF, definite diagnoses of end-stage lung (honeycombing without ground-glass opacity) or active alveolitis (ground-glass opacity) can be made on the basis of HRCT findings.

Müller et al. (27) reported 12 patients with IPF in whom disease activity, assessed by CT, was correlated with the open lung biopsy findings. In this study, the CT finding of air-space opacification (ground-glass opacity) was used to diagnose alveolitis and activity. Two independent observers correctly identified the 5 patients with marked-disease activity and 5 out of 7 patients with low-disease activity. In another study, of 14 patients with idiopathic pulmonary fibrosis who showed ground-glass opacity on HRCT, 12 (86%) had inflammation on biopsy which indicated the presence of active disease (25).

Lee et al. (41) correlated the extent of ground-glass opacity at presentation with the improvement in pulmonary function following treatment with corticosteroids in 19 patients with IPF. The extent of ground-glass opacity on CT correlated significantly with the improvement in the forced vital capacity ($r = 0.7$, $p < 0.001$) and in gas transfer as assessed by the carbon monoxide diffusing capacity ($r = 0.67$, $p < 0.002$) after treatment. Wells et al. (42) assessed whether CT could predict response to treatment and prognosis in 76 patients with IPF. The CT abnormalities were categorized as consisting predominantly of ground-glass opacity ($n = 8$), a mixed pattern ($n = 18$), or predominantly a reticular pattern ($n = 50$). Response to treatment was seen in approximately 80% of patients who had ground-glass opacity as the predominant abnormality compared to only 20% of patients with a mixed pattern and 4% of patients with a predominant reticular pattern. Overall the prognosis in the patients was poor with a 50% 4-year survival. All eight patients with predominant ground-glass opacity at presentation were alive after 4 years compared to only 40% of patients with mixed pattern and 20% of patients with a predominant reticular pattern at presentation (42).

Wells et al. (20) also performed serial CT scans in 21 patients with IPF. They demonstrated that improvement with treatment was associated with a decrease in the extent of ground-glass opacity. Deterioration on follow-up was associated with an increase in the extent of ground-glass opacity or an increase in the extent of reticular abnormalities (20). It has also been shown that areas of ground-glass opacity visible on HRCT precede and predict development of a reticular pattern or honeycombing in the same location (19,43) (Fig. 4-13). It should be emphasized, however, that the majority of patients with IPF have a predominantly reticular pattern at presentation; these do not respond to treatment and show little change on follow-up HRCT (19,20,42,43).

These various studies have demonstrated that HRCT can be helpful in predicting potential response to treatment and long-term prognosis in patients with idiopathic pulmonary fibrosis (42). CT is also helpful in determining the optimal site for lung biopsy, if this procedure is considered necessary. As pointed out by Carrington and Gaensler (17), at the time of open lung biopsy, the surgeon must attempt to obtain diagnostic tissue by avoiding areas of extensive honeycombing. This can be difficult in cases of IPF because the most severe honeycombing is typically subpleural in location. An important role for CT in the assessment of patients with IPF is to help the surgeon choose the best area for biopsy. Areas of honeycombing can be avoided and less abnormal areas, or areas of ground-glass attenuation, can be sought. Disease distribution cannot be adequately assessed from the conventional radiographs, but it can be easily determined using CT (44); CT scans may demonstrate areas of abnormal lung that are not apparent on chest radiographs (26).

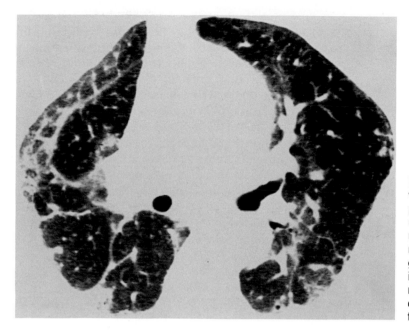

FIG. 4-18. Ground-glass opacity in a 63-year-old woman with mixed connective tissue disease and pulmonary fibrosis. HRCT shows bilateral asymmetric areas of ground-glass opacity and interlobular septal thickening, which have a predominantly subpleural distribution. Areas of ground-glass opacity are characteristic of active alveolitis in UIP. The combination of disease activity and mild fibrosis suggests that the patient has early disease. The appearance is indistinguishable from that of IPF.

Collagen–Vascular Diseases

Each of the collagen-vascular diseases can involve the respiratory system and cause focal or diffuse pulmonary disease; however, the frequency of lung abnormalities varies among the different diseases (6,45). Most collagen-vascular diseases can cause chronic interstitial pneumonia with clinical, radiologic, HRCT, and pathologic features indistinguishable from those of IPF (Figs. 4-18– 4-22) (Table 4-2) (6,13,22,33). Pleural thickening and pleural effusion are also common. The two most common conditions associated with interstitial fibrosis are rheumatoid arthritis and progressive systemic sclerosis (scleroderma).

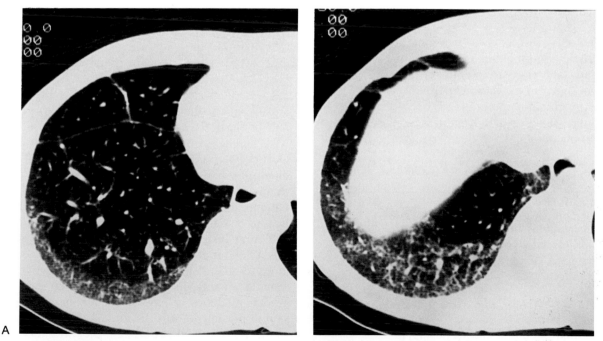

FIG. 4-19. Mixed connective tissue disease with pulmonary fibrosis. **A,B:** HRCT at two levels shows a fine reticular pattern posteriorly, which reflects septal thickening and intralobular interstitial fibrosis. Mild honeycombing is probably present.

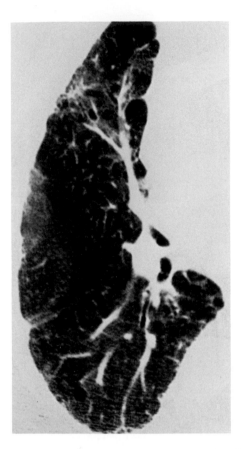

FIG. 4-20. Systemic lupus erythematosus and mild pulmonary fibrosis in a 65-year-old woman. HRCT through the right lung base shows patchy distribution of reticular and ground-glass opacities.

Rheumatoid Arthritis

Rheumatoid arthritis (RA) is commonly associated with thoracic abnormalities (46), including interstitial pneumonitis and fibrosis, pleural effusion or pleural thickening, necrobiotic nodules, BOOP, bronchiectasis, and bronchiolitis obliterans (47).

Pulmonary function abnormalities consistent with interstitial pneumonia have been reported in as many

TABLE 4-2. *HRCT findings in collagen-vascular disease[a,b]*

1. **Findings of Fibrosis**
   Honeycombing, Intralobular Interstitial Thickening, Irregular Interfaces, Traction Bronchiectasis
2. Irregular Interlobular Septal Thickening
3. **Ground-glass Opacity**
4. *Peripheral and Subpleural Predominance of Abnormalities*
5. *Lower and Posterior Lung Zone Predominance*
6. *Pleural Thickening*
7. *Esophageal Dilatation in PSS or MCTD*

[a] Most common findings in boldface.
[b] Findings most helpful in differential diagnosis in boldface italics.

as 40% of patients with RA (48,49), but in more than half of these patients, the chest radiograph is normal (46,49). The prevalence of radiologically detectable interstitial disease in patients with rheumatoid arthritis is probably around 10% (46,48,49). Histologically, radiologically, and on HRCT, the appearance of RA with interstitial fibrosis is usually indistinguishable from that of IPF (Figs. 3-15,3-28,4-18) (46,50–53). Clinical evidence of arthritis precedes the development of pulmonary fibrosis in about 90% of patients, and 90% have a positive serum rheumatoid factor.

HRCT findings reported in patients with rheumatoid arthritis (47) include nodules 3 mm to 3 cm in diameter that are predominantly subpleural in location (22%), bronchial abnormalities and bronchiectasis in the absence of fibrosis (21%), ground-glass opacity (14%), pulmonary fibrosis with or without honeycombing (10%), consolidation (6%), enlarged lymph nodes (9%), and pleural abnormalities (16%). Findings which were more frequent in symptomatic patients included honeycombing, bronchiectasis, nodules, and ground-glass opacity. In patients with rheumatoid arthritis, the presence of ground-glass opacity, consolidation, and fibrosis likely reflect the presence of interstitial pneumonia, while the small and large nodules probably represent necrobiotic (rheumatoid) nodules. Bronchiectasis in RA can be associated with chronic infection, which has an increased incidence in rheumatoid patients, or bronchiolitis obliterans (Fig. 3-91). The occurrence of bronchiolitis obliterans in patients with rheumatoid arthritis is discussed in Chapter 7.

HRCT can be useful in demonstrating lung disease in RA patients with pulmonary function abnormalities who have normal chest radiographs (45,54). Fujii et al. (55) reviewed the chest radiographic and HRCT findings of 91 patients with rheumatoid arthritis. On HRCT, 43 patients had findings of UIP with fibrosis, 5 had findings consistent with bronchiolitis obliterans, and 43 patients had a normal HRCT. In approximately half of these 91 patients, chest radiographic findings were similar to those shown on HRCT. However, 17 (37%) of 46 patients thought to have normal chest radiographs had HRCT abnormalities consistent with rheumatoid lung disease. Furthermore, 14 (33%) of 43 patients thought to have abnormal chest radiographs, had no evidence of significant lung disease on HRCT.

Pleural disease, either pleural effusion or pleural thickening, is common in patients with RA, being seen in up to 40% of patients at autopsy. However, symptomatic pleural disease is less common, and radiographic evidence of pleural thickening or pleural effusion is present in only 5% to 20% of patients (45,46). In the study by Fujii et al. (55), pleural thickening was visible on HRCT in 33% of the 91 patients studied and in 44% of the patients who had HRCT findings of interstitial pneumonia.

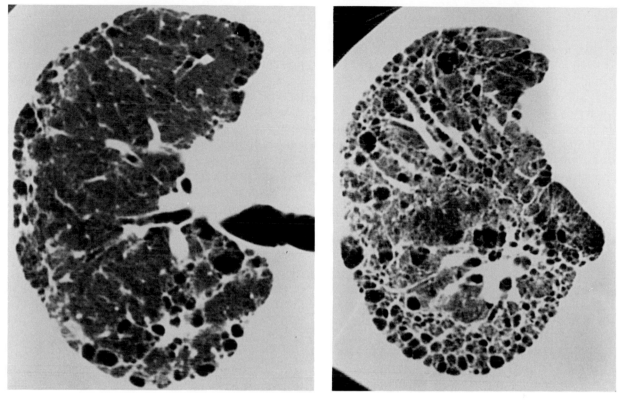

FIG. 4-21. Rheumatoid arthritis and end-stage UIP with honeycombing in a 60-year-old man. **A:** HRCT at the level of the tracheal carina shows subpleural honeycombing and interlobular septal thickening indistinguishable from IPF. **B:** HRCT through the right lung base shows diffuse honeycombing and septal thickening.

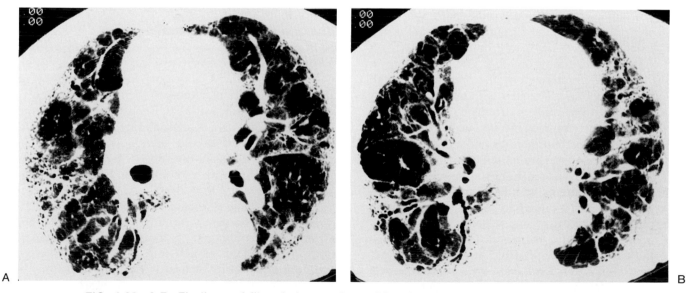

FIG. 4-22. A,B: Findings of fibrosis in a patient with scleroderma. Subpleural honeycombing, traction bronchiectasis, and some irregular interlobular septal thickening are the predominant features. These abnormalities closely mimic the appearance of IPF.

Progressive Systemic Sclerosis (Scleroderma)

Progressive systemic sclerosis (PSS) leads to some degree of UIP in nearly all cases (56,57). As many as 75% patients with PSS have evidence of lung disease at autopsy, although only 1% present with symptoms of pulmonary dysfunction (57). As with RA, chest radiographs may appear normal despite abnormal pulmonary function tests. The incidence of radiographically recognizable interstitial disease is probably around 25%, although various studies quote an incidence ranging from 10% to 80% (56,57). In addition to UIP, PSS is commonly associated with pulmonary vasculitis and pulmonary hypertension.

The radiographic and HRCT findings of interstitial fibrosis in PSS are quite similar to those of IPF (Fig. 4-19) (50–52,58). Schurawitzki et al. (52) studied 23 patients with PSS using plain radiographs and HRCT. Chest radiographs were abnormal in only 15 (65%), but HRCT showed evidence of interstitial lung disease in 21 (91%); the authors concluded that HRCT was clearly superior to chest radiographs for detecting minimal lung disease. HRCT findings in their patients included subpleural lines (74%), septal thickening or "parenchymal bands" (43%), and honeycombing or subpleural cysts (43%). Honeycombing had a uniform or peripheral distribution. Parenchymal abnormalities had upper-lung to middle-lung to lower-lung distribution ratios of 1 to 2.4 to 3.8, confirming the typical lower-lung zone predominance of abnormalities in this disease.

Remy-Jardin et al. (59) reviewed the HRCT, pulmonary function test, and bronchoalveolar lavage (BAL) results of 53 patients with PSS, emphasizing the frequency of honeycombing and ground-glass opacity in these subjects. Among the 32 patients with abnormal HRCT findings, 26 (81%) had ground-glass opacities and 19 (59%) had honeycombing. Honeycombing in PSS is usually characterized by the presence of small irregular cysts, often associated with areas of ground-glass opacity. In the study by Remy-Jardin et al., all patients with honeycombing also showed ground-glass opacity (59). These abnormalities had a distinct basal, posterior, and peripheral predominance. Small nodules with or without associated honeycombing have also been reported in patients with PSS, and are presumed to represent focal lymphoid hyperplasia, a common finding in progressive systemic sclerosis (59,60). However, nodules are not a prominent feature of this disease. In patients with PSS, HRCT findings of ground-glass opacity is often associated with a reduction in diffusing capacity, while honeycombing generally indicates a reduction in both lung volumes and diffusing capacity (59).

Other findings on CT in patients with PSS include diffuse pleural thickening seen in one-third of cases (59), asymptomatic esophageal dilatation present in 40% to 80% of cases (58,61), and enlarged mediastinal nodes seen in approximately 60% of cases (61). The presence of esophageal dilatation may be helpful in the differential diagnosis of PSS from other diffuse interstitial lung diseases. The coronal luminal diameter of the esophagus in patients with PSS, as shown on CT, has been reported to range from 12 to 40 mm (mean 23 mm), a finding that was not seen in any of a control group of 13 patients with a variety of other parenchymal and airway abnormalities (61).

Wells et al. (62) assessed the potential role of HRCT as a predictor of lung histology on open lung biopsy specimens in patients with PSS. In this study CT discriminated correctly between inflammatory and fibrotic histologic appearances in 16 of 20 (80%) of biopsy specimens. Predominant ground-glass opacities often correlated with the presence of inflammation; the presence of a predominantly reticular pattern on HRCT correlated closely with the presence of fibrosis on the pathologic specimens (62). Although, Remy-Jardin et al. (59), did not find a strong correlation between HRCT findings and the results of bronchoalveolar lavage in patients with PSS, BAL is less valid than biopsy as a predictor of activity.

UIP associated with progressive systemic sclerosis follows a less progressive course and has a better long-term prognosis than UIP associated with idiopathic pulmonary fibrosis (42,62). Improvement following treatment, similar to that seen in patients with IPF, is more frequent in patients with a prominent ground-glass component than in those with predominant reticular abnormalities (42).

Mixed Connective Tissue Disease

Mixed connective tissue disease (MCTD) is associated with clinical and laboratory findings overlapping those of PSS, systemic lupus erythematosus, and polymyositis-dermatomyositis. It is characterized by the presence of high titers of a circulating antinuclear, anti-ribonucleoprotein antibody which is uncommon in other connective tissue diseases (63). MCTD is commonly associated with radiologic and functional evidence of interstitial lung disease and/or pleural effusion; several studies indicate a prevalence of up to 80% (45,63,64). Pulmonary vasculitis with pulmonary hypertension and pulmonary hemorrhage are also associated with MCTD.

Pleural effusion or pleural thickening is present in less than 10% of cases of MCTD (63). More than two-thirds of patients with MCTD have abnormal pulmonary function tests, but chest radiographic abnormalities are less frequent, visible in about 20% (63). The interstitial lung disease of MCTD appears identical to that of UIP or IPF on histologic examination, radiographs, and in the few cases in which HRCT findings have been reported (Figs. 4-20, 4-21) (54,63).

Systemic Lupus Erythematosus

Systemic lupus erythematosus (SLE) is commonly associated with pleural and pulmonary abnormalities. Pleuritis or pleural fibrosis is present in up to 85% of cases at autopsy, and pleural effusion is often visible on chest radiographs in patients with SLE (65). More than 50% of patients with SLE have lung disease at some time (45), but interstitial pneumonia and fibrosis similar to that seen in other connective tissue diseases is relatively rare in SLE, with a prevalence of only a few percent (Fig. 4-22) (65). More common pulmonary abnormalities include pneumonia, lupus pneumonitis, and pulmonary hemorrhage. Each of these can be associated with HRCT findings of ground-glass opacity (54).

Polymyositis–Dermatomyositis

Polymyositis-dermatomyositis (PM-DM) is less commonly associated with pulmonary involvement than other connective tissue diseases. The reported incidence of pulmonary function abnormalities is about 30%, while approximately 5% of patients show chest radiographic abnormalities (45,64,66). The pattern of involvement is typically that of UIP or BOOP/COP (67).

Ankylosing Spondylitis

Extensive upper zonal pulmonary fibrosis may appear in patients with ankylosing spondylitis, usually 10 years or more after the onset of the disease (45,68). The precise frequency of pulmonary involvement is not known, and a range of 0% to 30% has been reported. The largest single series indicates a frequency of about 1% (69). Radiologically, the process begins as apical pleural involvement, and then an apical infiltrate develops and progresses to cyst formation. Generally, the disease begins unilaterally and becomes bilateral. The chest radiograph may mimic tuberculosis closely. Symptoms are usually absent, but the cavities become secondarily infected, most commonly by *Aspergillus fumigatus*, although a variety of other organisms may also infect the cavities. The histologic lesions consist of nonspecific inflammation and fibrosis. Bronchiolitis obliterans, together with a distal lipid pneumonia, is commonly present.

DRUG-INDUCED LUNG DISEASE

Many drugs can be associated with lung disease, but the highest incidence of adverse effects occurs with cytotoxic agents (70,71). Drugs can result in a variety of pathologic reactions in the lung parenchyma, including diffuse alveolar damage, interstitial pneumonitis with fibrosis, pulmonary edema, the adult respiratory distress syndrome, eosinophilic pneumonia, bronchiolitis obliterans organizing pneumonia/cryptogenic organizing pneumonia (BOOP/COP), pulmonary hemorrhage, and granulomatous lesions (70–72). Prompt recognition of pulmonary drug complications is important because early abnormalities may resolve completely when treatment with the drug is discontinued (73).

CT has been shown to be superior to chest radiography in the detection of abnormalities associated with pulmonary drug toxicity. Padley et al. (74) reviewed the chest radiographs and HRCT scans of 23 patients and 5 normal controls. Two independent observers detected abnormal findings on chest radiographs consistent with drug-induced lung disease in 17 (74%) of the 23 patients, while all 23 patients were considered to have abnormal HRCT studies. Bellamy et al. (73) reviewed the chest radiographs and CT scans in 100 patients receiving bleomycin. Pulmonary abnormalities due to bleomycin were detected on 15% of the chest radiographs and 38% of CT scans. These authors also demonstrated significant correlation between the extent of abnormalities on CT and changes in lung volume ($p > 0.01$).

Four primary patterns of drug-related lung injury have been described. These are (i) chronic pneumonitis and fibrosis, (ii) hypersensitivity lung disease, (iii) noncardiogenic pulmonary edema including the adult respiratory distress syndrome, and (iv) bronchiolitis obliterans (70,71,75). Each of these four patterns is characteristically associated with a different group of drugs, although many drugs can result in more than one type of lung reaction. HRCT findings associated with these four patterns have been reported (74).

Chronic Pneumonitis and Fibrosis

Both UIP and DIP have been associated with drug injury. A long list of drugs have been implicated in the development of chronic pneumonitis (70,71) but this pattern is most commonly the result of cytotoxic chemotherapeutic agents such as bleomycin, busulfan, vincristine, methotrexate, Adriamycin, and carmustine (BCNU). Nitrofurantoin, amiodarone, gold, and penicillamine are noncytotoxic drugs which can also result in this type of reaction. Plain radiographs in patients with chronic pneumonitis and fibrosis typically show a mixture of reticulation and consolidation.

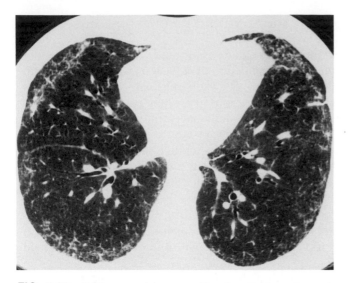

FIG. 4-23. A 61-year-old man with chronic lymphocytic leukemia developed shortness of breath after 5 months of treatment with chlorambucil. HRCT at the level of the inferior pulmonary veins demonstrates bilateral irregular reticular opacities involving predominantly the subpleural lung regions. The findings are similar to those seen in usual interstitial pneumonia (UIP).

TABLE 4-3. *HRCT findings in drug-induced lung disease associated with chronic pneumonitis and fibrosis (UIP/DIP)[a,b]*

1. **Findings of fibrosis**
   Honeycombing, Intralobular Interstitial Thickening, Irregular Interfaces, Traction Bronchiectasis
2. Ground-glass Opacity, Consolidation
3. **Peripheral and Subpleural Predominance of Abnormalities**[b]
4. **Lower and Posterior Lung Zone Predominance**[b]

[a] Most common findings in boldface.
[b] Findings most helpful in differential diagnosis in italics.

In the study by Padley et al. (74), the most common pattern seen on HRCT in patients with drug-induced lung injury was that of fibrosis, with or without associated consolidation (Table 4-3) (74). This pattern was visible in 12 of the 23 patients, and was characterized by the presence of irregular reticular opacities, honeycombing, architectural distortion, traction bronchiectasis, and/or areas of consolidation. Of the 12 examples of this pattern, 4 were the result of bleomycin, 4 resulted from nitrofurantoin toxicity, and the remaining cases were caused by amiodarone, busulfan, and gold. HRCT findings were similar to those seen in usual interstitial pneumonia (UIP) (Fig. 4-23) (70,71,73,74, 76–78).

HRCT abnormalities were usually bilateral and symmetric, with predominant lower-lung zone involvement (74). A peripheral and subpleural distribution of abnormalities was common, particularly in patients with bleomycin toxicity. In some patients, findings of fibrosis were patchy in distribution and predominantly peribronchovascular; this pattern was most common in patients receiving nitrofurantoin (74). The extent of abnormalities depends on the severity of lung damage. Mild damage is often limited to the posterior subpleural lung regions of the lower-lung zones. In patients with more severe abnormalities, there is greater involvement of the remaining lung parenchyma (73).

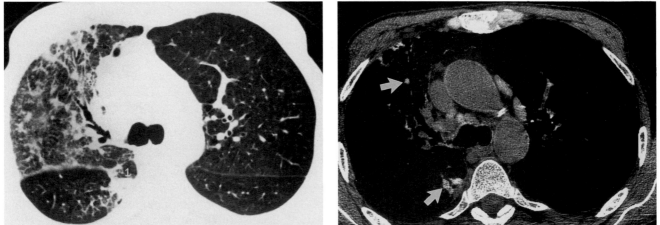

FIG. 4-24. A 61-year-old man with amiodarone lung. **A:** HRCT at the level of the tracheal carina demonstrates irregular linear opacities in the right upper lobe with associated traction bronchiectasis and architectural distortion as well as areas of ground-glass opacity. A localized area of consolidation is present in the right lower lobe. **B:** Corresponding soft-tissue windows demonstrate increased attenuation of the lung parenchyma (*arrows*). The attenuation of the area of consolidation in the right lower lobe measured 135 HU compared to 23 HU for the soft tissues of the chest wall. Also note increased attenuation of the mediastinal lymph nodes.

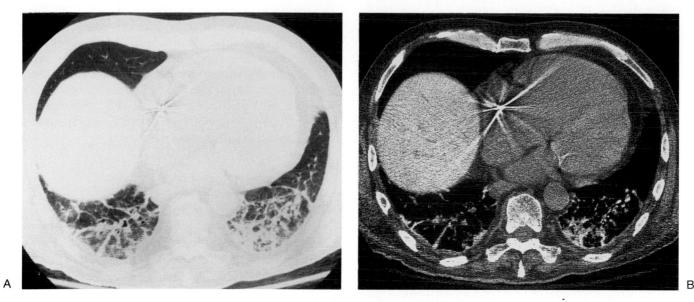

FIG. 4-25. A 68-year-old man with amiodarone lung. **A:** HRCT through the lung bases demonstrates a reticular pattern with associated traction bronchiectasis and ground-glass opacity. **B:** Corresponding mediastinal windows demonstrate increased attenuation of the lung parenchyma and of the liver. Also note cardiomegaly and presence of a pacemaker.

An interstitial pneumonitis having some characteristics of DIP or bronchiolitis obliterans organizing pneumonia/cryptogenic organizing pneumonia (BOOP/COP) has been described with several of the drugs described above, including nitrofurantoin, amiodarone, bleomycin, and busulfan (79). Like other causes of DIP or BOOP/COP, this reaction is characterized by the presence of consolidation that may have a patchy or nodular distribution, or may be predominantly peribronchial or subpleural in location (79).

Although the majority of drug reactions have a somewhat nonspecific pattern on CT, amiodarone-related lung toxicity can be readily recognized by the presence of lung attenuation greater than that of soft tissue, due to the tissue accumulation of this iodinated compound (74,76) (Figs. 3-70,4-24). Amiodarone is used in the treatment of refractory cardiac tachyarrhythmias. It accumulates in the liver and lung where it becomes entrapped in macrophage lysosomes. Patients with amiodarone pulmonary toxicity almost always show increased liver attenuation on CT, although this finding is also present in patients treated with amiodarone in the absence of drug toxicity (74,76,78) (Fig. 4-25). The patterns of pulmonary reaction to amiodarone include focal or diffuse areas of consolidation, reticular opacities and, less commonly, conglomerate masses (Fig. 3-70) (74,76,78).

Hypersensitivity Lung Disease

Hypersensitivity lung disease can be attributed to a large number of drugs, but is most commonly due to methotrexate, nitrofurantoin, bleomycin, procarbazine, BCNU, cyclophosphamide, and sulfonamides (70,71,74,80). Cough and dyspnea, with or without fever, can be acute in onset or progress over a period of several months following institution of treatment, and is unrelated to the cumulative drug dose. A peripheral eosinophilia is present in up to 40% (70,71). This reaction is characterized on HRCT by the presence of patchy areas of ground-glass attenuation, sometimes associated with small areas of consolidation (74). This pattern is similar to that seen with eosinophilic pneumonia or hypersensitivity pneumonitis, described in detail in Chapter 6 (Table 6-1). In the study by Padley (74), this pattern was visible in 7 of the 23 patients, and was due to methotrexate, nitrofurantoin, bleomycin, BCNU, and cyclophosphamide.

Pulmonary Edema

Pulmonary edema and the adult respiratory distress syndrome (ARDS) can be caused by a variety of drugs, most typically cytotoxic agents, aspirin, and narcotics (70,71). Although the mechanism of lung injury is unclear, it is likely due to increased capillary permeability. Onset is usually sudden, and within a few days of the onset of chemotherapy (70,71,74,75). On HRCT this reaction is characterized by the presence of extensive bilateral parenchymal consolidation that may be more marked in the dependent lung regions (Fig. 6-43) (74). Other than a temporal relationship to chemotherapy, there are no clinical or HRCT findings of drug-induced edema or ARDS that allow it to be distinguished from other causes. The prognosis of drug-related pulmonary edema is related to the severity of the lung injury. Two patients in the study by Padley et al. (74) developed ARDS as a result of mitomycin-C and busulfan therapy. Both these patients died.

Bronchiolitis Obliterans

The least common lung reaction to drugs is bronchiolitis obliterans, a finding which has been described primarily in association with penicillamine therapy for rheumatoid arthritis (Fig. 7-45) (70,71,81). However, the role of penicillamine is controversial, as bronchiolitis obliterans can be seen in patients with rheumatoid arthritis who have not been treated using this drug (82). Bronchiolitis obliterans has also been seen in patients treated with sulfasalazine (70). The abnormalities seen on HRCT in these patients consist of bronchial wall thickening and a pattern of mosaic perfusion, similar to that seen with other causes of bronchiolitis obliterans (Table 7-10) (74,83).

RADIATION PNEUMONITIS AND FIBROSIS

The development and appearance of radiation lung injury depend on a number of factors, including the volume of lung irradiated, shape of the radiation fields, radiation dose, number of fractions of radiation given, the time period over which the radiation is delivered, whether or not chemotherapy is also employed, and individual susceptibility (84,85). Generally speaking, radiation is best tolerated by the patient if given in smaller doses, over a long period of time, and to a single lung or a small lung region. For unilateral radiation with fractionated doses, radiographic findings of radiation pneumonitis are seldom detected with doses below 3000 cGy (centiGray), are variably present with doses between 3000 and 4000 cGy, and are nearly always visible at doses of 4000 cGy (85). Radiographic findings of radiation pneumonitis are usually unassociated with symptoms, although low-grade fever, cough, and dyspnea may be present in some patients.

Pulmonary abnormalities related to radiation injury have been divided into early and late manifestations. The early stage of radiation lung injury, referred to as radiation pneumonitis, occurs within 1 to 3 months after radiation therapy is completed, and is most severe from 3 to 4 months following treatment (84—86). Radiation pneumonitis is associated with histological findings of diffuse alveolar damage, intra-alveolar proteinaceous exudates, and hyaline membranes. Depending on the severity of lung injury, these abnormalities may resolve completely, but more often undergo progressive organization, leading eventually to fibrosis (84).

The late stage of radiation-induced lung injury, termed *radiation fibrosis*, develops gradually in patients with radiation pneumonitis when complete resolution does not occur (84). Radiation fibrosis evolves within the previously irradiated field, 6 to 12 months following radiation therapy, and usually becomes stable within 2 years of treatment (87). Histologically, dense fibrosis with obliteration of lung architecture and bronchiectasis are present.

CT and HRCT Findings

The hallmark of radiation pneumonitis on CT is the presence of increased lung attenuation corresponding closely to the location of the radiation ports. On CT, radiation pneumonitis can be associated with three patterns. These are:

1. Homogeneous ground-glass opacity uniformly involving the irradiated portions of lung (Fig. 4-26),
2. Patchy consolidation contained within the irradiated lung but not conforming to the shape of the radiation ports, and
3. Discrete consolidation conforming to the shape of the radiation ports, but not uniformly involving the irradiated lung parenchyma (88,89).

The first two patterns likely represent the presence of diffuse or patchy radiation pneumonitis, while the third pattern is thought to indicate the presence of progressive organization and early fibrosis (Table 4-4) (84,85,88). Abnormalities are typically nonanatomic, and do not tend to respect normal lung boundaries such as lobar fissures or lung segments (Fig. 4-26). Volume loss or pleural thickening can be seen in some cases (90). On CT, these abnormalities can be seen as early as 4 weeks following treatment (85,88).

Although findings of radiation pneumonitis are characteristically confined to areas of irradiated lung, relatively mild abnormalities may also be detected outside of the radiation portal, perhaps related to a hypersensi-

TABLE 4-4. *HRCT findings in radiation pneumonitis*

EARLY (Radiation Pneumonitis)
1. **Patchy or Dense Consolidation**
2. **Ground-glass Opacity**
3. *Abnormalities Largely Limited to Radiation Port*

LATE (Radiation Fibrosis)
1. **Streaky Opacities**
2. **Dense Consolidation with Volume Loss**
3. **Traction Bronchiectasis in Abnormal Regions**
4. *Abnormalities Largely Limited to Radiation Port*

a Most common findings in boldface.
b Findings most helpful in differential diagnosis boldface italics.

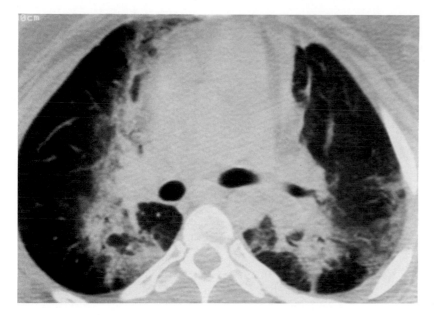

FIG. 4-26. Radiation pneumonitis in a patient who had mediastinal and hilar radiation. Bilateral, ill-defined regions of consolidation and ground-glass opacity correspond closely to the radiation ports, although increased opacity is also visible in the peripheral nonirradiated lung. (Courtesy of Joseph Cherian, M.D., Al-Sabah Hospital, Kuwait.)

tivity reaction (Fig. 4-26) (89,90). In a prospective study of CT findings in 54 irradiated patients, Mah et al. (90) demonstrated that 2 patients had minor extension of radiation injury beyond the boundaries of the radiation field. Ikezoe et al. (89) demonstrated CT findings of radiation pneumonitis beyond the radiation portals in 4 of 17 patients. The abnormalities seen in these 4 patients consisted of subtle areas of ground-glass opacity or patchy or homogeneous consolidation. The severity of the abnormalities seen outside the radiation ports in these patients was less severe than that seen within the radiation ports (89).

Progression of CT abnormalities more than 9 months after treatment likely indicates fibrosis (84). The development of radiation fibrosis can be recognized on CT by the appearance of streaky opacities, progressive volume loss, progressive dense consolidation, traction bronchiectasis, or pleural thickening within the irradiated lung (84) (Fig. 4-27). Fibrosis and volume loss typically result in a sharper demarcation between normal and irradiated lung regions than is seen in patients with radiation pneumonitis. This gives the abnormal lung regions a characteristically straight and sharply defined edge (84) (Table 4-4) (Fig. 4-28). Libshitz

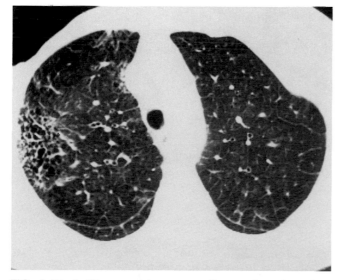

FIG. 4-27. A 78-year-old woman after undergoing right mastectomy and tangential beam radiation for breast carcinoma. HRCT 2 years later demonstrates marked fibrosis with honeycombing and traction bronchiectasis involving, predominantly the axillary region of the right lung.

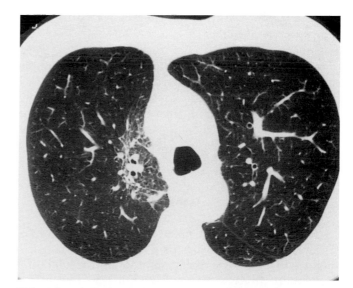

FIG. 4-28. A 67-year-old man after undergoing radiation therapy for carcinoma of the lung. HRCT scan performed 1 year later demonstrates reticular pattern and ground-glass opacity in the medial aspect of the right upper lobe. Note traction bronchiectasis due to fibrosis and sharp demarcation between normal and irradiated lung.

(85,88) has reported that patients with radiation fibrosis generally show dense consolidation, conforming to and totally involving the irradiated portions of lung, and containing ectatic air-bronchograms. However, in some patients linear opacities at the margins of the radiation port, reticular opacities similar to those seen in patients with UIP, or discrete consolidation conforming to the shape of the radiation portals but not uniformly involving the irradiated lung, can be seen.

Utility of CT and HRCT

CT is more sensitive than radiographs in detecting radiation- induced lung damage (89,91). Ikezoe et al. (89) performed serial CT scans in 17 patients and detected abnormalities on CT in 15 cases, most of which were present within 4 weeks of radiation therapy. In 3 of their patients, abnormalities were detected on CT but not on chest radiographs. In 3 other patients radiation pneumonitis was detected earlier on CT than on the radiographs. Similarly, Bell et al. (91) demonstrated that CT allowed detection of radiation pneumonitis in patients with normal chest radiographs. Preliminary results (89,92) indicate that HRCT is superior to conventional CT in the assessment of radiation-induced lung injury (89,92). CT can also be "extremely helpful" in detecting tumor recurrence within the irradiated field (85). Evidence of a mass or increased opacity developing within the irradiated field, particularly if it does not contain air-bronchograms, should suggest tumor recurrence (85,93).

ASBESTOSIS AND ASBESTOS-RELATED DISEASE

Asbestos exposure in the workplace, and to a lesser degree in the general population, is a major public health concern in the United States. Inhalation of asbestos fibers has been known to cause pulmonary and pleural fibrosis for more than 80 years. Asbestos-related abnormalities include asbestosis, asbestos-related rounded atelectasis, and asbestos-related pleural disease.

Asbestosis

The lung disease associated with asbestos fiber inhalation is known as "asbestosis" (94,95). Asbestosis is defined in pathologic terms, quite simply, as interstitial pulmonary fibrosis associated with the presence of intrapulmonary asbestos bodies or asbestos fibers (96,97).

After inhalation, asbestos fibers are first deposited in the respiratory bronchioles and alveolar ducts, but with longer and more extensive exposure, they also accumulate in a subpleural location (96–99). In patients with asbestosis, the earliest changes of fibrosis occur in the peribronchiolar region of the lobular core (98–100). As the fibrosis progresses, it involves the alveolar walls throughout the lobule, and eventually, the interlobular septa. Honeycombing can be seen in advanced cases. Visceral pleural thickening often overlies areas of parenchymal fibrosis. In asbestosis, abnormalities are usually most severe in the lower lungs, the posterior lungs, and in a subpleural location (99).

It is uncommon in clinical practice to obtain histologic proof of asbestosis; this diagnosis is usually presumptive and based on indirect evidence (97,101–103). The expression "clinical diagnosis of asbestosis" has been adopted by the American Thoracic Society to refer to a diagnosis based on a combination of chest radiographic abnormalities, restrictive abnormalities on pulmonary function tests, appropriate physical findings, and known exposure to asbestos (Table 4-5) (102–104). Although none of these clinical or radiographic criteria is specific, the presence of multiple abnormal findings in an individual with significant asbestos exposure is taken as presumptive evidence of asbestosis. A diagnosis of asbestosis is difficult to make and is probably inappropriate when only a few physical or functional abnormalities are present. Limitations in the accuracy of these criteria have been pointed out, and interstitial fibrosis in asbestos-exposed patients does not always reflect asbestosis; in one study, 5% of patients with biopsy-proven interstitial lung disease and asbestos exposure had a disease other than asbestosis on lung biopsy (105).

Symptoms and physical findings are present in only a small minority of patients with asbestosis unless the disease is relatively advanced (94,97,102). Similarly, reductions in lung volumes and diffusing capacity, which are typical of restrictive lung disease, are insensitive for detecting early or mild degrees of dysfunction

TABLE 4-5. *Criteria for a clinical diagnosis of asbestosis*

1. A reliable history of exposure to asbestos.
2. An appropriate time interval between exposure and detection.
3. Chest radiographic evidence of ILO type s, t, or u (small irregular) opacities with a profusion (severity) of 1/1 or greater.
4. Restrictive lung impairment with a forced vital capacity below the lower limit of normal.
5. A diffusing capacity below the lower limit of normal.
6. Bilateral late or paninspiratory crackles at the posterior lung base, not cleared by coughing.

Modified from Schwartz et al. (102), McLoud (103), and the American Thoracic Society (104).

in patients with asbestosis. The chest radiograph is often relied upon to help in diagnosis, but is quite limited in its ability to detect early disease. Clinical symptoms and radiographic findings of asbestosis are not usually detected until 10 years after exposure, and this latent period is sometimes as long as 40 years (97,102,104). Gallium scintigraphy can be of value in patients with early disease (100,106).

Plain Radiographs in Diagnosing Asbestosis

The International Labor Organization (ILO) classification of pneumoconiosis radiographs provides a method for objectively recording and quantitating the parenchymal and pleural abnormalities seen in patients with asbestos-related diseases (102,103,107,108). Although certain ILO abnormalities (Table 4-5) are often assumed to be diagnostic of asbestosis in patients who have been exposed to asbestos, numerous authors have stressed the limitations of chest radiographs in detecting or making a confident diagnosis of this disease (97,102,103,107–111).

Chest radiographs are relatively insensitive in detecting the presence of asbestosis. In a study performed by Epler and associates (18), of 58 patients with asbestosis diagnosed on lung biopsy, 6 (10%) had normal chest radiographs according to ILO standards. Recently, Kipen and coworkers (110) found that 25 (18%) of 138 asbestos-exposed patients with histologic proof of pulmonary fibrosis had no radiographic findings of this disease. Furthermore, 80% of the cases that were graded as less than 1/0 according to ILO standards had moderate or severe histologic grades of fibrosis.

It is also clear that the ILO classification of radiographs lacks specificity for diagnosing asbestosis (107,108); there are no plain radiographic findings which are pathognomonic of this disease. Epstein and associates (112) found that 36 (18%) of 200 screening chest radiographs showed small opacities that were consistent with pneumoconiosis using the ILO classification system; of these 36, 22 (61%) had no known occupational exposure to asbestos. In other studies, it has been suggested that cigarette smoking results in radiographic abnormalities indistinguishable from those produced by asbestosis, but this is controversial (103,107,113).

HRCT Techniques in Asbestos-Exposed Subjects

In patients with asbestos exposure, it has been recommended that scans should be obtained both supine and prone at each level (97,101,114), or in the prone position only (95,115). It is particularly important to scan asbestos-exposed individuals in the prone position, because the posterior lung is typically involved earlier and to a greater degree than the anterior lung (95). Unless prone scans are obtained, it may be impossible to distinguish normal dependent lung collapse from fibrosis in the posterior lung (Fig. 4-29).

In evaluating patients with asbestos exposure, several authors have indicated that a limited number of scans should be sufficient for the diagnosis of lung disease (95,97,101,111,114,115). Because of the typical basal distribution of asbestosis, obtaining 4 or 5 scans near the lung bases, with the most cephalad scan obtained at the level of the carina, should be sufficient

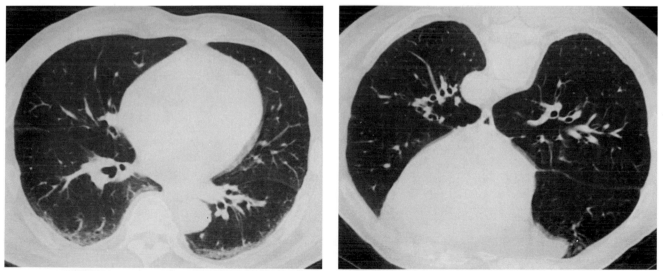

FIG. 4-29. Dependent lung opacity (collapse) in a patient with asbestos exposure. **A:** In the supine position, ill-defined areas of increased opacity are visible posteriorly. Irregularity of the costal pleural surfaces reflects pleural thickening and plaques. **B:** In the prone position, the lungs are normal in appearance. There is no evidence of septal thickening or fibrosis. The pleural irregularity, particularly within the posterior lung, remains visible.

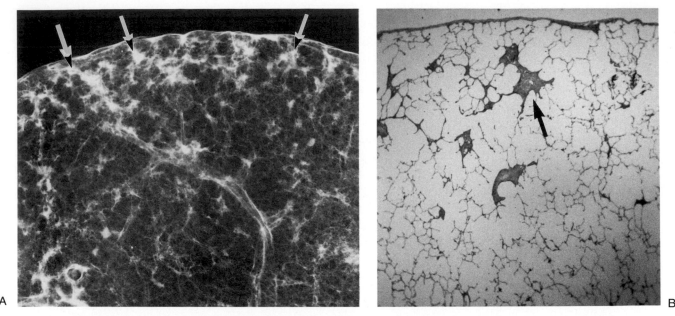

FIG. 4-30. Subpleural dot-like opacities in asbestosis. Radiograph (**A**) and histologic section (**B**) of an inflation-fixed lung obtained from a patient with early asbestosis. Small nodular opacities (*arrows*) are visible in the subpleural lung regions, representing peribronchiolar fibrosis. (Courtesy of Masanori Akira, M.D., National Kinki Chuo Hospital for Chest Disease, Osaka, Japan.) (From Akira et al., ref. 119, with permission.)

for detection of an abnormality, if present. Indeed, this approach has proven to have good sensitivity in patients with suspected asbestosis, and would be appropriate for screening groups of asbestos-exposed individuals (116). In an individual patient with asbestos exposure and suspected lung disease, however, the most appropriate protocol is to obtain HRCT at 2-cm intervals, both prone and supine. This technique allows a more complete assessment of abnormal findings, including lung masses, emphysema, and pleural abnormalities (95), allows a more accurate diagnosis of the type of lung disease present, and is more accurate in distinguishing fibrotic lung disease from emphysema, which can have similar symptoms.

HRCT Findings of Asbestosis

On HRCT, asbestosis can result in a variety of findings, depending on the severity of the disease (95,97,98,101,103,111,114,117,118). In general, HRCT findings reflect the presence of interstitial fibrosis, and are similar to those seen in patients with IPF. Although none of these findings are specific for asbestosis, the presence of parietal pleural thickening in association with lung fibrosis is highly suggestive (Table 4-6).

The earliest abnormal findings recognizable on HRCT in patients with asbestosis reflect the presence of centrilobular, peribronchiolar fibrosis (Table 4-6) (98,119). In one study (98), "dot-like" opacities were visible in the subpleural lung in patients with early as-

bestosis, forming clusters and subpleural curvilinear opacities when confluent; these correlated with the presence of peribronchiolar fibrosis extending to involve the contiguous airspaces and alveolar interstitium (Fig. 4-30). In a subsequent study (119), subpleural nodular opacities or "dots" were visible in 21 of 23 patients with early asbestosis, reflecting peribronchiolar fibrosis. These nodules are typically visible several millimeters from the pleural surface (Figs. 4-30,4-31). The presence of peribronchiolar fibrosis can also result in an abnormal prominence of the centrilobular arteries, giving rise to an increased reticulation in the peripheral lung (98,101).

As pulmonary fibrosis extends from the peribronchiolar regions to involve the remainder of the pulmonary

TABLE 4-6. HRCT findings in asbestosis

1. **Findings of Fibrosis**
   Irregular Interlobular Septal Thickening, Irregular Interfaces, Honeycombing, Traction Bronchiectasis
2. **"PARENCHYMAL Bands"**
3. **Subpleural Dot-like Opacities (Peribronchiolar Fibrosis)**
4. **Subpleural Lines**
5. **Parietal Pleural Thickening or Plaques**
6. Earliest Abnormalities Posterior and Basal
7. Ground-glass Opacity

---

a Most common finding(s) in boldface.
b Finding(s) most helpful in differential diagnosis in boldface italics.

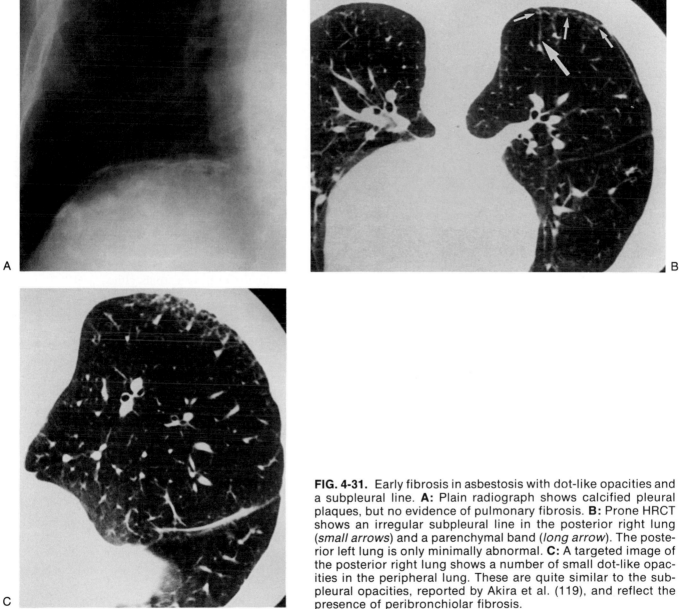

FIG. 4-31. Early fibrosis in asbestosis with dot-like opacities and a subpleural line. **A:** Plain radiograph shows calcified pleural plaques, but no evidence of pulmonary fibrosis. **B:** Prone HRCT shows an irregular subpleural line in the posterior right lung (*small arrows*) and a parenchymal band (*long arrow*). The posterior left lung is only minimally abnormal. **C:** A targeted image of the posterior right lung shows a number of small dot-like opacities in the peripheral lung. These are quite similar to the subpleural opacities, reported by Akira et al. (119), and reflect the presence of peribronchiolar fibrosis.

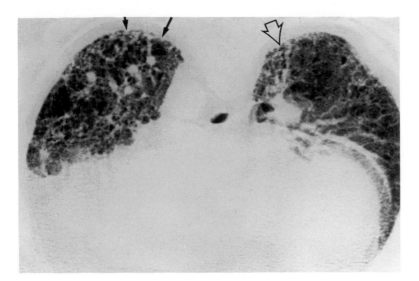

FIG. 4-32. Fibrosis in asbestosis. On a prone scan, an irregular subpleural line is present on the left (*arrows*). Subpleural dot-like opacities are visible bilaterally. Irregular septal thickening is also seen. Some subpleural lucencies (*open arrow*) may represent traction bronchiolectasis.

lobule, other findings of fibrosis can be recognized. Thickening of interlobular septa, intralobular interstitial thickening, traction bronchiectasis, architectural distortion, and findings of honeycombing can all be seen in patients with asbestosis, depending on the severity of their disease (Figs. 4-32–4-34) (97,98, 101,111). Interlobular septal thickening is common in early disease (Fig. 4-35) (97,114,120), but is less fre-

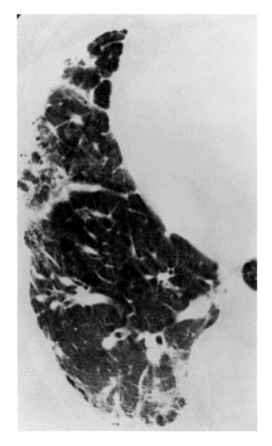

FIG. 4-33. Asbestosis. HRCT shows irregular septal thickening and early honeycombing.

quent in patients with severe disease because of superimposed honeycombing (121). Honeycombing typically predominates in the peripheral and posterior lung and is common in advanced asbestosis. In a study of patients with end-stage lung disease (121), subpleural honeycombing was present in 100% of patients with asbestosis.

"Parenchymal bands" have been reported as common in patients with asbestosis (Figs. 3-18,4-35,4-36) (97,98,101,115,120), and reflect thickening of septa marginating several lobules, fibrosis along the bronchovascular sheath (98), coarse scars, or areas of atelectasis adjacent to pleural plaques (Figs. 4-35,4-36). Parenchymal bands can be seen in a number of fibrotic diseases, but are particularly common in patients with asbestosis. In one study (97) multiple parenchymal bands were seen in 66% of asbestos-exposed patients, while parenchymal bands were much less frequent in a control group of patients without asbestos exposure. In another study, it was found that parenchymal bands were present in 79% of patients with asbestosis, as compared to only 11% of patients with idiopathic pulmonary fibrosis (122). In a study of patients with histologically proven asbestosis (120), parenchymal bands were visible on HRCT in 76%. Often, in patients with asbestos-related disease, parenchymal bands are associated with areas of thickened pleura and have a basal predominance (97,123).

Subpleural lines can reflect early fibrosis occurring in patients with asbestosis (Fig. 4-31) (98,124); this finding has been associated with the presence of peribronchiolar fibrosis and associated lung fibrosis resulting in collapse and flattening of alveoli (98). In patients with more severe fibrosis, a subpleural line can reflect honeycombing (Fig. 4-34) (124). Subpleural lines can also reflect atelectasis; in asbestos-exposed individuals, subpleural lines representing atelectasis have a propensity to occur adjacent to plaques (115).

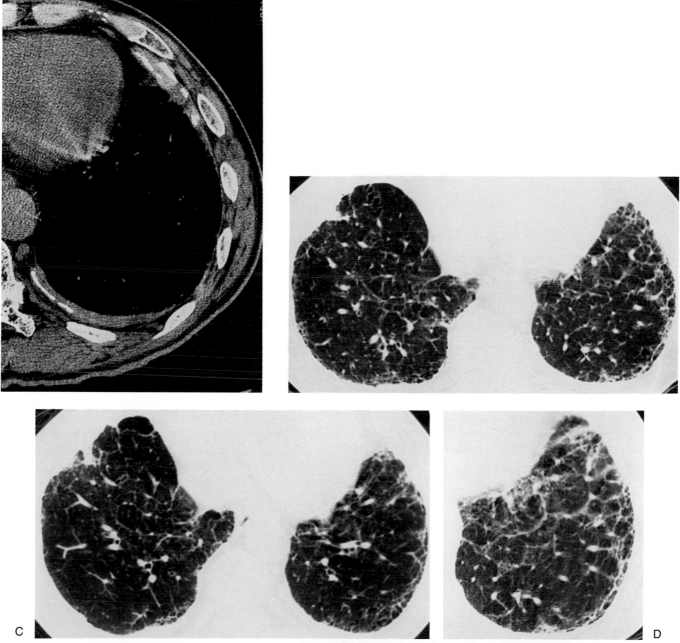

FIG. 4-34. Asbestosis with honeycombing in a 66-year old man. **A:** Calcified pleural plaques are visible, typical of asbestos exposure. **B,C:** HRCT at two levels through the lung bases shows thickening of interlobular septa and the intralobular interstitium. **D:** A targeted image shows septal thickening and early subpleural honeycombing.

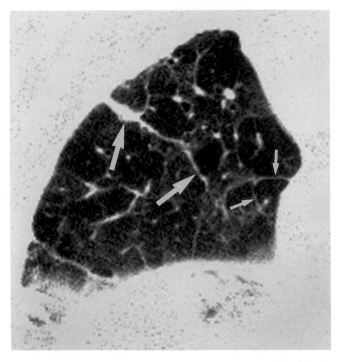

FIG. 4-35. Interlobular septal thickening and parenchymal bands in a patient with early asbestosis. View of the posterior lower lobe on a prone scan shows interlobular septal thickening (*small arrows*) and a thicker parenchymal band (*large arrows*). The parenchymal band at least partially corresponds to thickened septa.

Ground-glass opacity is uncommon in patients with asbestosis (122), but when present, correlates with the presence of mild alveolar wall and interlobular septal fibrosis or edema (98). This finding is much more frequent in association with idiopathic pulmonary fibrosis or other causes of interstitial pneumonia, than it is in patients with asbestosis (122).

A scoring system for use with HRCT, analogous to the ILO system, has recently been proposed (125). The HRCT scoring system was found to have better interobserver repeatability than the ILO system, although both HRCT and the ILO system scored correlated to a similar degree with impairment of lung function. Gamsu et al. (120) assessed the relative accuracies of a subjective semiquantitative scoring system for HRCT and a method of scoring based on cumulation of HRCT findings in patients with proven asbestosis; similar results were found for both scoring systems.

It should be kept in mind that patients with asbestosis usually show a number of HRCT findings indicative of lung fibrosis, and the abnormalities are usually bilateral and often somewhat symmetrical. The presence of focal or unilateral HRCT abnormalities should not be considered sufficient for making this diagnosis. In fact, in a recent study, three abnormal findings indicative of interstitial disease were required before a definite diagnosis could be made (120). Furthermore, although asbestosis can be present in the absence of visible pleural plaques, a diagnosis of asbestosis should be considered questionable unless pleural thickening is visible on HRCT.

Utility of HRCT in the Diagnosis of Asbestosis

In patients with significant asbestos exposure, who have no evidence of asbestosis on chest radiographs, it has been reported that as many as 20% to 30% will have some abnormal HRCT findings consistent with this disease (i.e., findings of pulmonary fibrosis) (101,109); however, other studies report the percentage of asbestos-exposed patients with normal chest radiographs and abnormal HRCT studies to be as low as

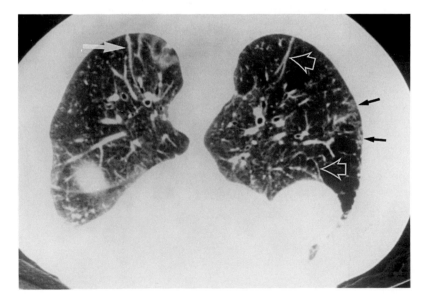

FIG. 4-36. Parenchymal bands in asbestosis. On a prone scan, areas of peripheral lung fibrosis are evident, particularly in the right lung (*small arrows*). Parenchymal bands are visible posteriorly on both sides. One of these bands (*large arrow*) is associated with a bronchus, perhaps representing fibrosis along the bronchovascular sheath, associated with atelectasis or coarse scaring. Other bands (*open arrows*) appear to represent thickened interlobular septa.

5% (111,115). Although the precise figures may vary depending on the population studied, it is universally conceded that HRCT is more sensitive than chest radiographs in detecting this disease. As stated above, from 10% to 20% of patients with asbestosis diagnosed histologically have normal chest radiographs (18,110).

Certainly, chest films underestimate the presence of histologic "asbestosis" (18,110), but what is the significance of HRCT abnormalities in asbestos-exposed patients with normal chest radiographs?

This question was addressed in a study of 169 asbestos-exposed workers with normal chest radiographs (ILO 0/0 or 0/1) who also had HRCT (109). In this group, HRCT scans were read as normal or nearly normal in 76 (45%), abnormal and suggestive of asbestosis in 57 (34%), or abnormal but not suggestive of pulmonary fibrosis in 36 (21%). Comparing the two groups in which HRCT was interpreted as normal or suggestive of asbestosis, the group considered to be abnormal on HRCT had significantly lower vital capacity (percent predicted) and diffusing capacity (percent predicted) than did the normal group; these are functional findings typically associated with asbestosis (109). On the other hand, there was no difference between the groups in a number of other clinical and functional parameters, including smoking history and measures of airway obstruction. Thus, based on this study, it appears as if HRCT is able to discriminate between groups of patients with normal and abnormal lung function, and indicates the significance of the abnormalities identified on HRCT. In another study, HRCT findings were found to correlate better with pulmonary function abnormalities in patients with early asbestosis than did chest radiographs (126).

HRCT can also be valuable for eliminating the diagnosis of asbestosis in patients who have chest radiographic findings which suggest this disease, but have some other abnormality. Friedman et al. (115) reported that approximately 20% of patients suspected of having interstitial disease on the basis of plain radiographs, were shown by HRCT to have emphysema, prominent vessels, pleural disease, or bronchiectasis as the cause of their abnormal plain film findings. Many asbestos-exposed patients with respiratory disability are smokers who have emphysema; HRCT can allow some estimation of the relative contribution of emphysema and fibrosis to the patients respiratory difficulties.

On the other hand, a normal HRCT cannot exclude the presence of asbestosis. In a study by Gamsu et al. (120) of 25 cases of histologically proven asbestosis, 5 had normal HRCT and 4 had abnormalities thought unlikely to represent asbestosis. Thus, in this group, only 64% had scans suggestive of this diagnosis.

HRCT need not be performed in all patients with asbestos exposure; if significant chest film abnormalities are present in the appropriate clinical setting (Table 4-5), CT is not necessary (106). It would seem most appropriate to limit the use of HRCT in asbestos-exposed patients to those who have:

1. Equivocal chest radiographic findings of asbestosis,
2. Pulmonary function abnormalities or symptoms, who have normal chest radiographs, and
3. Extensive pleural abnormalities in whom the differentiation of pleural and parenchymal abnormalities may be difficult.

In each of these three settings, the absence of findings of fibrosis on HRCT can be taken to mean that clinically significant asbestosis is not present, while the presence of fibrosis can lend strong support to the diagnosis.

Rounded Atelectasis and Focal Fibrotic Masses

Focal mass-like lung opacities can be seen in patients with asbestos exposure, reflecting the presence of rounded atelectasis or focal subpleural fibrosis (115,123). In one study (123), such masses were visible in about 10% of patients. It is important to distinguish these masses from lung cancer, which has an increased incidence in asbestos-exposed individuals.

The term *rounded atelectasis* refers to the presence of focal lung collapse, with or without folding of the lung parenchyma. It occurs in the presence of a variety of abnormalities, but is typically associated with pleural disease, and thus is a common finding in patients with asbestos exposure; in one study, 86% of cases were associated with asbestos (127). In patients with asbestos exposure, rounded atelectasis can represent the sequela of a preexisting exudative effusion, or can be the result of adjacent pleural fibrosis (127). In some patients with asbestos exposure, these masses are largely fibrotic.

In order to suggest the diagnosis of rounded atelectasis on the basis of HRCT, the opacity should be (i) round or oval in shape, (ii) peripheral in location and abutting the pleural surface, (iii) associated with curving of pulmonary vessels or bronchi into the edge of the lesion, and (iv) associated with an ipsilateral pleural abnormality, either effusion or pleural thickening (128). Rounded atelectasis is most common in the posterior lower lobes, and is sometimes bilateral or symmetrical (127,128). It may have acute or obtuse angles where it contacts the pleura.

Since rounded atelectasis represents collapsed lung parenchyma, it can show significant enhancement following the intravenous injection of contrast agents (129). In a recent study of dynamic CT following contrast infusion, a significant increase in attenuation of rounded atelectasis was consistently found, with a minimum attenuation increase of 200% (130). Although lung cancers can opacify to some degree following contrast injection (131), uniform dense opacification as seen in these patients has not been reported as a feature of lung cancer.

If the criteria for rounded atelectasis listed above are met, a confident diagnosis can usually be made. However, atypical cases are frequently encountered, having appearances best described as lenticular, wedge-shaped, or irregular (123). Furthermore, they may not be associated with curving of adjacent vessels, particularly if small in size. If these lesions can be shown to be unchanged in size over a year or more, they are likely benign; if not, needle biopsy may be necessary.

Asbestos-Related Pleural Disease

Benign exudative pleural effusion can be an early manifestation of asbestos exposure, being the only finding present in the first 10 years after exposure, and the most common finding present in the first 20 years following exposure (132). Asbestos-related pleural effusions can be unilateral or bilateral, and may be persistent or recurrent (95). CT in such patients sometimes shows the presence of pleural thickening or plaques invisible on chest radiographs, which are typical of asbestos exposure. However, the diagnosis of benign asbestos-related effusion is by exclusion; malignant mesothelioma must be considered in the differential diagnosis.

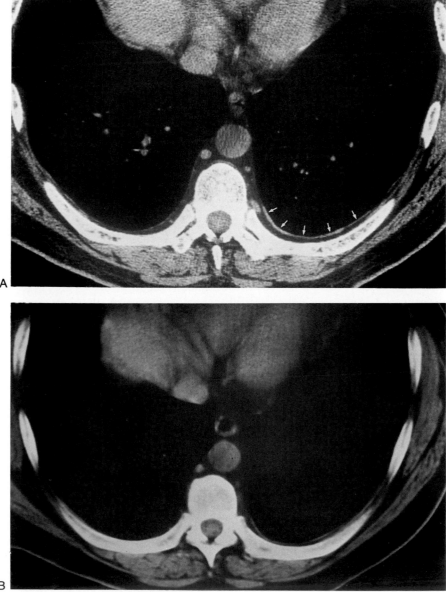

FIG. 4-37. Pleural thickening internal to a rib in asbestos exposure. **A:** HRCT shows a distinct white line (*arrows*) internal to a left posterior rib, representing pleural thickening. Extrapleural fat separates the thickened parietal pleura from the rib. Minimal pleural thickening is present on the right. The paravertebral line is normal. **B:** This finding is much more difficult to appreciate with 1-cm collimation and conventional CT technique.

Parietal pleural thickening occurs commonly in patients with occupational asbestos exposure (97,101, 103,111,115,133). In fact, the combination of pleural thickening and interstitial lung disease is most frequent in patients with asbestos exposure. Parietal pleural plaques are the most common manifestation, and the most characteristic radiographic feature, of asbestos exposure. They represent focal and discrete regions of pleural thickening, and predominate along the postero-lateral costal pleural surfaces, and along the surface of the diaphragm, but typically spare the apices and costophrenic sulci.

HRCT Findings of Pleural Thickening

On HRCT, parietal pleural thickening is easiest to see internal to visible rib segments; only the pleura, extrapleural fat, and endothoracic fascia pass internal to ribs (Fig. 2-16), and in most normal patients these are too thin to recognize on HRCT. Thickened pleura measuring as little as 1 to 2 mm can be readily diagnosed in this location (Fig. 4-37). Although the normal innermost intercostal muscle is visible on HRCT as a 1- to 2-mm-thick, opaque stripe between adjacent rib segments (Fig. 2-17), it does not pass internal to them, and should not be confused with pleural thickening. Pleural thickening is also easy to recognize in the paravertebral regions. In the paravertebral regions, the intercostal muscles are anatomically absent (Fig. 2-18), and any distinct stripe of density indicates pleural thickening (Figs. 4-38,4-39).

The HRCT diagnosis of pleural thickening is made easier in many locations by the presence of a distinct layer of extrapleural fat, usually measuring from 1 to 4 mm in thickness, which separates the thickened pleura from adjacent structures of the chest wall, such as rib, innermost intercostal muscle, intercostal vein, or subcostalis muscle (Figs. 4-37,4-39,4-40) (134). This layer of extrapleural fat represents the normal fatty connective tissue present external to the parietal pleura, and is likely thickened in patients with asbestos exposure as a result of pleural inflammation. Extrapleural fat allows the thickened pleura to be seen on HRCT as a discrete linear opacity, even when the pleural thickening is minimal.

Asbestos-related pleural thickening has a typical appearance on HRCT (97,101,111,134). The pleural thickening appears smooth and sharply defined, and can be recognized when measuring only 1 or 2 mm in thickness (Figs. 4-37–4-40) (134). Early pleural thickening is discontinuous and abnormal areas can be easily contrasted with adjacent normal regions. Areas of pleural thickening or plaques of thickened pleura are commonly visible adjacent to the inner surfaces of ribs or vertebral bodies (Figs 4-37,4-38). The presence of bilateral pleural plaques or focal pleural thickening is strongly suggestive of asbestos exposure, particularly when calcification is also visible (Fig. 4-41). Pleural calcification is visible on HRCT in about 15% of patients (Figs. 4-34,4-41) (114,115). In one study (101), calcification was identified with HRCT in 20% of 100 subjects, but it was seen in only 16% with conventional CT, and in 13% with chest radiographs. Often, even when not grossly calcified, asbestos-related areas of pleural thickening appear slightly denser than adjacent intercostal muscles (Figs. 4-38,4-40).

The diaphragmatic pleura is commonly involved in patients with asbestos-related pleural disease (Fig. 4-41). However, the diaphragm lies roughly in the plane

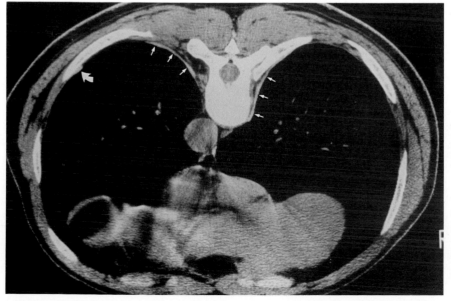

FIG. 4-38. Paravertebral pleural thickening in asbestos exposure. Prone HRCT shows 2- to 3-mm-thick lines (*arrows*) in both paravertebral regions, representing parietal pleural thickening. A small focus of pleural thickening internal to a rib (*large arrow*) is also seen.

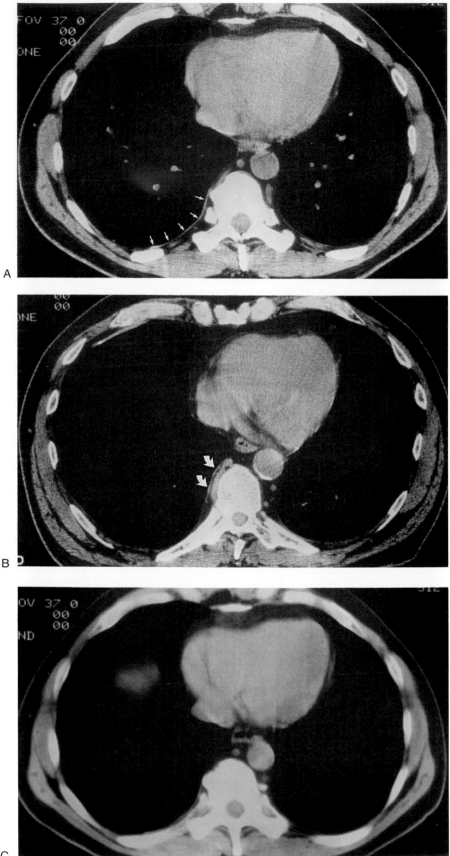

FIG. 4-39. Paravertebral pleural thickening in asbestos exposure. **A,B:** HRCT at two levels showing thickening of the right paravertebral line (*small arrows*). At one level, the thickened pleura (*large arrows*, B) is separated from the adjacent intercostal vein by fat. **C:** With 1-cm collimation and conventional CT technique these findings are difficult to see.

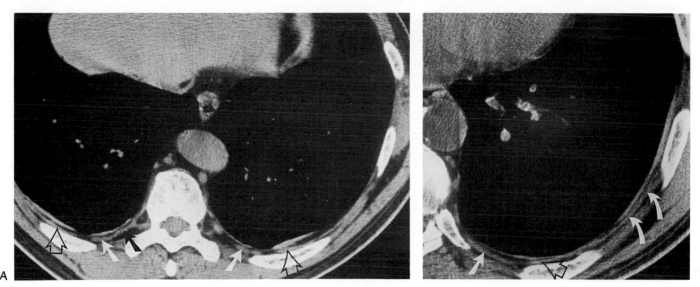

FIG. 4-40. Pleural thickening in asbestos exposure. **A,B:** HRCT in two different patients shows thickened pleura separated from intercostal vein (*arrows*), subcostalis muscle (*open arrows*), and intercostal muscle (*curved arrows*, B) by a layer of fat.

of the scan, and the detection of uncalcified pleural plaques on the diaphragmatic surface can be difficult with HRCT. In some patients, however, diaphragmatic pleural plaques are visible deep in the posterior costophrenic angle, below the lung base; in this location, the pleural disease can be localized with certainty to the parietal pleura because only parietal pleura is present below the lung base.

Pleural plaques along the mediastinum have been considered unusual in patients with asbestos-related pleural disease but are visible on CT scans in about 40% of patients (97,101,111,133,134). Paravertebral pleural thickening is commonly seen on HRCT (134).

Although it is unusual, pleural thickening can involve a fissure and result in a localized intrapulmonary pleural plaque. These may simulate a lung nodule on CT unless the plane of the fissure is identified. In patients who also have pulmonary fibrosis, visceral pleural thickening with irregularity of the pleural surface, can also be seen at soft-tissue window settings.

Diffuse pleural thickening is another common manifestation of asbestos exposure (133). Diffuse pleural thickening represents a synthesis and fusion of thickened visceral and parietal pleural layers, and it is usually related to the presence of prior asbestos-related benign pleural effusion. On CT, diffuse pleural thicken-

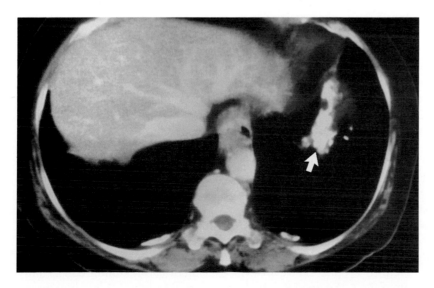

FIG. 4-41. Pleural plaques in a patient with asbestos exposure. CT shows calcified plaques posteriorly, and on the dome of the left hemidiaphragm (*arrow*).

ing is defined by the presence of a sheet of thickened pleura at least 5 cm in lateral dimension and 8 cm in craniocaudal dimension (101). Diffuse pleural thickening was found by Aberle and coworkers (101) in 7 of 100 exposed individuals. Because of visceral pleural thickening or associated lung fibrosis, the thickened pleura may appear ill-defined or irregular. Extensive calcification is uncommon. Diffuse pleural thickening is associated with significant impairment of pulmonary function; pulmonary function in patients with pleural plaques is normal or slightly reduced (135,136).

There is a significant correlation between the presence and severity of pleural disease and the presence and severity of asbestosis (97). In one study, HRCT findings of parenchymal fibrosis were visible in 14% of exposed patients without evidence of pleural thickening, 56% of those with focal plaques, and in 88% of those with diffuse pleural thickening (136). It is important to note, however, that pleural thickening and plaques commonly occur in the absence of pulmonary fibrosis (137), and asbestosis can sometimes be seen in the absence of visible pleural plaques (136), although this is more unusual.

Utility of HRCT in Diagnosing Asbestos-Related Pleural Disease

Pleural thickening is frequently seen on plain radiographs in patients with asbestos exposure (Fig. 4-31), but CT and particularly HRCT are much more sensitive in detecting pleural disease (97,101,111). Aberle and colleagues (101) studied the detection of pleural plaques and calcification with conventional radiographs, conventional CT, and HRCT in 100 subjects occupationally exposed to asbestos. Although HRCT was obtained only at selected levels, it was more sensitive in detecting plaques than the other two modalities (Figs. 4-37,4-39). Plaques were identified in 64 persons with HRCT, in 56 with conventional CT, and in 49 with chest radiographs. In another study (134) of 13 patients with evidence of asbestos-related pleural disease visible on HRCT, conventional CT showed some evidence of pleural abnormality in only 11; however, in all 13, some abnormal areas visible on HRCT were not seen with conventional CT. Similar results have been reported by others (111,138).

Furthermore, HRCT is much more accurate than plain films or conventional CT in distinguishing true pleural disease from extrapleural fat pads, which can closely mimic the appearance of pleural thickening (Fig. 4-42). In one study of patients with low levels of asbestos exposure, posteroanterior and right anterior oblique radiographs were thought to show pleural thickening in all, while HRCT showed true pleural

plaques in only 13% to 26% (139); most of the false-positive interpretations on chest radiographs were due to the presence of extrapleural fat.

Differential Diagnosis and Mimics of Parietal Pleural Thickening

Parietal pleural thickening or pleural effusion in association with lung disease can also be seen in patients with rheumatoid arthritis (53), lymphangiomyomatosis (140,141), coal worker's pneumoconiosis (142), tuberculosis (143), nontuberculous mycobacteria, and lymphangitic spread of carcinoma (58).

Normal extrapleural fat can be seen on HRCT internal to ribs in several locations, and can mimic pleural thickening (Fig. 4-42) (115). The normal layer of extrapleural fat between the parietal pleura and the endothoracic fascia is notably thicker adjacent to the lateral ribs than in other sites (134,144,145). It is most abundant over the posterolateral fourth to eighth ribs and can result in fat pads several millimeters thick which extend into the intercostal spaces (144,145). In normal subjects, these costal fat pads can be difficult to distinguish from pleural thickening or plaques when extended window settings (width 2000 H) are used, but are very low in attenuation and difficult to see with soft-tissue window settings (134).

The transversus thoracis and subcostalis muscles can also mimic pleural thickening in some patients. Anteriorly, at the level of the heart and adjacent to the lower sternum or xiphoid process, the transversus thoracis muscles are nearly always visible internal to the anterior ends of ribs or costal cartilages (Fig. 4-43) (134). Posteriorly, at the same level, a 1- to 2-mm-thick line is sometimes seen internal to one or more ribs, representing the subcostalis muscle; this muscle is present in only a small percentage of patients (Fig. 4-42) (134). In contrast to pleural thickening, these muscles are smooth, uniform in thickness, and symmetric bilaterally.

Segments of intercostal veins are commonly visible in the paravertebral regions, and can mimic focal pleural thickening (Fig. 4-43). Continuity of these opacities with the azygos or hemiazygos veins can sometimes allow them to be correctly identified (134). Furthermore, when viewed using lung window settings, intercostal vein segments do not indent the lung surface; pleural plaques of the same thickness certainly would.

Visceral pleural thickening, i.e., thickening of the subpleural interstitium, can be seen on HRCT in a number of lung diseases that produce pulmonary fibrosis. However, visceral pleural thickening can usually be distinguished from parietal pleural thickening by its

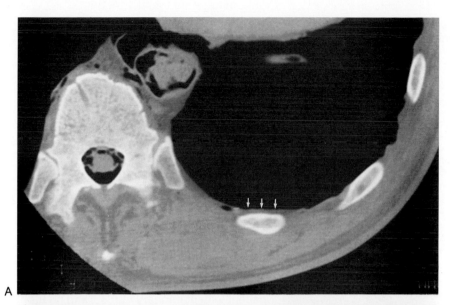

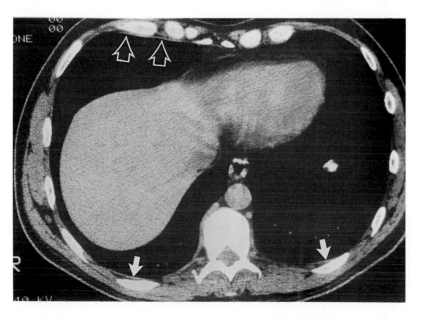

FIG. 4-42. Normal extrapleural fat pad in a cadaver. **A:** With a wide-window setting, soft tissue (*arrows*) is visible internal to the posterior rib segment. This appearance mimics pleural thickening. **B:** At a mediastinal window setting, the low density of the fat is apparent. (From Im et al., ref. 134, with permission.)

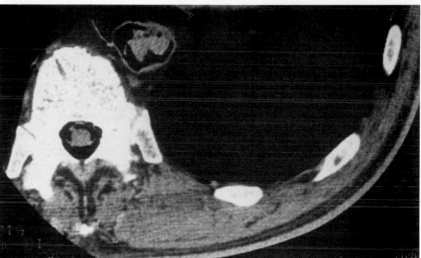

FIG. 4-43. Normal transversus thoracis and subcostalis muscles. HRCT in a normal subject shows the right transversus thoracis muscle internal to the anterior rib and costal cartilage (*open arrows*). Posteriorly, the subcostalis muscles (*solid arrows*) are visible bilaterally, anterior to ribs. Prominent intercostal veins are visible in the paravertebral regions.

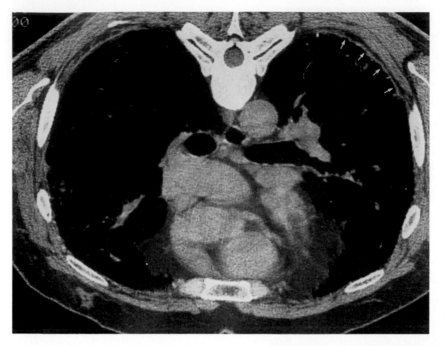

FIG. 4-44. Visceral pleural thickening in a patient with pulmonary fibrosis and no history of asbestos exposure. The pleural opacity (*arrows*) visible on prone HRCT appears very irregular.

irregular appearance; visceral pleural thickening usually appears very irregular at soft-tissue or wide-window settings (Fig. 4-44) because of abnormal lung reticulation and the "interface sign." Because its presence reflects an interstitial abnormality, visceral pleural thickening is usually localized to areas where the underlying lung is abnormal; this is not true of asbestos-related parietal pleural thickening.

Confluent subpleural nodules, so-called pseudoplaques (142,146), can be seen in patients with silicosis, coal worker's pneumoconiosis, or sarcoidosis (Fig. 3-42). These can mimic the appearance of parietal pleural plaques occurring in patients with asbestos exposure, but are associated with lung nodules rather than findings of fibrosis.

THE DIFFERENTIAL DIAGNOSIS OF "END-STAGE LUNG"

So-called end-stage lung represents the final common pathway of a number of chronic infiltrative lung diseases, characterized by acute and chronic inflammation. It is characterized by the presence of fibrosis, alveolar dissolution, bronchiolectasis, and disruption of normal lung architecture. Generally speaking, end-stage lung is considered to be present in patients who have morphologic evidence of honeycombing, extensive cystic changes, or conglomerate fibrosis (147–150).

Based on the analysis of chest radiographs and fragmentary lung histology obtained at open lung biopsy, it had been assumed that the morphologic appearance of end-stage lung lacked specificity, with the observed findings being similar regardless of etiology (121,148). Although significant overlap can occur between the HRCT appearances of different fibrotic diseases, Primack et al. (121) recently demonstrated, that the pattern and distribution of abnormalities seen on HRCT in patients with end-stage lung are determined, at least in part, by the underlying disease, and that in most cases, a specific diagnosis can be made on HRCT.

Primack et al. (121) reviewed the HRCT scans of 61 consecutive patients with end-stage lung. Two independent observers, without knowledge of the clinical or pathologic data, listed the three most likely diagnoses and recorded the degree of confidence in their first-choice diagnosis on a three-point scale. On the average, the two observers made a correct first-choice diagnosis in 87% of cases. A correct first-choice diagnosis was made most often in silicosis (100%), pulmonary histiocytosis X (100%), asbestosis (90%), usual interstitial pneumonia (88%), hypersensitivity pneumonitis (87%), and sarcoidosis (83%). The observers had a high degree of confidence in their first-choice diagnosis in 62% of the interpretations, and when they were confident in their diagnosis, they were correct in 100% of the cases. The most common conditions leading to end-stage lung disease in the study by Primack et al. (121) included usual interstitial pneumonia (43%), sarcoidosis (15%), pulmonary histiocytosis X (13%), asbestosis (8%) and hypersensitivity pneumonitis (extrinsic allergic alveolitis) (6%).

Usual interstitial pneumonia was characterized by predominant involvement of the lower-lung zones and subpleural regions, with peripheral honeycombing being the most common finding (Figs. 4-4–4-10). The abnormalities in patients with sarcoidosis involved mainly the upper-lung zones and had a peribronchovascular distribution (Figs. 3-53,5-18,5-20). End-stage fibrosis in sarcoidosis was associated with three different patterns: (i) subpleural honeycombing, (ii) central cystic changes due to markedly ectatic bronchi, and (iii) conglomerate fibrosis. In the six patients with sarcoidosis who had conglomerate fibrosis, bronchi could be seen within the areas of fibrosis. Pulmonary histiocytosis X was characterized in all cases by an upper-lung zone predominance of randomly distributed cystic spaces with relative sparing of the lung bases (Figs. 7-1 and 7-2). Asbestosis had an appearance identical to that of usual interstitial pneumonia, except that all five patients with asbestosis also had pleural plaques or diffuse pleural thickening (Fig. 4-34). Parenchymal bands are also much more common in patients with asbestosis (Fig. 4-35) (122). The abnormalities in end-stage hypersensitivity pneumonitis involved all lung zones to a similar degree in three patients, and had an upper-lung zone predominance in one. Honeycombing was predominantly subpleural in three cases, but unlike UIP, in chronic hypersensitivity pneumonitis there was relative sparing of the lung bases (Figs. 6-5,6-6). All patients with hypersensitivity pneumonitis had associated extensive areas of ground-glass attenuation in a random distribution.

The ability to make a confident correct specific diagnosis on HRCT in the majority of patients with end-stage lung may be of significant clinical utility, as open lung biopsy is not usually diagnostic in patients with this pattern of abnormalities, and its use is not recommended (151). Gaensler and Carrington (151) reviewed their experience with open lung biopsy in 502 patients with chronic diffuse infiltrative lung disease. Nonspecific "honeycombing," or end-stage lung, was the only diagnosis possible in 3.4% of patients. Based on their experience, they do not consider it advisable to perform lung biopsy in patients with radiographic evidence of extensive honeycombing "because in such patients, biopsy has made no contribution from either the diagnostic or the therapeutic standpoint" (151). Overall, the diagnostic yield in this study (151) was 92%, with a mortality rate of 0.3%, and a 2.5% rate of significant complications such as empyema, respiratory insufficiency, and myocardial ischemia. If end-stage lung disease is the only abnormality seen on CT, open lung biopsy is not likely warranted. The diagnosis in those patients can be based on clinical history, and the pattern and distribution of findings on HRCT.

REFERENCES

1. Liebow AA. New concepts and entities in pulmonary disease. In: *The Lung*. Baltimore: Williams & Wilkins; 1968:332–365.
2. Liebow AA, Carrington CB. Diffuse pulmonary lymphoreticular infiltration associated with dysproteinemia. *Med Clin North Am* 1973;57:809–843.
3. Steimlam CV, Rosenow EC, Divertie MB, Harrison EG. Pulmonary manifestations of Sjögren's syndrome. *Chest* 1976;70:354–361.
4. Joshi VV, Oleske JM, Minnefor AB, et al. Pathologic pulmonary findings in children with the acquired immunodeficiency syndrome. *Hum Pathol* 1985;16:241–246.
5. Grieco MH, Chinoy-Acharya P. Lymphoid interstitial pneumonia associated with the acquired immune deficiency syndrome. *Am Rev Respir Dis* 1985;131:952–955.
6. Colby TV, Carrington CB. Infiltrative lung disease. In: *Pathology of the Lung*. Stuttgart: Thieme Medical,1988.425–518.
7. Spencer H. *Pathology of the Lung*. Oxford: Pergamon Press: 1985:1025–1032.
8. Ohori NP, Sciurba FC, Owens GR, Hodgson MJ, Yousem SA. Giant-cell interstitial pneumonia and hard-metal pneumoconiosis. *Am J Surg Pathol* 1989;13:581–587.
9. Epler GR, Colby TV, McLoud TC, Carrington CG, Gaensler EA. Idiopathic bronchiolitis obliterans with organizing pneumonia. *N Engl J Med* 1985;312:152–159.
10. Müller NL, Guerry-Force ML, Staples CA, et al. Differential diagnosis of bronchiolitis obliterans with organizing pneumonia and usual interstitial pneumonia: clinical, functional, and radiologic findings. *Radiology* 1987;162:151–156.
11. Katzenstein AL, Myers JL, Prophet WD, Corley LS, Shin MS. Bronchiolitis obliterans and usual interstitial pneumonia: a comparative clinicopathologic study. *Am J Surg Pathol* 1986;10:373–381.
12. Chandler PW, Shin MS, Friedman SE, Myers JL, Katzenstein AL. Radiographic manifestations of bronchiolitis obliterans with organizing pneumonia vs usual interstitial pneumonia. *AJR* 1986;147:899–906.
13. Crystal RG, Fulmer JD, Roberts WC, Moss ML, Line BR, Reynolds HY. Idiopathic pulmonary fibrosis: clinical, histologic, radiographic, physiologic, scintigraphic, cytologic, and biochemical aspects. *Ann Intern Med* 1976;85:769–788.
14. Scadding JG, Hinson KFW. Diffuse fibrosing alveolitis (diffuse interstitial fibrosis of the lungs): correlation of histology at biopsy with prognosis. *Thorax* 1967;22:291–304.
15. Liebow AA, Steer A, Billingsley JG. Desquamative interstitial pneumonia. *Am J Med* 1965;38:369–404.
16. Hartman TE, Primack SL, Swensen SJ, Hansell D, McGuinness G, Müller NL. Desquamative interstitial pneumonia: thin-section CT findings in 22 patients. *Radiology* 1993;187:787–790.
17. Carrington CB, Gaensler EA, Coute RE, Fitzgerald MS, Gupta RG. Natural history and treated course of usual and desquamative interstitial pneumonia. *N Engl J Med* 1978;298:801–809.
18. Epler GR, McLoud TC, Gaensler EA, Mikus JP, Carrington CB. Normal chest roentgenograms in chronic diffuse infiltrative lung disease. *N Engl J Med* 1978;298:801–809.
19. Terriff BA, Kwan SY, Chan-Yeung MM, Müller NL. Fibrosing alveolitis: chest radiography and CT as predictors of clinical and functional impairment at follow-up in 26 patients. *Radiology* 1992;184:445–449.
20. Wells AU, Rubens MB, du Bois RM, Hansell DM. Serial CT in fibrosing alveolitis: prognostic significance of the initial pattern. *AJR* 1993;161:1159–1165.
21. Müller NL, Miller RR, Webb WR, Evans KG, Ostrow DN. Fibrosing alveolitis: CT-pathologic correlation. *Radiology* 1986;160:585–588.
22. Staples CA, Müller NL, Vedal S, Abboud R, Ostrow D, Miller RR. Usual interstitial pneumonia: correlation of CT with clinical, functional, and radiologic findings. *Radiology* 1987;162:377–381.
23. Nishimura K, Kitaichi M, Izumi T, Nagai S, Itoh H. Usual interstitial pneumonia: histologic correlation with high-resolution CT. *Radiology* 1992;182:337–342.
24. Remy-Jardin M, Giraud F, Remy J, Copin MC, Gosselin B, Duhamel A. Importance of ground-glass attenuation in chronic diffuse infiltrative lung disease: pathologic-CT correlation. *Radiology* 1993;189:693–698.
25. Leung AN, Miller RR, Müller NL. Parenchymal opacification in chronic infiltrative lung diseases: CT-pathologic correlation. *Radiology* 1993;188:209–214.

26. Vedal S, Welsh EV, Miller RR, Müller NL. Desquamative interstitial pneumonia: computed tomographic findings before and after treatment with corticosteroids. *Chest* 1988;93:215–217.
27. Müller NL, Staples CA, Miller RR, Vedal S, Thurlbeck WM, Ostrow DN. Disease activity in idiopathic pulmonary fibrosis: CT and pathologic correlation. *Radiology* 1987;165:731–734.
28. Crystal RG, Bitterman PB, Rennard SI, Hance AJ, Keogh BA. Interstitial lung diseases of unknown cause: disorders characterized by chronic inflammation of the lower respiratory tract. *N Engl J Med* 1984;310:154–166.
29. Stack BHR, Choo-King YF, Heard BE. The prognosis of crytogenic fibrosing alveolitis. *Thorax* 1972;27:535–542.
30. Watters LC, King TE, Schwarz MI, Waldron JA, Stanford RE, Cherniack RM. A clinical, radiographic and physiologic scoring system for the longitudinal assessment of patients with idiopathic pulmonary fibrosis. *Am Rev Respir Dis* 1986;133:97–103.
31. Wright PH, Heard BE, Steel SJ, Turner-Warwick W. Cryptogenic fibrosing alveolitis: assessment by graded trephine lung biopsy histology compared with clinical, radiographic and physiologic features. *Br J Dis Chest* 1981;75:61–70.
32. Livingstone JL, Lewis JG, Reid L, Jefferson KE. Diffuse interstitial pulmonary fibrosis: a clinical, radiological, and pathological study based on 45 patients. *Q J Med* 1964;33:71–103.
33. Turner-Warwick M, Burrows B, Johnson A. Cryptogenic fibrosing alveolitis: clinical features and their influence on survival. *Thorax* 1980;35:171–180.
34. Mathieson JR, Mayo JR, Staples CA, Müller NL. Chronic diffuse infiltrative lung disease: comparison of diagnostic accuracy of CT and chest radiography. *Radiology* 1989;171:111–116.
35. Strickland B, Strickland NH. The value of high definition, narrow section computed tomography in fibrosing alveolitis. *Clin Radiol* 1988;39:589–594.
36. Webb WR, Stein MG, Finkbeiner WE, Im JG, Lynch D, Gamsu G. Normal and diseased isolated lungs: high-resolution CT. *Radiology* 1988;166:81–87.
37. Zerhouni EA, Naidich DP, Stitik FP, Khouri NF, Siegelman SS. Computed tomography of the pulmonary parenchyma: part 2. interstitial disease. *J Thorac Imaging* 1985;1:54–64.
38. Zerhouni E. Computed tomography of the pulmonary parenchyma: an overview. *Chest* 1989;95:901–907.
39. Westcott JL, Cole SR. Traction bronchiectasis in end-stage pulmonary fibrosis. *Radiology* 1986;161:665–669.
40. Aquino SL, Webb WR, Zaloudek CJ, Stern EJ. Lung cysts associated with honeycombing: change in size on expiratory CT scans. *AJR* 1994;162:583–584.
41. Lee JS, Im JG, Ahn JM, Kim YM, Han MC. Fibrosing alveolitis: prognostic implication of ground-glass attenuation at high-resolution CT. *Radiology* 1992;184:415–454.
42. Wells AU, Hansell DM, Rubens MB, Cullinan P, Black CM, du Bois RM. The predictive value of appearances of thin-section computed tomography in fibrosing alveolitis. *Am Rev Respir Dis* 1993;148:1076–1082.
43. Akira M, Sakatani M, Ueda E. Idiopathic pulmonary fibrosis: progression of honeycombing at thin-section CT. *Radiology* 1993;189:687–691.
44. Miller RR, Nelems B, Müller NL, Evans KG, Ostrow DN. Lingular and right middle lobe biopsy in the assessment of diffuse lung disease. *Ann Thorac Surg* 1987;44:269–273.
45. Gamsu G. Radiographic manifestations of thoracic involvement by collagen vascular diseases. *J Thorac Imaging* 1992;7(3):1–12.
46. Shannon TM, Gale ME. Noncardiac manifestations of rheumatoid arthritis in the thorax. *J Thorac Imaging* 1992;7(2):19–29.
47. Remy-Jardin M, Remy J, Cortet B, Mauri F, Delcambre B. Lung changes in rheumatoid arthritis: CT findings. *Radiology* 1994;193:375–382.
48. Laitinen O, Nissila M, Salorinne Y, et al. Pulmonary involvement in patients with rheumatoid arthritis. *Scand J Respir Dis* 1975;56:297.
49. Frank ST, Weg JG, Harkleroad LE, Fitch RF. Pulmonary dysfunction in rheumatoid disease. *Chest* 1973;63:27–34.
50. Bergin CJ, Müller NL. CT of interstitial lung disease: a diagnostic approach. *AJR* 1987;148:9–15.
51. Bergin CJ, Müller NL. CT in the diagnosis of interstitial lung disease. *AJR* 1985;145:505–510.
52. Schurawitzki H, Stiglbauer R, Graninger W, et al. Interstitial lung disease in progressive systemic sclerosis: high-resolution CT versus radiography. *Radiology* 1990;176:755–759.
53. Steinberg DL, Webb WR. CT appearances of rheumatoid lung disease. *J Comput Assist Tomogr* 1984;8:881–884.
54. Meziane MA. High-resolution computed tomography scanning in the assessment of interstitial lung diseases. *J Thorac Imaging* 1992;7(3):13–25.
55. Fujii M, Adachi S, Shimizu T, Hirota S, Sako M, Kono M. Interstitial lung disease in rheumatoid arthritis: assessment with high-resolution computed tomography. *J Thorac Imaging* 1993;8:54–62.
56. Taorimina VJ, Miller WT, Gefter WB, Epstein DM. Progressive systemic sclerosis subgroups: variable pulmonary features. *AJR* 1981;137:277–285.
57. Arroliga AC, Podell DN, Matthay RA. Pulmonary manifestations of scleroderma. *J Thorac Imaging* 1992;7(2):30–45.
58. Grenier P, Chevret S, Beigelman C, Brauner MW, Chastang C, Valeyre D. Chronic diffuse infiltrative lung disease: determination of the diagnostic value of clinical data, chest radiography, and CT with Bayesian analysis. *Radiology* 1994;1994:383–390.
59. Remy-Jardin M, Remy J, Wallaert B, Bataille D, Hatron PY. Pulmonary involvement in progressive systemic sclerosis: sequential evaluation with CT, pulmonary function tests, and bronchoalveolar lavage. *Radiology* 1993;188:499–506.
60. Harrison NK, Myers AR, Corrin B, et al. Structural features of interstitial lung disease in systemic sclerosis. *Am Rev Respir Dis* 1991;144:706–713.
61. Bhalla M, Silver RM, Shepard JO, McLoud TC. *Chest* CT in patients with scleroderma: prevalence of asymptomatic esophageal dilatation and mediastinal lymphadenopathy. *AJR* 1993;161:269–272.
62. Wells AU, Hansell DM, Corrin B, et al. High resolution computed tomography as a predictor of lung histology in systemic sclerosis. *Thorax* 1992;47:508–512.
63. Prakash UBS. Lungs in mixed connective tissue disease. *J Thorac Imaging* 1992;7(2):55–61.
64. Hunninghake GW, Fauci AS. Pulmonary involvement in the collagen vascular diseases. *Am Rev Respir Dis* 1979;119:471–503.
65. Wiedemann HP, Matthay RA. Pulmonary manifestations of systemic lupus erythematosus. *J Thorac Imaging* 1992;7(2):1–18.
66. Schwarz MI. Pulmonary and cardiac manifestations of polymyositis-dermatomyositis. *J Thorac Imaging* 1992;7(2):46–54.
67. Tazelaar HD, Viggiano RW, Pickersgill J, Colby TV. Interstitial lung disease in polymyositis and dermatomyositis. clinical features and prognosis as correlated with histologic findings. *Am Rev Respir Dis* 1990;141:727–733.
68. Tanoue LT. Pulmonary involvement in collagen vascular disease: a review of the pulmonary manifestations of the Marfan syndrome, ankylosing spondylitis, Sjögren's syndrome, and relapsing polychondritis. *J Thorac Imaging* 1992;7(2):62–77.
69. Rosenow EC, Strimlan CV, Muhm JR, Ferguson RH. Pleuropulmonary manifestations of ankylosing spondylitis. *Mayo Clin Proc* 1977;52:641–649.
70. Cooper JAD, White DA, Matthay RA. Drug-induced pulmonary disease. Part 2: noncytotoxic drugs. *Am Rev Respir Dis* 1986;133:488–503.
71. Cooper JA Jr, White DA, Matthay RA. Drug-induced pulmonary disease. part 1: cytoxic drugs. *Am Rev Respir Dis* 1986;133:321–340.
72. Colby TV. Anatomic distribution and histopathologic patterns in interstitial lung disease. In: Schwarz MI, King TE Jr, eds. *Interstitial Lung Disease.* St. Louis: Mosby Year Book: 1993:59–77.
73. Bellamy EA, Husband JE, Blaquiere RM, Law MR. Bleomycin-related lung damage: CT evidence. *Radiology* 1985;156:155–158.

74. Padley SPG, Adler B, Hansell DM, Müller NL. High- resolution computed tomography of drug-induced lung disease. *Clin Radiol* 1992;46:232–236.

75. Pietra GG. Pathologic mechanisms of drug-induced lung disorders. *J Thorac Imaging* 1991;6(1):1–7.

76. Kuhlman JE, Teigen C, Ren H, Hurban RH, Hutchins GM, Fishman EK. Amiodarone pulmonary toxicity: CT findings in symptomatic patients. *Radiology* 1990;177:121–125.

77. Rimmer MJ, Dixon AK, Flower CD, Sikora K. Bleomycin lung: computed tomographic observations. *Br J Radiol* 1985; 58:1041–1045.

78. Kuhlman JE. The role of chest computed tomography in the diagnosis of drug-related reactions. *J Thorac Imaging* 1991; 6(1):52–61.

79. Rosenow EC, Myers JL, Swensen SJ, Pisani RJ. Drug-induced pulmonary disease: an update. *Chest* 1992;102:239–250.

80. Searles G, McKendry RJR. Methotrexate pneumonitis in rheumatoid arthritis: potential risk factors. four case reports and a review of the literature. *J Rheumatol* 1987;14:1164–1171.

81. Geddes DM, Corrin B, Brewerton DA, Davies RJ, Turner-Warwick M. Progressive airway obliteration in adults and its association with rheumatoid disease. *Q J Med* 1977;46:427–444.

82. Aquino SL, Webb WR, Golden J. Bronchiolitis obliterans associated with rheumatoid arthritis: findings on HRCT and dynamic expiratory CT. *J Comput Assist Tomogr* 1994;18: 555–558.

83. Morrish WF, Herman SJ, Weisbrod GL, Chamberlain DW. Bronchiolitis obliterans after lung transplantation: findings at chest radiography and high-resolution CT. *Radiology* 1991;179: 487–490.

84. Davis SD, Yankelevitz DF, Henschke CI. Radiation effects on the lung: clinical features, pathology, and imaging findings. *AJR* 1992;159:1157–1164.

85. Libshitz HI. Radiation changes in the lung. *Semin Roentgenol* 1993;28:303–320.

86. Maasilta P. Radiation-induced lung injury: from the chest physician's point of view. *Lung Cancer* 1991;7:367–384.

87. Gross NJ. The pathogenesis of radiation-induced lung damage. *Lung* 1981;159:115–125.

88. Libshitz HI, Shuman LS. Radiation-induced pulmonary change: CT findings. *J Comput Assist Tomogr* 1984;8:15–19.

89. Ikezoe J, Takashima S, Morimoto S, et al. CT appearance of acute radiation-induced injury in the lung. *AJR* 1988;150: 765–770.

90. Mah K, Poon PY, Van DJ, Keane T, Majesky IF, Rideout DF. Assessment of acute radiation-induced pulmonary changes using computed tomography. *J Comput Assist Tomogr* 1986; 10:736–743.

91. Bell J, McGivern D, Bullimore J, Hill J, Davies ER, Goddard P. Diagnostic imaging of post-irradiation changes in the chest. *Clin Radiol* 1988;39:109–119.

92. Ikezoe J, Morimoto S, Takashima S, Takeuchi N, Arisawa J, Kozuka T. Acute radiation-induced pulmonary injury: computed tomographic evaluation. *Semin Ultrasound CT MR* 1990; 11:409–416.

93. Bourgouin P, Cousineau G, Lemire P, Delvecchio P, Hebert G. Differentiation of radiation-induced fibrosis from recurrent pulmonary neoplasm by CT. *Can Assoc Radiol J* 1987;38: 23–26.

94. Becklake MR. Asbestos-related diseases of the lungs and pleura: current clinical issues. *Am Rev Respir Dis* 1982;126: 187–194.

95. Staples CA. Computed tomography in the evaluation of benign asbestos-related disorders. *Radiol Clin North Am* 1992;30: 1191–1207.

96. Kagan E. Current issues regarding the pathobiology of asbestosis: a chronologic perspective. *J Thorac Imaging* 1988;3(4):1–9.

97. Aberle DR, Gamsu G, Ray CS, Feuerstein IM. Asbestos-related pleural and parenchymal fibrosis: detection with high-resolution CT. *Radiology* 1988;166:729–734.

98. Akira M, Yamamoto S, Yokoyama K, et al. Asbestosis: high-resolution CT-pathologic correlation. *Radiology* 1990;176: 389–394.

99. Craighead JE, Abraham JL, Churg A, et al. The pathology of asbestos-associated disease of the lungs and pleural cavities: diagnostic criteria and proposed grading schema. *Arch Pathol Lab Med* 1982;106:544–596.

100. Bégin R, Ostiguy G, Filion R, Groleau S. Recent advances in the early diagnosis of asbestosis. *Semin Roentgenol* 1992;27: 121–139.

101. Aberle DR, Gamsu G, Ray CS. High-resolution CT of benign asbestos-related diseases: clinical and radiographic correlation. *AJR* 1988;151:883–891.

102. Schwartz A, Rockoff SD, Christiani D, Hyde J. A clinical diagnostic model for the assessment of asbestosis: a new algorithmic approach. *J Thorac Imaging* 1988;3:29–35.

103. McLoud TC. The use of CT in the examination of asbestos-exposed persons [Editorial]. *Radiology* 1988;169:862–863.

104. American Thoracic Society. The diagnosis of nonmalignant diseases related to asbestos. *Am Rev Repir Dis* 1986;134:363–368.

105. Gaensler EA, Jederlinic PJ, Churg A. Idiopathic pulmonary fibrosis in asbestos-exposed workers (see comments). *Am Rev Respir Dis* 1991;144:477–478.

106. Klaas VE. A diagnostic approach to asbestosis, utilizing clinical criteria, high resolution computed tomography, and gallium scan. *Am J Ind Med* 1993;23:801–809.

107. Gefter WB, Conant EF. Issues and controversies in the plain-film diagnosis of asbestos-related disorders in the chest. *J Thorac Imaging* 1988;3:11–28.

108. Rockoff SD, Schwartz A. Roentgenographic underestimation of early asbestosis by International Labor Organization classification: analysis of data and probabilities. *Chest* 1988;93: 1088–1091.

109. Staples CA, Gamsu G, Ray CS, Webb WR. High resolution computed tomography and lung function in asbestos-exposed workers with normal chest radiographs. *Am Rev Respir Dis* 1989;139:1502–1508.

110. Kipen HM, Lilis R, Suzuki Y, Valciukas JA, Selikoff IJ. Pulmonary fibrosis in asbestos insulation workers with lung cancer: a radiological and histopathological evaluation. *Br J Ind Med* 1987;44:96–100.

111. Friedman AC, Fiel SB, Fisher MS, Radecki PD, Lev-Toaff AS, Caroline DF. Asbestos-related pleural disease and asbestosis: a comparison of CT and chest radiography. *AJR* 1988;150: 268–275.

112. Epstein DM, Miller WT, Bresnitz EA, Levine MS, Gefter WB. Application of ILO classification to a population without industrial exposure: findings to be differentiated from pneumoconiosis. *AJR* 1984;142:53–58.

113. Blanc PD, Gamsu G. The effect of cigarette smoking on the detection of small radiographic opacities in inorganic dust diseases. *J Thorac Imaging* 1988;3:51–56.

114. Gamsu G, Aberle DR, Lynch D. Computed tomography in the diagnosis of asbestos-related thoracic disease. *J Thorac Imaging* 1989;4:61–67.

115. Friedman AC, Fiel SB, Radecki PD, Lev-Toaff AS. Computed tomography of benign pleural and pulmonary parenchymal abnormalities related to asbestos exposure. *Semin Ultrasound CT MR* 1990;11:393–408.

116. Murray K, Gamsu G, Webb WR, Salmon CJ, Egger MJ. High-resolution CT sampling for detection of asbestos-related lung disease. *Acad Radiol* 1995;2:111–115.

117. Aberle DR, Balmes JR. Computed tomography of asbestos-related pulmonary parenchymal and pleural diseases. *Clin Chest Med* 1991;12:115–131.

118. Aberle DR. High-resolution computed tomography of asbestos-related diseases. *Semin Roentgenol* 1991;26:118–131.

119. Akira M, Yokoyama K, Yamamoto S, et al. Early asbestosis: evaluation with high-resolution CT. *Radiology* 1991;178: 409–416.

120. Gamsu G, Salmon CJ, Warnock ML, Blanc PD. CT quantification of interstitial fibrosis in patients with asbestosis: a comparison of two methods. *AJR* 1995;164:63–68.

121. Primack SL, Hartman TE, Hansell DM, Müller NL. End-stage lung disease: CT findings in 61 patients. *Radiology* 1993;189: 681–686.

122. Al-Jarad N, Strickland B, Pearson MC, Rubens MB, Rudd RM. High-resolution computed tomographic assessment of asbesto-

sis and cryptogenic fibrosing alveolitis: a comparative study. *Thorax* 1992;47:645–650.

123. Lynch DA, Gamsu G, Ray CS, Aberle DR. Asbestos-related focal lung masses: manifestations on conventional and high-resolution CT scans. *Radiology* 1988;169:603–607.

124. Yoshimura H, Hatakeyama M, Otsuji H, et al. Pulmonary asbestosis: CT study of subpleural curvilinear shadow. work in progress. *Radiology* 1986;158:653–658.

125. Al-Jarad N, Wilkinson P, Pearson MC, Rudd RM. A new high resolution computed tomography scoring system for pulmonary fibrosis, pleural disease, and emphysema in patients with asbestos related disease. *Br J Ind Med* 1992;49:73–84.

126. Dujic Z, Tocilj J, Saric M. Early detection of interstitial lung disease in asbestos exposed non-smoking workers by mid-expiratory flow rate and high resolution computed tomography. *Br J Ind Med* 1991;48:663–664.

127. Hillerdal G. Rounded atelectasis: clinical experience with 74 patients. *Chest* 1989;95:836–941.

128. McHugh K, Blaquiere RM. CT features of rounded atelectasis. *AJR* 1989;153:257–260.

129. Taylor PM. Dynamic contrast enhancement of asbestos-related pulmonary pseudotumours. *Br J Radiol* 1988;61:1070–1072.

130. Westcott JL, Hallisey MJ, Volpe JP. Dynamic CT of round atelectasis. *Radiology* 1991;181(P):182.

131. Swensen SJ, Morin RL, Schueler BA, et al. Solitary pulmonary nodule: CT evaluation of enhancement with iodinated contrast material—a preliminary report. *Radiology* 1992;182:343–347.

132. Epler GR, McLoud TC, Gaensler EA. Prevalence and incidence of benign asbestos pleural effusion in a working population. *JAMA* 1982;247:617–622.

133. McLoud TC, Woods BO, Carrington CB, Epler GR, Gaensler EA. Diffuse pleural thickening in an asbestos-exposed population: prevalence and causes. *AJR* 1985;144:9–18.

134. Im JG, Webb WR, Rosen A, Gamsu G. Costal pleura: appearances at high-resolution CT. *Radiology* 1989;171:125–131.

135. Hillerdal G, Malmberg P, Hemmingsson A. Asbestos-related lesions of the pleura: parietal plaques compared to diffuse thickening studied with chest roentgenography, computed tomography, lung function, and gas exchange. *Am J Ind Med* 1990;18:627–639.

136. Schwartz DA, Galvin JR, Dayton CS, Stanford W, Merchant JA, Hunninghake GW. Determinants of restrictive lung function in asbestos-induced pleural fibrosis. *J Appl Physiol* 1990; 68:1932–1937.

137. Ren H, Lee DR, Hruban RH, et al. Pleural plaques do not predict asbestosis: high-resolution computed tomography and pathology study. *Mod Pathol* 1991;4:201–209.

138. Al-Jarad N, Poulakis N, Pearson MC, Rubens MB, Rudd RM. Assessment of asbestos-induced pleural disease by computed tomography—correlation with chest radiograph and lung function. *Respir Med* 1991;85:203–208.

139. Ameille J, Brochard P, Brechot JM, et al. Pleural thickening: a comparison of oblique chest radiographs and high-resolution computed tomography in subjects exposed to low levels of asbestos pollution. *Int Arch Occup Environ Health* 1993;64: 545–548.

140. Rappaport DC, Weisbrod GL, Herman SJ, Chamberlain DW. Pulmonary lymphangioleiomyomatosis: high-resolution CT findings in four cases. *AJR* 1989;152:961–964.

141. Sherrier RH, Chiles C, Roggli V. Pulmonary lymphangioleiomyomatosis: CT findings. *AJR* 1989;153:937–940.

142. Remy-Jardin M, Degreef JM, Beuscart R, Voisin C, Remy J. Coal worker's pneumoconiosis: CT assessment in exposed workers and correlation with radiographic findings. *Radiology* 1990;177:363–371.

143. Im J-G, Webb WR, Han MC, Park JH. Apical opacity associated with pulmonary tuberculosis: high-resolution CT findings. *Radiology* 1991;178:727–731.

144. Vix VA. Extrapleural costal fat. *Radiology* 1974;112:563–565.

145. Sargent EN, Boswell WD, Ralls PW, Markovitz A. Subpleural fat pads in patients exposed to asbestos: distinction from non-calcified pleural plaques. *Radiology* 1984;152:273–277.

146. Remy-Jardin M, Beuscart R, Sault MC, Marquette CH, Remy J. Subpleural micronodules in diffuse infiltrative lung diseases: evaluation with thin-section CT scans. *Radiology* 1990;177: 133–139.

147. Hogg JC. Benjamin Felson lecture. Chronic interstitial lung disease of unknown cause: a new classification based on pathogenesis. *AJR* 1991;156:225–233.

148. Genereux GP. The end-stage lung: pathogenesis, pathology, and radiology. *Radiology* 1975;116:279–289.

149. Snider GL. Interstitial pulmonary fibrosis. *Chest* 1986; 89(Suppl):115–121.

150. Fulmer JD, Crystal RG. Interstitial lung disease. *Curr Pulmonol* 1979;1:1–65.

151. Gaensler EA, Carrington CB. Open biopsy for chronic diffuse infiltrative lung disease: clinical, roentgenographic, and physiologic correlations in 502 patients. *Ann Thorac Surg* 1980;30: 411–426.

FIVE

Diseases Characterized Primarily by Nodular or Reticulonodular Opacities

On plain radiographs, the finding of "reticulonodular" opacities is quite nonspecific and its correlation with histology is often poor (1). This radiographic pattern can reflect the presence of true nodules occurring in association with reticular interstitial thickening or the radiographic summation of purely nodular or purely reticular opacities (2–4).

Because the presence of pulmonary nodules can be of great value in differential diagnosis, it is important to distinguish between true nodular disease and disease that merely appears nodular on chest radiographs. On HRCT, the presence of small nodules can be accurately diagnosed, even in patients with extensive associated reticular opacities. Thus the presence of nodular or reticulonodular interstitial disease can be much more precisely defined using HRCT than is possible on plain films. Furthermore, because of the absence of summation artifacts, the presence, size, and number of small nodular opacities can be more accurately assessed using HRCT than with chest radiographs (3–7).

Diseases in which HRCT can identify the presence of small nodules include neoplastic processes such as lymphangitic spread of carcinoma, hematogenous metastases, bronchioloalveolar carcinoma, and Kaposi's sarcoma; sarcoidosis; silicosis and coal worker's pneumoconiosis; and mycobacterial and fungal infections. In patients with lymphangitic spread of carcinoma and sarcoidosis, nodules are often associated with reticular opacities, whereas with the other entities nodules usually predominate.

PULMONARY LYMPHANGITIC CARCINOMATOSIS

Pulmonary lymphangitic carcinomatosis (PLC) is a term that refers to tumor growth in the lymphatic sys-

tem of the lungs. It occurs most commonly in patients with carcinomas of the breast, lung, stomach, pancreas, prostate, cervix, or thyroid, and in patients with metastatic adenocarcinoma from an unknown primary site (8,9). PLC usually results from hematogenous spread to lung, with subsequent interstitial and lymphatic invasion, but can also occur because of direct lymphatic spread of tumor from mediastinal and hilar lymph nodes (9). Symptoms of shortness of breath are common and can predate radiographic abnormalities.

The radiographic manifestations of pulmonary lymphangitic carcinomatosis include reticular opacities, septal lines, hilar and mediastinal lymphadenopathy, and pleural effusion (5,10). However, these findings are nonspecific. In one study, an accurate chest radiographic diagnosis was made in only 20 of 87 (23%) patients with PLC (11). Furthermore, in about 50% of cases of pathologically proven PLC, the chest radiograph is normal (11,12).

The pulmonary lymphatics, involved in patients with PLC, are located in the axial interstitial compartment (the peribronchovascular and centrilobular interstitium) and in the peripheral interstitial compartment (within the interlobular septa and in the subpleural regions) (1). Tumor growth in the lymphatics located within these compartments, and associated edema, result in the characteristic HRCT findings of PLC (13,14). As discussed in Chapter 3, this distribution of abnormalities has been termed *lymphatic* or *perilymphatic* (15,16).

HRCT Findings

Pulmonary lymphangitic carcinomatosis is characterized on HRCT by reticular opacities, which sometimes have a nodular appearance (Figs. 3-11,3-47,3-48,5-1,5-2). Specific findings include:

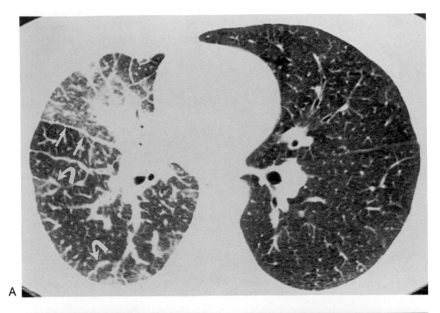

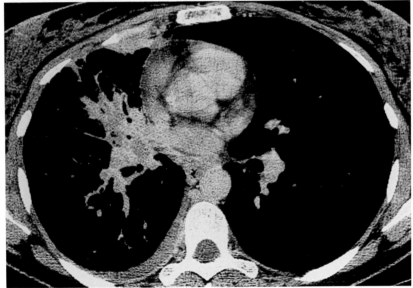

FIG. 5-1. Septal thickening in unilateral lymphangitic carcinomatosis. **A:** HRCT at a lung window setting in a 44-year-old woman with adenocarcinoma, demonstrates thickening of the interlobular septa (*curved arrows*) and major fissure (*straight arrows*), which is both smooth and nodular or "beaded." Intralobular vessels appear abnormally prominent because of centrilobular interstitial thickening. There is also parahilar peribronchovascular interstitial thickening, as evidenced by apparent thickening of the bronchial wall and increased diameter of the hilar vessels. Note that even though there is septal thickening, there is no distortion of pulmonary architecture, as would be typical of pulmonary fibrosis. **B:** A mediastinal window setting demonstrates nodular thickening of the right peribronchovascular interstitium, right anterior pleural thickening, and a small right pleural effusion.

1. Thickening of the peribronchovascular interstitium surrounding vessels and bronchi in the parahilar lung,
2. Interlobular septal thickening and subpleural interstitial thickening that is smooth, or nodular and "beaded,"
3. Thickening of the peribronchovascular axial interstitium in the centrilobular regions, and
4. A preservation of normal lung architecture at the lobular level, despite the presence of these findings (13,14,17–19) (Table 5-1).

Peribronchovascular interstitial thickening or "peribronchial cuffing" is commonly visible on HRCT in the parahilar lung and can be diffuse, focal, or asymmetric (Figs. 5-1–5-4) (13,20,21). The thickened peribronchovascular interstitium may be smooth and concentric,

closely mimicking the appearance of bronchial wall thickening (Fig. 3-4), or it can be nodular (Fig. 3-48) (13); in both instances, the thickened interstitium is sharply marginated from the adjacent aerated lung. In patients with peribronchovascular interstitial thickening from PLC, pulmonary artery branches adjacent to the bronchi also appear larger than normal, and "nodular" (13); in other words, the size relationship of the "thick-walled bronchi" and adjacent vessels is maintained.

Stein et al. (18) performed an extensive analysis of the CT patterns of lymphangitic carcinomatosis and found a localized or diffuse increase in reticular opacities and an increase in the number and thickness of interlobular septa (so-called peripheral lines or peripheral arcades) in all patients with PLC (Figs. 5-1 to 5-4). In patients with PLC, interlobular septal thickening

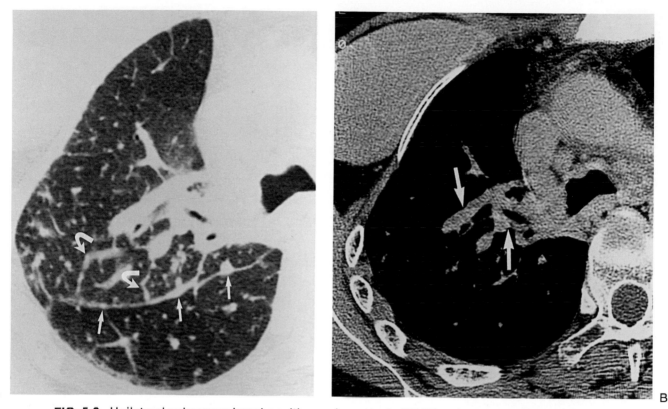

FIG. 5-2. Unilateral pulmonary lymphangitic carcinomatosis. HRCT at the level of the aortic arch in a 44-year-old woman with a previous right mastectomy for adenocarcinoma now presenting with unilateral right pulmonary lymphangitic carcinomatosis. **A:** Lung windows demonstrate nodular thickening of the interlobular septa (*curved arrows*) and interlobar fissure (*straight arrows*). **B:** Mediastinal windows show mediastinal lymphadenopathy and nodular thickening of the central peribronchovascular interstitium (*arrows*). Incidental note is made of right breast implant and right paratracheal lymphadenopathy.

is often most pronounced in the peripheral lung regions. In the study by Stein et al., thickened septa appeared 1 to 2 cm in length, usually contacted the pleural surface, and were more numerous and thicker than similar septa (or "peripheral lines") seen in healthy

---

TABLE 5-1. *HRCT findings in lymphangitic spread of carcinoma*[a,b]

1. ***Smooth or Nodular Peribronchovascular Interstitial Thickening ("Peribronchial Cuffing")***
2. ***Smooth or Nodular Interlobular Septal Thickening***
3. **Smooth or Nodular Thickening of Fissures**
4. ***Normal Lung Architecture; No Distortion***
5. Prominence of Centrilobular Structures
6. Diffuse, Patchy, or Unilateral Distribution
7. Lymph Node Enlargement
8. *Pleural Effusion*

---

[a] Most common findings in boldface.
[b] Findings most helpful in differential diagnosis in italics.

control subjects. In lymphatic spread of carcinoma, the thickened septa often have a "beaded" appearance resulting from tumor growth in the lymphatics, but can also appear smooth in contour, as contrasted with the irregular septal thickening seen in patients with fibrosis (Figs. 3-11,3-47,3-48,5-1–5-3) (13,14). In an HRCT study of postmortem lung specimens, 19 of 22 cases with interstitial pulmonary metastases showed the appearance of beaded or nodular septal thickening. The beaded septa corresponded directly to the presence of tumor growing in pulmonary capillaries, lymphatics, and the septal interstitium (14). Smooth or nodular thickening of the subpleural interstitium is also commonly seen; this is easiest to recognize adjacent to the fissures.

Stein et al. (18) observed septal thickening that outlined distinct pulmonary lobules ("polygonal arcades") in approximately 50% of patients with PLC (Fig. 5-3). These lobules usually contained a visible central branching opacity or dot, representing the intralobular artery branch, or branches, surrounded by the thickened axial interstitium. This appearance is one of the most characteristic HRCT features of PLC

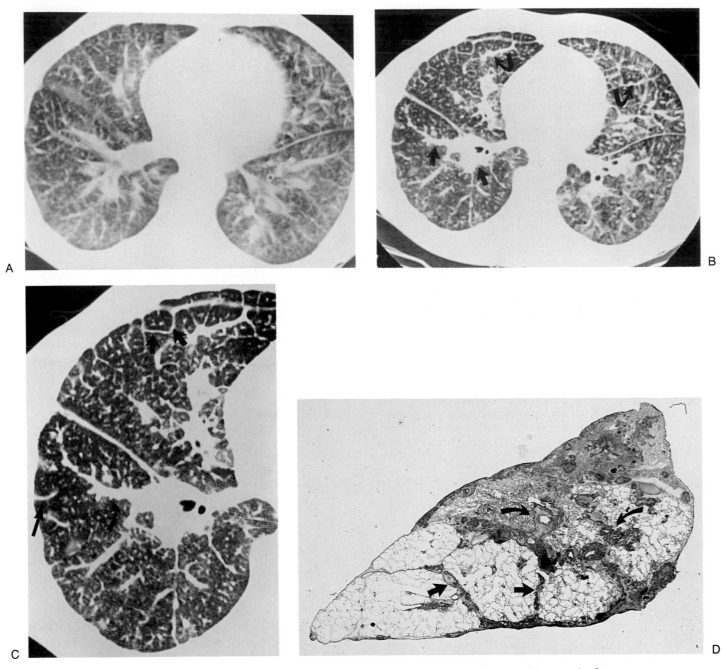

FIG. 5-3. Lymphangitic carcinomatosis and septal thickening in a 52-year-old man. **A:** Conventional 10-mm collimation CT scan shows prominence of the peribronchovascular interstitium and an ill-defined increase in the attenuation of both lungs. The appearance mimics that of congestive heart failure. **B:** A 1.5-mm collimation scan (standard algorithm) at the same level demonstrates numerous "polygonal arcades" representing thickened interlobular septa. In several areas the thickening is nodular (*curved arrows*). Thickening of the peribronchovascular interstitium ("bronchovascular bundles") is also present, particularly on the right side (*straight arrows*). **C:** HRCT (bone algorithm, targeted to right lung) more clearly defines septal thickening (*long arrows*), "polygonal arcades" (*short arrows*), and nodular thickening of the peribronchovascular interstitium (*curved arrow*). The nodular thickening is most suggestive of tumor. **D:** Scanning micrograph of open lung biopsy specimen shows thickening of the interlobular septa (*arrows*) and peribronchovascular interstitium (*curved arrows*) largely due to tumor deposits rather than fibrous tissue or edema. (From Munk et al., ref. 13, with permission.)

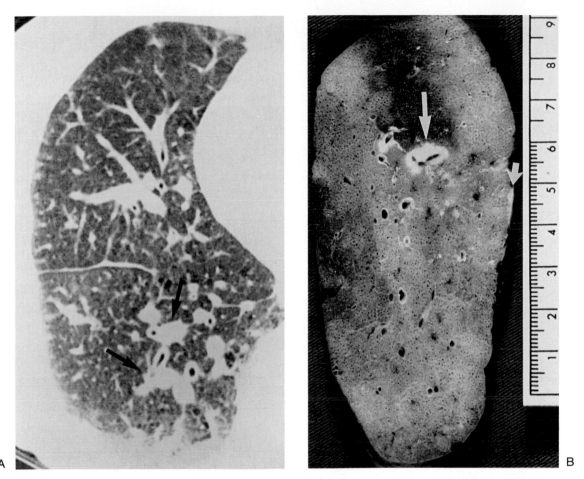

FIG. 5-4. Pulmonary lymphangitic carcinomatosis. **A:** HRCT in a patient with lymphangitic carcinomatosis shows thickening of the peribronchovascular interstitium (*arrows*) and interlobular septa. **B:** Pathologic specimen in a different patient with localized lymphangitic carcinomatosis. Note thickening of the peribronchovascular interstitium (*long arrow*) and subpleural interstitium (*short arrow*) due to lymphatic spread of tumor. (From Munk et al., ref. 13 with permission.)

(13,14,17–19). Prominence of the centrilobular dot (artery) is commonly seen in regions of lung in which septal thickening is seen. In a distinct minority of patients with PLC, the centrilobular interstitial thickening predominates (Fig. 3-31) (22).

Five factors account for thickening of the peribronchovascular interstitium, interlobular septa, and centrilobular axial interstitium that is seen on HRCT in patients with PLC:

1. tumor-filling pulmonary vessels or lymphatics,
2. the presence of tumor within the interstitium,
3. distention of vessels or lymphatic channels distal to central vascular or lymphatic tumor emboli,
4. interstitial pulmonary edema secondary to tumor obstruction of the lymphatics, and
5. interstitial fibrosis secondary to the presence of interstitial tumor or secondary to long-standing interstitial edema (1,5,13,14).

In patients with HRCT findings of PLC, pathologic studies (13,14) have shown that the visible thickening of the interlobular septa and peribronchovascular interstitium was caused mainly by interstitial tumor growth, rather than by vascular distension, edema, or fibrosis, although these abnormalities were also present (13,14).

In approximately 50% of patients, the abnormalities of PLC appear focal or unilateral rather than diffuse. Focal disease may involve mainly or exclusively the axial interstitium, leading to thickening of the bronchovascular bundles or it may involve mainly the peripheral interstitium leading to thickening of the interlobular septa (21).

It is characteristic of PLC that lung architecture appears normal despite the presence of abnormal reticular opacities; pulmonary lobules surrounded by thick septa are easily identified because the lobules appear normal in size and shape. There is no distortion of lobular size or dimensions in PLC as is typically seen in patients with interstitial fibrosis. The importance of this finding cannot be overemphasized; if there is lung distortion associated with findings that would otherwise be typical of PLC, another diagnosis should be considered.

Hilar lymphadenopathy is visible on CT in only 50% of patients with PLC, supporting the supposition that PLC is often the result of hematogenous spread of tumor to the interstitium rather than central lymphatic obstruction with retrograde spread of tumor or edema (18). In a study by Grenier et al. (23), lymphadenopathy was visible in 38% to 54% of patients with lymphangitic carcinomatosis. Mediastinal lymph node enlargement can also be seen. Lymph node enlargement can be symmetrical or asymmetrical. Pleural effusion may also be present.

Utility of HRCT

In patients with PLC, characteristic HRCT findings can be seen in patients with normal chest radiographs. In such cases the HRCT findings tend to be focal and more pronounced in peripheral lung regions not well visualized on chest radiographs (18). Furthermore, conventional CT is not adequate for assessing the lung parenchyma in patients with PLC; findings such as interlobular septal thickening, which are characteristic of PLC, are not often visible on scans obtained with 10-mm collimation (Fig. 5-3) (13,18).

In a patient with a known tumor, who has symptoms of dyspnea, HRCT findings typical of PLC are usually considered diagnostic, and in clinical practice a lung biopsy is usually not performed. In patients without a known neoplasm, HRCT can be helpful in directing lung biopsy to the most productive sites, as PLC is often focal (13). Also, since transbronchial biopsy is usually positive in PLC, typical HRCT findings can also serve to suggest this as the most appropriate procedure.

Differential Diagnosis

Although, peribronchovascular interstitial thickening and smooth septal thickening, as are often seen in patients with PLC, can also be seen in association with pulmonary edema, the differentiation of these entities can usually be made on clinical grounds. Nodular or beaded interstitial thickening is characteristic of PLC, but not pulmonary edema. In the study by Ren et al. (14), nodular septal thickening was not noted in any pathologic specimens of patients with pulmonary edema, fibrosis, or in normal lungs.

However, it is clear that the presence of nodular septal thickening is a nonspecific finding that reflects a perilymphatic distribution of abnormalities, also commonly seen in patients with sarcoidosis (13,14) and coal worker's pneumoconiosis or silicosis (7). In sarcoidosis and coal worker's pneumoconiosis, although nod-

ules are commonly seen, the septal thickening is usually less extensive than that seen in patients with lymphatic spread of tumor. Moreover, in sarcoidosis and coal worker's pneumoconiosis (CWP), distortion of lung architecture and secondary pulmonary lobular anatomy is common, particularly if septal thickening is present; this distortion is not seen in patients with PLC (24). On the other hand, the presence of pleural effusion would be more in keeping with PLC than sarcoidosis or silicosis. The differentiation of PLC, sarcoidosis, and silicosis and CWP are discussed in greater detail in the discussion of sarcoidosis, below.

In pulmonary fibrosis, nodular septal thickening is uncommon, and the margins of the thickened interlobular septa are irregular. Distortion of the lung architecture and lung destruction (honeycombing) are common in patients with fibrosis (19,25).

HEMATOGENOUS METASTASES

In many patients, hematogenous tumor metastases to the lung results in the presence of localized tumor nodules rather than interstitial invasion, as occurs in PLC. Hematogenous metastases typically result in multiple, large, well-defined nodules; in patients with this appearance, plain radiographic diagnosis is not difficult. In some patients, however, widespread hematogenous metastasis is associated with the presence of numerous small nodules, mimicking the appearance of a diffuse interstitial disease on chest radiographs. In such patients, HRCT may be obtained to define the "lung disease" that is present, and may be valuable in suggesting the correct diagnosis.

HRCT Findings

In patients with hematogenous metastases, HRCT typically shows small discrete nodules that have a peripheral and basal predominance when limited in number (9); in patients who have innumerable metastases, a uniform distribution throughout the lung can be seen (Fig. 5-5) (Table 5-2) (26). Typically, hematogenous

---

TABLE 5-2. *HRCT findings in hematogenous metastases*[a,b]

1. ***Smooth, Well-defined Nodules with a Random and Uniform Distribution***
2. ***Some Nodules Visible in Relation to Vessels or Pleural Surfaces***
3. **Features of Lymphangitic Spread of Carcinoma May Be Present**

[a] Most common findings in boldface.
[b] Findings most helpful in differential diagnosis in boldface italics.

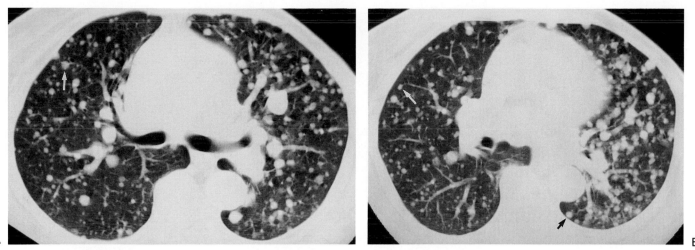

FIG. 5-5. A,B: Hematogenous metastases. The nodules are sharply defined. Although some nodules (*arrows*) appear to be related to small vascular branches, most nodules lack a specific relationship to lobular structures and appear to be random in distribution. Subpleural nodules are visible. Septal thickening is absent.

metastases lack the specific relationship to lobular structures and interlobular septa that is seen in patients with PLC. Nodules tend to appear evenly distributed with respect to lobular anatomy, or "random" in distribution. Some nodules, however, may be seen to be related to small branches of pulmonary vessels, and this finding can be helpful in diagnosis. Although, interlobular septal thickening, and peribronchovascular interstitial thickening, common findings in PLC, are typically lacking, some overlap between the appearances of PLC and hematogenous metastases is not uncommon.

To elucidate the HRCT characteristics of pulmonary metastatic nodules, Murata et al. (26) compared HRCT and pathology in 5 lungs obtained at autopsy from patients with metastatic neoplasms. The relationship of metastatic nodules to lobular structures was studied using HRCT, specimen radiographs, and stereomicroscopy. Nodules were widely distributed throughout pulmonary lobules as seen on HRCT, and no predominance in specific lobular regions was noted. Eleven percent of small nodules (less than 3 mm in diameter) appeared centrilobular, 68% were intralobular, and 21% were seen in relation to interlobular septa.

Utility of CT and HRCT

Although HRCT may be used in order to characterize the distribution and morphology of lung nodules visible on chest radiographs in patients with hematogenous pulmonary metastases, conventional CT techniques, with contiguous thick slices, are of more value in detecting pulmonary metastases in patients with normal chest films (9). Furthermore, conventional CT is clearly more sensitive than plain radiographs in detecting lung metastases (9). In one study (27), plain radiographs, CT, and surgery were compared as to the number of nodules detected in 100 lungs from 84 patients with previously treated extrathoracic malignancies who showed new lung nodules. Of 237 nodules resected, 173 (73%) were identified with CT. Chest radiography disclosed all resected nodules in 44% of cases, whereas CT disclosed all nodules in 78%. Two hundred seven (87%) of the resected nodules were of metastatic origin, 21 (9%) were benign, and nine (4%) were bronchogenic carcinomas. Of those nodules seen with CT and not with radiography of the chest, 84% were of metastatic origin.

BRONCHIOLOALVEOLAR CARCINOMA

Bronchioloalveolar carcinoma (BAC) can present as a solitary nodule or mass (43% of patients), as an area of focal or diffuse consolidation (30%), or as a diffuse abnormality characterized by ill-defined nodules (27%) (28). Solitary nodules have a typical spiculated appearance, and may contain air-bronchograms or cystic lucencies (29).

Areas of consolidation associated with BAC can represent the presence of intra-alveolar tumor growth and mucin and fluid produced by the tumor; air-bronchograms are commonly visible (29,30). Also, because fluid and mucus produced by the tumor is of low attenuation, if CT is performed with contrast infusion, the "CT angiogram sign" can be seen; the "CT angiogram sign" is said to be present if contrast-enhanced pulmonary vessels appear denser than surrounding opacified lung. In a study by Im et al. (31), the CT scans of 12

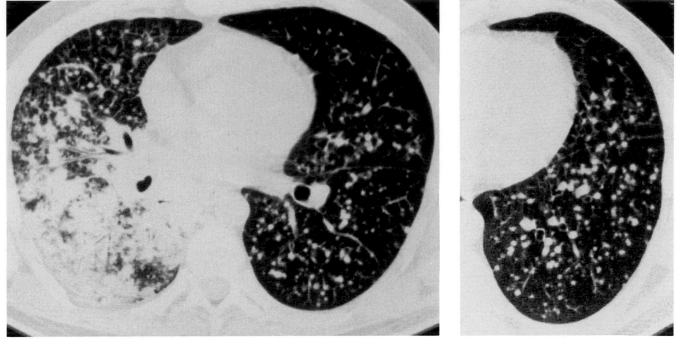

A   B

FIG. 5-6. Bronchioloalveolar carcinoma in a 34-year-old man. **A:** HRCT demonstrates areas of consolidation in the right lower lobe, ill-defined nodules, some of which appear to be centrilobular, and multiple, small, well-defined nodules. **B:** Targeted view of the left lung shows numerous small nodules, particularly in the left lower lobe. At least some of these nodules show a random distribution, similar to hematogenous metastases. Note the presence of subpleural nodules.

patients with lobar or segmental BAC were reviewed; the CT angiogram sign was seen in nearly all. Although this sign can be seen in association with other consolidative processes, and is dependent on the volume of

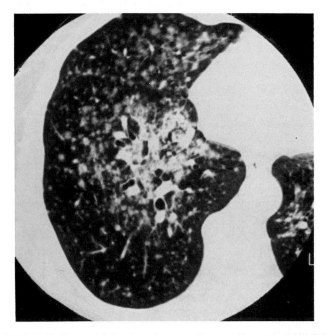

FIG. 5-7. Bronchioloalveolar carcinoma. Targeted HRCT image through the right lung. Ill-defined nodules are visible throughout the lung, and most appear centrilobular in location. Transbronchial biopsy was diagnostic.

contrast infused, in this study, its specificity was 92% in diagnosing BAC (31).

Patients with diffuse lung involvement from BAC can show (i) patchy areas of consolidation that are peribronchovascular and contain air-bronchograms or air-filled cystic spaces (Fig. 5-6) (32), (ii) extensive centrilobular air-space nodules (Figs. 5-6,5-7), or (iii) diffuse small nodules mimicking the appearance of hematogenous metastases (Fig. 5-6) (Table 5-3) (29).

CT can play a crucial role in the initial evaluation of patients with BAC, who appear to have limited and potentially resectable lesions, based on their plain radiographic appearance. CT can show the presence of diffuse disease, when unrecognizable on plain films,

TABLE 5-3. *HRCT findings in bronchioloalveolar carcinoma[a,b]*

1. ***Diffuse, Patchy, or Multifocal Consolidation***
2. **CT Angiogram Sign on Enhanced Scan**
3. ***Ill-defined Centrilobular Nodules***
4. ***Combination of 1 and 3.***
5. **Features of Hematogenous Metastases**

[a] Most common findings in boldface.
[b] Findings most helpful in differential diagnosis in boldface italics.

indicating unresectability (33). However, as pointed out by Zwirewich and other (34), CT is only 65% sensitive in detecting multiple adenocarcinomas.

KAPOSI'S SARCOMA

Approximately 15% to 20% of patients with AIDS develop Kaposi's sarcoma (KS). KS is much more common among subjects who acquire AIDS through sexual contact; almost all cases occur in homosexual or bisexual men, and KS in intravenous-drug users or hemophiliacs is less frequent (35).

Pulmonary involvement occurs in about 20% of AIDS patients with KS. Chest radiographs typically show bilateral and diffuse abnormalities characterized by the presence of interstitial opacities that are predominantly peribronchovascular, poorly defined nodules which can be several centimeters in diameter, and ill-defined areas of consolidation (35). Pleural effusions, which are usually bilateral, are seen in 30% of cases. Hilar or mediastinal lymph node enlargement is apparent on the chest radiograph in approximately 10% of patients.

CT and HRCT Findings

Pathologically, pulmonary involvement in KS is patchy, but has a distinct relationship to vessels and bronchi in the parahilar regions (35). Typical CT features of KS include irregular and ill-defined nodules that often predominate in the peribronchovascular regions, peribronchovascular interstitial thickening, interlobular septal thickening, pleural effusion, and lymphadenopathy (Figs. 5-8,5-9) (Table 5-4) (36).

TABLE 5-4. *HRCT findings in Kaposi's sarcoma[a,b]*

1. ***Irregular and Ill-defined Peribronchovascular Nodules***
2. ***Peribronchovascular Interstitial Thickening***
3. **Interlobular Septal Thickening**
4. **Pleural Effusions**
5. **Lymphadenopathy**

[a] Most common findings in boldface.
[b] Findings most helpful in differential diagnosis in boldface italics.

In a comparison study (37) of radiographs and CT in 24 patients with intrathoracic KS, 22 (92%) of 24 had radiographic findings of bilateral parahilar opacities. CT scans, obtained in 16 patients, confirmed the presence of parahilar opacities in 14 (88%), with extension into the lung parenchyma along the peribronchovascular interstitium (Figs. 5-8,5-9). In a separate CT study of 13 patients with KS (38), all had multiple "flame-shaped" or nodular lesions with ill-defined margins, which were usually symmetric (11 of 13) and peribronchovascular and parahilar in distribution (9 of 13). Ten also had pleural effusion, which was bilateral in 9. Five had mediastinal adenopathy, and 2 had hilar adenopathy. In a study by Hartman et al. (36) of 26 patients with KS, the most common CT findings included nodules (85%), a peribronchovascular distribution of disease (81%), lymphadenopathy (50%), interlobular septal thickening (38%), consolidation (35%) or ground-glass opacity (23%), and pleural effusion (35%).

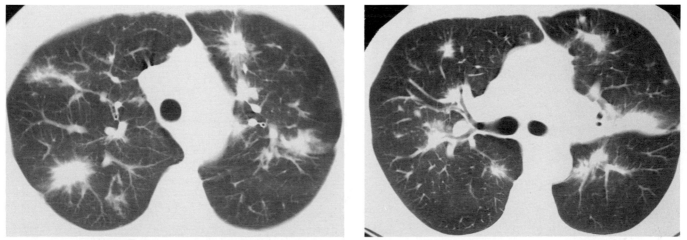

FIG. 5-8. Kaposi's sarcoma. CT in an AIDS patient with KS shows typical findings of ill-defined and irregular or "flame-shaped" nodules occurring predominantly in the parahilar and peribronchovascular regions. Several nodules surround bronchi or contain air-bronchograms. There is also evidence of peribronchovascular interstitial thickening.

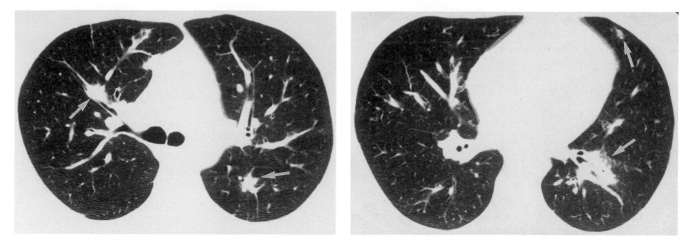

FIG. 5-9. Kaposi's sarcoma. HRCT in an AIDS patient with KS shows ill-defined nodules (*arrows*) in the parahilar and peribronchovascular regions. This appearance and distribution is typical of KS.

Utility of HRCT

In most patients, the presence of typical nodules on CT and a parahilar distribution of abnormalities allow KS to be distinguished from other thoracic complications of AIDS. In the study by Hartman et al. (36), which included 102 patients with thoracic complications of AIDS, the accuracy of CT in diagnosing KS was assessed in a blinded fashion. In patients with KS, this diagnosis was listed first in 83% of cases, and was listed among the top three choices in 92% (36). However, a number of other diseases in AIDS patients can be associated with the presence of pulmonary nodules, including lymphoma (Fig. 5-10), bronchogenic carcinoma, *Pneumocystis carinii* pneumonia, tuberculosis, nontuberculous mycobacterial infection, bacterial, fungal, or viral infections (36,39).

SARCOIDOSIS

Sarcoidosis is a systemic disorder of unknown cause, characterized by the presence of noncaseating granulomas. These may resolve spontaneously or progress to fibrosis (40). Sarcoidosis may involve almost any organ, but most morbidity and mortality is the result of pulmonary disease (41). Pulmonary manifestations are present in 90% of patients, 20% to 25% of whom have permanent functional impairment (41).

Pathologically, the most characteristic feature of sarcoidosis is the presence of noncaseating granulomas in a lymphatic or perilymphatic distribution (15). The granulomas are well formed, with histiocytes centrally, surrounded by a collarette of lymphocytes and mononuclear cells (40,42). Although some investigators believe that alveolitis is the initial pathologic lesion in

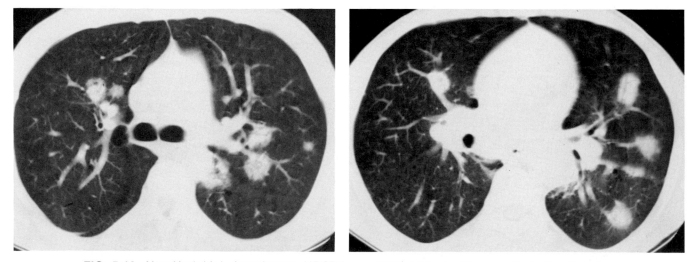

FIG. 5-10. Non-Hodgkin's lymphoma. HRCT in an AIDS patient with non-Hodgkin's lymphoma shows ill-defined nodules, many of which are parahilar and peribronchovascular, or contain air-bronchograms. This appearance mimics that of KS.

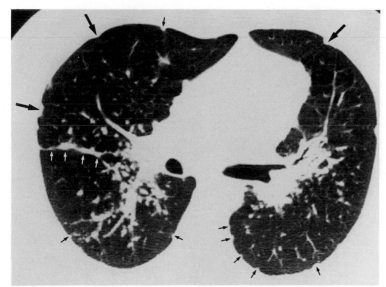

FIG. 5-11. Sarcoidosis with a "perilymphatic" distribution of nodules. Numerous small nodules are seen in relation to the parahilar, bronchovascular interstitium. Bronchial walls appear irregularly thickened. Subpleural nodules (*small arrows*) are seen bordering the costal pleural surfaces and right major fissure. This appearance is virtually diagnostic of sarcoidosis. Clusters of subpleural granulomas (*large arrows*) have been termed pseudoplaques.

sarcoidosis, and that alveolitis is essential to the development of sarcoid granulomas and lung fibrosis in these patients (42–45), this hypothesis is based primarily on indirect evidence from findings on bronchoalveolar lavage and gallium scintigraphy (44,45). The lung parenchyma between granulomas is usually normal in patients with sarcoidosis, and although there may be a mononuclear infiltrate in the alveolar walls immediately adjacent to a granuloma, there is no discernible evidence of a diffuse alveolitis (46).

Approximately 60% to 70% of patients with sarcoidosis have characteristic radiologic findings. These consist of symmetric bilateral hilar and paratracheal lymphadenopathy, with or without concomitant parenchymal abnormalities (47–49). In 25% to 30% of cases, however, the radiologic findings are nonspecific or atypical, and in 5% to 10% of patients, the chest radiograph is normal (40,41,47–51).

Sarcoid granulomas, which are the hallmark of this disease, are distributed primarily along the lymphatics in the peribronchovascular interstitial space (both in the parahilar regions and lobular core), and, to a lesser extent, in the interlobular septa and subpleural interstitial space. This characteristic "perilymphatic" distribution of sarcoid granulomas is difficult to recognize on plain radiographs, but is clearly seen on HRCT (Figs. 3-43,5-11–5-13) and in macroscopic illustrations of the pathology of this disease (16,40,42,52–55). The perilymphatic distribution of granulomas is one of the features of sarcoidosis that is most helpful in making a pathologic diagnosis and is also responsible for the high rate of success of diagnosis by bronchial and transbronchial biopsy (40). Although sarcoid granulomas are microscopic in size, they often coalesce to form macroscopic nodules several millimeters in diameter.

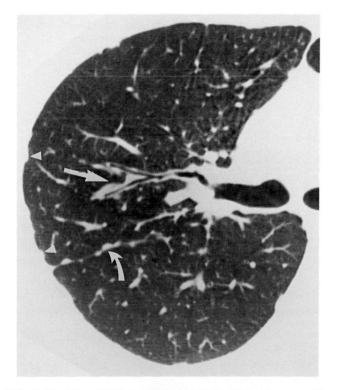

FIG. 5-12. Interstitial nodules in a 41-year-old man with sarcoidosis. HRCT at the level of the right upper-lobe bronchus shows nodular thickening of the peribronchovascular interstitium (*straight arrow*) and right major fissure (*curved arrow*). Also visible are numerous subpleural nodules (*arrowheads*). (From Müller et al., ref. 52, with permission.)

HRCT Findings

The most characteristic HRCT abnormality in patients with sarcoidosis consists of small nodules that are visible:

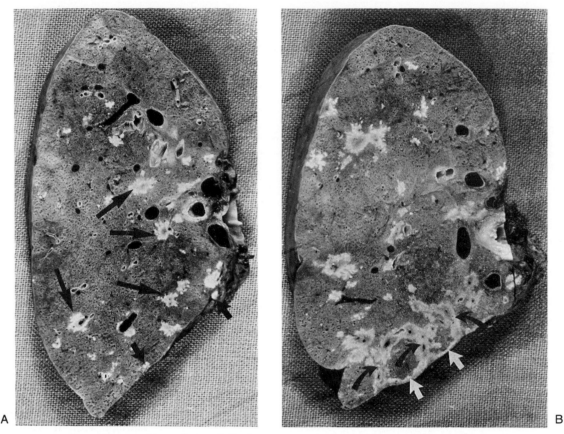

FIG. 5-13. Sarcoidosis with nodules. **A,B:** Gross pathologic specimen, cut in the transverse plane, at two levels through the right upper lobe in a 55-year-old woman with sarcoidosis. Noncaseating sarcoid granulomas are located within the peribronchovascular interstitium (*long arrows*), subpleural regions (*short arrows*), and to a lesser extent in relation to interlobular septa containing veins (*curved arrows*) in B. (From Müller et al., refs. 52 and 53, with permission.)

1. in the peribronchovascular regions, adjacent to the parahilar vessels and bronchi,
2. adjacent to the major fissures,
3. in the costal subpleural regions,
4. within the interlobular septa, and
5. in the centrilobular regions (Figs. 3-43,3-44,5-11,5-12) (24,51,52,55–58) (Table 5-5).

Nodules visible on HRCT can appear as small as a few millimeters in diameter; they tend to be sharply defined despite their small size. In most cases, these nodules represent coalescent groups of microscopic granulomas (Figs. 3-5,3-43,5-13) (57,59), although nodules visible on HRCT can also represent nodular areas of fibrosis (57). The nodules may be numerous and distributed throughout both lungs. However, in up to 50% of patients, the nodularity may be scanty or focal, localized to small areas in one or both lungs (Fig. 5-14). An upper lobe predominance is common.

Sarcoid granulomas frequently cause nodular thickening of the parahilar, peribronchovascular intersti-

TABLE 5-5. *HRCT findings in sarcoidosis[a,b]*
1. ***Smooth or Nodular Peribronchovascular Interstitial Thickening ("Peribronchial Cuffing")***
2. ***Small, Well-defined Nodules in Relation to the Pleural Surfaces, Interlobular Septa, Centrilobular Structures***
3. ***Peribronchovascular Distribution of Nodules in the Central Lung and Upper Lobes***
4. **Large Nodules (>1 cm) or Consolidation**
5. Ground-glass Opacity
6. **Findings of Fibrosis: Septal Thickening, Traction Bronchiectasis,** Honeycombing
7. ***Conglomerate Masses Associated with Bronchiectasis***
8. Patchy Distribution
9. **Lymph Node Enlargement, Usually Symmetrical**
[a] Most common findings in boldface. [b] Findings most helpful in differential diagnosis in boldface italics.

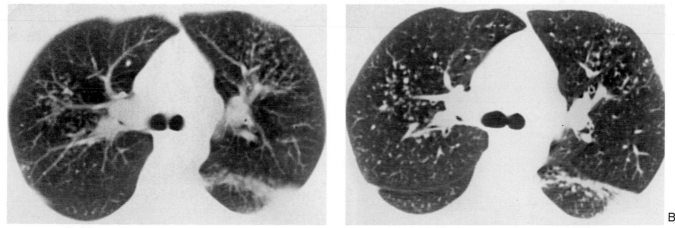

FIG. 5-14. Sarcoidosis in a 28-year-old man. **A:** A 10-mm collimation scan at the level of the tracheal carina shows bilateral hilar lymphadenopathy and nodules in a predominantly peribronchovascular distribution. **B:** A 1.5-mm collimation scan (standard algorithm) at the same level. The peribronchovascular distribution of the nodules is more difficult to appreciate, but the individual nodules are more clearly seen. Note the patchy distribution of the abnormalities. An area of increased attenuation in the superior segment of the left lower lobe is presumably due to conglomeration of subpleural granulomas. (From Müller et al., ref. 52, with permission.)

tium as seen on HRCT, and extensive peribronchovascular nodularity is characteristic and highly suggestive of this disease (Figs. 3-5,5-11,5-12,5-14). Subpleural nodules are also typical of sarcoidosis (16,52). Irregular or nodular interlobular septal thickening is apparent in the majority of patients (Fig. 5-15), but is usually not extensive (51,53). Granulomas in relation to the peribronchovascular interstitium in the lobular core can be seen as centrilobular nodules on HRCT, but these are not usually a predominant feature of sarcoidosis (Fig. 3-43) (22).

Confluence of granulomas may result in large opac-

ities with ill-defined contours, or areas of frank consolidation (Figs. 5-14,5-15). Large nodules, measuring from 1 to 4 centimeter in diameter were seen in 15% to 25% of patients in several studies (Figs. 3-45,3-52) (52,56,59,60). Grenier et al. (61) reported the presence of confluent nodules greater than 1 cm in 53% of patients with sarcoidosis. In our experience these predominate in the upper lobes and the peribronchovascular regions. Air-bronchograms may be seen within these nodules. Large nodules can also cavitate, but this is uncommon; Grenier et al. (61) report this finding in only 3% of cases.

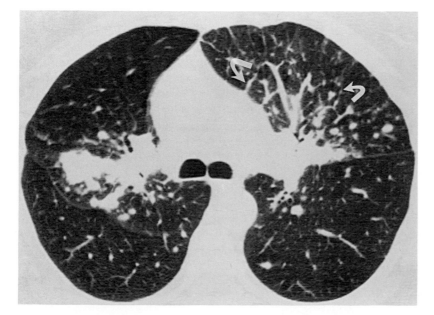

FIG. 5-15. Septal thickening in a 68-year-old woman with sarcoidosis. HRCT at the level of the tracheal carina shows bilateral hilar lymphadenopathy and nodules in a central peribronchovascular distribution. Nodular thickening of the interlobular septa is present, particularly on the left side (*arrows*).

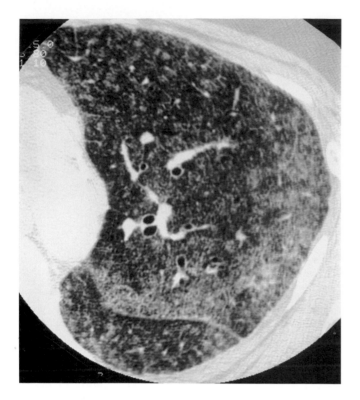

FIG. 5-16. Sarcoidosis with small nodules and ground-glass opacity. Very small nodules are present diffusely. Within the lung periphery, ground-glass opacity likely reflects the presence of confluence of multiple small nodules.

Patients with sarcoidosis sometimes show patchy areas of ground- glass opacity on HRCT (Figs. 5-16–5-18), which may be superimposed on a background of interstitial nodules or fibrosis. One study (57) indicated that areas of ground-glass opacity are associated with disease activity as assessed by ^{67}Ga scintigraphy. Correlation of ground-glass opacity in patients with sarcoidosis with pathologic specimens has been obtained in a small number of patients (52,59,62). The results of these correlations suggest that areas of ground-glass opacity usually are due to the presence of extensive interstitial sarcoid granulomas rather than alveolitis. Leung et al. (62) correlated CT findings with findings in pathologic specimens in 29 patients with chronic infiltrative lung disease. Their study included two patients with sarcoidosis in whom ground-glass opacity was present in an area in which open lung biopsy was performed. At pathologic examination, extensive interstitial sarcoid granulomas were the only finding in one patient, and fine honeycombing and diffuse sarcoid granulomas were found in the other. In neither case was there evidence of alveolitis. The absence of alveolitis in two other patients with sarcoidosis who underwent lobectomy because of concomitant bronchogenic carcinoma, was also reported by Müller et al. (52). Nishimura et al. (59) reviewed the CT and pathologic findings in eight patients with sarcoidosis. The most frequent feature on CT was the presence of small nodules along bronchi, vessels, and subpleural regions and thickening of the bronchovascular bundles. Pathologically these findings were shown to be due to granulomas. Areas of ground-glass opacity were present in six cases (75%). Open lung biopsy in an area of ground-glass opacity was obtained in one of these cases. Histopathologic analysis demonstrated only interstitial granulomas.

In patients with sarcoidosis, who have been followed using HRCT, areas of nodularity, consolidation, and ground-glass opacity tend to decrease over time (Fig. 5-19). Although fibrosis need not occur with healing of granulomatous lesions, findings of fibrosis tend to become more prominent over time. As fibrosis develops, irregular reticular opacities, including irregular septal thickening, often become a prominent feature (Figs. 3-14,5-17,5-18). Reticular opacities, as with the nodules, are frequently seen along the parahilar bronchovascular bundles (52,56,63). The most common early HRCT finding of fibrosis with lung distortion is posterior displacement of the main and upper lobe bronchi (Figs. 3-53,5-18); this finding indicates loss of volume in the posterior segments of the upper lobes (24).

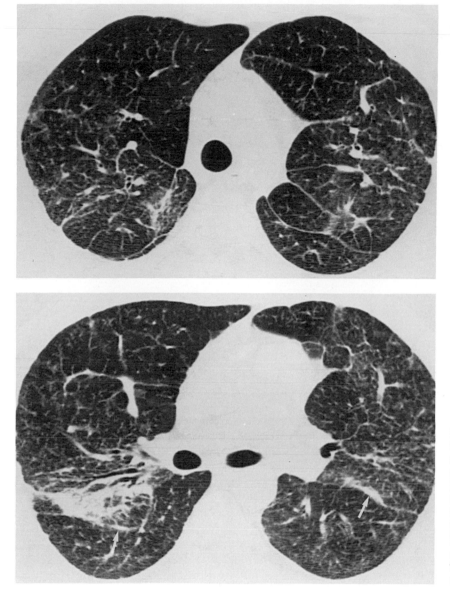

FIG. 5-17. Pulmonary sarcoidosis and findings of pulmonary fibrosis in a 32-year-old man. HRCT at the level of the tracheal carina shows extensive irregular or nodular septal thickening (*arrows*), irregular interfaces, and traction bronchiectasis. Posterior displacement of the upper lobe bronchi is an early sign of lung distortion. Extensive bilateral ground-glass opacities correlated with increased ⁶⁷Ga uptake reflecting the presence of active inflammation.

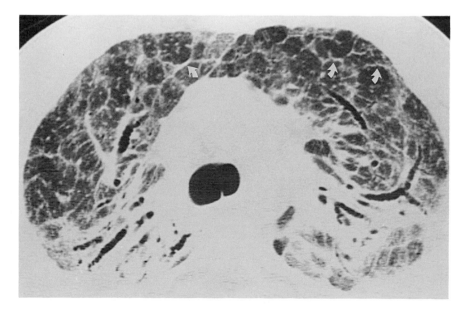

FIG. 5-18. Pulmonary sarcoidosis and findings of pulmonary fibrosis in a 32-year-old man. HRCT at the level of the tracheal carina shows extensive irregular or nodular septal thickening (*arrows*), irregular interfaces, and traction bronchiectasis. Posterior displacement of the upper lobe bronchi is an early sign of lung distortion. Extensive bilateral ground-glass opacities correlated with increased ⁶⁷Ga uptake.

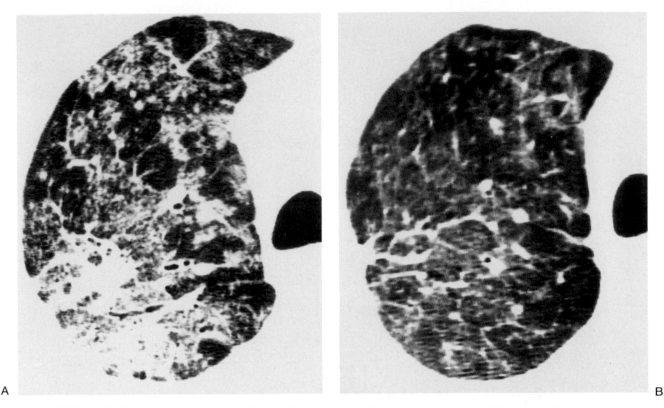

A   B

FIG. 5-19. Sarcoidosis before and after treatment. **A:** Before treatment, multiple nodules, areas of ground-glass opacity, and dense consolidation are present. **B:** After treatment, there has been a significant decrease in nodularity and consolidation. Ground-glass opacity, septal thickening, and parenchymal bands persist. At least some of these findings reflect residual fibrosis.

Progressive fibrosis also leads to abnormal central conglomeration of parahilar bronchi and vessels, associated with masses of fibrous tissue, typically most marked in the upper lobes (Figs. 3-53,5-20) (51,57). This finding is frequently associated with bronchial dilation, a finding referred to as traction bronchiectasis (25,64), and is typical of sarcoidosis; the only other diseases that commonly result in this appearance are silicosis, tuberculosis, and talcosis.

Honeycombing or lung cysts can be present in patients with sarcoidosis, but is less common than in other fibrotic lung diseases such as idiopathic pulmonary fibrosis. The cysts vary in diameter from 3 mm to 2 cm, with walls less than 1 mm in thickness, and are invariably subpleural in location (57). Honeycombing is usually limited to patients with severe fibrosis and central conglomeration of bronchi (57). The honeycombing seen in patients with sarcoidosis involves mainly the middle- and upper-lung zones, with relative sparing of the lung bases (65).

CT has also been shown to be helpful in assessing the presence and extent of some complications of sarcoidosis (50). Even though true cavitary sarcoidosis is rare, pseudocavities representing bullae or bronchiectasis are common in patients with extensive fibrosis. Superimposed bacterial infection and saprophytic fun-

gal infection with mycetoma formation can be readily detected with CT (50).

HRCT demonstrates the characteristic symmetric hilar and paratracheal lymphadenopathy better than plain chest radiographs, despite the spacing of scans (Fig. 5-21). Lymph node calcification is not uncom-

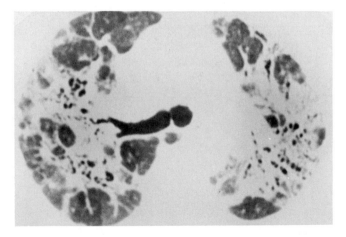

FIG. 5-20. Extensive pulmonary fibrosis due to sarcoidosis. A 1.5-mm collimation CT scan (standard algorithm) at the level of the right upper-lobe bronchus shows central conglomeration of ectatic bronchi typical of sarcoidosis.

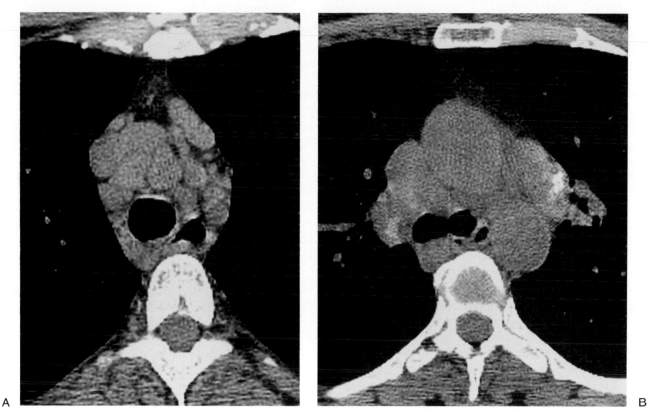

FIG. 5-21. A,B: Extensive mediastinal and hilar lymph node enlargement with calcification, seen on HRCT in a patient with sarcoidosis.

mon, and can be "egg-shell" in appearance (Figs. 5-21,5-22). On CT, lymph node enlargement is often seen in other locations including anterior mediastinum, ax-illa, internal mammary chain and retrocrural region (50). HRCT may be useful in detecting hilar lymphade-nopathy in lungs distorted by fibrosis.

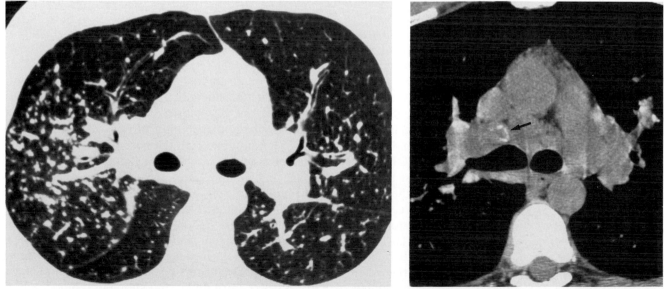

FIG. 5-22. Lung window (**A**) and soft-tissue window (**B**) scans in a patient with sarcoidosis, lung nodules, and hilar and mediastinal lymph node enlargement and calcification. **A:** Small, well-defined nodules are visible with a distribution characteristic of sarcoidosis. Nodules are patchy in distribution. **B:** Hilar lymph node calcification is easily seen. One lymph node (*arrow*) shows egg-shell calcification.

Clinical Utility of HRCT

High-resolution CT can show parenchymal abnormalities in patients with normal chest radiographs and in patients in whom only hilar adenopathy is apparent (52). HRCT has also been shown to be superior to chest radiographs in demonstrating early fibrosis and distortion of the lung parenchyma in patients with sarcoidosis (60). However, CT cannot be used to rule out parenchymal involvement; HRCT can be normal in patients with pulmonary involvement by sarcoidosis proved by transbronchial biopsy or lobectomy (52,57,66).

In patients with sarcoidosis as in those with other chronic infiltrative lung diseases, ground-glass opacity usually reflects the presence of active, potentially treatable, or reversible disease (59,60,62,67). Serial CT scans performed in patients with pulmonary sarcoidosis, both with and without treatment, have demonstrated that nodules, ground-glass opacity, consolidation, and interlobular septal thickening usually represent potentially treatable or reversible disease (58,60,67). However, Remy-Jardin et al. (58) did not find a significant correlation between the presence or extent of HRCT abnormalities and changes in disease activity measured using serum angiotensin converting enzyme or the percentage of T lymphocytes in bronchoalveolar lavage fluid. Irregular lines reticular opacities are usually irreversible but may occasionally improve or resolve (67). Architectural distortion and honeycombing represent irreversible disease (58,60,67).

Although CT provides a superior pictorial assessment of disease pattern, extent, and distribution, it is controversial whether it correlates better than chest radiographs with clinical and functional impairment in patients with sarcoidosis (68). In a review of 27 patients with sarcoidosis, Müller et al. (69) demonstrated that CT and radiographic assessment of disease extent had similar correlations with the severity of dyspnea ($r = 0.61$ and 0.58, respectively, $p < 0.001$), total lung capacity ($r = -0.54$ and -0.62, respectively, $p < 0.01$), and with gas transfer as assessed by the carbon monoxide diffusing capacity (DLCO) ($r = -0.62$ and -0.52, respectively, $p < 0.01$). In a prospective HRCT study of 44 patients, Brauner et al. (24) found that the CT visual score had a lower correlation than did the radiographic score with total lung capacity (TLC) ($r = -0.30$ and -0.49, respectively), forced expiratory volume at one second (FEV1.0 sec) ($r = -0.41$ and -0.40, respectively) and DLCO ($r = -0.41$ and -0.46, respectively). Bergin et al. (56), on the other hand, found that the CT scores of disease correlated better with functional impairment (all $r > 0.49$) than the radiographic scores (all $r < 0.15$). The discrepancy between these different results is difficult to explain, but may be due to a difference in patient groups as

well as differences in data analysis. Most investigators believe that HRCT has a very limited role, if any, in assessing or predicting pulmonary function in patients with sarcoidosis (68).

Remy-Jardin et al. (58), also have reported low, but statistically significant correlations between the HRCT extent of various findings of sarcoidosis, with the exception of nodules, and pulmonary function test results. The best correlations were between the overall extent of abnormalities seen on HRCT, and FVC ($r = -0.40$), FEV1 ($r = -0.37$), TLC ($r = -0.48$), and DLCO ($r = -0.49$), all p values < 0.0001. Specific HRCT findings having the best correlations with pulmonary function tests were consolidation, ground-glass opacity, and lung distortion, although these correlations were generally low.

Carrington et al. (55) have suggested that poor correlation between the radiographic severity of disease and the functional impairment in patients with sarcoidosis may be due to the fact that the nodular lesions, although easily seen and quantitated, cause minimal dysfunction. This situation is similar to that seen in patients with silicosis, in whom the severity of interstitial fibrosis rather than the number or size of nodules is responsible for impaired function (55). Indeed, in the study by Müller et al. (69) patients with predominantly irregular reticular opacities had more severe dyspnea and lower-lung volumes than patients with predominantly nodular opacities ($p < 0.05$). Also, as indicated above, Remy-Jardin et al. (58) found that the extent of nodular opacities seen on HRCT in patients with sarcoidosis lacked a significant correlation with pulmonary function tests.

Differential Diagnosis

Conditions that most closely mimic the HRCT appearance of sarcoidosis are pulmonary lymphangitic carcinomatosis, silicosis, coal worker's pneumoconiosis (CWP), and berylliosis. Each of these can result in a perilymphatic distribution of nodules, with nodules being seen in relation to the perihilar peribronchovascular interstitium, interlobular septa, the subpleural regions, and lobular core. However, the predominant distribution of each of these in relation to these compartments is somewhat different.

In sarcoidosis, nodules tend to predominate in the peribronchovascular and subpleural regions; in PLC, nodules are most frequently septal and peribronchovascular (18,57,70); in silicosis and CWP nodules usually appear centrilobular and subpleural in location on HRCT (7,16,71–73). In patients with silicosis and CWP, nodules tend to appear bilaterally symmetric and uniformly distributed through the lung, findings that are much less frequent with sarcoidosis.

When septal thickening is present in patients with sarcoidosis, it is usually less extensive than that seen in patients with PLC and is often associated with distortion of lobular architecture, a finding indicative of fibrosis that is not seen with PLC (52,74). Conglomerate masses and other evidence of fibrosis such as honeycombing can be seen with either sarcoidosis or with silicosis and CWP (51), but are not seen in PLC. In some patients with sarcoidosis, however, the pattern of parenchymal involvement may be quite similar to that of lymphatic spread of tumor (52,70).

BERYLLIUM DISEASE (BERYLLIOSIS)

Berylliosis is a chronic granulomatous lung disease resulting from occupational exposure to beryllium, which is indistinguishable from sarcoidosis histologically (75,76). Exposure to beryllium can occur in the ceramics industry, in nuclear weapons production, or in fluorescent lamp manufacture. Berylliosis is characterized by a beryllium-specific, cell-mediated immune response, which can be diagnosed in its early stages by the use of a blood test, called the beryllium lymphocyte transformation test (BeL T) (75).

HRCT findings in patients with berylliosis are similar to those reported in patients with sarcoidosis. The most common findings are parenchymal nodules (57%) and interlobular septal thickening (50%). As in patients with sarcoidosis, nodules often predominate in the peribronchovascular regions or along interlobular septa. Other HRCT findings include ground-glass opacity (32%), honeycombing (7%), conglomerate masses (7%), bronchial wall thickening (46%), and hilar or mediastinal lymphadenopathy (39%) (75). In a study of 28 patients (75) with berylliosis detected using BeL T, and confirmed by lung biopsy, chest radiographs were abnormal in 54%, while HRCT showed at least one abnormality in 89%. Although HRCT did not detect abnormalities in all patients, many subjects in this study had preclinical disease without symptoms of respiratory dysfunction.

SILICOSIS AND COAL WORKER'S PNEUMOCONIOSIS

Silicosis and coal worker's pneumoconiosis (CWP) are distinct diseases, with differing histology, resulting from the inhalation of different inorganic dusts. However, the radiographic and HRCT appearances of silicosis and coal worker's pneumoconiosis are quite similar, and they cannot be easily or reliably distinguished in individual cases.

Silicosis is caused by inhalation of dust-containing, crystallized silicon dioxide (77,78). In North America, heavy-metal mining and hard-rock mining are the occupations most frequently associated with chronic silicosis. The diagnosis of silicosis requires the combination of an appropriate history of silica exposure and characteristic findings on the chest radiograph. Pathologically, the pulmonary lesions seen in patients with silicosis are centrilobular, peribronchiolar nodules consisting of layers of laminated connective tissue. The nodules measure a few millimeters in diameter and are scattered diffusely throughout the lungs, although they are usually most numerous in the upper lobes and parahilar regions. Focal emphysema (also known as focal-dust emphysema) surrounding the nodule is common.

As indicated by its name, coal worker's pneumoconiosis results from inhalation of coal dust. Since a small amount of silica is present in coal-mine dust, it was long assumed that CWP represented a form of silicosis, but this is not usually the case (79). CWP can be seen in workers exposed to washed coal, which is nearly free of silica, and a very similar pneumoconiosis occurs with inhalation of pure carbon. As with silicosis, a history of significant exposure (10 years or more) is necessary in order to consider the diagnosis (78,79). Histologically, the characteristic lesion of CWP is the so-called coal macule, which consists of a focal accumulation of coal dust surrounded by a small amount of fibrous tissue (79); however, the amount of fibrosis is much less than that seen with silicosis (78). As the disease progresses, coal macules are surrounded by small areas of focal emphysema. As in patients with silicosis, these abnormalities tend to surround respiratory bronchioles in the lobular core and are therefore primarily centrilobular in location (78,79).

The characteristic radiologic abnormality seen in patients with both silicosis and CWP consists of small well-circumscribed nodules usually measuring 2 to 5 mm in diameter, but ranging from 1 to 10 mm, mainly involving the upper and posterior lung zones (78–80); although there is a tendency for the nodules of silicosis to be better defined than those of CWP, this is not necessarily true in individual cases. These small nodules indicate the presence of "simple" or uncomplicated silicosis or CWP.

The appearance of large opacities, also known as conglomerate masses or progressive massive fibrosis, indicates the presence of complicated silicosis or complicated CWP. A "large" opacity is considered to be greater than 1 cm in diameter (78,79). These masses tend to develop in the midportion or periphery of the upper-lung zones and migrate toward the hila, leaving overinflated emphysematous spaces between the conglomerate mass and the pleura (81). Although the appearance of the conglomerate masses seen in silicosis and CWP are quite similar, their histology is different. In patients with silicosis, these masses represent a conglomeration of numbers of silicotic nodules associated with fibrous tissue; in CWP, they consist of an amorphous black mass surrounded by fibrous tissue. In both silicosis and CWP, these masses can undergo necrosis and cavitation.

Although simple silicosis and simple CWP cause few symptoms and little clinical impairment, the development of complicated silicosis or complicated CWP are associated with the appearance of respiratory symptoms and a deterioration of lung function (78,79). However, patients with silicosis usually have greater respiratory impairment for a given degree of radiographic abnormality than do patients with CWP. Furthermore, the complicated form of silicosis has a poorer prognosis than does simple silicosis, but this is not necessarily the case with CWP (79,82). In patients with silicosis, the size of the conglomerate masses is often related to the severity of symptoms.

Hilar lymphadenopathy is present in many patients. The lymph nodes are often calcified. A characteristic peripheral "egg-shell" calcification is seen in approximately 5% of cases of silicosis and is virtually pathognomonic of this entity (80). When egg-shell calcification is seen in a patient with CWP, it reflects the presence of silica in the coal dust (78).

CT and HRCT Findings

On CT, as on the radiograph, the most characteristic feature of either simple silicosis or simple CWP is the presence of small nodules (Figs. 3-46,5-23,5-24) that are centrilobular or subpleural (Figs. 3-46,5-24) in location (Table 5-6) (6,7,16,72,73,83). The nodules vary in

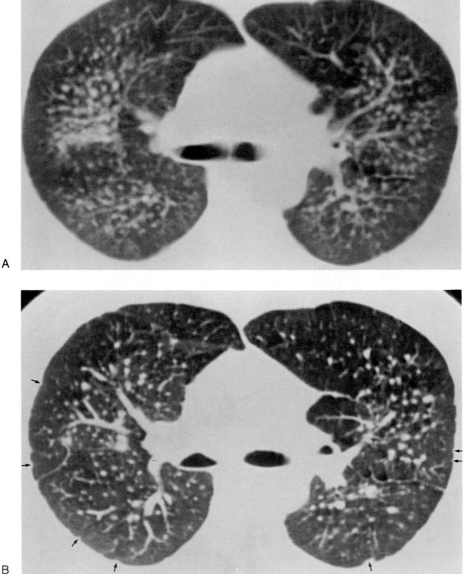

FIG. 5-23. Silicosis and nodules in a 50-year-old man. **A:** Conventional 10-mm collimation CT scan shows numerous lung nodules bilaterally, with relative sparing of the lung periphery. **B:** HRCT at the same level. The HRCT more clearly defines the presence of subpleural nodules (*small arrows*). The nodules are smoothly marginated and sharply defined. Nodule profusion is more easily evaluated on the conventional CT.

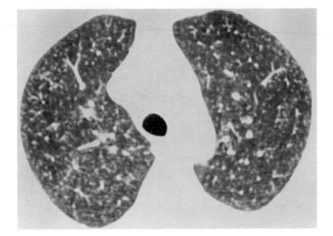

FIG. 5-24. Coal worker's pneumoconiosis in a 56-year-old man. HRCT at the level of the aortic arch shows numerous small nodules. The nodules are less well defined than those seen in silicosis. These involve both lungs diffusely at this level. A diffuse distribution is more typical of CWP or silicosis than it is of sarcoidosis.

size but usually measure 2 to 5 mm in diameter as seen on HRCT, and can be calcified. Nodules occurring in relation to thickened interlobular septa, as are seen in patients with PLC or sarcoidosis, are few or lacking. The nodules seen in patients with silicosis tend to be more sharply defined than those seen in CWP (Figs. 5-23,5-24).

Nodules are present diffusely and bilaterally, but in patients with mild silicosis or CWP, they may be seen only in the upper lobes. A posterior predominance of nodules is also often visible on CT (Fig. 3-46) (7,73) (Table 5-6). More severe silicosis is characterized on CT by an increase in the number and size of nodules. Nodules often appear to be uniformly distributed throughout the involved lung regions, rather than being clustered (Fig. 5-23).

Akira et al. (71) reviewed the HRCT scans in 90 patients with pneumoconiosis who had small, rounded opacities on chest radiographs; 61 of these 90 had silicosis, and 12 had CWP. The 90 patients were divided into three groups on the basis of the type of opacity

that was visible. The first group consisted of 55 patients whose radiographs predominantly showed International Labor Organization (ILO) type p rounded opacities (nodules < 1.5 mm in diameter), including 32 patients with silicosis; 6 patients with coal worker's pneumoconiosis; and 17 patients with talcosis, welder's lung, and graphite pneumoconiosis. The second group consisted of 29 patients whose radiographs showed predominantly ILO type q rounded opacities (nodules 1.5 to 3 mm in diameter), including 23 patients with silicosis and 6 patients with coal worker's pneumoconiosis. The third group consisted of 6 patients with silicosis whose radiographs showed predominantly ILO type r rounded opacities (nodules < 3 mm in diameter).

In those patients with radiographic type p pneumoconiosis, HRCT showed ill-defined centrilobular, peribronchiolar opacities (Fig. 5-24), sometimes having the appearance of small branching structures or a few closely spaced dots (71). In 21 of the 55 patients, Akira et al. (71) also demonstrated small intralobular areas of abnormally low attenuation. CT-pathologic correlation in two postmortem specimens showed that the small branching opacities and the areas of low attenuation corresponded, respectively, to areas of irregular fibrosis around and along the respiratory bronchioles and to focal areas of associated centrilobular emphysema.

Opacities of the q and r types were characterized by sharply demarcated, rounded nodules or irregular, contracted nodules (71). Appearances with CT differed among the three types of opacities, but no differences were noted between the CT appearances of silicosis and the other pneumoconioses with the same size of nodules. Focal centrilobular emphysema was more commonly found with type p pneumoconiosis than with these two types.

In studies by Remy-Jardin et al. (7,16) of 86 patients with CWP, parenchymal nodules 7 mm or less in diam-

TABLE 5-6. *HRCT findings in silicosis and CWP[a,b]*

1. **Small Nodules, 2–5 mm in Diameter, Ill-defined or Well-defined, Centrilobular and Subpleural**
2. **Reticular Opacities Inconspicuous**
3. **Diffuse Distribution, with Upper-lobe and Posterior Predominance**
4. **Conglomerate Masses, Irregular in Shape, Containing Areas of Necrosis**
5. **Focal Centrilobular Emphysema**
6. Irregular or Cicatricial Emphysema in Silicosis
7. Lymph Node Enlargement

[a] Most common findings in boldface.
[b] Findings most helpful in differential diagnosis in boldface italics.

eter were seen on CT and HRCT in 81% of patients with CWP; in 3% the nodules were calcified. In half of the patients, the nodules were low in attenuation; they usually had irregular borders. Subpleural nodules were frequently seen (Fig. 5-25), representing macules or focal areas of visceral pleural thickening (7,16). Coalescence of subpleural nodules into ''pseudoplaques'' was visible in some; pseudoplaques can mimic the appearance of an asbestos-related pleural plaque.

Increased reticular opacities are not a prominent feature of silicosis or CWP. However, Remy-Jardin et al. (7,16) reported the occurrence of lower-lobe honeycombing in 8% of 86 patients with CWP they studied. The significance of this finding is unclear.

Progressive massive fibrosis is always associated with a background of small nodules visible on HRCT (7). In the patients with CWP reported by Remy-Jardin

et al. (7), conglomerate masses were usually oval in shape and nearly all had irregular borders (Fig. 5-26). Distortion of lung architecture and vascular anatomy were also evident. The most prominent CT feature of the progressive massive fibrosis associated with silicosis is mass-like consolidation associated with apical parenchymal scarring and adjacent bullous changes (irregular or cicatricial emphysema) (Figs. 3-54,5-26); emphysema seems to be more conspicuous in patients with silicosis than in those with CWP (7). Calcification in association with conglomerate masses is common. In patients with CWP, conglomerate masses larger than 4 cm always contained areas of necrosis, visible as low attenuation, with or without cavitation (7). Thickening of extrapleural fat adjacent to peripheral conglomerate masses was also reported by Remy-Jardin et al. (7).

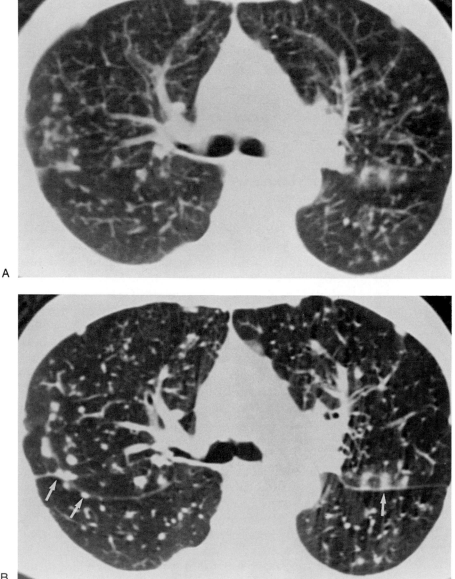

FIG. 5-25. Silicosis in a 60-year-old man. **A:** Conventional 10-mm collimation CT scan at the level of the right upper-lobe bronchus shows nodules bilaterally. A few subpleural nodules are also visible. Groups of subpleural nodules (so-called pseudoplaques) mimic the appearance of the pleural plaques that occur in patients with asbestos exposure. **B:** HRCT at the same level better delineates the nodule margins as well as nodular thickening of the subpleural interstitium adjacent to the major fissures (*arrows*).

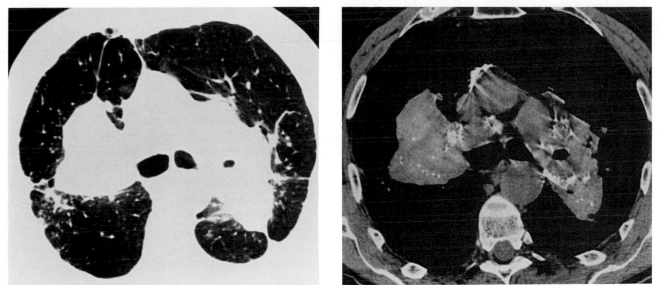

A
B

FIG. 5-26. Progressive massive fibrosis due to silicosis in a 70-year-old man. **A:** HRCT using a lung window setting, at the level of the main bronchi, shows bilateral conglomerate masses and emphysema. **B:** Mediastinal window setting at the same level shows areas of calcification within the conglomerate masses, hila, and mediastinal nodes.

Hilar and/or mediastinal lymph node enlargement was visible in 15% to 38% of patients with silicosis studied by Grenier et al. (23). Egg-shell calcification can sometimes be seen (Fig. 5-27).

Utility of CT and HRCT

High-resolution CT has been shown to be superior to both conventional CT and chest radiography in the detection of small nodules in patients with silicosis (6)

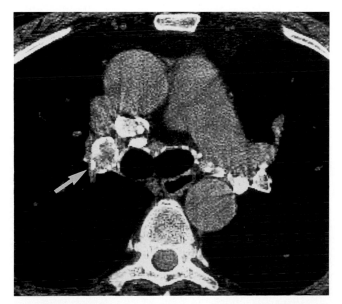

FIG. 5-27. Egg-shell calcification (*arrow*) on HRCT in a patient with silicosis.

and coal worker's pneumoconiosis (7,73). Bégin et al. (6) compared HRCT to conventional CT and chest radiographs in the detection of early silicosis in 49 patients and two normal controls. All patients had been exposed to silica dust for an average of 29 ± 2 years and had chest radiograph scores of 0 or 1 as determined by the International Labor Office (ILO) criteria.

In this study, chest radiographs were interpreted as normal in 32 patients, indeterminate in 6, and abnormal in 13. Thirteen (41%) of the 32 cases interpreted as normal on radiographs had evidence of silicosis on CT or HRCT. Furthermore, in 10% of the patients with silicosis, abnormalities were visible only on HRCT (6); in the remaining cases, abnormalities were more clearly defined using HRCT than on the conventional CT studies. Remy-Jardin et al. (7) reviewed the chest radiographs and CT scans in miners exposed to coal dust. Nodules were detected on HRCT in 11 out of 48 patients (23%) with no evidence of pneumoconiosis on chest radiographs (ILO profusion score < 1/0). Inter-reader agreement in the assessment of lung opacities, as assessed by kappa statistics, is also significantly better for the readings of CT scans than chest radiographs (*p* < 0.001) (6).

CT and HRCT also can provide significant information regarding the stage of the disease in patients with silicosis and CWP, because they can detect coalescence of nodules and the development of conglomerate masses that may not be apparent on plain radiographs (72,73). Also, in some patients who appear to have this finding on chest radiographs, HRCT shows that progressive massive fibrosis is not present (7).

It has been shown that in patients with silicosis, pulmonary function abnormalities correlate more closely with the severity of emphysema than the profusion of small nodules. A major advantage of CT relative to chest radiographs is the evaluation of emphysema extent. Chest radiographs may detect large bullae but are notably insensitive in detecting more diffuse emphysema. In the ILO classification, the presence of bullae is denoted by the symbol "bu," but there is no system for quantitating bullous changes. CT, on the other hand, allows quantitation of the severity and extent of emphysema seen in association with silicotic nodules.

For example, Bergin et al. (73) compared the qualitative and quantitative CT assessment of silicosis with chest radiographs and pulmonary function tests in 17 patients with silicosis and in 6 controls. The CT scans were visually graded as to the extent of silicosis, mean attenuation values were measured, and the extent of any associated emphysema was determined. Significant correlation was found between the ILO category of nodule profusion recorded from the radiograph and both the mean attenuation values ($r > 0.62$, $p < 0.001$) and the visual CT scores ($r > 0.84$, $p < 0.001$) for extent. Although, there was poor correlation between the pulmonary function tests results and the nodule profusion determined using the chest radiographs and CT, there was a significant correlation between the CT emphysema score and measurements of airflow obstruction and impairment of gas transfer. Emphysema associated with silicosis was easily detected on CT but not on the radiographs.

Also, Kinsella et al. (84) reviewed pulmonary function testing and chest CT scans in 30 subjects with silicosis. The extent of emphysema was the strongest independent predictor of pulmonary function impairment; the extent of small nodules was also an independent predictor of pulmonary function impairment, albeit a weaker one. It was also shown in this study, that in the absence of progressive massive fibrosis, smokers had more extensive emphysema and more severe functional impairment than did nonsmokers (84). In the absence of progressive massive fibrosis, silicosis was not associated with significant emphysema.

To investigate the relationship of lung function, airflow limitation, and lung injury in silica-exposed workers, Begin et al. (85) analyzed the clinical, functional, and radiologic data of 94 long-term workers exposed in the granite industry or in foundries. In those workers with coalescence of nodules and conglomerate masses seen on chest radiographs or CT scans, there was a significant loss of lung volume, impairment in gas exchange, and increased airflow obstruction as compared to patients who did not show this finding. Furthermore, in 40% of the patients with conglomeration this finding was visible only on CT.

Differential Diagnosis

As indicated above, patients with silicosis can show HRCT findings similar to those seen with sarcoidosis and pulmonary lymphangitic carcinomatosis (73), although the diseases can usually be distinguished on the basis of history and a careful examination of the scans. The HRCT features that suggest sarcoidosis include a central clustering of nodules in relation to parahilar vessels and bronchi and the presence of focal or multifocal abnormalities intermixed with normal or almost normal areas of lung; in silicosis and CWP, nodules usually appear bilaterally symmetric and more uniformly distributed. Also the development of reticular opacities is much less common with silicosis than with sarcoidosis. Beaded septa as seen in patients with PLC and sarcoidosis are generally lacking in patients with silicosis.

DIFFUSE PARENCHYMAL AMYLOIDOSIS

Primary pulmonary amyloidosis is a rare disease, occurring in three forms. It can predominantly involve the tracheobronchial tree (tracheobronchial amyloidosis), result in large discrete lung nodules or masses (nodular parenchymal amyloidosis), or can involve the lung diffusely (diffuse parenchymal or alveolar septal amyloidosis). In diffuse parenchymal or alveolar septal amyloidosis, amyloid deposition in the lung is often widespread, involving small blood vessels and the lung interstitium. Multiple small nodules of amyloid may be present.

The diffuse parenchymal or alveolar septal form of amyloidosis, is least common, but is most significant clinically. Patients with diffuse parenchymal amyloidosis are more likely to die of respiratory failure than are patients with the two other forms of the disease (86). The most common presenting complaint in patients with diffuse parenchymal amyloidosis is progressive dyspnea. Physiologic assessment demonstrates a pattern of restrictive lung disease, but progressive worsening of pulmonary function tests does not occur until late in the course of the disease (86).

Radiologically, diffuse parenchymal amyloidosis results in nonspecific diffuse interstitial or alveolar opacities that, once established, change very little over time (87). The abnormal areas can calcify or, rarely, show frank ossification (87); calcification is more common in the large nodular form of disease (88). Diffuse parenchymal amyloidosis may appear predominantly as small nodules, thus simulating miliary tuberculosis, silicosis, or sarcoidosis, but patchy or diffuse inhomogeneous opacities may also be seen.

HRCT Findings

A single patient with diffuse parenchymal amyloidosis has been reported (89). This patient presented with dyspnea, pulmonary function evidence of restrictive lung disease, and reduced diffusing capacity, and was treated for suspected idiopathic pulmonary fibrosis. The diagnosis of amyloidosis was initially suggested because of HRCT findings of small interstitial nodules associated with dense calcification.

HRCT findings in this patient included abnormal reticular opacities, interlobular septal thickening, small, well-defined nodules 2 to 4 mm in diameter, and confluent consolidative opacities that predominated in the subpleural regions of the mid and lower-lung zones (Figs. 3-49,5-28). Some nodules were densely calcified and some of the areas of consolidation contained punctate foci of calcification. These calcifications were not visible on chest radiographs. A follow-up HRCT (Fig. 5-28) performed 16 months after the initial examination (Fig. 3-49) showed progression of the diffuse parenchymal disease, including an increase in the reticular opacities, septal thickening, the size and number of nodules and consolidative opacities, and an increase in the size and number of the multiple calcifications.

HRCT findings in this case correlated closely with open lung biopsy findings typical of amyloidosis (89). Amyloid deposits were located in the walls of arteries, veins, and airways, and in the perivascular interstitium; some of these deposits were nodular in appearance. Interlobular septal thickening by amyloid was also present, and extensive amyloid deposits were present beneath the visceral pleura. Foci of calcification and metaplastic ossification were widely scattered throughout the amyloid material.

Calcification of small interstitial nodules on HRCT has a limited differential diagnosis. Multifocal lung calcification, often associated with lung nodules, has also been reported in association with infectious granulomatous diseases such as tuberculosis (90), sarcoidosis (16), silicosis and coal worker's pneumoconiosis (7,16), talcosis (91), fat embolism associated with ARDS (92), metastatic calcification (93), and alveolar microlithiasis (94,95).

MYCOBACTERIAL INFECTIONS

Although the prevalence of tuberculosis has declined since the advent of modern chemotherapy, pulmonary tuberculosis remains an important cause of disease worldwide, especially in nonwhite, immigrant, or debilitated patients (96). Despite effective chemotherapy, the incidence of tuberculosis has risen steadily since 1985, at least partially as result of the AIDS epidemic (97–100); also of concern is the increasing prevalence of multidrug resistant tuberculosis (MDR-TB). The frequency of pulmonary infection resulting from nontuberculous mycobacteria has also increased during this period (101–106).

Tuberculosis

Traditionally, TB infection has been considered in two stages—primary infection and reactivation or postprimary disease. In fact, however, in individual

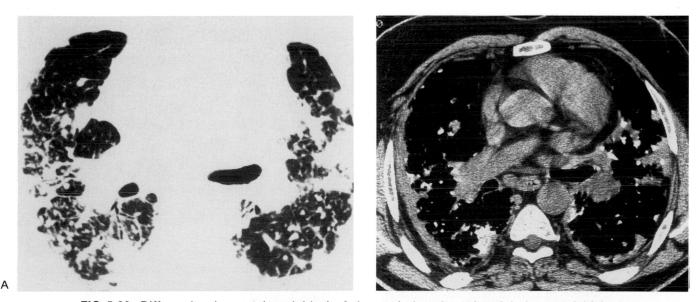

A

B

FIG. 5-28. Diffuse alveolar septal amyloidosis. **A:** Lung window shows interlobular septal thickening, small, well-defined nodules, and subpleural masses. **B:** Soft-tissue window setting shows the subpleural masses to best advantage. Many small nodules are calcified. This study was performed 16 months after that shown in Fig. 3-49.

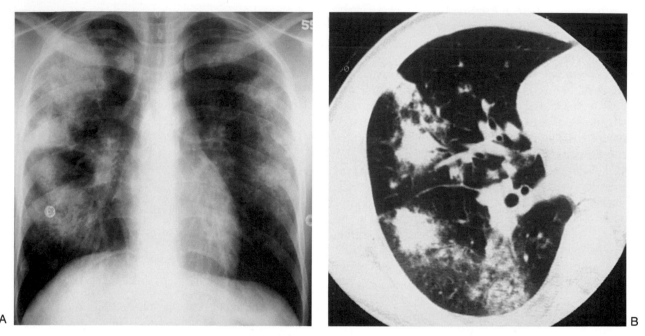

FIG. 5-29. Primary tuberculosis with patchy consolidation. **A:** Posteroanterior chest radiograph shows the presence of bilateral peripheral areas of consolidation. Initially, this pattern suggested the possibility of chronic eosinophilic pneumonia. **B:** Targeted reconstructed HRCT image through the right lower lobe shows patchy and nodular consolidation both centrally and peripherally. Transbronchial biopsy proved tuberculosis.

cases, a clear distinction between these two types of disease may be impossible to make in the absence of prior chest radiographs or, more importantly, a recent history of exposure or skin-test conversion (107–110). Nonetheless, given the widespread use of these terms, awareness of their definitions remains important.

Primary pulmonary tuberculosis (TB) is acquired by the inhalation of airborne organisms. The initial site of lung infection is variable, but often, the middle and lower-lung zones are first involved (107,111–113). A focal pneumonitis typically results, with subsequent caseous necrosis and lymphatic spread of organisms

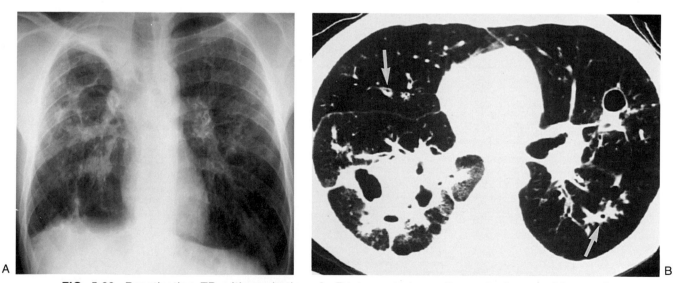

FIG. 5-30. Reactivation TB with cavitation. **A:** Posteroanterior radiograph shows evidence of significant volume loss in the right upper lobe associated with cavitation. Although there is a suggestion of cavitation in the middle and lower lobes bilaterally, precise delineation of the number and extent of cavities is difficult. **B:** HRCT through the mid-lung zones shows both thick- and thin-walled cavities bilaterally, associated with focal areas of air-space consolidation. The number and appearance of these are much more easily evaluated in cross-section as is bronchiectasis (*arrows*).

to hilar and mediastinal lymph nodes. In 90% to 95% of subjects, development of immunity results in healing of the lesions, with development of pulmonary and hilar granulomas. Hematogenous spread of infection also occurs in patients with primary TB, but these organisms are inactivated as immunity develops.

Radiographically, in a series reported by Woodring et al. (107), primary TB was associated with consolidation (50% of patients) that often involved the middle or lower lobes (Fig. 5-29), cavitation (29%), segmental or lobar atelectasis (18%), hilar and mediastinal lymphadenopathy (35%), and miliary disease (6%). These findings may occur alone or in combination, but in up to 15% of patients with documented TB, chest radiographs may be normal (107,110).

In most subjects, the primary infection is localized and clinically inapparent. However, in 5% to 10% of patients with primary TB, the infection is poorly contained and dissemination occurs; this is termed *pro-*

gressive primary tuberculosis. Extensive cavitation of the tuberculous pneumonia can occur with endobronchial spread of the infection; rupture of necrotic lymph nodes into the bronchi can also result in endobronchial dissemination (111,113). Hematogenous spread can also occur as a result of progressive primary TB.

With the development of delayed hypersensitivity, pulmonary granulomas heal with fibrosis. However, viable organisms often survive, and reactivation of lung disease (reactivation or postprimary TB) may occur at a later date (113). Patients with reactivation or postprimary TB characteristically show radiographic evidence of apical abnormalities, identifiable in up to 90% of cases. The apical predominance of reactivation TB is usually attributed to the oxygen-rich environment existing in the lung apices, but may in fact result from diminished apical lymphatic drainage (106). In patients with postprimary TB described by Woodring et

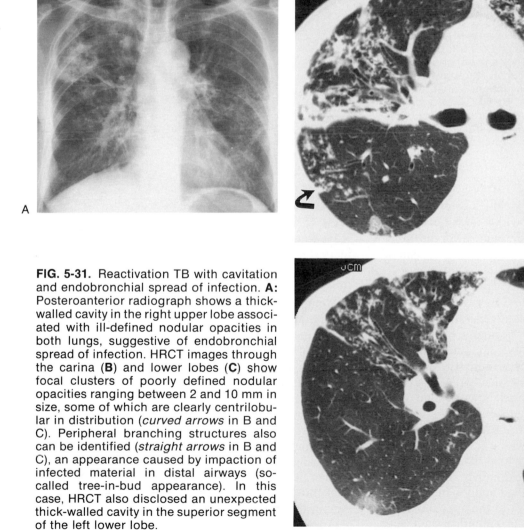

FIG. 5-31. Reactivation TB with cavitation and endobronchial spread of infection. **A:** Posteroanterior radiograph shows a thick-walled cavity in the right upper lobe associated with ill-defined nodular opacities in both lungs, suggestive of endobronchial spread of infection. HRCT images through the carina (**B**) and lower lobes (**C**) show focal clusters of poorly defined nodular opacities ranging between 2 and 10 mm in size, some of which are clearly centrilobular in distribution (*curved arrows* in B and C). Peripheral branching structures also can be identified (*straight arrows* in B and C), an appearance caused by impaction of infected material in distal airways (so-called tree-in-bud appearance). In this case, HRCT also disclosed an unexpected thick-walled cavity in the superior segment of the left lower lobe.

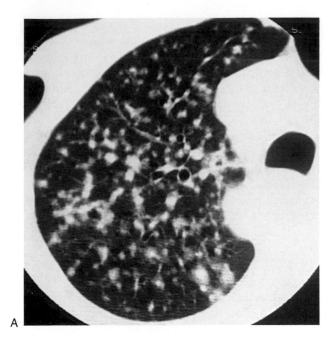

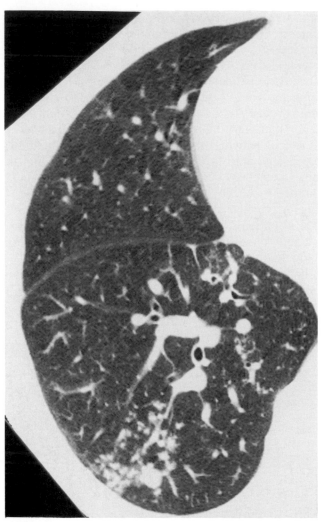

FIG. 5-32. Endobronchial spread of tuberculosis in reactivation TB. **A:** Targeted HRCT through the right upper lobe shows numerous, diffuse, poorly defined nodules typical of endobronchial spread of infection, some appearing perivascular and centrilobular in location. Chest radiographs (not shown) showed this process to be present diffusely throughout both lungs, without evidence of cavitation. Transbronchial biopsy proved tuberculosis. **B:** HRCT through the right lower lobe in a different patient shows clusters of small nodules with a focal distribution. These are also typical of endobronchial spread of infection.

al. (107), radiographic findings included patchy consolidation and/or streaky opacities (100% of patients), primarily in the apical and posterior segments of the upper lobes (91%), cavitation (45%), bronchogenic spread of disease with ill-defined nodules (21%), evidence of fibrosis (29%), and pleural effusion (18%) (Fig. 5-30).

Radiographic signs of active TB, regardless of its stage, include focal consolidation, generally apical or, less commonly, in the superior segments of the lower lobes and cavitation (Figs. 5-30–5-32). Endobronchial spread of infection also indicates activity, and may occur in the absence of radiographically demonstrable cavitation. Endobronchial spread is associated with poorly defined pulmonary nodules varying between 5 and 10 mm in size, so-called air-space or acinar nodules. Disease activity may also be inferred in those patients treated empirically in whom radiographic resolution can be documented. Although radiographic findings cannot generally be relied upon to indicate inactive disease, a lack of change in the appearance of opacities on radiographs over a 6-month period, has

proved valuable in determining disease to be inactive (114).

Pleural effusions are common in patients with primary TB, being seen in as many as 25% of patients; these effusions are thought to represent a hypersensitivity reaction to TB proteins, and organisms are uncommonly isolated from the fluid. The effusions may be large, unilateral, and unassociated with obvious parenchymal disease on chest radiographs (107).

Pleural effusion is also associated with postprimary TB; although it is less frequent than in primary TB; pleural effusion has been reported in 18% of patients with postprimary TB (107). Pleural effusion can be caused by rupture of a tuberculous cavity into the pleural space, causing empyema. Bronchopleural fistula can also result leading to a pleural air-fluid level.

In many cases of advanced cavitary tuberculosis, extensive pleural abnormalities are present, with pleural thickening and calcification being most common. Pleural thickening has been reported in up to 41% of patients with postprimary TB studied (107). Usually,

TABLE 5-7. *HRCT findings in active tuberculosis*[a,b]

1. **Patchy Unilateral or Bilateral Air-space Consolidation, Frequently Peribronchial in Distribution**

2. **Cavitation, Thin- or Thick-walled**

3. **Scattered Air-space (Acinar) Nodules, Centrilobular Branching Structures, "Tree-in-Bud"**

4. *Superimposition of Findings 1, 2, and 3*

5. Miliary Disease—Small, Well-defined Nodules

6. Pleural Effusion, Broncho-pleural Fistula, Empyema Necessitatis

7. **Low-density Hilar/Mediastinal Lymph Nodes**

[a] Most common findings in boldface.
[b] Findings most helpful in differential diagnosis in boldface italics.

pleural abnormalities represent the sequelae of underlying parenchymal disease and are apical in location; in occasional cases, pleural thickening is attributable to prior pneumothorax therapy.

CT and HRCT Findings

The CT and HRCT findings seen in association with tuberculosis are numerous and varied and reflect the protean manifestations of this disease (90,111,112, 115–120) (Table 5-7). Findings include air-space consolidation of varying degrees (Fig. 5-29), cavitation (Figs. 5-30,5-31), ill-defined air-space nodules that reflect endobronchial spread of infection (Figs. 5-31–5-33), small, well-defined nodules that indicate miliary or hematogenous spread of infection (Figs. 3-41, 5-34), pleural effusion, and lymph node enlargement with central necrosis (Fig. 5-35) (90,115,121). A combination of these findings is most helpful in making a diagnosis of tuberculosis; most commonly, TB is associated with poorly defined nodular opacities, parenchymal consolidation, and/or cavitation (Figs. 5-29–5-31). Although most tuberculous cavities are thick-walled, thin-walled cavities are frequently seen as well, especially in patients undergoing treatment.

Im et al. (90) reported the HRCT findings in 41 patients with newly diagnosed active TB (29 patients) or recent reactivation of disease (12 patients). In the 29 patients with newly diagnosed active TB, HRCT findings included cavitary nodules (69%), lobular consolidation (52%), interlobular septal thickening (34%), bronchovascular distortion (17%), bronchial impaction (17%), and fibrotic bands (17%). Mediastinal lymph node enlargement was seen in 9 (31%) of patients with newly diagnosed disease. Patients having follow-up HRCT during treatment showed a gradual decrease in lobular consolidation. On the other hand, bronchovascular distortion, emphysema, fibrosis, and bronchiectasis increased on follow-up scans, indicating the presence of fibrosis (90). In most cases parenchymal

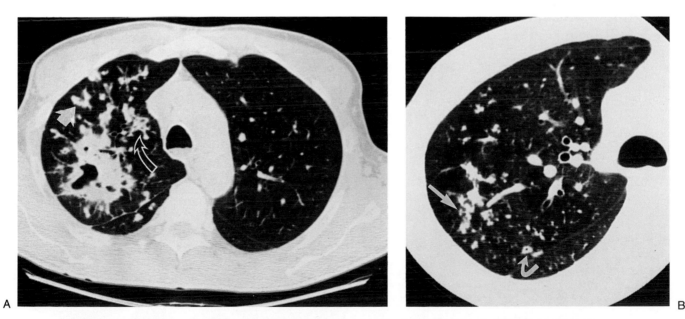

FIG. 5-33. Cavitary tuberculosis with endobronchial spread of infection. **A:** HRCT shows an irregular, thick-walled cavity in the posterior segment of the right upper lobe. Scattered nodules and clusters of nodules (*curved arrow*) are typical of endobronchial spread of infection. Branching opacities in the peripheral lung (*straight arrow*) are typical of dilated bronchioles filled with infected material, so-called tree-in-bud. **B:** Targeted reconstruction shows clustered nodules (*straight arrow*). A small nodular opacity with a central lucency (*curved arrow*) may represent a cavitary nodule, or bronchiolectasis with surrounding inflammation.

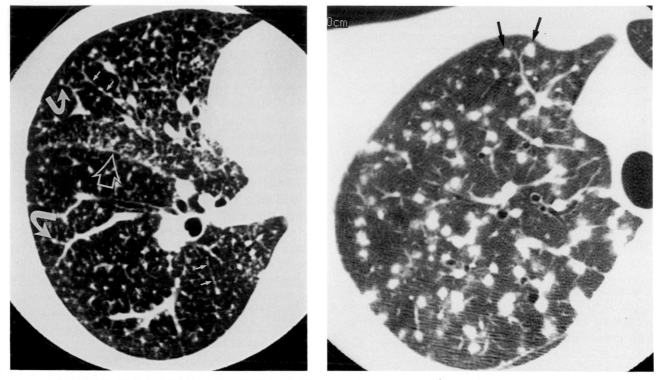

FIG. 5-34. Miliary tuberculosis. **A:** HRCT with targeted reconstruction through the right lower lobe shows numerous, well-defined, 1- to 2-mm nodules that are diffuse in distribution. Some nodules appear septal (*arrows*) or subpleural (*open arrow*), while others appear to be associated with small, feeding vessels, suggesting a hematogenous origin (*curved arrows*). Transbronchial biopsy proved tuberculosis. **B:** Miliary TB in another patient shows larger nodules, but the same distribution is noted as that seen in A. Nodules appear uniformly distributed and of similar size. Some nodules appear septal, subpleural, or associated with small vessels (*arrows*). Bronchial abnormalities and tree-in-bud appearance are absent.

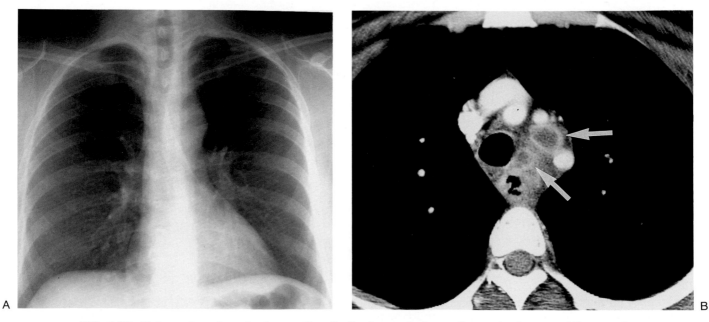

FIG. 5-35. Tuberculous lymphadenopathy. **A:** Posteroanterior radiograph shows subtle prominence of the mediastinum. **B:** Contrast-enhanced CT at the level of the great vessels shows several low-density, rim-enhancing lymph nodes (*arrows*) typical of mycobacterial infection. In this case, the diagnosis of *Mycobacterium tuberculosis* was established by transbronchial needle aspiration of subcarinal nodes (not shown).

abnormalities have a clearly segmental distribution. In a study of 71 patients with TB, Ikezoe et al. (119) found that a pattern of segmental distribution of abnormalities was present in 97% of cases. In addition, satellite lesions were identified in 93% of cases while single cavities were seen in 95%.

In the 12 patients with reactivation of disease reported by Im et al. (90), CT findings of distortion of bronchovascular structures (58%), bronchiectasis (58%), emphysema (50%), and fibrotic bands (50%) were more frequent than in the patients with newly diagnosed disease, and indicative of prior infection with scarring. Lobular consolidation was less common in this group than in patients with newly diagnosed active disease.

Of greatest import in making an accurate HRCT diagnosis of active TB, are findings of endobronchial spread of infection (90,118,122,123). On HRCT, endobronchial spread of TB can result in:

1. Poorly defined nodules or rosettes of nodules, 2 to 10 mm in diameter, which can often be identified as centrilobular, and/or
2. Branching centrilobular opacities, appropriately described as mimicking a "tree-in-bud" (Figs. 3-36,5-31–5-33) (90).

Pathologically, the centrilobular nodules reflect the presence of intra- and peribronchiolar inflammatory exudate, while the branching trees-in-bud correlate with the presence of solid caseous material filling or surrounding terminal or respiratory bronchioles or alveolar ducts (Fig. 3-36) (90). With more extensive disease, coalescence of the centrilobular opacities occurs, resulting in focal areas of bronchopneumonia. In the study by Im et al. (90), the earliest HRCT findings of endobronchial dissemination were the presence of centrilobular nodules, 2 to 4 mm in diameter (Figs. 5-31,5-32), or centrilobular branching structures, "trees-in-bud" (Figs. 5-31,5-33). These findings invariably resolved within 5 to 9 months of beginning treatment, and thus indicated reversible disease.

Im et al. (90) stress the high frequency of HRCT findings of endobronchial spread of infection in their patients with newly diagnosed active TB or recent reactivation of disease. Of the 29 patients with newly diagnosed active TB (90), 28 (97%) had HRCT findings of endobronchial spread of infection, with centrilobular nodules or centrilobular branching structures (97%) or a "tree-in-bud" appearance (72%), bronchial wall thickening (79%) with or without bronchiectasis, or poorly defined nodules 5 to 8 mm in diameter (69%). Findings of bronchogenic spread were also seen in 11 (92%) of 12 patients with reactivation; these findings included centrilobular nodules or visible centrilobular branching structures (92% of patients) or a "tree-in-bud" (67%), bronchial wall thickening (58%) with or

without bronchiectasis, and poorly defined nodules 5 to 8 mm in diameter (42%). Importantly, findings of bronchogenic spread were present even in the absence of cavitation, which was identified in only 24 of 41 (58%) patients (90).

On HRCT, miliary TB results in a very fine, nodular or reticulonodular pattern, with nodules evenly distributed throughout the lung (90,115,118) (Figs. 3-41,5-34). This appearance reflects the presence of uniformly-sized, individual, 1- to 3- or 4-mm nodules involving the intralobular interstitium, interlobular septa, and the subpleural, and perivascular regions (Fig. 5-34). Miliary nodules, present in one patient in Im's study (90), could be distinguished from nodules seen in association with endobronchial spread, because of their smaller size, uniform diameter, even distribution throughout the lung, and because they were unassociated with evidence of bronchial wall thickening (Fig. 3-41).

Hilar and mediastinal lymph node enlargement is commonly seen on HRCT in patients with active TB. In the study by Im et al. (90), mediastinal lymph node enlargement was seen on HRCT in 9 of 29 patients with newly diagnosed disease, and in 2 of 12 patients with reactivation. Right paratracheal and tracheobronchial nodes preponderate (121). In another study by Im et al. (121) of patients with active TB, nodes larger than 2 cm in diameter invariably showed central areas of low attenuation on contrast-enhanced CT, with peripheral rim enhancement; this finding is considered strongly suggestive of active TB (Fig. 5-35). As further documented by Pastores et al. (124), rim-enhancing lymph nodes can be identified in nearly 85% of AIDS patients and 67% of HIV(+) patients with culture or histologically verified TB. Other mediastinal abnormalities visible using CT include fibrosing mediastinitis and endotracheal or endobronchial disease (111).

Pleural abnormalities are also common on HRCT. In patients with active TB, pleural effusions can be small or large, and are often associated with parietal pleural thickening visible on CT; associated visceral pleural thickening may indicate empyema, while air collections within the pleural fluid indicate the presence of bronchopleural fistula and empyema. Empyema necessitatis with chest wall involvement can also result. In patients with long-standing pleural thickening, calcification may be present; residual loculated pleural fluid collections identified with CT in patients with chronic pleural thickening frequently harbor viable bacilli (125). Apical pleural thickening and extrapleural fat thickening is common in patients with post-primary TB and apical lung abnormalities (117)

Utility of HRCT and Clinical Indications

Chest radiographs play a major role in the diagnosis and management of patients with tuberculosis infection, but have limitations (107–112). Radiographic misdiagnosis of primary TB is frequent, occurring in over 30% of cases (107). Also, findings of reactivation or postprimary TB are frequently overlooked on chest radiographs. In the study by Woodring et al. (107), reactivation TB was correctly diagnosed in only 59% of cases.

CT and HRCT can be valuable in several settings. CT is more sensitive than chest radiography in the detection and characterization of both subtle parenchymal (90,112,118) and mediastinal disease (121,124). In patients clinically suspected of having TB, with normal or equivocal radiographic abnormalities, the increased sensitivity of CT may allow prompt diagnosis prior to results of culture (124).

CT and HRCT are especially efficacious in detecting small foci of parenchymal cavitation, both in areas of confluent pneumonia and in areas of dense fibrocalcific disease, associated with distortion of the underlying lung parenchyma (Figs. 5-30,5-31) (111,112). In one study of 41 patients with active TB (90), HRCT showed cavities in 58%, while chest radiographs showed cavities in only 22%. HRCT is also helpful in distinguishing parenchymal cavities from areas of cystic bronchiectasis occurring in association with lung fibrosis (64). Although there is no specific correlation between the radiographic or CT appearance of tuberculous cavities and disease activity (96), CT is an especially effective method for determining the stability of cavities when present. Cavities in patients with tuberculosis usually disappear following chemotherapy; however, "healed" cavities may sometimes persist.

CT and particularly HRCT may also be of value in detecting the presence of diffuse lung involvement when corresponding chest radiographs are normal, or show minimal or limited disease (90,111,112,115). It has been shown that CT and HRCT are more sensitive than plain radiographs in detecting endobronchial spread of TB, a finding which, in our experience and that of others, invariably indicates the presence of activity (Fig. 5-31). In one series, endobronchial tuberculosis was identifiable by CT alone in 40% of cases (112). Occasionally, endobronchial spread is so extensive and diffuse that the appearance mimics diffuse malignancy, especially that resulting from disseminated bronchoalveolar cell carcinoma. Although in most cases the clinical history and course are sufficiently different to avoid confusion, the correct diagnosis may require histologic verification.

CT can also be of value in identifying other forms of diffuse lung disease. In select cases, CT can clarify otherwise misleading chest radiographs, expediting an accurate diagnosis. More important, it has been documented that CT can reveal miliary disease when the chest radiograph is normal (112,118). It should be emphasized, however, that a number of disease entities, in addition to tuberculosis, can result in miliary disease, especially in immunocompromised patients (126). These include both fungal and viral infections. Less commonly, miliary nodules may be the primary finding in HIV(+) patients with *Pneumocystis carinii* pneumonia.

CT more accurately defines the presence and extent of lymph node disease than does routine chest radiography (Fig. 5-35). In particular, the finding of low-attenuation necrotic lymph nodes, with rim enhancement following contrast infusion, strongly suggests a diagnosis of mycobacterial infection, both in immunocompetent patients and in patients who are HIV-positive (36,121,124,127). This appearance is more easily seen on contrast-enhanced CT than on HRCT obtained without contrast enhancement. Although a similar appearance may be seen in patients with fungal infections, especially cryptococcosis and histoplasmosis, this appearance is less frequent in patients with lymphadenopathy secondary to metastatic neoplasm, Kaposi's sarcoma, or lymphoma, and in our experience almost always indicates the presence of a treatable infection (37). In some cases CT can serve as a guide for determining the best sites for node biopsy, and can help determine whether mediastinoscopy or parasternal mediastinotomy is most appropriate. Other mediastinal abnormalities have also been described, including fibrosing mediastinitis as well as endotracheal or bronchial lesions (111). These too are generally easily identified with CT.

CT can be valuable in such cases in which pleural disease is not visible on plain films (125). Residual loculated pleural fluid collections may be identified with CT; these frequently harbor viable bacilli (125). CT can also be valuable in diagnosing bronchopleural fistula.

Complications associated with tuberculosis, including intracavitary mycetoma, and pleural disease such as empyema and bronchopleural fistulas can also be diagnosed using CT. Mycetomas (fungus balls) are common in patients with cavitary tuberculosis, and colonization of cavities by *Aspergillus* species is most frequent. Conventional CT and HRCT are far more efficacious than are chest radiographs in detecting intracavitary mycetoma (Fig. 5-36), and its HRCT appearance has been well described (128). A mature fungus ball is easily identified as a well-circumscribed intracavitary mass or opacity, associated with an air-crescent sign (Fig. 5-36). Typically the position of the intracavitary opacity (and therefore the air-crescent) changes when the patient is scanned in prone and supine positions. As described by Roberts et al. (128), immature or developing aspergillomas can have a somewhat different appearance. In distinction to well-formed fungus balls, immature mycetomas are identifiable as an irregular spongework of soft tissue containing airspaces and obliterating the cavity (Fig. 5-37).

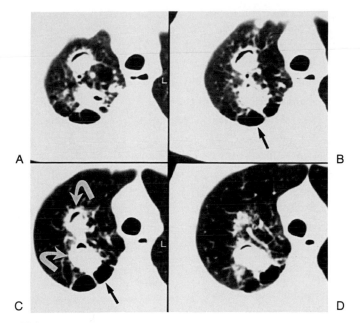

FIG. 5-36. Cavitary tuberculosis associated with an aspergilloma. **A–D:** Enlargements of sequential HRCT images obtained through the right upper lobe, from above-downwards in a patient whose chest radiograph (not shown) suggested the presence of a poorly defined nodule or mass. Two separate cavities can be identified; within both, discrete filling defects can be seen (*curved arrows*, D). Note that these do not represent air-fluid levels. Posteriorly, several bullae can be identified as well, easily distinguished from the adjacent cavities (*straight arrows*, C,D). Subsequent scans obtained in the prone position (not shown) confirmed that the filling defects were free-moving. These findings are characteristic of intracavitary fungus balls. Aspergillomas were subsequently documented bronchoscopically.

Presumably this appearance reflects the presence of irregular fronds of fungal mycelia mixed with some residual intracavitary air. Furthermore, thickening of the wall of a tuberculous cavity can be a finding of superim-

posed fungal infection prior to the development of a fungus ball. In select cases, these findings may lead to earlier and hence more efficacious therapy, including the localization of cavities prior to surgical resection.

Nontuberculous (Atypical) Mycobacterial Infections

Nontuberculous, or atypical, mycobacteria (NTMB) are ubiquitous in the environment, being found in soil, lakes, streams, various food sources, and in domestic animals. Unlike tuberculosis, which is transmitted by person to person contact, NTMB infection is thought to occur because of environmental exposure. Pulmonary infection results predominantly from inhalation of organisms along with dust or aerosolized water droplets. In patients with AIDS, organisms can be acquired through the gastrointestinal tract, with resultant bacteremia and secondary lung involvement (106,129).

A number of species of NTMB have been identified, but pulmonary disease is usually the result of *M. kansasii* or organisms classified as belonging to the *M. avium-intracellulare* complex (MAC) (106,113,129). Because NTMB cultured from the sputum can be a contaminant rather than a pathogen, or can reflect the presence of inconsequential airway colonization in patients with morphologic abnormalities such as bronchiectasis, emphysema, or pneumoconiosis, criteria for the diagnosis of true NTMB infection have been established by the American Thoracic Society (130). In general terms, the ATS criteria for NTMB infection require:

1. In patients with radiographic evidence of cavitation, two or more cultures positive for NTMB, with moderate to heavy growth of organisms,
2. In patients without radiographic evidence of cavitation, two or more cultures positive for *M. kan-*

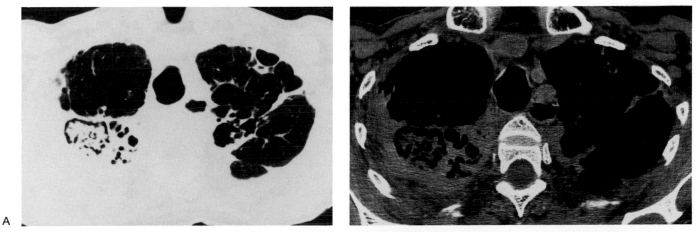

FIG. 5-37. Developing aspergilloma. Lung (**A**) and soft tissue (**B** window scans in a patient with end-stage sarcoidosis and upper lobe cystic disease. A developing aspergilloma in the right upper lobe shows a typical, irregular, sponge-like appearance.

sasii or MAC, with moderate to heavy growth of organisms, and persistent positive cultures after two weeks of treatment, or

3. A diagnostic lung biopsy (106,130).

Nontuberculous mycobacterial infection can be associated with a variety of clinical and radiographic presentations, but two common patterns are seen in immunocompetent individuals (106,129). The first of these, so-called classical NTMB infection, closely resembles tuberculosis; the second form of infection, which has been termed the "nonclassical" form of NTMB, has distinct radiographic and clinical features (106).

Classical NTMB infection is seen predominantly in men, most commonly in their 50s, 60s, and 70s, and many patients have an underlying lung disease, such as COPD, or other risk factors such as smoking or alcohol abuse (106,131). Symptoms are often insidious, and include cough, hemoptysis, and weight loss; fever is present in a minority of patients. Radiographs typically show apical opacities that are nodular or consolidative, and are associated with scarring and volume loss (106,129,131,132). As seen on chest radiographs, cavitation occurs in the large majority (90%) of cases, and is frequently associated with pleural thickening (40%), or endobronchial spread of infection (60%) (131,132). Pleural effusion and lymph node enlargement are less common. Disseminated infection with an appearance mimicking miliary TB is uncommon, being seen in a few percent of cases (129).

The second form of NTMB occurs in 20% to 30% of immunocompetent patients with NTMB, and is typically produced by infection with MAC (106). Patients generally lack predisposing conditions. Women constitute about 80% of cases, and many are in their 70s. As with classical NTMB, the onset of disease is insidious, with chronic cough and hemoptysis being the most

TABLE 5-8. *HRCT findings in nontuberculous mycobacterial infection[a,b]*
1. **Bronchiectasis**
2. **Small or Large Nodules**
3. ***Combination of 1 and 2***
4. **Patchy Unilateral or Bilateral Air-space Consolidation**
5. Cavitation, Thin- or Thick-walled
6. Scattered Air-space (Acinar) Nodules, Centrilobular Branching Structures, "Tree-in-Bud"
7. Scarring and Volume Loss
8. Pleural Effusion or Thickening
9. Hilar/Mediastinal Lymph Node Enlargement

[a] Most common findings in boldface.
[b] Findings most helpful in differential diagnosis in boldface italics.

common symptoms. Fever is uncommon (106). Typical radiographic findings include multiple, bilateral, poorly defined nodules, which involve the lung in a patchy fashion, and lack the upper lobe predominance seen in patients with classical disease. Patchy bronchiectasis is commonly visible radiographically, being most common in the middle lobe and lingula.

CT and HRCT Findings

The CT appearance of pulmonary NTMB infection has been reported by several authors (106,120, 133–135), and varies with the form of disease. As would be expected, the CT appearance of "classical" NTMB mimics that seen in patients with TB. Findings

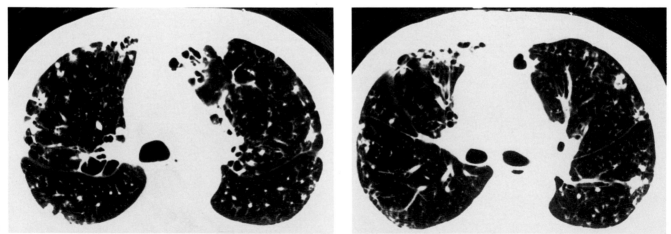

FIG. 5-38. *Mycobacterium avium-intracellulare* complex (MAC) infection. **A,B:** HRCT at two levels in a 63-year-old man shows findings of bronchiectasis and small nodules and clusters of nodules in the peripheral lung. This combination of findings is suggestive of MAC infection.

include apical opacities, cavities that may be smooth or irregular in appearance, bronchiectasis in regions of severe lung damage, pleural thickening adjacent to abnormal lung regions, and small nodules (0.5 to 2.0 cm) in areas of lung distant to the dominant focus of infection (106), probably representing endobronchial spread of infection.

The CT appearance of "nonclassical" NTMB infection caused by *Mycobacterium avium-intracellulare* complex (MAC) has been reported by several authors (133–135). Although patients with atypical mycobacterial infections can show a variety of CT findings, there is a propensity for such patients to have bronchiectasis in combination with small nodules, although not necessarily in the same lobe (Fig. 5-38) (Table 5-8) (120,133,134). In a study by Hartman et al. (133), CT scans were reviewed in 62 patients with positive MAC cultures. Of the 62 patients, 60 had pulmonary opacities, which were nodular in 39, and 40 had bronchiectasis. Most significant, all 35 patients with small nodular infiltrates also had bronchiectasis. None of these

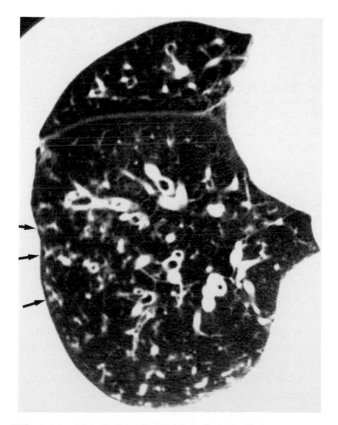

FIG. 5-39. *Mycobacterium avium-intracellulare* complex (MAC). Targeted HRCT through the right lower lobe of an elderly white female with a chronic cough, shows focal areas of bronchiectasis associated with scattered, poorly defined centrilobular nodular and tubular branching structures (*arrows*). Not infrequently, as in this case, these HRCT findings are the first to suggest possible infection by a nontuberculous mycobacterium. Subsequent sputum samples revealed heavy growth of MAC.

35 patients were immunocompromised, and 29 (83%) of them were women, with a mean age of 66 years. Of the 27 patients without small nodular infiltrates and bronchiectasis, 25 had underlying malignancy or immunocompromise. In a study (120) comparing the frequency of bronchiectasis in patients with tuberculosis to that seen with MAC infection, bronchiectasis was found to be significantly more common in patients with MAC (94% vs. 27% for patients with TB).

Moore (134) reviewed the CT and HRCT findings in 40 patients with cultures positive for atypical mycobacteria. Common findings included bronchiectasis (80%), consolidation or ground-glass opacity (73%), nodules (70%), and evidence of scarring and/or volume loss (28%). Less commonly observed were cavities, lymphadenopathy, and pleural disease. Both small (< 1 cm) well-defined nodules and large and ill-defined nodules were seen; some small nodules were centrilobular and associated with a tree-in-bud appearance (Figs. 5-39,5-40). In some patients, bronchiectasis was seen to develop in previously normal lung regions, suggesting that this finding results from the mycobacterial infection, and does not represent a preexisting or predisposing condition. She concluded that some combination of bronchiectasis, consolidation, and nodules on CT scans should raise the possibility of atypical mycobacterial infection; thirty of the 40 patients showed 2 or 3 of these findings. As reported by Hartman et al. (133), most (65%) patients were women, with a mean age of 68 years.

Swensen et al. (135) tested the hypothesis that bronchiectasis and multiple small lung nodules seen on chest CT are indicative of MAC infection or colonization by reviewing the CT scans of 100 patients with a CT diagnosis of bronchiectasis; 24 of these 100 patients also had multiple pulmonary nodules visible on CT. Mycobacterial cultures were performed in 15 of the 24 patients with lung nodules seen in combination with bronchiectasis and 48 of the 76 patients who had bronchiectasis without lung nodules. Of the 15 patients with bronchiectasis and lung nodules, 8 (53%) had cultures positive for MAC, as did 2 of the 48 (4%) patients with no CT evidence of lung nodules. Thus, the authors found that CT findings of small lung nodules in association with bronchiectasis had a sensitivity of 80%, a specificity of 87%, and an accuracy of 86% in predicting positive cultures for MAC.

Mycobacterial Infections in AIDS Patients

Mycobacterial infections occur in about 10% of AIDS patients (35). In patients with AIDS and TB infection, although evidence suggests reactivation is the most likely mechanism of disease, the radiographic appearance is more typical of primary TB. Noncavitary

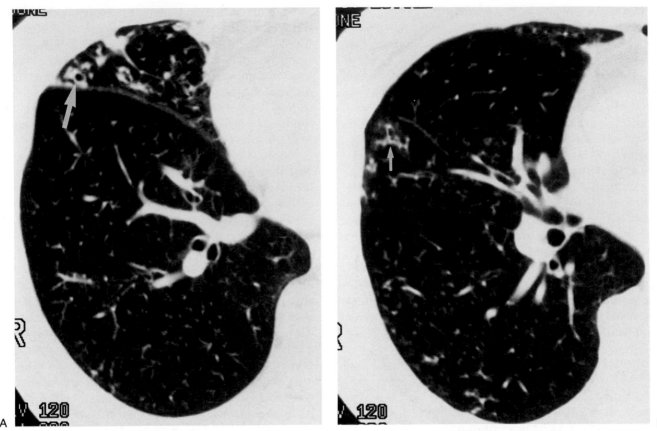

FIG. 5-40. *Mycobacterium avium-intracellulare* complex (MAC). **A,B:** HRCT in an elderly white female shows focal bronchiectasis (*large arrow*) associated with a tree-in-bud appearance (*small arrow*) and small centrilobular nodules. These abnormalities are largely limited to the right middle lobe.

areas of consolidation distributed equally in upper and lower-lung regions and hilar and mediastinal lymphadenopathy are common. MAC infection is also commonly seen, and is usually widely disseminated at the time of diagnosis.

Tuberculosis in the HIV(+) Patient

The incidence of *M. tuberculosis* in the United States has dramatically increased as a result of the AIDS epidemic. TB is now defined as an AIDS indicator disease in HIV(+) patients with CD4 cell counts below 200 cells mm³ (136).

The diagnosis of TB especially in patients with AIDS is frequently problematic (100). The tuberculin skin test remains positive in only about one-third of AIDS patients while positive acid-fast sputum smears occur in less than 50% of HIV(+) patients with active tuberculosis (137,138). Additionally, the likelihood of a positive smear has been shown to be independent of both the presence of parenchymal cavitation on chest radiographs and the CD4 cell count (138,139). Bronchoalveolar lavage is only positive in approximately 20% of cases.

The radiographic manifestations of TB in HIV(+) patients reflect the extent of cellular immune compromise (100,103,138,140,141). Early in the course of infection, especially in patients with CD4 cell counts greater than 200/mm³, tuberculosis is usually indistinguishable from that which occurs in non-HIV(+) patients. Cutaneous reactivity to tuberculin is generally preserved, and radiographic manifestations include upper lobe cavitary infiltrates (100,102,103). In contrast, in more severely immunocompromised patients, sputum culture is more likely to be positive, and radiographs are usually suggestive of primary infection. Long et al. (103), found that a pattern typical of primary TB was identified on chest radiographs in 80% of AIDS patients as compared to 30% of HIV(+) patients without clinical AIDS, and only 11% of HIV(−) patients with TB. In a study of 97 HIV-infected patients with TB, Jones et al. (141) found that mediastinal adenopathy was noted in 20 (34%) of 58 patients with CD4 counts < 200 cells/mm³ compared with only 4 (14%) of 29 patients with CD4 counts > 200 cells/mm³.

Dissemination of infection is also more common in patients with greater degrees of immunocompromise. As documented by Hill et al. (142) in a study of 51

AIDS patients with disseminated disease, chest radiographs showed evidence of miliary disease in nearly half and intrathoracic lymphadenopathy in one-third.

Up to 85% of HIV(+) patients with documented tuberculosis have abnormal radiographs. These findings have led the Centers for Disease Control and Prevention (CDC) to recommend routine radiographic screening of all HIV-seropositive patients (143). In addition, as delay in diagnosis may cause a significant increase in mortality in this population, it has been suggested that empiric therapy be initiated in all patients with chest radiographic findings suggestive of TB (144).

Despite a close correlation between radiographic findings and the level of immunocompromise, a normal radiograph does not preclude active disease. Normal chest radiographs have been reported in as many as 15% of cases with documented sputum culture positive tuberculosis, even in patients with CD4 counts < 200 mm^3 (138,145). In a retrospective study of 133 AIDS patients with culture positive tuberculosis, chest radiographs failed to suggest the correct diagnosis in 32% of cases (138). In this study, the failure to diagnose TB resulted when radiographs appeared normal (13% of cases), showed "minimal" radiographic abnormalities such as linear opacities or calcified granulomas, or showed atypical patterns of disease, such as diffuse reticulonodular infiltrates mimicking infection with *Pneumocystis carinii* pneumonia (138).

Evaluation of this population is further complicated by the increasing frequency of multidrug resistant organisms (MDR-TB). The result either of initial infection with a drug-resistant organism (primary resistance) or inadequate treatment (secondary resistance), infection with drug-resistance organisms frequently results in rapidly progressive disease in the absence of appropriate therapy. Although patients with MDR-TB are more likely to have infiltrates and cavities, these findings are nonspecific. Nonetheless, it has been suggested that chest radiographs may play an indispensable role in the early diagnosis of drug-resistance by confirming a lack of response to routine antituberculous chemotherapy. As reported by Lessnau et al. (145) in a study of 72 patients, 33 with sensitive MTB, and 39 with single-drug resistant (3) or multidrug resistant MTB (36), initial radiographs were of little value in distinguishing these groups. However, after 2 weeks of therapy, 20 of 35 (57%) patients with MDR-TB showed progression of disease, while this was not the case in patients with sensitive MTB. Based on these data, the authors suggested that pending drug sensitivity results, evidence of worsening on chest radiographs following 2 weeks of routine antituberculous therapy could be interpreted as presumptive evidence of MDR-TB (145). On the other hand, as documented by others, disease progression on treatment may not indicate MDR-TB but coexistent infection. Small et al., for example, in a study of 33 HIV(+) patients with tuberculosis found that while all 25 patients with pulmonary TB alone exhibited radiographic improvement after appropriate therapy, in 8 patients, radiographic evidence of progression was found to correlate with a newly acquired nontuberculous pulmonary disease.

Nontuberculous Mycobacterial Infection in the HIV(+) Patient

Although less commonly identified as a cause of pulmonary disease than *M. tuberculosis*, the incidence of nontuberculous mycobacterial infections, especially MAC, is increasing, especially in HIV(+) homosexual men (146). Because the main portal of infection in patients with MAC is the gastrointestinal tract, infection is typically disseminated at the time of diagnosis. Intrathoracic involvement typically occurs late in the course of infection, with significant chest radiographic changes occurring in only 5% of cases. Unfortunately, radiographic findings are indistinguishable from those caused by *M. tuberculosis*, and include intrathoracic adenopathy, pulmonary infiltrates, nodules and miliary disease. In most cases, these findings probably represent secondary infection in patients with already documented disseminated disease. In addition to MAC, patients with AIDS also may become infected with other nontuberculous mycobacteria (147–150). In particular, *M. kansasii* may result in treatable pulmonary disease that otherwise resembles reactivation tuberculosis. As shown by Levine and Chaisson (147), 14 of 19 patients with documented *M. kansasii* infection had exclusive pulmonary disease. Nine of these showed marked improvement following initiation of antituberculous chemotherapy while autopsies performed on another three treated patients showed no evidence of residual infection.

CT and HRCT in HIV(+) Patients

Among 16 AIDS patients with TB or MAC infections (36), CT findings included lymphadenopathy (75%), nodules (38%), pleural effusion (38%), consolidation (19%), masses (25%), ground-glass opacity (19%). As in immunocompetent patients with TB, CT and HRCT can be valuable in diagnosis when plain radiographs are nonspecific. On CT in these patients, mycobacterial infection was suggested as the first choice diagnosis in 44%, and among the top 3 choices in 77%.

Only a few reports of CT findings in AIDS patients with nontuberculous mycobacterial infections have been published (36,150). Of particular note, unlike patients with TB, low-density lymphadenopathy appears to occur infrequently, identified in one series in only 3 of 11 patients with documented adenopathy and infection with MAC (36).

FUNGAL DISEASE AND INVASIVE ASPERGILLOSIS

Most fungal diseases result in CT and HRCT patterns of disease indistinguishable from those described for mycobacterial infections, including both focal and diffuse parenchymal infiltrates, cavitation, nodules, hilar and mediastinal adenopathy, and pleural disease. This, of course, reflects the similar pathology of tuberculous and most fungal infections. For example, small centrilobular nodules similar to those seen with endobronchial spread of tuberculosis have been reported with endobronchial spread of cryptococcal pneumonia (122,123). In general, the accurate diagnosis of a fungal infection requires confirmation by histologic examination of a biopsy specimen or culture.

One possible exception is the diagnosis of invasive pulmonary aspergillosis in immunocompromised patients. In patients with invasive pulmonary aspergillosis, CT can show characteristic findings that strongly suggest the diagnosis early in the course of disease (151,152). Clinically, this diagnosis may be extremely difficult to make, and transbronchial or open lung biopsies are frequently hazardous in immunosuppressed patients because of profound bone marrow suppression. This problem is further compounded by the potentially severe side effects associated with routine antifungal therapy.

Typically, radiographic findings of invasive pulmonary aspergillosis are nonspecific until healing of the lesion or lesions has begun; during healing, cavitary nodules with air-crescents characteristically develop, reflecting the presence of a necrotizing pneumonia.

Invasive pulmonary aspergillosis commonly results in scattered foci of pulmonary parenchymal inflammation, infarction, and necrosis, which reflect hematogenous dissemination of the fungal organism associated with vascular obstruction. As documented by Kuhlman et al. (152) in patients with acute leukemia who have early invasive aspergillosis, CT predictably shows a "halo" of opacity surrounding focal dense parenchymal nodules. The halo surrounding the nodule is characteristically lower in attenuation than the nodule itself; in other words the halo is of ground-glass opacity. This appearance has been termed the *halo sign.* Many of these characteristic lesions are associated with vessels (Fig. 5-41).

Hruban et al. (153) have obtained radiologic-pathologic correlation in patients with documented invasive pulmonary aspergillosis, and have clarified the etiology of the halo sign. In their patients the halo and central nodule reflected, respectively, a rim of coagulation necrosis or hemorrhage surrounding a central fungal nodule or infarct; an association of the halo sign with hemorrhagic nodules has been confirmed by others (154).

Some authors (152,153) have concluded that, in an appropriate population, the CT appearance of early invasive aspergillosis with a visible halo sign, is sufficiently characteristic to justify an presumptive diagnosis and treatment. In one study, a halo sign was seen in 5 of 21 bone marrow transplantation patients with a fungal infection (155). However, others have emphasized that this finding can be associated with a variety of infectious and noninfectious processes. The halo sign has been reported in association with tuberculosis (156), candidiasis, Legionella pneumonia, cytomegalovirus, herpes simplex, Wegener's granulomatosis, metastatic angiosarcoma, and Kaposi's sarcoma (154).

The utility of CT in assessing immunosuppressed patients with fever has been stressed by several investigators; in this setting CT is more sensitive in detecting nodules suggestive of fungal infection and in characterizing their appearance. In a study (155), of febrile bone marrow transplant recipients, nodules were visible on

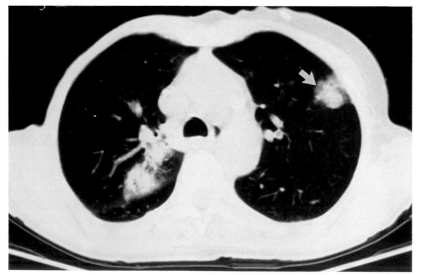

FIG. 5-41. Invasive pulmonary aspergillosis. HRCT section at the level of the carina in a severely immunocompromised patient following a right mastectomy. Focal, somewhat nodular areas of consolidation are present bilaterally, some of which are adjacent to areas of ground-glass opacification (*arrow*). It has been shown that this finding corresponds histologically with the presence of hemorrhage and edema and is particularly suggestive of the diagnosis of early invasive aspergillosis.

CT in 20 of 21 patients with fungal infections, and CT also showed cavitation ($n = 7$), the halo sign ($n = 4$), ill-defined margins ($n = 5$), air-bronchograms ($n = 2$), or a cluster of fluffy nodules ($n = 1$). Chest radiographs showed nodules in only 17, and cavitation in only 5. In none of the nine episodes of fever resulting from bacteremia were there opacities on chest radiographs or CT studies. The authors concluded that CT studies demonstrating complicated nodules in febrile BMT patients strongly suggest a fungal infection, whereas negative CT studies suggest bacteremia or infection of nonpulmonary origin.

In AIDS patients, CT can also be of value in the diagnosis of fungal infections (36). Fungal infections, however, are relatively uncommon in this setting, being seen in less than 5% of patients (35). Fungal infections in AIDS patients usually accompany disseminated disease. CT findings reported in AIDS patients include lymphadenopathy, nodules, masses, and consolidation (36).

SEPTIC EMBOLISM AND INFARCTION

Septic pulmonary emboli, with or without infarction, generally result in diffuse parenchymal abnormalities; only rarely do they present as solitary lesions within the lungs. The correct radiographic diagnosis usually is suggested by the finding of well-defined, bilateral peripheral nodules with various degrees of cavitation, especially in the setting of known intravenous-drug abuse, or some other known source of sepsis. In a sig-

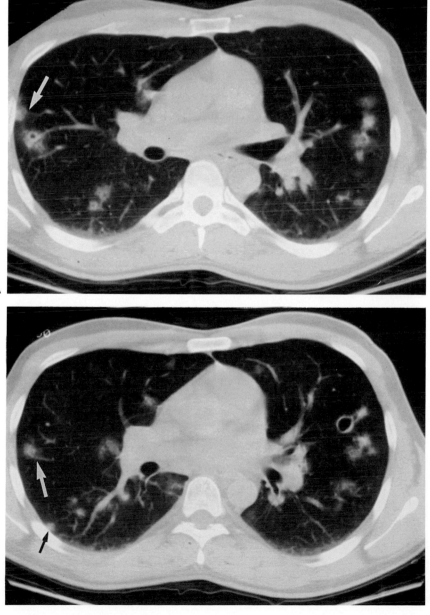

FIG. 5-42. Septic pulmonary emboli. **A,B:** CT sections through the midlungs of a known intravenous-drug abuser show scattered, mostly peripheral, poorly defined foci of air-space consolidation, many of which contain varying degrees of cavitation. Note that a number of these appear to be associated with "feeding" vessels (*arrows*, A,B), suggesting a hematogenous origin. Subsequent blood cultures confirmed staphylococcal septicemia.

TABLE 5-9. HRCT findings in septic embolism and infarction[a,b]

1. **Bilateral Peripheral Nodules in Varying Stages of Cavitation**

2. **Peripheral Wedge-shaped Triangular Opacities Abutting Pleural Surfaces, with or without Cavitation**

3. **Relationship of Opacities to Vessels**

4. *Superimposition of Findings 1, 2, and 3*

5. Associated Pleural and/or Pericardial Effusions

6. Indwelling Venous Catheters

[a] Most common findings in boldface.
[b] Findings most helpful in differential diagnosis in boldface italics.

nificant percentage of cases, however, these findings may not be readily apparent on the radiograph (157). Cavitary parenchymal nodules presumably result from septic occlusion of small, peripheral pulmonary arterial branches, resulting in the development of metastatic lung abscesses. The finding of triangular, wedge-shaped regions most likely results from infarction complicated by infection, presumably caused by larger emboli than those that result in simple nodular lung abscesses.

CT and HRCT Findings

The CT appearance of septic pulmonary emboli and infarcts has been well described (Table 5-9) (157–160). In patients with septic embolism, peripheral nodules in varying stages of cavitation are often present, presumably due to intermittent seeding of the lungs by infected material. Especially characteristic is the finding of identifiable feeding vessels in association with peripheral nodules (Fig. 5-42); this was visible in 10 (67%) of 15 cases studied by Huang et al. (157). Similar findings have been reported by Kuhlman et al. (159) in a series of 18 patients with documented septic pulmonary emboli; these authors found nodules associated with vessels in 67% of cases.

CT can be helpful in suggesting the diagnosis of septic embolism. Compared with plain radiographs, CT scans provided useful additional information in 8 of 15 cases (53%) in one study (157). Furthermore, the diagnosis of septic embolism was first suggested on CT in 7 of 15 cases, and in 6 of 18 cases (157,159).

Septic emboli may also result in pulmonary infarction. An infarction is recognizable as a triangular, wedge-shaped opacity with its base oriented at the pleural surface. Following the administration of a bolus of intravenous-contrast medium, the perimeter of an infarct characteristically enhances, possibly owing to collateral blood flow from adjacent bronchial arteries, while the center of the lesion remains lucent. Cystic changes within an area of infarction may signify either necrosis or infection. Unfortunately, this appearance is not entirely diagnostic, because pneumonias may occasionally have a similar appearance. As suggested by Balakrishnan et al. (160), in a CT- pathologic correlative study of 12 proven pulmonary infarcts in 10 patients, specificity increases when a vessel can be identified at the apex of the infarct.

It should be noted that especially septic emboli, but rarely the appearance of pulmonary infarcts, may be mimicked either by a vasculitis, such as Wegener's granulomatosis, or even cavitary metastases. In these cases, however, confusion with septic emboli, in particular, is rare because of the differences in clinical presentation.

REFERENCES

1. Trapnell DH. The radiological appearance of lymphangitic carcinomatosis of the lung. *Thorax* 1964;19:251–260.
2. Heitzman ER. Pattern recognition in pulmonary radiology. In: *The Lung: Radiologic-Pathologic Correlations*, 2nd ed. St. Louis: Mosby; 1984:70–105.
3. Genereux GP. Pattern recognition in diffuse lung disease: a review of theory and practice. *Med Radiogr Photog* 1985;61: 2–31.
4. Carstairs LS. The interpretation of shadows in a restricted area of a lung field on the chest radiograph. *Proc r Soc Med* 1961; 54:1961.
5. Heitzman ER. *The Lung: Radiologic-Pathologic Correlations*, 2nd ed. St. Louis: Mosby; 1984:413–421.
6. Bégin R, Ostiguy G, Fillion R, Colman N. Computed tomography scan in the early detection of silicosis. *Am Rev Respir Dis* 1991;3:1.
7. Remy-Jardin M, Degreef JM, Beuscart R, Voisin C, Remy J. Coal worker's pneumoconiosis: CT assessment in exposed workers and correlation with radiographic findings. *Radiology* 1990;177:363–371.
8. Spencer H. *Pathology of the Lung*. Oxford: Pergamon Press; 1985:1085–1090.
9. Davis SD. CT evaluation for pulmonary metastases in patients with extrathoracic malignancy. *Radiology* 1991;180:1–12.
10. Janower ML, Blennerhasset JB. Lymphangitic spread of metastatic tumor to lung. *Radiology* 1971;101:267–273.
11. Goldsmith SH, Bailey HD, Callahan EL, Beattie EJ. Pulmonary metastases from breast carcinoma. *Arch Surg* 1967;94: 483–488.
12. Sadoff F, Grossman J, Weiner N. Lymphangitic pulmonary metastasis secondary to breast cancer with normal chest x-rays and abnormal perfusion lung scans. *Oncology* 1975;31:164–171.
13. Munk PL, Müller NL, Miller RR, Ostrow DN. Pulmonary lymphangitic carcinomatosis: CT and pathologic findings. *Radiology* 1988;166:705–709.
14. Ren H, Hruban RH, Kuhlman JE, et al. Computed tomography of inflation-fixed lungs: the beaded septum sign of pulmonary metastases. *J Comput Assist Tomogr* 1989;13:411–416.
15. Colby TV. Anatomic distribution and histopathologic patterns in interstitial lung disease. In: Schwarz MI, King TE Jr, eds. *Interstitial Lung Disease*. St. Louis: Mosby Year Book; 1993: 59–77.
16. Remy-Jardin M, Beuscart R, Sault MC, Marquette CH, Remy J. Subpleural micronodules in diffuse infiltrative lung diseases: evaluation with thin-section CT scans. *Radiology* 1990;177: 133–139.

17. Zerhouni EA, Naidich DP, Stitik FP, Khouri NF, Siegelman SS. Computed tomography of the pulmonary parenchyma: part 2. interstitial disease. *J Thorac Imaging* 1985;1:54–64.
18. Stein MG, Mayo J, Müller N, Aberle DR, Webb WR, Gamsu G. Pulmonary lymphangitic spread of carcinoma: appearance on CT scans. *Radiology* 1987;162:371–375.
19. Meziane MA, Hruban RH, Zerhouni EA, et al. High resolution CT of the lung parenchyma with pathologic correlation. *Radiographics* 1988;8:27–54.
20. Webb WR. High-resolution CT of the lung parenchyma. *Radiol Clin North Am* 1989;27:1085–1097.
21. Johkoh T, Ikezoe J, Tomiyama N, et al. CT findings in lymphangitic carcinomatosis of the lung: correlation with histologic findings and pulmonary function tests. *AJR* 1992;158:1217–1222.
22. Gruden JF, Webb WR, Warnock M. Centrilobular opacities in the lung on high-resolution CT: diagnostic considerations and pathologic correlation. *AJR* 1994;162:569–574.
23. Grenier P, Chevret S, Beigelman C, Brauner MW, Chastang C, Valeyre D. Chronic diffuse infiltrative lung disease: determination of the diagnostic value of clinical data, chest radiography, and CT with Bayesian analysis. *Radiology* 1994;194:383–390.
24. Brauner MW, Grenier P, Mompoint D, Lenoir S, de Cremoux H. Pulmonary sarcoidosis: evaluation with high-resolution CT. *Radiology* 1989;172:467–471.
25. Webb WR, Stein MG, Finkbeiner WE, Im JG, Lynch D, Gamsu G. Normal and diseased isolated lungs: high-resolution CT. *Radiology* 1988;166:81–87.
26. Murata K, Takahashi M, Mori M, et al. Pulmonary metastatic nodules: CT-pathologic correlation. *Radiology* 1992;182:331–335.
27. Peuchot M, Libshitz HI. Pulmonary metastatic disease: radiologic-surgical correlation. *Radiology* 1987;164:719–722.
28. Hill CA. Bronchioloalveolar carcinoma: a review. *Radiology* 1984;150:15–20.
29. Adler B, Padley S, Miller RR, Müller NL. High-resolution CT of bronchioloalveolar carcinoma. *AJR* 1992;159:275–277.
30. Hommeyer SH, Godwin JD, Takasugi JE. Computed tomography of air-space disease. *Radiol Clin North Am* 1991;29:1065–1084.
31. Im JG, Han MC, Yu EJ, et al. Lobar bronchioloalveolar carcinoma: "angiogram sign" on CT scans. *Radiology* 1990;176:749–753.
32. Naidich DP, Zerhouni EA, Hutchins GM, Genieser NB, McCauley DI, Siegelman SS. Computed tomography of the pulmonary parenchyma: part 1. distal air-space disease. *J Thorac Imaging* 1985;1:39–53.
33. Metzger RA, Multhern CB, Arger PH, Coleman BG, Epstein DM, Gefter WB. CT differentiation of solitary from diffuse bronchioloalveolar carcinoma. *J Comput Assist Tomogr* 1981;5:830–833.
34. Zwirewich CV, Miller RR, Müller NL. Multicentric adenocarcinoma of the lung: CT-pathologic correlation. *Radiology* 1990;176:185–190.
35. Naidich DP, McGuinness G. Pulmonary manifestations of AIDS: CT and radiographic correlations. *Rad Clin North Am* 1991;29:999–1017.
36. Hartman TE, Primack SL, Müller NL, Staples CA. Diagnosis of thoracic complications in AIDS: accuracy of CT. *AJR* 1994;162:547–553.
37. Naidich DP, Tarras M, Garay SM, Birnbaum B, Rybak BJ, Schinella R. Kaposi sarcoma: CT-radiographic correlation. *Chest* 1989;96:723–728.
38. Wolff SD, Kuhlman JE, Fishman EK. Thoracic Kaposi sarcoma in AIDS: CT findings. *J Comput Assist Tomogr* 1993;17:60–62.
39. Gruden JF, Klein JS, Webb WR. Percutaneous transthoracic needle biopsy in AIDS: analysis in 32 patients. *Radiology* 1993;189:567–571.
40. Colby TV, Carrington CB. Infiltrative lung disease. In: *Pathology of the Lung*. Stuttgart: Thieme Medical; 1988:425–518.
41. Crystal RG, Bitterman PB, Rennard SI, Hance AJ, Keogh BA. Interstitial lung diseases of unknown cause: disorders characterized by chronic inflammation of the lower respiratory tract. *N Engl J Med* 1984;310:154–166.
42. Thomas PD, Hunninghake GW. Current concepts of the pathogenesis of sarcoidosis. *Am Rev Respir Dis* 1987;135:747–760.
43. Rosen Y, Athanassiades TJ, Moon S, Lyons HA. Nongranulomatous interstitial pneumonitis in sarcoidosis. *Chest* 1978;74:122–125.
44. Crystal RG, Gadek JE, Ferrans VJ, Fulmer JD, Line BR, Hunninghake GW. Interstitial lung disease: current concepts of pathogenesis, staging and therapy. *Am J Med* 1981;70:542–568.
45. Keogh BA, Hunninghake GW, Line BR, Crystal RG. The alveolitis of pulmonary sarcoidosis: evaluation of natural history and alveolitis-dependent changes in lung function. *Am Rev Resp Dis* 1983;128:256–265.
46. Müller NL, Miller RR. Ground-glass attenuation, nodules, alveolitis, and sarcoid granulomas [editorial]. *Radiology* 1993;189:31–32.
47. Hillerdal G, Neu E, Osterman K, Schmekel B. Sarcoidosis: epidemiology and prognosis, a 15-year European study. *Am Rev Respir Dis* 1984;130:29–32.
48. McLoud TC, Epler GR, Gaensler EA, Burke GW, Carrington CB. A radiographic classification for sarcoidosis: physiologic correlation. *Invest Radiol* 1982;17:129–138.
49. Scadding JG, Mitchell DN, eds. *Sarcoidosis*, 2nd ed. London: Chapman and Hall Medical; 1985:101–180.
50. Hamper UM, Fishman EK, Khouri NF, Johns CJ, Wang KP, Siegelman SS. Typical and atypical CT manifestations of pulmonary sarcoidosis. *J Comput Assist Tomogr* 1986;10:928–936.
51. Dawson WB, Müller NL. High-resolution computed tomography in pulmonary sarcoidosis. *Semin Ultrasound CT MR* 1990;11:423–429.
52. Müller NL, Kullnig P, Miller RR. The CT findings of pulmonary sarcoidosis: analysis of 25 patients. *AJR* 1989;152:1179–1182.
53. Müller NL, Miller RR. Computed tomography of chronic diffuse infiltrative lung disease: part 2. *Am Rev Respir Dis* 1990;142:1440–1448.
54. Heitzman ER. Sarcoidosis. In: *The Lung: Radiologic-Pathologic Correlations*. St. Louis: Mosby; 1984:294–310.
55. Carrington CB, Gaensler EA, Mikus JP, Schachter AW, Burke GW, Goff AM. Structure and function in sarcoidosis. *Ann N Y Acad Sci* 1976;278:265–283.
56. Bergin CJ, Bell DY, Coblentz CL, et al. Sarcoidosis: correlation of pulmonary parenchymal pattern at CT with results of pulmonary function tests. *Radiology* 1989;171:619–624.
57. Lynch DA, Webb WR, Gamsu G, Stulbarg M, Golden J. Computed tomography in pulmonary sarcoidosis. *J Comput Assist Tomogr* 1989;13:405–410.
58. Remy-Jardin M, Giraud F, Remy J, Wattinne L, Wallaert B, Duhamel A. Pulmonary sarcoidosis: role of CT in the evaluation of disease activity and functional impairment and in prognosis assessment. *Radiology* 1994;191:675–680.
59. Nishimura K, Itoh H, Kitaichi M, Nagai S, Izumi T. Pulmonary sarcoidosis: correlation of CT and histopathologic findings. *Radiology* 1993;189:105–109.
60. Brauner MW, Lenoir S, Grenier P, Cluzel P, Battesti JP, Valeyre D. Pulmonary sarcoidosis: CT assessment of lesion reversibility. *Radiology* 1992;182:349–354.
61. Grenier P, Valeyre D, Cluzel P, Brauner MW, Lenoir S, Chastang C. Chronic diffuse interstitial lung disease: diagnostic value of chest radiography and high-resolution CT. *Radiology* 1991;179:123–132.
62. Leung AN, Miller RR, Müller NL. Parenchymal opacification in chronic infiltrative lung diseases: CT-pathologic correlation. *Radiology* 1993;188:209–214.
63. Bergin CJ, Müller NL. CT of interstitial lung disease: a diagnostic approach. *AJR* 1987;148:9–15.
64. Westcott JL, Cole SR. Traction bronchiectasis in end-stage pulmonary fibrosis. *Radiology* 1986;161:665–669.
65. Primack SL, Hartman TE, Hansell DM, Müller NL. End-stage lung disease: CT findings in 61 patients. *Radiology* 1993;189:681–686.
66. Nakata H, Kimoto T, Nakayama T, Kido M, Miyazaki N, Harada S. Diffuse peripheral lung disease: evaluation by high-resolution computed tomography. *Radiology* 1985;157:181–185.

67. Murdoch J, Müller NL. Pulmonary sarcoidosis: changes on follow-up CT examinations. *AJR* 1992;159:473–477.
68. Austin JHM. Pulmonary sarcoidosis: what are we learning from CT? *Radiology* 1989;171:603–604.
69. Müller NL, Mawson JB, Mathieson JR, Abboud R, Ostrow DN, Champion P. Sarcoidosis: correlation of extent of disease at CT with clinical, functional, and radiographic findings. *Radiology* 1989;171:613–618.
70. Mathieson JR, Mayo JR, Staples CA, Müller NL. Chronic diffuse infiltrative lung disease: comparison of diagnostic accuracy of CT and chest radiography. *Radiology* 1989;171: 111–116.
71. Akira M, Higashihara T, Yokoyama K, et al. Radiographic type p pneumoconiosis: high-resolution CT. *Radiology* 1989;171: 117–123.
72. Bégin R, Bergeron D, Samson L, Boctor M, Cantin A. CT assessment of silicosis in exposed workers. *AJR* 1987;148: 509–514.
73. Bergin CJ, Müller NL, Vedal S, Chan Yeung M. CT in silicosis: correlation with plain films and pulmonary function tests. *AJR* 1986;146:477–483.
74. Bergin C, Roggli V, Coblentz C, Chiles C. The secondary pulmonary lobule: normal and abnormal CT appearances. *AJR* 1988;151:21–25.
75. Newman LS, Buschman DL, Newell JD, Lynch DL. Beryllium disease: assessment with CT. *Radiology* 1994;190:835–840.
76. Harris KM, McConnochie K, Adams H. The computed tomographic appearances in chronic berylliosis. *Clin Radiol* 1993; 47:26–31.
77. Seaton A. Silicosis. In: *Occupational Lung Diseases*, 2nd ed. Philadelphia: WB Saunders; 1984:250–294.
78. Sargent EN, Morgan WKC. Silicosis. In: *Induced Disease. Drug, Irradiation, Occupation*. New York: Grune & Stratton; 1980:297–315.
79. Sargent EN, Morgan WKC. Coal workers' pneumoconiosis. In: *Induced Disease. Drug, Irradiation, Occupation*. New York: Grune & Stratton; 1980:275–295.
80. Fraser RG, Paré JAP. The pneumoconioses and chemically-induced lung diseases. In: *Diagnosis of Diseases of the Chest*. Philadelphia: WB Saunders; 1977:1484–1502.
81. Pendergrass EP. Caldwell Lecture 1957: silicosis and a few of the other pneumoconioses: observations of certain aspects of the problem, with emphasis on the role of the radiologist. *AJR* 1958;80:1–41.
82. Parkes WR. Diseases due to free silica. In: *Occupational Lung Disorders*, 2nd ed. London: Butterworth; 1982:134–158.
83. Bégin R, Ostiguy G, Groleau S, Filion R. Computed tomographic scanning of the thorax in workers at risk of or with silicosis. *Semin Ultrasound CT MR* 1990;11:380–392.
84. Kinsella N, Müller NL, Vedal S, Staples C, Abboud RT, Chan-Yeung M. Emphysema in silicosis: a comparison of smokers with nonsmokers using pulmonary function testing and computed tomography. *Am Rev Respir Dis* 1990;141:1497–1500.
85. Bégin R, Ostiguy G, Cantin A, Bergeron D. Lung function in silica-exposed workers: a relationship to disease severity assessed by CT scan. *Chest* 1988;94:539–545.
86. Thompson PJ, Citron KM. Amyloid and the lower respiratory tract. *Thorax* 1983;38:84–87.
87. Hui AN, Koss MN, Hochholzer L, Wehnut WD. Amyloidosis presenting in the lower respiratory tract: clinicopathologic, radiologic, immunohistochemical and histochemical studies on 48 cases. *Arch Pathol Lab Med* 1986;110:212–218.
88. Ayuso MC, Gilabert R, Bombi JA, Salvador A. CT appearance of localized pulmonary amyloidosis. *J Comput Assist Tomogr* 1987;11:197–199.
89. Graham CM, Stern EJ, Finkbeiner WE, Webb WR. High-resolution CT appearance of diffuse alveolar septal amyloidosis. *AJR* 1992;158:265–267.
90. Im JG, Itoh H, Shim YS, et al. Pulmonary tuberculosis: CT findings—early active disease and sequential change with anti-tuberculous therapy. *Radiology* 1993;186:653–660.
91. Padley SPG, Adler BD, Staples CA, Miller RR, Müller NL. Pulmonary talcosis: CT findings in three cases. *Radiology* 1993; 186:125–127.
92. Hamrick-Turner J, Abbitt PL, Harrison RB, Cranston PE. Diffuse lung calcification following fat emboli and adult respiratory distress syndromes: CT findings. *J Thorac Imaging* 1994;9: 47–50.
93. Hartman TE, Müller NL, Primack SL, et al. Metastatic pulmonary calcification in patients with hypercalcemia: findings on chest radiographs and CT scans. *AJR* 1994;162:799–802.
94. Cluzel P, Grenier P, Bernadac P, Laurent F, Picard JD. Pulmonary alveolar microlithiasis: CT findings. *J Comput Assist Tomogr* 1991;15:938–942.
95. Korn MA, Schurawitzki H, Klepetko W, Burghuber OC. Pulmonary alveolar microlithiasis: findings on high-resolution CT. *AJR* 1992;158:981–982.
96. Centers for Disease Control. Tuberculosis, final data: United States, 1986. *MMWR* 1988;36:817–820.
97. Buckner CB, Leithiser RE, Walaker CW, Allison JW. The changing epidemiology of tuberculosis and other mycobacterial infections in the United States: implications for the radiologist. *AJR* 1991;156:255–264.
98. Hass DW, Des Prez RM. Tuberculosis and acquired immunodeficiency syndrome: a historical perspective on recent developments. *Am J Med* 1994;96:439–450.
99. Modilevsky T, Sattler FR, Barnes PF. Mycobacterial disease in patients with human immunodeficiency virus infection. *Arch Int Med* 1989;149:2201–2205.
100. Barnes PF, Bloch AB, Davidson PT, Snider DE. Tuberculosis in patients with human immunodeficiency virus infection. *N Engl J Med* 1991;324:1644–1650.
101. Louie E, Rice LB, Holzman RS. Tuberculosis in non-Haitian patients with acquired immunodeficiency syndrome. *Chest* 1986;90:542–545.
102. Pitchenik AE, Rubinson HA. The radiographic appearance of tuberculosis in patients with the acquired immune deficiency syndrome (AIDS) and Pre-Aids. *Am Rev Respir Dis* 1985;131: 393–396.
103. Long R, Maycher B, Scalcini M, Manfreda J. The chest roentgenogram in pulmonary tuberculosis patients seropositive for human immunodeficiency virus type 1. *Chest* 1991;99:123–127.
104. Macher AM, Kovacs JA, Vee G, et al. Bacteremia due to Mycobacterium avium-intracellulare in the acquired immunodeficiency syndrome. *Ann Int Med* 1983;99:782–785.
105. Marinelli DL, Albelda SM, Williams TM, Kern JA, Iozzo RV, Miller WT. Nontuberculous mycobacterial infection in AIDS: clinical, pathologic, and radiographic features. *Radiology* 1986; 160:77–82.
106. Miller WT Jr. Spectrum of pulmonary nontuberculous mycobacterial infection. *Radiology* 1994;191:343–350.
107. Woodring JH, Vandiviere HM, Fried AM, Dillon ML, Williams TD, Melvin IG. Update: the radiographic features of pulmonary tuberculosis. *AJR* 1986;146:497–506.
108. Buckner CB, Walker CW. Radiologic manifestations of adult tuberculosis. *J Thorac Imaging* 1990;5:28–37.
109. Leung AN, Müller NL, Pineda PR, FitzGerald JM. Primary tuberculosis in childhood: radiographic manifestations. *Radiology* 1992;182:87–91.
110. Krysl J, Korzeniewska-Koesela M, Müller NL, FitzGerald JM. Radiologic features of pulmonary tuberculosis: an assessment of 188 cases. *Can Assoc Radiol J* 1994;45:101–107.
111. Kuhlman JE, Deutsch JH, Fishman EK, Siegelman SS. CT features of thoracic mycobacterial disease. *Radiographics* 1990;10:413–431.
112. Naidich DP, McCauley DI, Leitman BS, Genieser NB, Hulnick DH. Computed tomography of pulmonary tuberculosis. In: Siegelman SS, ed. *Contemporary Issues in Computed Tomography*. New York: Churchill Livingstone; 1984:175–217.
113. Haque AK. The pathology and pathophysiology of mycobacterial infections. *J Thorac Imaging* 1990;5:8–16.
114. American Thoracic Society. Diagnostic standards and classification of tuberculosis. *Am Rev Resp Dis* 1990;142:725–735.
115. Lee KS, Song KS, Lim TH, Kim PN, Kim IY, Lee BH. Adult-onset pulmonary tuberculosis: findings on chest radiographs and CT scans. *AJR* 1993;160:753–758.
116. Lee KS, Kim YH, Kim WS, Hwang SH, Kim PN, Lee BH.

Endobronchial tuberculosis: CT features. *J Comput Assist Tomogr* 1991;15:424–428.

117. Im J-G, Webb WR, Han MC, Park JH. Apical opacity associated with pulmonary tuberculosis: high-resolution CT findings. *Radiology* 1991;178:727–731.

118. McGuinness G, Naidich DP, Jagirdar J, Leitman B, McCauley DI. High resolution CT findings in miliary lung disease. *J Comput Assist Tomogr* 1992;16:384–390.

119. Ikezoe J, Takeuchi N, Johkoh T, et al. CT appearance of pulmonary tuberculosis in diabetic and immunocompromised patients: comparison with patients who had no underlying disease. *AJR* 1992;159:1175–1179.

120. Primack SL, Logan PM, Hartman TE, Lee KS, Müller NL. Pulmonary tuberculosis and Mycobacterium avium-intracellulare: a comparison of CT findings. *Radiology* 1995;194:413–417.

121. Im J-G, Song KS, Kang HS, et al. Mediastinal tuberculous lymphadenitis: CT manifestations. *Radiology* 1987;164:115–119.

122. Murata K, Itoh H, Todo G, et al. Centrilobular lesions of the lung: demonstration by high-resolution CT and pathologic correlation. *Radiology* 1986;161:641–645.

123. Murata K, Khan A, Herman PG. Pulmonary parenchymal disease: evaluation with high-resolution CT. *Radiology* 1989;170:629–635.

124. Pastores SM, Naidich DP, Aranda CP, McGuinness G, Rom WN. Intrathoracic adenopathy associated with pulmonary tuberculosis in patients with human immunodeficiency virus infection. *Chest* 1993;103:1433–1437.

125. Hulnick DH, Naidich DP, McCauley DI. Pleural tuberculosis evaluated by computed tomography. *Radiology* 1983;149:759–765.

126. Wasser LS, Brown E, Talavera W. Miliary PCP in AIDS. *Chest* 1989;96:693–695.

127. Naidich DP, Garay SM, Goodman PC, Ryback BJ, Kramer EL. Pulmonary manifestations of AIDS. In: *Radiology of Acquired Immune Deficiency Syndrome*. New York: Raven Press; 1988:47–77.

128. Roberts CM, Citron KM, Strickland B. Intrathoracic aspergilloma: role of CT in diagnosis and treatment. *Radiology* 1987;165:123–128.

129. Woodring JH, Vandiviere HM. Pulmonary disease caused by nontuberculous mycobacteria. *J Thorac Imaging* 1990;5:64–76.

130. American Thoracic Society. Diagnosis and treatment of disease caused by nontuberculous mycobacteria. *Am Rev Respir Dis* 1990;142:940–953.

131. Christensen EE, Dietz GW, Ahn CH, et al. Pulmonary manifestations of Mycobacterium intracellularis. *AJR* 1979;133:59–66.

132. Christensen EE, Dietz GW, Ahn CH, Chapman JS, Murry RC, Hurst GA. Radiographic manifestations of pulmonary Mycobacterium kansasii infections. *AJR* 1978;131:985–993.

133. Hartman TE, Swensen SJ, Williams DE. Mycobacterium avium-intracellulare complex: evaluation with CT. *Radiology* 1993;187:23–26.

134. Moore EH. Atypical mycobacterial infection in the lung: CT appearance. *Radiology* 1993;187:777–782.

135. Swensen SJ, Hartman TE, Williams DE. Computed tomography in diagnosis of Mycobacterium avium-intracellulare complex in patients with bronchiectasis. *Chest* 1994;105:49–52.

136. Centers for Disease Control. 1993 revised classification system for HIV infection and expanded surveillance case definition for AIDS among adolescents and adults. *MMWR* 1992;41:1–11.

137. FitzGerald JM, Grzybowski S, Allen EA. The impact of human immunodeficiency virus infection on tuberculosis and its control. *Chest* 1991;100:191–200.

138. Greenberg SD, Frager D, Suster B, Walker S, Stavropoulos C, Rothpearl A. Active pulmonary tuberculosis in patients with AIDS: spectrum of radiographic findings (including a normal appearance). *Radiology* 1994;193:115–119.

139. Smith RL, Yew K, Berkowitz KA, Aranda CP. Factors affecting the yield of acid-fast sputum smears in patients with HIV and tuberculosis. *Chest* 1994;106:684–686.

140. Goodman PC. Pulmonary tuberculosis in patients with acquired immunodeficiency syndrome. *J Thorac Imaging* 1990;1990:38–45.

141. Jones BE, Young SMM, Antoniskis D, Davidson PT, Kramer F, Barnes PF. Relationship of the manifestations of tuberculosis to CD4 cell counts in patients with human immunodeficiency virus infection. *Am Rev Resp Dis* 1993;148:1292–1297.

142. Hill AR, Somasundaram P, Brustein S, et al. Disseminated tuberculosis in the acquired immunodeficiency syndrome. *Am Rev Res Dis* 1991;144:1164–1170.

143. Centers for Disease Control. Screening for tuberculosis and tuberculous infection in high risk populations and the use of preventive therapy for tuberculous infection in the United States: recommendations of the Advisory Committee for Elimination of Tuberculosis. *MMWR* 1990;39:1–12.

144. Kramer F, Modilevsky T, Waliany AR, Leedom JM, Barnes PF. Delayed diagnosis of tuberculosis in patients with human immunodeficiency virus infection. *Am J Med* 1990;89:451–456.

145. Lessnau KD, Gorla M, Talavera W. Radiographic findings in HIV-positive patients with sensitive and resistant tuberculosis. *Chest* 1994;106:687–689.

146. Katz MH, Hessol NA, Buchbinder SP, Hirozawa A, O'Malley P, Holmberg SD. Temporal trends of opportunistic infections and malignancies in homosexual men with AIDS. *J Infect Dis* 1994;170:198–202.

147. Levine B, Chaisson RE. Mycobacterium kansasii: a cause of treatable pulmonary disease associated with advanced human immunodeficiency virus (HIV) infection. *Ann Int Med* 1991;114:861–868.

148. Bamberger DM, Driks MR, Gupta MR, et al. Mycobacterium kansasii among patients infected with human immunodeficiency virus in Kansas City. *Clin Infect Dis* 1994;18:395–400.

149. Barber TW, Craven DE, Farber HW. Mycobacterium gordonae: a possible opportunistic respiratory tract pathogen in patients with advanced human immunodeficiency virus, type 1 infection. *Chest* 1991;100:716–720.

150. Rigsby MO, Curtis AM. Pulmonary disease from nontuberculous mycobacteria in patients with human immunodeficiency virus. *Chest* 1994;106:913–919.

151. Kuhlman JE, Fishman EK, Burch PA, Karp JE, Zerhouni EA, Siegelman SS. CT of invasive pulmonary aspergillosis. *AJR* 1988;150:1015–1020.

152. Kuhlman JE, Fishman EK, Burch PA, Karp JE, Zerhouni EA, Siegelman SS. Invasive pulmonary aspergillosis in acute leukemia: the contribution of CT to early diagnosis and aggressive management. *Chest* 1987;92:95–99.

153. Hruban RH, Meziane MA, Zerhouni EA, Wheeler PS, Dumler JS, Hutchins GM. Radiologic-pathologic correlation of the CT halo sign in invasive pulmonary aspergillosis. *J Comput Assist Tomogr* 1987;11:534–536.

154. Primack SL, Hartman TE, Lee KS, Müller NL. Pulmonary nodules and the CT halo sign. *Radiology* 1994;190:513–515.

155. Mori M, Galvin JR, Barloon TJ, Gingrich RD, Stanford W. Fungal pulmonary infections after bone marrow transplantation: evaluation with radiography and CT. *Radiology* 1991;178:721–726.

156. Gaeta M, Volta S, Stroscio S, Romeo P, Pandolfo I. CT "halo sign" in pulmonary tuberculoma. *J Comput Assist Tomogr* 1992;16:827–828.

157. Huang RM, Naidich DP, Lubat E, Schinella R, Garay SM, McCauley DI. Septic pulmonary emboli: CT-radiographic correlation. *AJR* 1989;153:41–45.

158. Müller-Leisse C, Klosterhalfen B, Hauptmann S, et al. Computed tomography and histologic results in the early stages of endotoxin-injured pig lungs as a model for adult respiratory distress syndrome. *Invest Radiol* 1993;28:39–45.

159. Kuhlman JE, Fishman EK, Teigen C. Pulmonary septic emboli: diagnosis with CT. *Radiology* 1990;174:211–213.

160. Balakrishnan J, Meziane MA, Siegelman SS, Fishman EK. Pulmonary infarction: CT appearance with pathologic correlation. *J Comput Assist Tomogr* 1989;13:941–945.

SIX

Diseases Characterized Primarily by Parenchymal Opacification

The diseases reviewed in this chapter produce ground-glass opacity or air-space consolidation as primary HRCT abnormalities. Ground-glass opacity is defined as an ill-defined or hazy increase in lung attenuation that does not obscure underlying vessels; if vessels within the area of abnormality are obscured, the term consolidation is used (1).

Ground-glass opacity results from morphologic abnormalities below the resolution of HRCT, and can reflect minimal thickening of the pulmonary interstitium or alveolar walls, or the presence of cells or fluid within the alveolar airspaces (2–7). Ground-glass opacity is the main abnormality seen in patients with hypersensitivity pneumonitis (extrinsic allergic alveolitis or EAA), desquamative interstitial pneumonia (DIP), alveolar proteinosis, in diffuse pneumonias, such as *Pneumocystis carinii* pneumonia, in immunocompromised patients, and in acute interstitial pneumonia (AIP).

Parenchymal consolidation is seen most commonly in patients with bronchiolitis obliterans organizing pneumonia/cryptogenic organizing pneumonia (BOOP/COP), chronic eosinophilic pneumonia, and in bacterial pneumonias (8). Parenchymal opacification ranging from ground-glass opacity to consolidation may also be seen with pulmonary edema (5,9–11); adult respiratory distress syndrome (12–14); viral, tuberculous, and fungal pneumonias (14,15); radiation pneumonitis (16,17); infarction (14); and bronchioloalveolar carcinoma (14,18). The clinical findings and plain radiographic appearances of many of these diseases are sufficient for diagnosis. However, in selected cases HRCT may contribute to patient management by detecting abnormalities when corresponding chest radiographs are normal, clarifying confusing or equivocal radiographic findings, or by delineating the extent of disease. As will be discussed, HRCT can play an especially important role in detecting infections in immunocompromised patients.

HYPERSENSITIVITY PNEUMONITIS (EXTRINSIC ALLERGIC ALVEOLITIS)

Hypersensitivity pneumonitis (HP), also known as extrinsic allergic alveolitis (EAA), is an allergic lung disease caused by the inhalation of antigens contained in a variety of organic dusts (19). Farmer's lung, which is the best-known HP syndrome, results from the inhalation of fungal organisms (thermophilic actinomycetes) that grow in moist hay. Many other HP syndromes also result from fungi, but as with farmer's lung, they are usually named after the setting in which exposure occurs or the organic substance involved; several examples are bird breeder's lung, mushroom worker's lung, malt worker's lung, maple-bark disease, and hot-tub lung. Acute exposure of susceptible individuals to an offending antigen produces fever, chills, dry cough, and dyspnea; long-term exposure can produce progressive shortness of breath with few or minimal systemic symptoms (20). Recurrent acute episodes are common with recurrent exposure.

The radiographic and pathologic abnormalities that are seen in patients with HP are quite similar, regardless of the organic antigen responsible (Fig. 6-1); these abnormalities can be classified into acute, subacute, and chronic stages. In the acute stage, heavy exposure to the inciting antigen can cause diffuse ill-defined air-space consolidation visible on radiographs; this reflects alveolar filling by neutrophils, eosinophils, lymphocytes, and large mononuclear cells or obstructive pneumonitis (19,21). It should be recognized, however, that not all patients with clinical symptoms of HP show acute radiographic abnormalities of air-space disease. Ill-defined "acinar" or air-space nodules can also be seen with acute exposure.

After resolution of the acute abnormalities, which may take several days, or between episodes of acute exposure, a fine nodular pattern is often visible on ra-

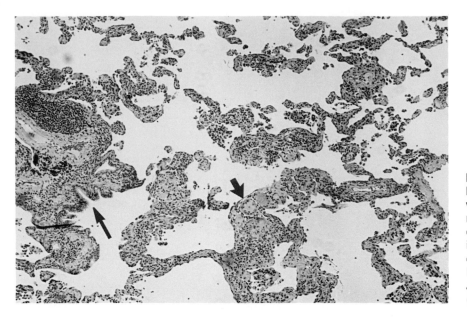

FIG. 6-1. Microscopic view of an open lung biopsy specimen from a patient with subacute hypersensitivity pneumonitis. A diffuse interstitial mononuclear cell infiltrate is present. This interstitial infiltrate accounts for the ground-glass opacity seen on HRCT. Also noted are localized areas of bronchiolitis (*large arrow*) and small ill-defined granulomas (*small arrow*).

diographs. This pattern is characteristic of the subacute stage of HP, but, as with acute disease, it is not always seen (22). The nodular appearance correlates with the presence of alveolitis, interstitial infiltrates, small granulomas, and cellular bronchiolitis; histologic abnormalities are usually most severe in a peribronchiolar distribution (20,23). Unlike the granulomas seen in patients with sarcoidosis, the granulomas in HP are irregular in shape and poorly defined (20).

The chronic stage of HP is characterized by the presence of fibrosis, which may develop months or years after the initial exposure (22). The fibrosis can be patchy in distribution, and radiographically and pathologically can mimic the appearance of idiopathic pulmonary fibrosis (IPF) with honeycombing (24).

The radiographic appearance of recurrent, transient, ill-defined consolidation superimposed on a pattern of small nodules is considered typical and highly suggestive of HP (20). However, it should be emphasized that the plain radiologic findings seen in this disease are nonspecific, and there have been conflicting reports as to the radiologic pattern and distribution of disease (22,25). Also, repeated exposure to the offending antigen can lead to a confusing superimposition of different radiographic patterns and stages of the disease process—acute and subacute changes and chronic fibrosis can all be present at the same time.

It is commonly believed that the chronic stage of hypersensitivity pneumonitis is characterized by fibrosis that mainly involves the upper-lung zones (22,26). This conclusion, however, is based on the radiographic findings in a small number of cases, most of them from a single study (26), and in most cases, radiographic findings of fibrosis appear to predominate in the middle lung zones (26,27).

HRCT Findings

The HRCT findings of HP depend on the stage of disease. Silver et al. (23) described the HRCT findings in two patients with acute HP. Both of these had bilateral air-space consolidation and small (1 to 3 mm in diameter), ill-defined, rounded opacities on both radiographs and on HRCT. In these two patients, the HRCT and radiographic findings were considered to be identical, and HRCT added no further information.

Much more commonly, HRCT is performed in the subacute stage of HP, weeks to months following first exposure to the antigen. Typical findings include patchy ground-glass opacity (Figs. 3-62,6-2,6-3) and small ill-defined nodules that are usually centrilobular in distribution (Fig. 6-4) (Table 6-1). In the study by Silver et al. (23), three of the patients had clinically subacute HP at the time of their CT study. Their symptoms had been present for 3 to 7 months prior to CT. These three patients had poorly defined nodules, 1 to 5 mm in diameter, visible on their chest radiographs and CT scans. CT also showed bilateral areas of ground-glass opacity (Figs. 6-2–6-4) that were not apparent on the radiograph. The ground-glass opacity was seen in the same distribution as the small, rounded opacities. Correlation with pathologic specimens demonstrated that the findings on HRCT reflected the presence of mononuclear cell bronchiolitis, mononuclear cell interstitial infiltrates, and scattered, poorly defined, non-necrotizing granulomas (23).

Hansell and Moskovic (28) reviewed the HRCT findings in 15 patients with subacute HP. The most common abnormality on HRCT was the presence of diffuse bilateral ground-glass opacity, present in 11 (73%) of the patients. The diffuse ground-glass opacity was rec-

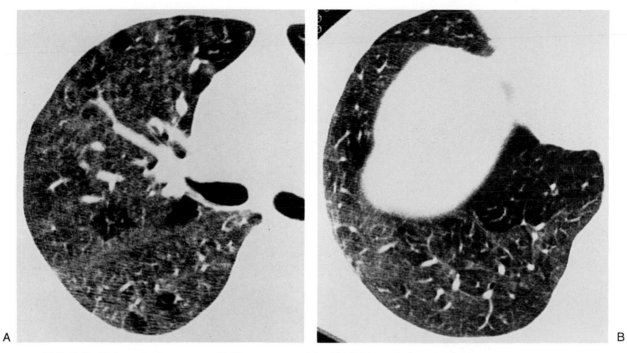

FIG. 6-2. Subacute hypersensitivity pneumonitis. HRCT in a 68-year-old woman with subacute extrinsic allergic alveolitis, at the levels of the right upper-lobar bronchus (**A**) and at the right base (**B**). Patchy ground-glass opacities are seen at both levels. At level A, some individual lobules appear spared.

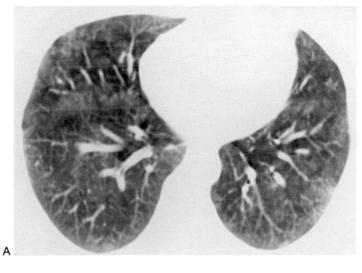

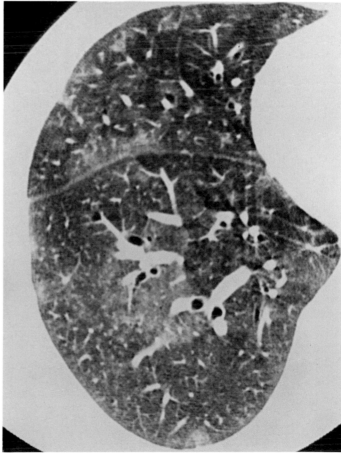

FIG. 6-3. Subacute hypersensitivity pneumonitis. **A:** Conventional CT (10-mm collimation) in a 50-year-old man shows bilateral ground-glass opacity. **B:** HRCT through the right lung at the same level better defines the patchy areas of ground-glass opacity. The intervening areas of lung appear normal.

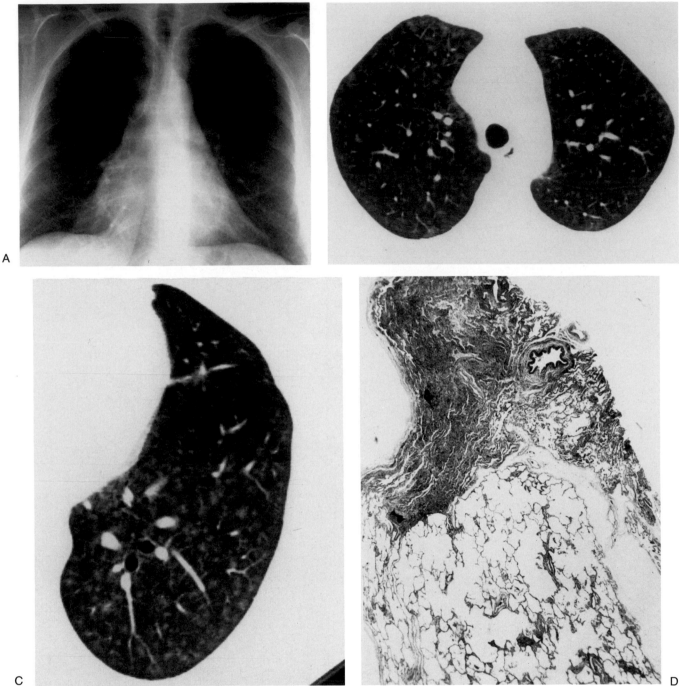

FIG. 6-4. Subacute hypersensitivity pneumonitis in a bird fancier. **A:** Chest radiograph is normal despite progressive shortness of breath. **B:** HRCT through the upper lobes shows diffuse ill-defined nodules of ground-glass opacity. **C:** HRCT in the left lower lobe shows that many of the nodules surround or are associated with small vascular branches, a finding which indicates their centrilobular location. This appearance is frequently seen in patients with subacute hypersensitivity pneumonitis. **D:** Open lung biopsy specimen shows a focal area of infiltration, corresponding to a centrilobular nodule. A small bronchiole is visible in the region of abnormality.

TABLE 6-1. *HRCT findings in hypersensitivity pneumonitis*[a,b]

SUBACUTE

1. **Patchy Ground-glass Opacity**
2. **Small Nodular Opacities, Often Centrilobular**
3. *Superimposition of Findings 1 and 2*
4. Findings of Fibrosis

CHRONIC

1. **Findings of Fibrosis**
   Intralobular interstitial thickening, Irregular interfaces, Irregular interlobular septal thickening, Visible intralobular bronchioles, Honeycombing, Traction bronchiectasis
2. **Superimposed Ground-glass Opacity**
3. *Patchy or Random Distribution of Abnormalities*
4. *No Zonal Predominance of Fibrosis, Relative Sparing of the Costophrenic Angles*

[a] Most common findings in boldface.
[b] Findings most helpful in differential diagnosis in boldface italics.

ognized on HRCT by the presence of abnormally prominent bronchial walls and a marked contrast between the attenuation of the lung parenchyma and the air in the major airways. Although the ground-glass opacity was diffuse, it was most marked in the middle- and lower-lung zones. The second most common finding, present in six patients (40%) was the presence of poorly defined nodules measuring approximately 4 mm in diameter and being most numerous in the middle- and lower-lung zones.

Remy-Jardin et al. (29) reviewed the HRCT findings in 21 patients with subacute bird-breeder's HP. The most common finding, seen in 16 (76%) of the patients was the presence of nodules. These measured less than 5 mm in diameter, were bilateral, and involved all three lung zones to a comparable degree. The nodules were poorly defined and were usually peribronchiolar or centrilobular in distribution (Fig. 6-4). The second most common finding, seen in 11 (52%) of the patients was the presence of areas of ground-glass opacity. The ground-glass opacity was seen in conjunction with nodules or, less commonly, as an isolated finding. The ground-glass opacity involved all three lung zones but was slightly more marked in the lower-lung zones. It was patchy in distribution in eight patients and diffuse in three patients.

Chronic HP is characterized by the presence of fibrosis, although findings of active disease are often superimposed. Silver et al. (23) described the HRCT findings in six patients with subacute symptoms superimposed on chronic HP. In these patients, symptoms had been present for 1 to 6 years. The chest radiographs and CT scans in these six patients showed irregular reticular opacities representing fibrosis (Figs. 6-5,6-6). The CT

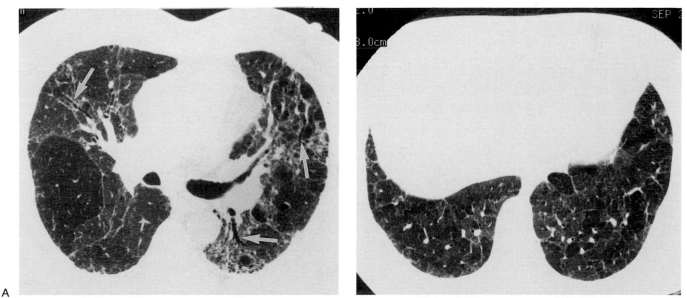

A   B

FIG. 6-5. A 54-year-old man with recurrent episodes of hypersensitivity pneumonitis over 10 years. **A:** HRCT at the level of the bronchus intermedius demonstrates evidence of fibrosis with irregular reticular opacities, traction bronchiectasis (*arrows*), and architectural distortion. Localized honeycombing is present in the subpleural lung regions of the left lower lobe. Also noted are bilateral areas of ground-glass opacity in a patchy distribution. These may represent subacute hypersensitivity pneumonitis superimposed on chronic fibrosis. **B:** HRCT scan through the lung bases shows areas of ground-glass opacity in a patchy distribution but no definite evidence of fibrosis.

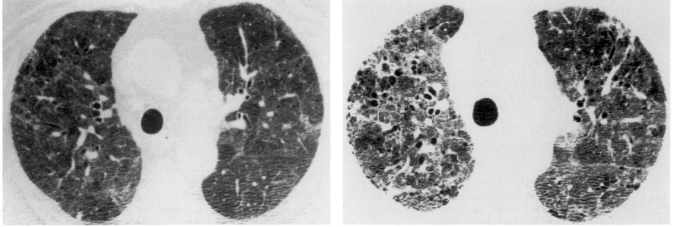

A   B

FIG. 6-6. Progression of hypersensitivity pneumonitis. **A:** HRCT at the level of the upper lobes shows patchy ground-glass opacity, but findings of reticulation and fibrosis are minimal. **B:** On a HRCT obtained 1 year later, there is extensive evidence of fibrosis with irregular reticular opacities, traction bronchiectasis, and some areas of honeycombing. Patchy ground-glass opacity remains visible, particularly in the left lung.

scans also showed patchy bilateral areas of ground-glass opacity (Figs. 6-5,6-6) and scattered, small nodules (Fig. 6-7).

Adler et al. (30) reviewed the HRCT scans in 16 patients with chronic HP. All patients showed findings of fibrosis with irregular opacities and distortion of the

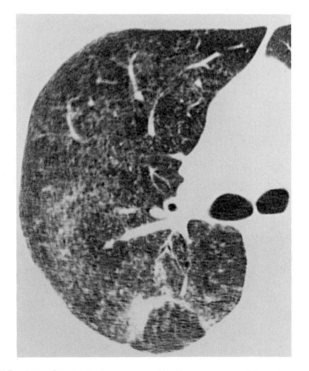

FIG. 6-7. Chronic hypersensitivity pneumonitis with superimposed subacute disease. HRCT at the level of the tracheal carina in a 31-year-old man shows ill-defined small nodular opacities and ground-glass opacities. Mild fibrosis is present posteriorly due to intermittent chronic exposure to the antigen.

lung parenchyma. The distribution of the fibrosis in the transverse plane was variable, being patchy in distribution in some cases, and predominantly subpleural or peribronchovascular in others. Honeycombing, when present, was usually subpleural in distribution (30). In a study by Grenier et al. (31), honeycombing was seen in 23% of patients with HP. Other findings in the patients studied by Adler et al. (30), indicative of active disease, included poorly defined, small nodular opacities seen in 10 (62%) and areas of ground-glass opacity seen in 15 (94%) of the cases. The nodules and areas of ground-glass opacity involved mainly the mid and lower-lung zones. In another study (32) of six patients with chronic hypersensitivity pneumonitis, HRCT revealed ill-defined nodular centrilobular and peribronchiolar opacities in all six cases, and areas of ground-glass density in four; in patients with HP, these findings are usually indicative of active disease.

Findings of fibrosis in patients with chronic HP most often show a mid-lung zone predominance or are evenly distributed throughout the upper, mid, and lower-lung zones (30). Relative sparing of the lung bases, seen in a majority of cases of chronic HP, can sometimes allow distinction of this entity from idiopathic pulmonary fibrosis, in which the fibrosis usually predominates in the lung bases. It should be noted, however, that 2 of the 16 cases reported by Adler et al. (30) showed a lower-lung zone predominance of abnormalities. Furthermore, Grenier et al. (31) report a lower lobe predominance of disease in 31% of patients with HP. Therefore, in some patients with chronic HP, HRCT findings are identical to those of IPF. In clinical practice, the differential diagnosis of HP and IPF is facilitated by the clinical history and laboratory findings.

Utility of HRCT

Several studies have demonstrated that HRCT is more sensitive than chest radiographs in the assessment of patients with HP (Fig. 6-4), although the sensitivity of HRCT is not 100%. In a study by Remy-Jardin et al. (29), seven of 21 patients with subacute HP (33%) had normal chest radiographs and all patients had abnormal HRCT scans. Lynch et al. (33) assessed the sensitivity of HRCT and chest radiographs in the detection of HP diagnosed in a population of swimming pool employees. The diagnosis of HP was based on two or more work-related signs or symptoms, abnormal results on transbronchial biopsies, or abnormal lymphocytosis on bronchoalveolar lavage fluid. Only one of 11 subjects (9%) had abnormal findings on the chest radiographs while five (45%) had abnormal HRCT findings. The abnormality on HRCT in each case consisted of small, poorly defined centrilobular nodules. This population-based study allowed assessment of patients with relatively mild disease. Pulmonary function tests were either normal or only minimally abnormal in all cases. It should be pointed out that in this study, HRCT scans were performed at 4-cm slice intervals so that mild localized abnormalities might have been missed on HRCT (33). It cannot be overemphasized that optimal assessment of infiltrative lung disease requires HRCT scans at 1-cm intervals in the supine position or at 2-cm intervals in both supine and prone positions. In another study (32), six patients with chronic hypersensitivity pneumonitis were examined using pulmonary function tests, bronchoalveolar lavage, lung biopsy, chest radiographs, and HRCT. The chest radiographs showed a variety of findings, including a mixed alveolar/interstitial pattern, peribronchiolar thickening, a diffuse granular pattern, or linear fibrosis. In general, HRCT showed more abnormalities than were apparent on the plain chest radiographs, and demonstrated findings of active disease not suggested on the chest radiographs.

In addition to its increased sensitivity, the pattern and distribution of lung abnormalities are better assessed on HRCT than on conventional CT or chest radiographs (23,28). The CT appearance of ill-defined centrilobular nodules less than 5 mm in diameter amid patchy areas of ground-glass opacity appears to be characteristic of the subacute stage of HP (23,28,33).

In HP, small nodules and areas of ground-glass opacity represent potentially treatable or reversible disease. Remy-Jardin et al. (29) performed sequential CT scans several months apart in 14 patients with subacute, and 13 patients with chronic bird-breeder's lung. After cessation of exposure to the avian antigen, the HRCT scans in patients with subacute HP showed marked improvement in the areas of ground-glass opacity or small nodules or returned to normal. Patients who continued to be exposed to the avian antigen showed no interval change in the HRCT scans. Similarly, in patients with chronic HP, there was improvement in the small nodules and in the areas of ground-glass opacity in patients who were no longer exposed to the avian antigen. Findings of fibrosis such as irregular linear areas of attenuation, architectural distortion, and honeycombing are irreversible.

In a patient presenting with a several-month history of dry cough, progressive shortness of breath, and a HRCT scan showing bilateral areas of ground-glass opacity, the differential diagnosis includes hypersensitivity pneumonitis (HP), desquamative interstitial pneumonia (DIP), and alveolar proteinosis (28,34–37). A careful clinical history and serologic testing can often confirm the diagnosis of HP thus precluding the need for open lung biopsy. DIP is rare, usually has a subpleural predominance of areas of ground-glass opacity, and is not associated with centrilobular nodules, as is HP (13,37). Alveolar proteinosis, also rare, is characterized by the presence of smoothly thickened interlobular septa within the areas of hazy increased opacity giving a "crazy-paving" appearance (34,35). It can be readily diagnosed by bronchoalveolar lavage.

DESQUAMATIVE INTERSTITIAL PNEUMONIA (DIP)

Desquamative interstitial pneumonia (DIP) represents a histologic pattern of lung injury first described by Liebow et al. (38) in 1965. DIP is characterized histologically by the presence of numerous macrophages filling the alveolar airspaces, mild inflammation of the alveolar walls, and minimal fibrosis (38,39). DIP has been associated with idiopathic pulmonary fibrosis, collagen-vascular diseases, histiocytosis X, asbestosis, drug reactions, and hard-metal pneumoconiosis. Although it is discussed in Chapter 4, it is reviewed here because of its propensity to be associated with ground-glass opacity on HRCT.

The relationship between DIP and UIP (usual interstitial pneumonia) is described in detail in Chapter 4. These entities probably represent different stages or degrees of lung injury associated with the same disease process, and both may be present in the same patient (40–44). However, there are significant pathologic and clinical differences between DIP and UIP. DIP is characterized by the presence of cellularity and mild fibrosis, while UIP is usually associated with fewer inflammatory cells, progressive lung fibrosis, and honeycombing. Patients with DIP also have milder symptoms, a better prognosis, and respond better to treatment with corticosteroids than do patients with UIP. Carrington et al. (45) reported a 5-year mortality of only 5% in patients with DIP, as compared to 45%

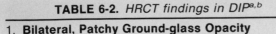

TABLE 6-2. *HRCT findings in DIP*[a,b]

1. **Bilateral, Patchy Ground-glass Opacity**
2. **Subpleural and Basal Predominance**
3. *Superimposition of Findings 1 and 2*
4. Findings of Mild Fibrosis

[a] Most common findings in boldface.
[b] Findings most helpful in differential diagnosis in boldface italics.

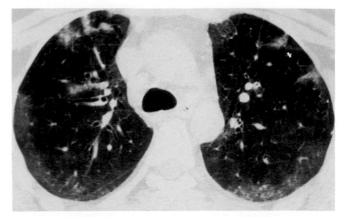

FIG. 6-9. A 45-year-old patient with DIP. HRCT at the level of the tracheal carina demonstrates bilateral areas of ground-glass opacity. The ground-glass opacity is most marked in the subpleural lung regions.

in patients with UIP. Because of these differences, a distinction between these two entities is important.

The most common finding on chest radiographs in patients with DIP is the presence of ground-glass opacities in the lower-lung zones (38,45,46). However, in 3% to 22% of patients with biopsy-proven DIP, the chest radiograph has been reported as being normal (38,45,47).

HRCT Findings

On HRCT, the predominant abnormality in patients with DIP is the presence of areas of ground-glass opacity (36,37) (Figs. 4-14–4-16) (Table 6-2). This is not surprising, considering that the predominant histologic findings in patients with DIP are filling of the alveolar airspaces with macrophages, relative preservation of the underlying pulmonary anatomy, and minimal fibrosis.

Hartman et al. (37) reviewed the HRCT scans in 22 patients with biopsy-proven DIP. The predominant abnormality in this group was the presence of areas of ground-glass opacity. The areas of ground-glass opac-

ity were seen mainly in the lower-lung zones in 16 patients (73%), the middle lung zones in three patients (14%), and the upper-lung zones in three patients (14%). The areas of ground-glass opacity had a predominantly peripheral distribution in 13 patients (59%), a patchy distribution in five patients (23%), and a diffuse distribution in four patients (18%) (Figs. 4-14–4-16,6-8,6-9).

Irregular linear opacities were seen in 13 (59%) of 22 patients. These were more marked in the lower-lung zones in 11 patients, middle lung zones in one patient, and upper-lung zones in one patient. In 11 of the 13 patients with irregular linear opacities, there was associated architectural distortion, indicating the presence of fibrosis. Honeycombing was identified in seven pa-

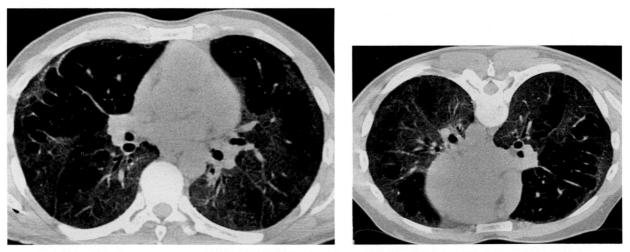

FIG. 6-8. HRCT scans from a 39-year-old man with biopsy-proven DIP. **A:** HRCT at the level of the superior segmental bronchi shows areas of ground-glass opacity in a predominantly subpleural distribution. **B:** HRCT obtained at the same level as in A with the patient in the prone position, shows that the ground-glass opacity is not secondary to dependent atelectasis. (From Hartman et al., ref. 37, with permission.)

tients. The honeycombing was present only in the lower-lung zones, was peripheral, and involved less than 10% of the lung bases.

The HRCT distribution of the abnormalities in DIP is similar to that reported in patients with UIP (37,48,49). However, the predominant pattern in DIP consists of areas of ground-glass opacity whereas the predominant pattern in UIP consists of irregular reticulation and honeycombing.

RESPIRATORY BRONCHIOLITIS AND RESPIRATORY BRONCHIOLITIS–INTERSTITIAL LUNG DISEASE

Respiratory bronchiolitis (RB) is a condition usually associated with cigarette smoking, although it can also occur in patients with a variety of occupational or environmental exposures; it probably represents a nonspecific reaction of lung to inhaled irritants (50). RB is often present as an incidental finding on lung biopsy in heavy smokers, and is usually unassociated with specific symptoms (51). However, smokers with findings of RB who are symptomatic have recently been described. These patients typically present with clinical findings mimicking those of interstitial lung disease, and are generally referred to as having "respiratory bronchiolitis-interstitial lung disease," or RB-ILD (52–54).

RB is characterized histologically by the presence of numerous macrophages filling respiratory bronchioles and adjacent alveolar ducts and alveoli. The macrophages contain periodic acid-Schiff (PAS)-positive brown pigment; this pigment represents particulate matter unique to cigarette smoke, contained within cytoplasmic phagolysosomes. A mixed cellular infiltrate may also be present, involving the peribronchiolar interstitium and nearby alveolar walls (50). In patients with symptomatic RB-ILD, peribronchiolar and alveolar wall inflammation are more pronounced than in patients who are asymptomatic (53). RB-ILD typically involves the lung parenchyma in a patchy fashion, with some areas spared while adjacent lobules may be severely involved.

Patients with RB-ILD are typically young, usually in their 20s, 30s, and 40s, and complain of chronic cough and progressive shortness of breath, often of 1- or 2-years duration (Fig. 6-10). Pulmonary function test results are variable, but usually show a restrictive abnormality. A reduced diffusing capacity, averaging 62% of predicted in the series reported by Yousem et al. (54), is the most consistent abnormality in patients with RB-ILD. Chest radiographs can be normal or can show nonspecific bilateral, irregular, opacities, usually with a lower zonal predominance (54).

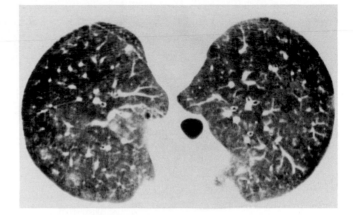

FIG. 6-10. Respiratory bronchiolitis-interstitial lung disease in a 29-year-old female smoker with 6 months of progressive dyspnea and cough. Prone HRCT shows patchy areas of ground-glass opacity, some of which appear nodular.

The prognosis of patients with RB-ILD is good; progression to pulmonary fibrosis, respiratory failure, or death have not been reported during follow-up periods of several years (54). Smoking cessation leads to amelioration of symptoms. Patients who continue to smoke may improve clinically, but those with persistent complaints may benefit from oral steroid therapy. Despite symptomatic regression, histologic changes may not resolve completely. Some authors have suggested that RB may be the precursor to chronic airway abnormalities or centrilobular emphysema in susceptible individuals.

HRCT Findings

The HRCT features demonstrated in patients with RB correlate well with the histologic abnormalities typical of this entity. Multifocal areas of ground-glass opacity, involving the lungs in a patchy fashion, are typically visible on HRCT in symptomatic patients with RB-ILD (Table 6-3) (Fig. 6-10), although HRCT can be normal in the presence of symptoms and an abnormal biopsy (55,56). Centrilobular predominance of the ground-glass opacities is sometimes visible (Fig.

TABLE 6-3. *HRCT findings in RB-ILD[a]*

1. **Patchy Unilateral or Bilateral Ground-glass Opacity[b]**
2. **Small Nodular Opacities, Often Centrilobular**
3. Findings of Fibrosis Absent

[a] Most common findings in boldface.
[b] Findings most helpful in differential diagnosis.

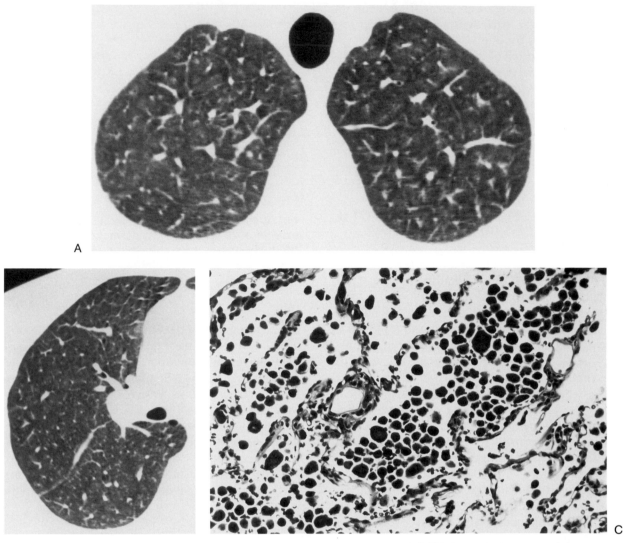

FIG. 6-11. Respiratory bronchiolitis-interstitial lung disease. **A:** HRCT through the upper lobes shows patchy areas of ground-glass opacity, many of which appear to be centrilobular, and surround small vascular branches. (From Gruden et al., ref. 99, with permission.) **B:** HRCT at a lower level also shows small, ill-defined areas of ground glass opacity. **C:** Open lung biopsy specimen shows numerous dark-pigmented macrophages filling alveoli, typical of respiratory bronchiolitis.

6-11). Findings of fibrosis and other HRCT abnormalities have been lacking in the patients studied.

Ground-glass opacity can also be seen in healthy smokers with normal pulmonary function (57), a finding which is probably related to RB. Patchy ground-glass opacity was present on HRCT in 21% of healthy smokers in one study (57), although in our experience, this finding is less common. In a subsequent comparison of HRCT and pathology in heavy smokers (51), ground-glass opacity was visible in 27% of patients, and was attributed to the presence of (i) intra-alveolar macrophages and alveolar wall inflammation or fibrosis, (ii) alveolar wall thickening, or (iii) organizing alveolitis.

ALVEOLAR PROTEINOSIS

Pulmonary alveolar proteinosis (PAP) is a disease characterized by filling of the alveolar spaces with a PAS-positive proteinaceous material, rich in lipid (58). The pathogenesis of this disease is poorly understood, and the majority of cases are considered to be idiopathic. Some cases result from exposure to dusts (particularly silica) or from immunologic disturbances due to immunodeficiency, hematologic and lymphatic malignancies, or chemotherapy (59–64).

In patients with PAP, men outnumber women by a ratio of 4 to 1. Patients range in age from a few months to more than 70 years, with two-thirds of patients being between 30 and 50 years old (44). Symptoms are usually mild and of insidious onset. They include nonproductive cough, fever, and mild dyspnea on exertion.

The prognosis of patients with pulmonary alveolar proteinosis has improved considerably since the advent of treatment using bronchoalveolar lavage (58,62,65). After lavage, many patients remain in remission, but others relapse; patients who relapse require retreatment every 6 to 24 months, and a few become refractory to treatment (66).

The usual radiographic manifestations of PAP are those of air-space consolidation or ground-glass opacity; air-bronchograms are rare. The typical radiograph shows a bilateral, patchy, diffuse, or perihilar ill-defined nodular or confluent air-space pattern, which is usually most severe in the lung bases (67–70). The radiographic appearance often resembles that of pulmonary edema except for the absence of cardiomegaly and pleural effusion.

HRCT Findings

Godwin et al. (35) reported the CT findings of nine patients with pulmonary alveolar proteinosis. Findings showed the air-space disease to have a variable appearance, which ranged from ill-defined nodular opacities (air-space nodules) to large areas of confluent air-space consolidation (Table 6-4). The air-space disease typically appears as ground-glass opacity, but dense consolidation can also be seen. In some patients, areas of ground-glass opacity or consolidation are sharply demarcated from the surrounding normal parenchyma, giving the abnormal areas a geographic appearance. In some of these cases, the sharp margination of areas of lung opacity reflect lobular or lobar boundaries; in other cases, there is no apparent anatomic reason to account for this sharp edge. The distribution of disease is variable (35), sometimes being mainly central and sometimes peripheral. CT, and particularly HRCT, commonly shows smooth thickening of the interlobular septa that is not apparent on the radiograph.

TABLE 6-4. *HRCT findings in alveolar proteinosis*[a,b]

1. **Bilateral Ground-glass Opacity**
2. **Smooth Septal Thickening in Abnormal Areas**
3. ***Superimposition of Findings 1 and 2, i.e., "Crazy-paving"***
4. Consolidation
5. Patchy or Geographic Distribution

[a] Most common findings in boldface.
[b] Findings most helpful in differential diagnosis in boldface italics.

A geographic distribution of consolidation or ground-glass opacity, and smooth thickening of the interlobular septa (Figs. 3-10,3-63,6-12) was visible on CT in all of six cases reported by Murch and Carr (34). The thickened interlobular septa were present only within areas of consolidation and were shown on open lung biopsy to reflect septal edema. Interstitial abnormalities characterized by the presence of alveolar wall infiltration by lymphocytes and macrophages, and interstitial edema, have also been reported in other studies. These findings probably reflect interstitial inflammation (69,71). Septal thickening can also represent interstitial accumulation of the proteinaceous material. It should be emphasized that in patients with alveolar proteinosis, septal thickening is usually visible only in regions of ground-glass opacity.

The demarcation of normal and abnormal lung regions and the demonstration of thickened interlobular septa are much better seen on high-resolution than on conventional CT. The combination of a geographic distribution of areas of ground-glass opacity with smoothly thickened interlobular septa within the areas of air-space disease, resulting in a "crazy-paving" appearance, is strongly suggestive of alveolar proteinosis (Figs. 3-10,3-63,6-12) (34), although this appearance can be seen in some other conditions associated with the presence of ground-glass opacity, including *Pneumocystis* and cytomegalovirus infections.

CT can also demonstrate focal pneumonia in patients with PAP that is not apparent on plain radiographs (35). Superimposed infection, often by *Nocardia asteroides*, is a common complication of alveolar proteinosis; on plain radiographs it can be difficult or impossible to distinguish infection from the air-space consolidation due to alveolar proteinosis. By detecting focal areas of dense consolidation or abscess formation, CT may confirm a clinical suspicion of superimposed infection (35). In early studies, infection with *Nocardia* was reported in as many as 8% of patients with alveolar proteinosis (62). It is now less common, presumably owing to the use of bronchoalveolar lavage in treatment of affected patients (60,65,67).

CHRONIC EOSINOPHILIC PNEUMONIA

Chronic eosinophilic pneumonia is an idiopathic condition characterized by extensive filling of alveoli by a mixed inflammatory infiltrate consisting primarily of eosinophils. A similar interstitial infiltrate is often present (20,72). Chronic eosinophilic pneumonia is usually associated with an increased number of eosinophils in the peripheral blood. Clinically, patients present with fever, cough, weight loss, malaise, and shortness of breath. Symptoms are often severe and last 3

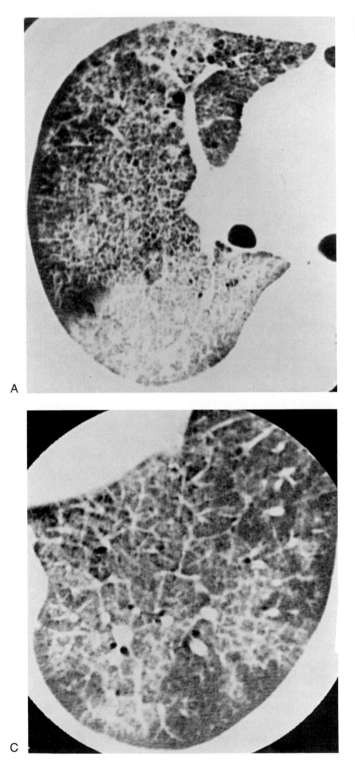

A

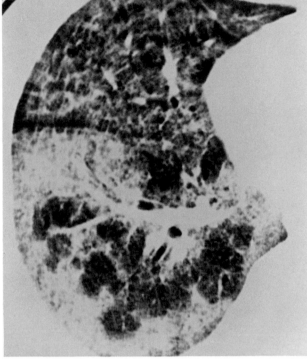

B

C

FIG. 6-12. Alveolar proteinosis. **A:** HRCT at the level of the bronchus intermedius in a 44-year-old man shows extensive ground-glass opacity. A reticular pattern is also apparent, presumably representing thickening of the interlobular septa. **B:** HRCT at the level of the right inferior pulmonary vein shows similar findings. **C:** HRCT through the left lower lobe shows ground-glass opacities and thickened interlobular septa. This is the typical "crazy-paving" appearance of alveolar proteinosis.

months or more (72–75). Life-threatening respiratory compromise may occur, but this is unusual (76).

Radiographically, chronic eosinophilic pneumonia is characterized by the presence of homogeneous peripheral air-space consolidation, "the photographic negative of pulmonary edema" (72). This pattern can re-

main unchanged for weeks or months unless steroid therapy is given; chronic eosinophilic pneumonia responds promptly to the administration of steroids.

The combination of blood eosinophilia, peripheral consolidation visible on the radiograph, and rapid response to steroid therapy are often sufficiently charac-

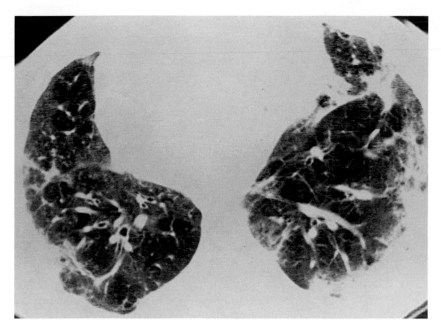

FIG. 6-13. Chronic eosinophilic pneumonia. HRCT through the lung bases in a 43-year-old woman shows subpleural air-space consolidation.

teristic to obviate the need for lung biopsy (72–75). The diagnosis, however, may be difficult in patients with minimal blood eosinophilia or in whom the peripheral distribution of infiltrates is not apparent. A recent study indicates that the classic radiologic picture may be seen in fewer than 50% of cases (75).

CT and HRCT Findings

Mayo et al. (77) reviewed the chest radiographs and CT scans in six patients with chronic eosinophilic pneumonia. All patients had patchy air-space consolidation (Figs. 3-66,6-13), and in five of the six cases, the consolidation was most marked in the middle and upper-lung zones (Table 6-5). In only one of the six patients was the classic pattern of air-space consolidation confined to the outer third of the lungs readily

apparent on the plain radiographs; however, in all six, a characteristic peripheral air-space consolidation was clearly demonstrated on CT. This study suggests that CT may be helpful in making the diagnosis of chronic eosinophilic pneumonia when the clinical findings are suggestive but the radiographic pattern is nonspecific.

Band-like subpleural opacities, which may be related to atelectasis in regions of abnormal lung can sometimes be seen. Such opacities have been previously reported on chest radiographs in patients with resolving eosinophilic pneumonia. Ground-glass opacity has also been observed on HRCT in patients with this disease.

An appearance identical to that of chronic eosinophilic pneumonia can be seen in patients with Loeffler's syndrome, an eosinophilic lung disease probably related to chronic eosinophilic pneumonia. Loeffler's syndrome, however, is usually self-limited and associated with pulmonary infiltrates that are transient or "fleeting" (8). With Loeffler's syndrome, areas of consolidation can appear and disappear within days; chronic eosinophilic pneumonia has a more protracted course, and areas of consolidation remain unchanged over weeks or months.

The presence of peripheral air-space consolidation can only be considered suggestive of chronic eosinophilic pneumonia in the appropriate clinical setting—that is, in patients with eosinophilia. An identical appearance of peripheral air-space consolidation can be seen in bronchiolitis obliterans with organizing pneumonia/cryptogenic organizing pneumonia (BOOP/

TABLE 6-5. *HRCT findings in eosinophilic pneumonia[a,b]*

1. **Patchy Unilateral or Bilateral Air-space Consolidation**
2. ***Peripheral, Middle and Upper-lung Predominance***
3. Ground-glass Opacity

[a] Most common findings in boldface.
[b] Findings most helpful in differential diagnosis in boldface italics.

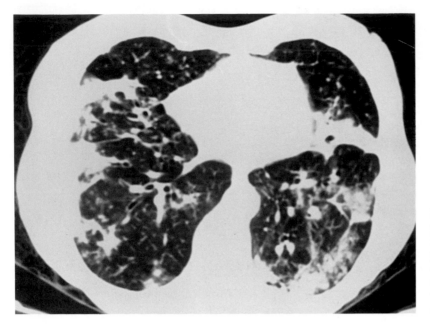

FIG. 6-14. Bronchiolitis obliterans organizing pneumonia/cryptogenic organizing pneumonia (BOOP/COP). The HRCT findings in a 64-year-old woman mimic the appearance of chronic eosinophilic pneumonia. A 1.5-mm collimation CT scan (standard algorithm) through the lower-lung zones shows peripheral air-space consolidation.

COP) (Figs. 3-65,6-14) (78). However, whereas virtually all cases of chronic eosinophilic pneumonia have a predominantly upper-lobe distribution, the consolidation in BOOP/COP often involves the lower-lung zones to a greater degree (78). On the other hand, some patients with lung disease have pathologic features of both chronic eosinophilic pneumonia and BOOP/COP (77,78). Therefore it is not surprising that they can have identical radiologic and CT findings (77–80). A peripheral distribution of disease, mimicking chronic eosinophilic pneumonia, can sometimes be seen in patients with sarcoidosis (81) and DIP.

BRONCHIOLITIS OBLITERANS ORGANIZING PNEUMONIA/ CRYPTOGENIC ORGANIZING PNEUMONIA

Bronchiolitis obliterans organizing pneumonia (BOOP) or cryptogenic organizing pneumonia (COP) is a disease characterized pathologically by the presence of granulation tissue polyps within the lumina of bronchioles and alveolar ducts and patchy areas of organizing pneumonia, consisting largely of mononuclear cells and foamy macrophages, in the surrounding lung (Fig. 6-15) (82,83). Most cases are idiopathic, but a

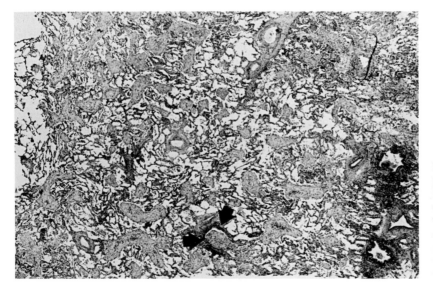

FIG. 6-15. Bronchiolitis obliterans organizing pneumonia/cryptogenic organizing pneumonia (BOOP/COP). A microscopic view of an open lung biopsy specimen from a patient with BOOP and findings of ground-glass opacity on HRCT. The specimen shows the presence of granulation tissue polyps in bronchioles and alveolar ducts (*arrows*) and areas of consolidation.

BOOP-like reaction may also be seen in patients with pulmonary infection, drug reactions, collagen-vascular diseases, Wegener's granulomatosis, and after toxic-fume inhalation (82,84–87).

Since its original description, a number of names have been used to describe this entity (83). "BOOP" is generally used in the United States. However, because the clinical, functional, radiologic, and HRCT findings in BOOP are primarily the result of an organizing pneumonia, it has been suggested that the term cryptogenic organizing pneumonia (COP) more accurately reflects the true nature of this disease (88–91); true bronchiolitis obliterans may not be present in up to one-third of cases with BOOP (44), and patients seldom present with clinical or functional abnormalities typical of bronchiolitis obliterans. Although each of these terms has its merits, it is simplest to consider them as equivalent (BOOP/COP), and we shall do so in this book. It should be noted, however, that strictly speaking, "cryptogenic organizing pneumonia" is synonymous with "idiopathic BOOP," while "BOOP" is synonymous with "organizing pneumonia" (83). Recently, the term "proliferative bronchiolitis" has also been used to describe the principal bronchiolar abnormality present in patients with BOOP/COP, and some authors have suggested that this term be used to describe this entity (92).

Patients with BOOP/COP typically present with a several-month history of nonproductive cough (80,91,93,94). They often have a low-grade fever, malaise, and shortness of breath. Pulmonary function tests characteristically show a restrictive pattern. Clinically and functionally, the findings may be similar to idiopathic pulmonary fibrosis, although the duration of symptoms in patients with BOOP/COP is shorter, systemic symptoms are more common, and finger clubbing is rarely seen (80,91,93,94). The patients usually respond well to corticosteroid therapy and have a good prognosis (93).

The characteristic radiologic features of BOOP/COP consist of patchy, nonsegmental, unilateral or bilateral areas of air-space consolidation (80,91,93,94). Irregular reticular opacities may be present, but they are rarely a major feature. Small nodular opacities may be seen as the only finding or, more commonly, are seen in association with areas of air-space consolidation.

Although the radiologic findings of BOOP/COP are nonspecific, in the majority of cases, the presence of areas of consolidation and the paucity or absence of reticular opacities allows an easy distinction of BOOP/COP from UIP (80,94). In a small percentage of patients, the consolidation may be peripheral, a pattern similar to that seen in chronic eosinophilic pneumonia (79,80).

HRCT Findings

The CT and HRCT findings in patients with BOOP/COP have been described in several studies (78,80,95,96). Typical HRCT features of this entity include:

1. Patchy consolidation (seen in 80% of cases) or ground-glass opacity (in 60% of cases), often with a subpleural and/or peribronchial distribution,
2. Small, ill-defined nodules (30% to 50% of cases) which may be peribronchial or peribronchiolar (Fig. 3-103), and
3. Bronchial wall thickening or dilatation in abnormal lung regions (Table 6-6).

Müller et al. (80) initially described the CT appearance of two patients with BOOP/COP. Both patients showed findings of consolidation; in one patient, the consolidation was patchy in distribution, and in the other, the consolidation was almost entirely subpleural, similar to that seen in chronic eosinophilic pneumonia (Figs. 3-65,6-14). Miki et al. (97) reported one case of BOOP/COP studied using HRCT. HRCT showed bilateral segmental air-space consolidation with air-bronchograms. In this case, HRCT was used to select a site for open lung biopsy. Follow-up CT after steroid therapy showed almost complete resolution.

Müller et al. (78) subsequently reviewed the radiographic and CT features of 14 patients with biopsy-proven BOOP/COP. All patients had areas of air-space consolidation or small nodules, or both (Figs. 6-16,6-17). Ten of the 14 patients had patchy unilateral or bilateral air-space consolidation, seven had small nodular opacities, and two had irregular linear opacities. A predominantly subpleural distribution of the air-space consolidation was apparent on CT in six patients (Figs.

TABLE 6-6. HRCT findings in BOOP/COP[a,b]
1. **Patchy Bilateral Air-space Consolidation (80%)**
2. **Ground-glass Opacity (60%)**
3. **Subpleural and/or Peribronchovascular Distribution**
4. **Bronchial Wall Thickening, Dilatation in Abnormal Areas**
5. Small Nodular Opacities, Often Peribronchiolar
6. *Combination of Findings 1 and 2*

[a] Most common findings in boldface.
[b] Findings most helpful in differential diagnosis in boldface italics.

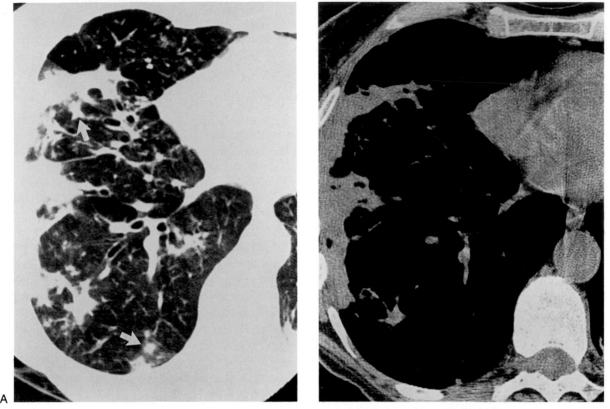

FIG. 6-16. BOOP/COP. **A:** HRCT through the right lower-lung zone in a 64-year-old woman shows air-space consolidation mainly in the subpleural regions. Some small nodules of consolidation are seen to be centrilobular (*arrows*). **B:** Mediastinal window settings better delineate the dense subpleural consolidation.

6-16,6-17), whereas this appearance was seen on radiographs in two. In some patients the air-space consolidation was more marked in a peribronchial distribution.

Nodular opacities, measuring 1 to 10 mm in diameter, were seen in 50% of patients; these nodules were

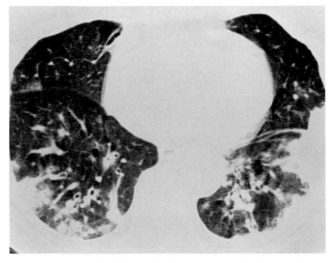

FIG. 6-17. BOOP/COP. HRCT through the lower-lung zones in a 68-year-old woman shows subpleural and peribronchial distribution of the air-space consolidation. Some areas of consolidation are nodular.

typically ill-defined (Figs. 3-103,6-16,6-17) (78). In two patients, these were more numerous along the bronchovascular bundles. On pathologic examination the parenchymal nodules were found to represent localized zones of organizing pneumonia, which were centered around abnormal bronchioles (Fig. 6-18) (78). Individual abnormal regions were separated from other involved areas by relatively normal parenchyma. Areas of ground-glass opacity were also seen (Figs. 6-19,6-20).

Bronchial wall thickening and dilatation was seen on HRCT in most patients with extensive consolidation and was usually restricted to these areas (Fig. 6-21) (78). This finding was felt to be nonspecific and not necessarily related to BOOP/COP. Follow-up CT was not performed in this study and therefore it is not known whether these bronchial abnormalities are reversible or whether they represent cylindrical bronchiectasis. Small pleural effusions are seen on CT in 30% of patients with BOOP/COP.

Nishimura and Itoh (98) described the findings on 5-mm collimation CT scans in eight patients with BOOP/COP and compared the CT findings with those on open lung biopsy. The CT findings consisted of a combination of ground-glass opacity and air-space consolidation. The abnormalities were panlobular, diffusely in-

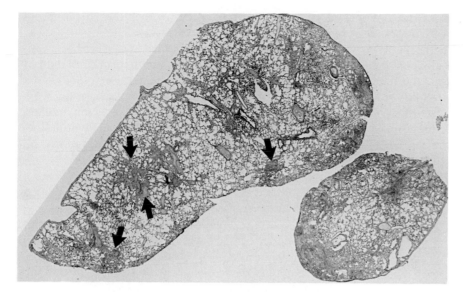

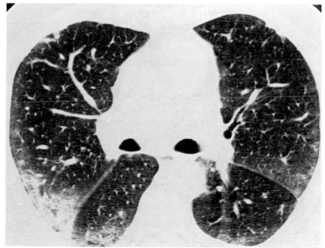

FIG. 6-18. Open lung biopsy specimen from a patient with BOOP/COP viewed at low power. In this patient, ill-defined nodular opacities were seen on HRCT. The pathologic specimen shows that the nodular opacities seen on HRCT are due to small localized areas of organizing pneumonia (*arrows*) surrounding areas of bronchiolitis obliterans.

FIG. 6-19. BOOP/COP in a 55-year-old man. HRCT shows patchy, bilateral ground-glass opacities and air-space consolidation mainly in the subpleural regions.

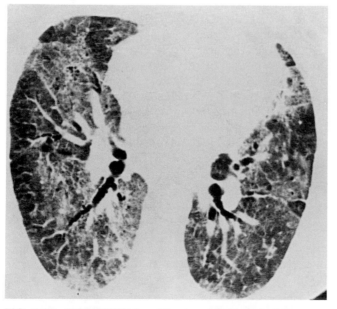

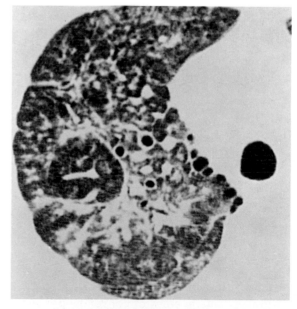

FIG. 6-20. BOOP/COP in a 65-year-old woman. Extensive bilateral ground-glass opacities show relative sparing of the subpleural region.

FIG. 6-21. BOOP/COP. HRCT through the right upper lobe in a patient with BOOP shows ground-glass opacities, bronchial wall thickening, and small nodules. Many of the nodules are centrilobular.

volving the secondary lobules. The authors did not specify the distribution of abnormalities in relation to the lung zones involved. Correlation with the pathologic specimens demonstrated that biopsies from areas of dense consolidation showed filling of the terminal air-spaces with branching granulation tissue buds. Biopsy from areas with ground-glass opacity demonstrated alveolar septal inflammation but little granulation tissue in the terminal air-spaces.

Recently, Lee et al. (96) reviewed the HRCT findings in 43 patients with biopsy-proven BOOP/COP (Table 6-6). The study included 32 immunocompetent and 11 immunocompromised patients. The most common pattern of abnormality seen was consolidation, which was present in 34 (79%) of 43 cases. It was present alone in nine and as part of a mixed pattern in 25 cases. In 32 cases, the consolidation was bilateral, with a nonsegmental, patchy distribution. The consolidation was predominantly subpleural in ten cases, predominantly peribronchovascular in ten cases (Fig. 6-22), and in seven had areas of both subpleural and peribronchovascular consolidation. Thus 27 (63%) of 43 cases had a predominantly subpleural and/or peribronchovascular distribution of consolidation. The consolidation had no zonal or anterior-posterior predominance. Consolidation was more common in immunocompetent patients being seen in 29 of 32 (91%) compared to 5 of 11 immunocompromised patients (45%) (p < 0.01).

Areas of ground-glass opacity were present in 26 (60%) of 43 cases. In all but two cases, the areas of ground-glass opacity were seen as part of a mixed pattern. The areas of ground-glass opacity were bilateral and random in distribution. Areas of ground-glass opacity were present in 8 of 11 (73%) immunocompro-

mised patients as compared to 18 of 32 (56%) immunocompetent patients (p < 0.25).

Nodules were present in 13 cases (30%). They were the only finding in four cases and part of a mixed pattern in nine cases. They were bilateral in ten cases and unilateral in three. The nodules were less than 5 mm in diameter in five cases and greater than 5 mm in diameter in eight. Most of the nodules had well-defined smooth margins. Nodules were more frequently observed in immunocompromised patients (6 of 11, 55%) than in immunocompetent patients (7 of 32, 22%) (p < 0.025). Nodules in BOOP/COP sometimes appear to be predominantly centrilobular (99).

In three cases (7%) (96), irregular lines were present. They were associated with consolidation and located in the subpleural region of the lower-lung zones. Mild honeycombing was present in two cases, in the subpleural region of the lower-lung zones.

Bronchial dilatation was present in association with areas of consolidation in 24 cases and with areas of ground-glass opacity and nodules in two cases each. Small pleural effusions were present in 15 cases (35%), including 14 immunocompetent and one immunocompromised patient. They were bilateral in ten cases and unilateral in five.

The CT and the plain film findings of BOOP/COP are nonspecific and may be seen in a variety of infections and neoplastic diseases. However, CT provides a better assessment of disease pattern and distribution than do chest radiographs and is therefore superior to plain film in determining optimal biopsy site. HRCT is recommended routinely as a guide to optimal biopsy site in all patients undergoing open lung biopsy.

LIPOID PNEUMONIA

Exogenous lipoid pneumonia results from the chronic aspiration or inhalation of animal, vegetable, or petroleum-based oils or fats. The degree of lung inflammation or fibrosis associated with the aspirated oil is related to the amount of free fatty acid which is present. Animal fats generally result in more inflammation and fibrosis than vegetable or mineral oils, because they are hydrolyzed by lung lipases, releasing fatty acids. A large quantity of oily material must usually be aspirated before symptoms develop. Lower lobe opacities or ill-defined masses are typical on chest radiographs (8,100).

CT and HRCT Findings

If a large amount of lipid has been aspirated, CT can show low-attenuation consolidation (−35 to −75 HU), which can mimic the appearance of ground-glass opacity (Fig. 6-23) (Table 6-7) (100); this appearance is most

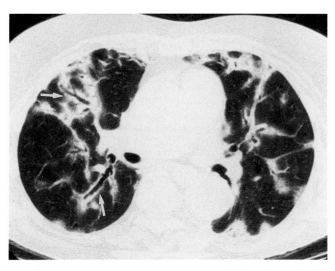

FIG. 6-22. An 81-year-old woman with BOOP/COP. HRCT demonstrates bilateral areas of consolidation. The consolidation is predominantly peribronchial in distribution. Note bronchial dilatation in the areas of consolidation (*arrows*).

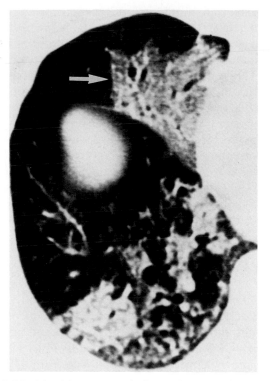

FIG. 6-23. Lipoid pneumonia from chronic mineral oil aspiration. HRCT at the right lung base shows patchy areas of consolidation. On the lung window scan, low-attenuation consolidation in the middle lobe (*arrow*) mimics the appearance of ground-glass opacity.

TABLE 6-7. HRCT findings in lipoid pneumonia[a,b]

1. **Patchy Unilateral or Bilateral Air-space Consolidation**
2. *Consolidation Low in Attenuation*
3. Ground-glass Opacity
4. *Lower-lung Predominance*

[a] Most common findings in boldface.
[b] Findings most helpful in differential diagnosis in boldface italics.

common in patients with chronic mineral oil aspiration. However, because inflammation or fibrosis may accompany the presence of the lipid material, the CT attenuation of the consolidation need not be low. In some patients, necrosis and cavitation may be present (101). Huggosson et al. (101) reported a series of nine infants, with a history of animal or vegetable fat intake, and a lung biopsy or bronchoalveolar lavage diagnosis of lipoid pneumonia. Eight had aspiration of animal fats. Pathological findings were an intense lymphocytic infiltration with scattered lipid-containing granulomas. Plain films and CT showed areas of consolidation in the medial-posterior parts of the lungs. CT attenuation measurements did not reveal fat.

Lee et al. (102) reviewed the chest radiographs and HRCT scans in six patients with proven lipoid pneumo-

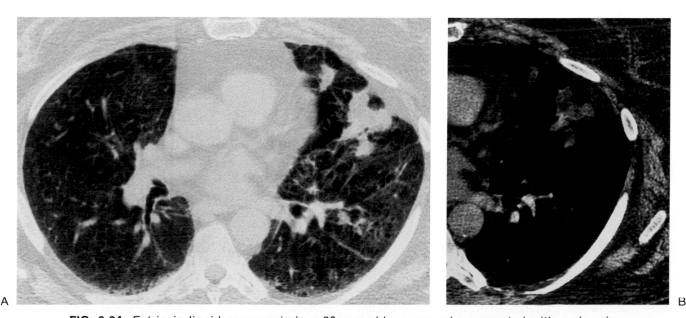

A   B

FIG. 6-24. Extrinsic lipoid pneumonia in a 66-year-old woman, who presented with a chronic cough. The chest radiograph demonstrated ill-defined bilateral infiltrates and a nodular opacity in the lingula. **A:** HRCT shows patchy areas of consolidation in the lingula and left lower lobe. **B:** Soft-tissue window setting scan shows the presence of fat in the areas of consolidation. Attenuation values range from −70 to −90 HU. A history of mineral oil ingestion was obtained following the CT.

nia. Lipoid pneumonia was related to the ingestion of mineral oil in three and shark liver oil (as a restorative) in three. Clinical symptoms included cough, mild fever, and chest discomfort. Chest radiographs demonstrated bilateral air-space consolidation in three patients, irregular mass-like opacities in two, and a reticular pattern in one.

CT and HRCT demonstrated diffuse parenchymal consolidation in three cases, localized areas of irregular consolidation in two, and subpleural pulmonary fibrosis and honeycombing in one case (102). The areas of consolidation primarily involved the lower-lung zones while the irregular areas of consolidation were in the lingula. In the three patients with consolidation, CT and HRCT demonstrated attenuation lower than that of chest wall musculature, but slightly higher than that of subcutaneous fat. These three cases were all related to the intake of large amounts of shark liver oil. The two cases of lipoid pneumonia appearing as irregular mass-like opacities on chest radiographs were shown on HRCT to represent localized areas of consolidation containing fat (Fig. 6-24). In these two patients, the mass-like lesions were surrounded by findings suggestive of fibrosis, including reticular opacities and architectural distortion. In one patient, with findings of subpleural fibrosis and honeycombing, no areas of low attenuation were visible on CT. It should be pointed out, however, that the diagnosis of lipoid pneumonia in this patient was based on history and transbronchial biopsy, and may not have been related to the findings of fibrosis seen on CT.

DIFFUSE PNEUMONIA

The CT and HRCT findings of various causes of pneumonia have been described (8,70,103–108). Generally, focal pneumonias, with the exception of multinodular diseases, are not assessed using CT, and plain radiographs in combination with clinical findings are sufficient for diagnosis. The appearances of mycobacterial and fungal infections appearing as lung nodules are described in Chapter 5.

Diffuse parenchymal opacification resulting from pneumonia can be seen with a variety of organisms. Diffuse pneumonia is most common in immunocompromised patients, including those with malignancy, acquired immunodeficiency syndrome (AIDS), and transplant recipients, but occasionally occur in subjects with normal immunity. Although the clinical and chest radiographic findings associated with different types of diffuse pneumonias have been extensively described, in many cases, a timely diagnosis proves elusive based on radiographs alone. On the other hand, many infectious processes have distinctive CT appearances, often allowing a presumptive diagnosis to be made, especially in the immunocompromised population (107,108). Also, in patients with an established diagnosis, CT may play an important role in assessing individual response to therapy. Lastly, identification of the varied manifestations of pulmonary infection is necessary to avoid confusion with noninfectious infiltrative diseases.

The use of CT to diagnose diffuse pulmonary infection has received relatively little attention (8,108). However, the CT appearances of some pneumonias, notably *Pneumocystis carinii* pneumonia and cytomegalovirus pneumonia have been well described, and it is important to be familiar with the typical CT appearances of these diseases.

Pneumocystis carinii Pneumonia (PCP)

Pneumocystis carinii pneumonia (PCP) affects approximately 65% of all HIV-infected patients at some point during the course of their disease, and accounts for nearly 25% of AIDS-related deaths (109–114). Although the incidence of PCP in patients with AIDS has diminished significantly as a result of effective prophylaxis using aerosolized pentamidine or trimethoprim-sulfamethoxazole, it remains the most common life-threatening pneumonia in this group (114). Currently, PCP prophylaxis is recommended in all HIV(+) patients with CD4+ T-lymphocyte counts < 200 cells/ mm^3 (113). In contradistinction, the incidence of PCP in immunocompromised patients who do not have AIDS has been increasing, with mortality in this population approaching 50% (112). A definitive diagnosis of PCP requires the demonstration of organisms in sputum or bronchoalveolar lavage fluid (109). Sputum induction has variously been reported to detect PCP in 50% to 90% of cases and is indicated in all patients considered at high risk for PCP.

Pathologically, PCP results in the presence of foamy, intra-alveolar exudates. Atypical patterns of presentation, however, are not unusual (115,116). As documented by Travis et al. (116), in a study of atypical pathologic findings in 123 lung biopsy specimens, PCP also may result in cavitation, vascular invasion, vasculitis, and even noncaseating, calcified granulomas.

Radiographically, PCP has been reported to cause diffuse bilateral interstitial and/or alveolar infiltrates in up to 85% of cases (109,117–119); however, it should be emphasized that, in as many as 15% of proven cases, radiographs remain normal (Fig. 6-25). The most characteristic appearance on chest radiographs is the finding of fine to medium reticular or nodular opacities, or ill-defined hazy consolidation; these appearances can be diagnostic in many cases (120). Atypical features include asymmetric and/or nodular infiltrates, apical disease, cavitary nodules and cysts, miliary nod-

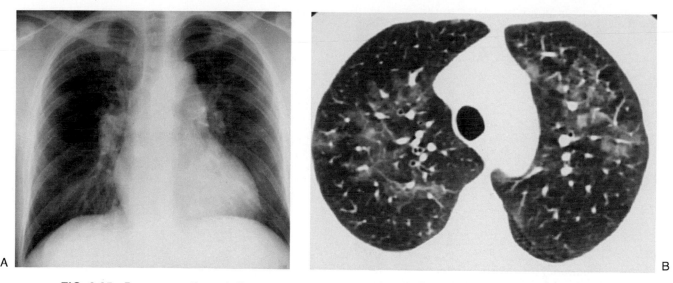

FIG. 6-25. *Pneumocystis carinii* pneumonia—acute phase. **A:** Posteroanterior chest radiograph shows no evidence of parenchymal consolidation. Hilar fullness bilaterally is secondary to enlarged pulmonary arteries in this patient with known pulmonary artery hypertension (PHT). An association between AIDS and PHT has been noted. **B:** HRCT section through the upper lobes in the same patient as in A, obtained at the same time, shows typical foci of ground-glass opacification bilaterally, compatible with the early intra-alveolar, exudative phase of infection. Note that despite the increased lung opacity, normal parenchymal architectural detail can still be identified. Transbronchial biopsy-proven PCP.

ules, adenopathy, effusions, and pneumothoraces (121–125).

Of particular interest is the frequency of cystic abnormalities and associated pneumothoraces in AIDS patients with PCP (121,122,126). It has been estimated that 10% or more of patients with PCP demonstrate either air-filled cysts or pneumatoceles, typically involving the upper lobes (121). Chow et al. (127), in a recent report of 100 patients with proven PCP, found radiographic evidence of cysts in 34 (34%) of patients. Of these, 32 had multiple cysts varying between 1 and 5 cm in diameter. Although present throughout the lungs, in more than 50% of patients, cysts predominated in the upper-lung zones. A clear association between cysts and pneumothorax was also shown, and 35% of the 34 patients with cysts developed pneumothorax. With therapy, cysts typically shrink or resolve entirely within 5 months (121,127). In most series, there is a greater tendency for patients receiving aerosolized pentamidine for prophylaxis to develop upper lobe infiltrates and cysts, but this is not always the case (127).

CT and HRCT Findings

CT findings in patients with PCP have been reported by several authors (Table 6-8) (107,108,128–130). Bergin et al. (130), in a study of 14 patients with *Pneumocystis carinii* pneumonia, showed that the predominant

CT finding was areas of ground-glass opacity and/or consolidation (Figs. 6-26,6-27). In many cases, in addition to diffuse, bilateral disease, a distinct "mosaic" pattern could be identified, with areas of normal lung intervening between scattered, focal areas of parenchymal involvement (Fig. 6-27). In seven cases, thickened septal lines were seen in association with areas of ground-glass opacity, presumably reflecting a combination of fluid and cellular debris within alveoli, as

---

TABLE 6-8. *HRCT findings in* P. carinii *pneumonia*[a,b]

1. **Patchy Bilateral Ground-glass Opacity, Often Central or Perihilar**

2. **Thick-walled, Irregular, Septated Cavities; Thin-walled Cysts, (+/−) Pneumothoraces**

3. ***Superimposition of Findings 1 and 2***

4. Centrilobular Nodular or Linear Branching Opacities

5. Bronchiectasis/Bronchiolectasis

6. Reticulation and Septal Thickening (Resolving Disease)

7. Conglomerate Nodules or Masses (Rare)

[a] Most common findings in boldface.
[b] Findings most helpful in differential diagnosis in boldface italics.

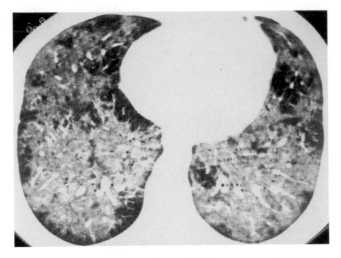

FIG. 6-26. *Pneumocystis carinii* pneumonia—acute phase. HRCT section through the lower lobes in a patient with documented PCP shows evidence of both diffuse ground-glass opacification and consolidation.

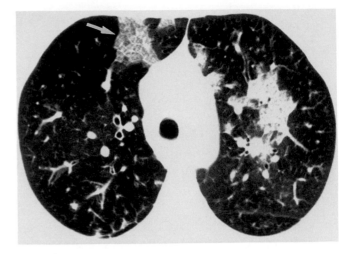

FIG. 6-28. Subacute *Pneumocystis carinii* pneumonia with septal thickening. HRCT section through the distal trachea shows focal areas of ground-glass opacification both upper lobes in a patient with documented PCP. Note that within these areas interlobular septal thickening is apparent (*arrow*), presumably resulting from the organization of acute intra-alveolar exudates.

well as thickening of the alveolar interstitium either by edema or cellular infiltration (Fig. 6-28) (130).

A similar spectrum of CT findings has also been described by Kuhlman et al. and Hartman et al. (107,129). In a retrospective study of 39 patients (129), Kuhlman et al. found three patterns of CT involvement, including a ground-glass pattern, a "patchwork" pattern, and

an interstitial or reticular pattern in 26%, 56% and 18% of cases, respectively. Associated CT findings included nodular densities in 18% of cases, adenopathy and/or effusions in another 18% of cases, and cystic abnormalities in 38% of cases (129). Hartman et al.

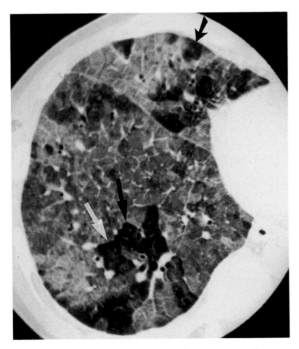

FIG. 6-27. *Pneumocystis carinii* pneumonia—acute phase. Retrospectively targeted HRCT section through the right lung in a patient with documented acute PCP shows a "mosaic" pattern of ground-glass opacification. Note that there is clear sparing of isolated secondary lobules (*arrows*).

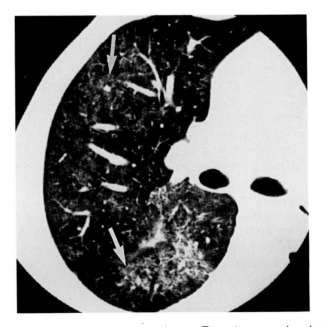

FIG. 6-29. PCP-subacute phase. Target reconstructed HRCT image through the right mid-lung in a patient receiving therapy for documented *P. carinii* pneumonia. Discrete foci of increased density can be seen, many of which have a slightly reticular configuration (*arrows*). These findings are compatible with organization of previous intra-alveolar exudates resulting in infiltration of the pulmonary interstitium.

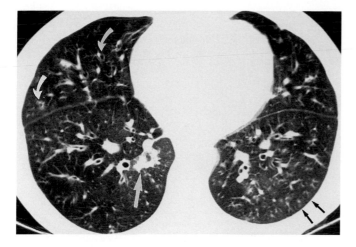

FIG. 6-30. *Pneumocystis carinii* pneumonia. HRCT section through the lower lobes in a patient with previously treated PCP. Note that in addition to residual areas of consolidation (*white arrow*), a few centrilobular opacities can be identified (*black arrows*) as well as mild bronchiectasis (*curved arrows*), presumably the result of bronchiolitis. These changes were not identifiable on the accompanying chest radiograph (not shown).

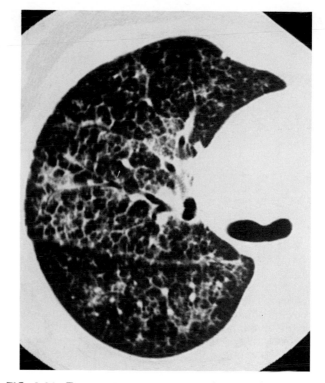

FIG. 6-31. Targeted HRCT image through the right lung shows diffuse, coarse reticulation in the central portions of the lung, in a patient with previously diagnosed and treated *P. carinii* pneumonia. In this case, infection with PCP has resulted in a pattern of diffuse fibrosis largely confined to the central portions of the lung.

(107) studied 24 patients with PCP; CT findings included ground-glass opacity in 92%, consolidation in 38%, cystic changes in 33%, nodules in 25%, lymphadenopathy in 25%, and pleural effusion in 17%. Interlobular septal thickening and reticular abnormalities were present in 17%. PCP may also result in poorly defined centrilobular nodules and branching opacities. These are presumably the result of distal airway involvement, and may account for the occasional presence of either bronchiectasis or bronchiolectasis (131). Occasionally, miliary nodules may be the primary finding in HIV(+) patients with PCP.

CT findings in patients with PCP reflect the stage of disease (130). Initially, scattered foci of ground-glass opacity or air-space consolidation can be identified, corresponding to the presence of intra-alveolar exudates as well as some degree of thickening of the alveolar septa; this can be termed the acute phase of PCP (Figs. 6-25–6-27). In our experience, CT is considerably more sensitive than routine chest radiographs for the detection of early parenchymal disease. Occasionally, areas of dense consolidation or coalescence may be identified, especially in patients with more extensive parenchymal inflammation (Fig. 6-25). With time, interstitial abnormalities predominate in patients with PCP. In treated patients with resolving or subacute infection, reticular opacities representing thickened interlobular septa and intralobular lines can be seen in association with ground-glass opacity (Figs. 6-28,6-29). Reticulation reflects organization of intra-alveolar exudates with resultant thickening of the pulmonary interstitium; it typically occurs in areas in which ground-

glass opacity was visible during the acute phase of disease.

Following therapy, residual changes generally can be appreciated on CT scans (Fig. 6-30). Rarely, infection with *P. carinii* results in diffuse parenchymal fibrosis (Fig. 6-31) (132). In our experience, this appearance is generally distinguishable from acute infection, due to the absence of CT evidence of air-space disease. Less frequently, PCP results in mild, peripheral bronchiectasis and/or bronchiolectasis, presumably the result of PCP bronchiolitis (131).

Cystic changes are frequently identified with CT in patients with PCP, with an incidence of about 35% in several studies (107,128,133,134). Kuhlman et al. (133) have also noted the appearance of premature bullous disease in AIDS patients. Using criteria previously established for the CT diagnosis of emphysema, these authors found bullous changes in 23 of 55 (42%) patients, despite an average age of only 37 years. In 70% of these cases, these changes were preceded by one or more documented episodes of infection (133). Gurney and Bates also have reported identifying upper lobe cystic disease both in AIDS patients as well as in intravenous-drug abusers (134). Frequently indistinguishable radiographically, bullous lung disease secondary to intravenous-drug abuse resulted in peripheral cystic

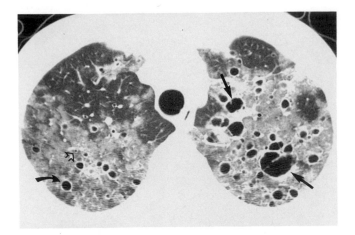

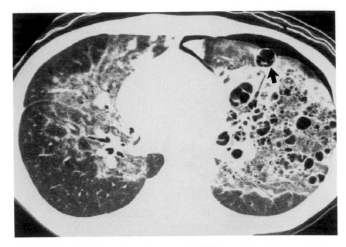

FIG. 6-32. PCP-cystic disease. HRCT section through the upper lobes shows extensive cystic changes throughout the lungs. These cysts are variable in size and are most often thick walled (*curved arrow*). Many are septated, probably the result of coalescence (*straight arrows*). Note that cystic changes occur only in areas of ground-glass opacification and that within these same areas there are also clearly dilated bronchi (*open arrow*). These findings suggest that many of the cysts probably represent pneumatoceles.

FIG. 6-34. PCP-cystic disease. HRCT section through the mid-lungs shows extensive cystic disease primarily within areas of ground-glass opacification. Note that one of these in the lung periphery is communicating with the pleural space resulting in a bronchopleural fistula (*arrow*). Not surprisingly, these often prove difficult to treat.

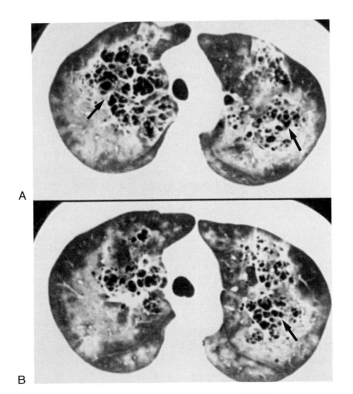

FIG. 6-33. PCP-cystic disease. **A,B:** HRCT images in a patient with documented PCP show the presence of innumerable cysts superimposed on a background of diffuse air-space consolidation, bilaterally. Note that many of the cysts are thick walled, and many have become confluent (*arrows*). In our experience, the finding of bizarre, multiseptated, thick-walled cysts scattered throughout the parenchyma arising in foci of air-space disease should strongly suggest the diagnosis of cystic *P. carinii* pneumonia.

abnormalities with sparing of the central portions of the lungs, while well-defined cysts randomly distributed throughout the lungs were more characteristic in patients with documented PCP (134).

Feuerstein et al. have described cystic lung disease in five patients with PCP in whom radiographic-CT/ pathologic correlation was obtained (135). In two patients *P. carinii* organisms and chronic inflammation were demonstrated in the walls of necrotic, thin-walled cavities. However, large apical and subpleural cysts lined by fibrous tissue could also be identified without evidence either of inflammation or infection. Importantly, cystic abnormalities were only identified by CT in 2 of 5 patients, even in retrospect (135). These findings suggest a spectrum of cystic changes in AIDS patients, with larger subpleural cysts potentially arising from rupture of intraparenchymal necrotizing cavities (136). In our experience, cystic changes in the lung appear to follow a predictable evolution. Initially, cysts appears as small foci in areas of parenchymal consolidation, often associated with clearly dilated, thick-walled bronchi (Figs. 6-32,6-33). With time, these coalesce to form bizarre-shaped, thick-walled cysts that often appear septated. There is a tendency for subpleural cysts to communicate with the pleura, accounting for the high incidence of pneumothoraces developing in these patients (Fig. 6-34). Following therapy these lesions eventually regress, resulting either in complete disappearance, or residual nodules and/or masses (Fig. 6-35). In addition to suggesting the proper diagnosis, CT can be of value in select cases by differentiating these lesions from those caused by other cavitary diseases potentially occurring in this population, especially septic emboli and fungal infections (137,138).

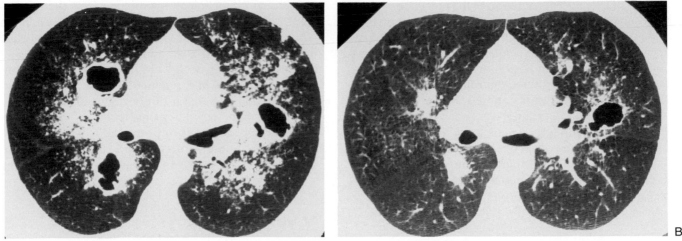

FIG. 6-35. PCP-cystic disease. **A:** HRCT section through the mid-lungs shows bilateral thick-walled cysts in association with ill-defined nodular opacities in a patient with documented PCP. This case is somewhat atypical in that cysts usually form within areas of ground-glass opacification or consolidation. **B:** Follow-up scan at the same level as A, obtained several weeks following initiation of successful therapy shows that the two cysts on the right have collapsed and are identifiable only as focal areas of dense consolidation. On the left side, the residual cyst is smaller and thinner walled. Previously identified nodular infiltrate has largely resolved.

Utility of CT

The accuracy of CT in the diagnosis of PCP and other pulmonary complications of AIDS was recently assessed by Hartman et al. (107). The CT and HRCT scans of 102 patients who had AIDS and proven thoracic complications were reviewed, along with those of 20 HIV-positive patients without active intrathoracic disease. The CT scans were independently assessed by two observers without knowledge of clinical or pathological data. Nineteen of the 20 cases without active disease were correctly identified by one observer, and 18 by the other. All 102 cases with active disease were correctly identified as abnormal by one observer, and 101 cases by the second observer. Furthermore, without benefit of clinical or pathologic information, a

confident diagnosis was achieved using CT in 48% of the cases, and this diagnosis was correct in 92% of these.

The most common pulmonary complication in the patients with AIDS studied by Hartman et al. was PCP, present in 35 cases. Based on the CT findings, the two observers made a confident diagnosis of PCP in 25 cases and this diagnosis was correct 94% of the time. The diagnosis of PCP in these cases was based on the presence of areas of ground-glass opacity. False-positive diagnoses in 6% of the cases were due to motion or poor inspiratory effort resulting in apparent areas of ground-glass opacity. Although the appearance of ground-glass opacity can be seen in immunosuppressed patients as a result of other pneumonias (Fig. 6-36), they are much less common.

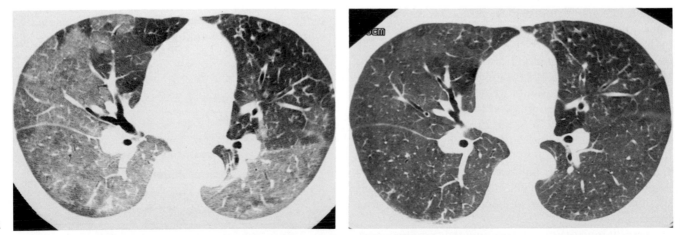

FIG. 6-36. Mycoplasma pneumonia with ground-glass opacity. **A:** HRCT section at the level of the middle-lobe bronchus demonstrates ground-glass opacification of the right lung and superior segment of the left lower lobe in a patient with proven mycoplasma pneumonia. **B:** Follow-up HRCT at the same level as in A shows only minimal residual ground-glass opacification.

Although in patients with AIDS the presence of areas of ground-glass opacity is most suggestive of PCP, in immunocompromised patients without AIDS, ground-glass opacity is a less specific finding. Brown et al. (139) compared the findings on HRCT with pathologic specimens in 33 immunocompromised patients with acute pulmonary complications. Fourteen patients without AIDS had ground-glass opacity as their main abnormality. In these 14 patients PCP accounted for the areas of ground-glass opacity in three cases, cytotoxic drug reaction in four, cryptogenic organizing pneumonia in four, lymphoma in two cases, and cytomegalovirus pneumonia in one.

Cytomegaloviral (CMV) Pneumonia

Cytomegaloviral (CMV) pneumonia frequently occurs in immunosuppressed patients, especially following organ transplantation (140–145). Following allogeneic bone marrow transplantation, for example, CMV pneumonitis characteristically causes fever, pulmonary infiltrates, and hypoxia resulting in the adult respiratory distress syndrome (140); it typically occurs more than 2 months following transplantation. Patients with severe graft-vs.-host disease are usually at highest risk. Crawford et al., in a study of 111 open lung biopsies performed on 109 marrow transplant recipients with diffuse pulmonary infiltrates, identified infection in 63% of cases; 90% of these proved to be due to cytomegaloviral infection (141). Bacterial or yeast infections were identified in only 4% of cases, while *Pneumocystis carinii* pneumonia was identified in only 6%. With the use of cytomegalovirus-negative blood products in patients lacking cytomegalovirus antibodies as well as the intravenous administration of CMV immune globulin and prophylactic administration of antiviral agents, including acyclovir or gancyclovir, the incidence of serious cytomegaloviral infection has been reduced. A similar approach is also now used in patients following heart-lung or lung transplantation (144).

Cytomegaloviral infection also has been frequently identified in renal transplantation patients. Moore et al. (145), in a study of patients treated with cyclosporin-prednisone immunosuppression following renal transplantation, found that CMV was present in 8 of 17 cases of pneumonia, including 5 of 6 patients with diffuse pulmonary infiltrates and all 6 patients with multiple-organism infections. It has been speculated that cytomegaloviral infection itself may compromise T-cell function causing further immunocompromise in this population.

Cytomegalovirus is well-recognized as the most common viral organism to be identified in patients with AIDS; however, there is considerable controversy concerning the clinical significance of this finding (146). CMV is frequently detected by cytology, histopathology or by culture in AIDS patients, without causing recognizable disease, and is present in up to 80% of patients at autopsy (147–149). Proven cases of clinically significant CMV pneumonitis are relatively uncommon, and have been rarely reported antemortem. However, with the increasing length of patient survival, largely the result of prophylaxis for PCP, CMV pneumonitis is more often being recognized in late-stage disease, especially in patients with CD4+ counts < 50/mm^3 (150).

CT and HRCT Findings

To date, little attention has been paid to CT findings in patients with CMV pneumonitis (144,151,152). In most studies, CMV has been reported to cause diffuse consolidation or ground-glass opacity, and nodular or reticulonodular opacities (Table 6-9). CMV pneumonitis should be included in the differential diagnosis of diffuse ground-glass opacification and/or consolidation, especially in AIDS patients unresponsive to therapy for *Pneumocystis carinii* pneumonia.

In a recent retrospective study of 21 AIDS patients with CMV pneumonitis, McGuinness et al. (153), reported a variety of CT abnormalities. Although ground-glass opacity and dense consolidation were frequently seen, occurring in 9 (42%) of 21 and 7 (33%) of 21 cases, respectively, ground-glass opacity was the predominant finding in only four cases while consolidation was the predominant finding in only one case (Fig. 6-37) (153). Pathologically, these changes corresponded primarily to the presence of diffuse alveolar damage. Similar to HRCT findings in patients with resolving PCP, reticular changes were identified in six cases, corresponding histologically to the presence of alveolar wall thickening, intralobular interstitial thickening, and interlobular septal thickening (Fig. 6-38). Most striking, in this same population, nodules (including one patient with diffuse miliary nodules) and/or masses were iden-

---

TABLE 6-9. *HRCT findings in CMV pneumonia^{a,b}*

1. **Patchy Bilateral Foci of Ground-glass Opacification and/or Consolidation**

2. **Scattered, Poorly Defined Nodules and/or Masses**

3. ***Superimposition of Findings 1 and 2***

4. Reticulation (resolving disease)

5. Small Nodules, Diffuse

---
^{a} Most common findings in boldface.
^{b} Findings most helpful in differential diagnosis in boldface italics.

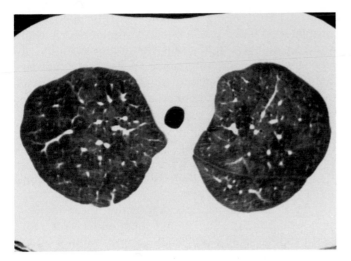

FIG. 6-37. CMV pneumonitis—acute phase. HRCT section through the upper lobes shows subtle diffuse ground-glass opacification in an AIDS patient with histologically documented CMV pneumonitis. Note that this appearance is indistinguishable from that caused by acute *P. carinii* pneumonia.

tified in 62% of cases, including five cases in which ground-glass opacification could be seen.

ACUTE INTERSTITIAL PNEUMONIA

Acute interstitial pneumonia (AIP) is a fulminant disease of unknown etiology that usually occurs in a previously healthy person and produces histologic findings of diffuse alveolar damage (154). There is often a prodromal illness associated with symptoms of a viral upper respiratory infection, followed by rapidly increasing dyspnea and respiratory failure. AIP was described in 1986 by Katzenstein et al. (154) in eight patients. The patients presented with symptoms of acute

TABLE 6-10. HRCT findings in AIP[a,b]
1. **Bilateral Ground-glass Opacity**
2. **Bilateral Consolidation**
3. **All Lung Zones**
4. *Superimposition of Findings 1 and 2*

[a] Most common findings in boldface.
[b] Findings most helpful in differential diagnosis in boldface italics.

respiratory failure and required mechanical ventilation within 1 to 2 weeks from the onset of symptoms. Seven of the eight patients died within six months, and one recovered. The pathologic abnormalities consisted of thickening of the alveolar walls due to edema, inflammatory cells, and active fibroblast proliferation but little mature collagen deposition. There was extensive alveolar damage with hyaline membrane formation. They emphasized that this condition, which they called acute interstitial pneumonia, is clinically and pathologically distinct from usual interstitial pneumonia (UIP) and desquamative interstitial pneumonia (DIP), which account for the majority of cases of idiopathic pulmonary fibrosis (154). Because the acute presentation and the histologic features are identical with those of ARDS, AIP has also been referred to as idiopathic ARDS (155).

Primack et al. (156) reviewed the radiographic and HRCT findings in nine patients with acute interstitial pneumonia (Table 6-10). Bilateral air-space opacification was present on the chest radiographs of all nine patients. The air-space opacification was diffuse in five patients (56%), involved mainly the upper-lung zones in two (22%), and involved mainly the lower-lung zones in two (22%). Honeycombing was identified on the radiographs in two patients.

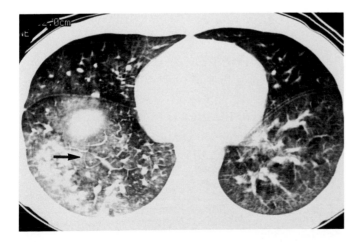

FIG. 6-38. CMV pneumonitis—subacute phase. HRCT section through the lung bases shows diffuse ground-glass opacification most marked in the right lower lobe in a patient with proven CMV pneumonitis. Thickened interlobular septa are clearly identifiable in the right lower lobe (*arrow*), consistent with dilated lymphatics resulting from organization of intra-alveolar exudates.

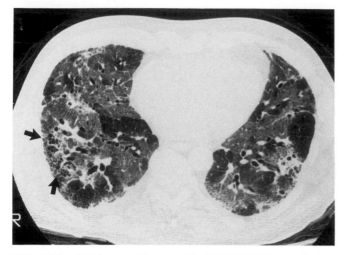

FIG. 6-39. A 74-year-old man with AIP. HRCT through the lung bases demonstrates extensive bilateral areas of ground-glass opacity. Also noted are a reticular pattern and fine honeycombing involving mainly the subpleural lung regions of the right lower lobe (*arrows*).

HRCT Findings

Bilateral, symmetric areas of ground-glass opacity were present on HRCT in all nine cases (Fig. 6-39). The areas of ground-glass opacity involved all lung zones to a similar extent in seven patients (78%) and had an upper-lung zone predominance in the other two patients. In six patients (67%), the areas of ground-glass opacity had a patchy distribution with focal areas of sparing, giving a geographic appearance, and three patients had diffuse involvement. In none of the cases did the areas of ground-glass opacity involve mainly the central or subpleural lung regions.

Bilateral areas of air-space consolidation were iden-

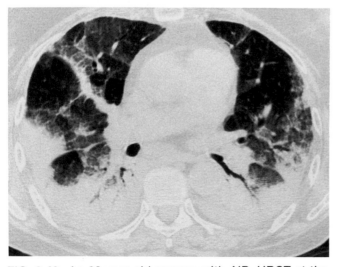

FIG. 6-40. An 83-year-old woman with AIP. HRCT at the level of the bronchus intermedius demonstrates extensive bilateral consolidation involving the dependent regions of the lower lobes. Patchy areas of ground-glass opacity are present anteriorly.

tified on HRCT in six of nine cases (Fig. 6-40). The consolidation had a predominantly basilar distribution in three patients, a diffuse distribution in two, and an upper-lung zone predominance in one. A predominantly subpleural distribution of consolidation was present in two cases; the distribution in the other four cases being random.

Subpleural honeycombing was seen at HRCT in three patients, including the two cases in which it was apparent on the radiographs. The areas of honeycombing involved less than 10% of the lung parenchyma.

Eight of the nine patients died within three months of presentation. The surviving patient underwent a follow-up HRCT study that showed only mild residual peripheral reticulation 2 months after the initial HRCT study. Repeat open lung biopsy at the time of the follow-up HRCT study in this case showed inactive fibrosis.

PULMONARY EDEMA AND THE ADULT RESPIRATORY DISTRESS SYNDROME

Patients with pulmonary edema, either hydrostatic (cardiogenic) or increased permeability (non-cardiogenic), and the adult respiratory distress syndrome (ARDS) are not generally imaged using HRCT, as their diagnosis is usually based on a combination of clinical and chest radiographic findings. However, a knowledge of their HRCT appearances can be helpful in avoiding misdiagnosis. Although hydrostatic and permeability edema cannot always be distinguished on the basis of plain film or CT findings (8,108), their appearances tend to differ.

TABLE 6-11. *HRCT findings in pulmonary edema*[a,b]

HYDROSTATIC EDEMA

1. **Smooth Interlobular Septal Thickening**
2. **Patchy Ground-glass Opacity**
3. **Smooth Peribronchovascular Interstitial Thickening**
4. **Smooth Subpleural or Fissural Thickening**
5. *Superimposition of Findings 1–4*
6. Centrilobular Nodules
7. Dependent, Parahilar, or Lower-lung Predominance May Be Seen

INCREASED PERMEABILITY EDEMA OR ARDS

1. **Diffuse or Patchy Ground-glass Opacity or Consolidation**
2. Centrilobular Opacities
3. **Peripheral Distribution**

[a] Most common findings in boldface.
[b] Findings most helpful in differential diagnosis in boldface italics.

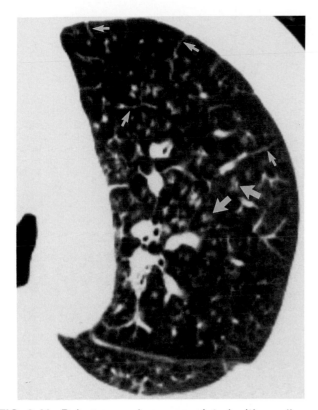

FIG. 6-41. Pulmonary edema associated with cardiomyopathy. Both interlobular septal thickening (*small arrows*) and ill-defined centrilobular opacities (*large arrows*) are visible. Also note thickening of the peribronchovascular interstitium, with peribronchial cuffing.

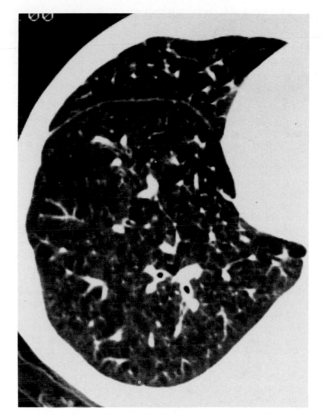

FIG. 6-42. Pulmonary edema in a patient with renal failure and chronic dyspnea. Hazy, ground-glass opacities are present, some of which are centrilobular in location. Despite the lack of thickened septa, pleural fluid, or prominent pulmonary vessels, open lung biopsy (not illustrated) showed only pulmonary edema. (From Gruden et al., ref. 99, with permission.)

Hydrostatic edema generally results in a combination of septal thickening and ground-glass opacity (Fig. 6-41), but septal thickening (Fig. 3-9) or ground-glass opacity (Fig. 6-42) can predominate in individual cases (Table 6-11) (10,157,158). In some patients, ill-defined, perivascular and centrilobular opacities can also be seen (Fig. 6-41) (99). There is a tendency for hydrostatic edema to have a perihilar and gravitational distribution (159), but this is not always visible. Thickening of the parahilar peribronchovascular interstitium (peribronchial cuffing), and fissural thickening are also common (Fig. 6-41). In a study of hydrostatic edema in isolated dog lungs (160), HRCT showed a predominantly central and peribronchovascular distribution of edema, associated with an increased thickness of bronchial walls.

Pulmonary edema occurring secondary to lung injury or ARDS is generally associated with ground-glass opacity or consolidation (Fig. 6-43). Opacities can be diffuse or patchy, affecting the lung in a geographic fashion, and sometimes predominate in the centrilobular regions (9,161). Interlobular septal thickening is less common than in hydrostatic edema, but can be seen (161). Depending on the etiology of the edema, opacities can predominate in the peripheral and subpleural regions, or can spare the lung periphery (9,161).

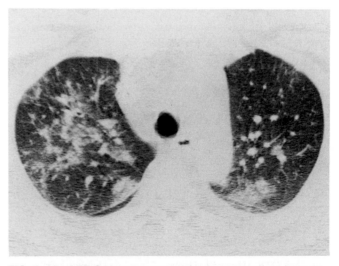

FIG. 6-43. ARDS due to cytotoxic drug reaction in a 44-year-old man. HRCT demonstrates patchy bilateral areas of consolidation and ground-glass opacity in the upper lobes. Diffuse consolidation was present in the lower lobes. The diagnosis was proven by open lung biopsy.

REFERENCES

1. Webb WR, Müller NL, Naidich DP. Standardized terms for high-resolution computed tomography of the lung: a proposed glossary. *J Thorac Imaging* 1993;8:167–185.
2. Wells AU, Hansell DM, Corrin B, et al. High resolution computed tomography as a predictor of lung histology in systemic sclerosis. *Thorax* 1992;47:508–512.
3. Wells AU, Hansell DM, Rubens MB, Cullinan P, Black CM, du Bois RM. The predictive value of appearances of thin-section computed tomography in fibrosing alveolitis. *Am Rev Respir Dis* 1993;148:1076–1082.
4. Wells AU, Rubens MB, du Bois RM, Hansell DM. Serial CT in fibrosing alveolitis: prognostic significance of the initial pattern. *AJR* 1993;161:1159–1165.
5. Remy-Jardin M, Remy J, Giraud F, Wattinne L, Gosselin B. Computed tomography assessment of ground-glass opacity: semiology and significance. *J Thorac Imaging* 1993;8:249–264.
6. Remy-Jardin M, Giraud F, Remy J, Copin MC, Gosselin B, Duhamel A. Importance of ground-glass attenuation in chronic diffuse infiltrative lung disease: pathologic-CT correlation. *Radiology* 1993;189:693–698.
7. Leung AN, Miller RR, Müller NL. Parenchymal opacification in chronic infiltrative lung diseases: CT-pathologic correlation. *Radiology* 1993;188:209–214.
8. Hommeyer SH, Godwin JD, Takasugi JE. Computed tomography of air-space disease. *Radiol Clin North Am* 1991;29:1065–1084.
9. Murata K, Herman PG, Khan A, Todo G, Pipman Y, Luber JM. Intralobular distribution of oleic acid-induced pulmonary edema in the pig: evaluation by high-resolution CT. *Invest Radiol* 1989;24:647–653.
10. Todo G, Herman PG. High-resolution computed tomography of the pig lung. *Invest Radiol* 1986;21:689–696.
11. Primack SL, Müller NL, Mayo JR, Remy-Jardin M, Remy J. Pulmonary parenchymal abnormalities of vascular origin: high-resolution CT findings. *Radiographics* 1994;14:739–746.
12. Greene R. Adult respiratory distress syndrome: acute alveolar damage. *Radiology* 1987;163:57–66.
13. Webb WR. High-resolution CT of the lung parenchyma. *Radiol Clin North Am* 1989;27:1085–1097.
14. Naidich DP, Zerhouni EA, Hutchins GM, Genieser NB, McCauley DI, Siegelman SS. Computed tomography of the pulmonary parenchyma: part 1. distal air-space disease. *J Thorac Imaging* 1985;1:39–53.
15. Meziane MA, Hruban RH, Zerhouni EA, et al. High resolution CT of the lung parenchyma with pathologic correlation. *Radiographics* 1988;8:27–54.
16. Ikezoe J, Morimoto S, Takashima S, Takeuchi N, Arisawa J, Kozuka T. Acute radiation-induced pulmonary injury: computed tomographic evaluation. *Semin Ultrasound CT MR* 1990;11:409–416.
17. Ikezoe J, Takashima S, Morimoto S, et al. CT appearance of acute radiation-induced injury in the lung. *AJR* 1988;150:765–770.
18. Adler B, Padley S, Miller RR, Müller NL. High-resolution CT of bronchioloalveolar carcinoma. *AJR* 1992;159:275–277.
19. Chryssanthopoulos C, Fink JN. Hypersensitivity pneumonitis. *J Asthma* 1983;20:285–296.
20. Fraser RG, Paré JAP, Paré PD, Fraser RS, Genereux GP. Diseases of altered immunologic activity. In: *Diagnosis of Diseases of the Chest.* Philadelphia: W. B. Saunders, 1989, 1177–1326.
21. Coleman A, Colby TV. Histologic diagnosis of extrinsic allergic alveolitis. *Am J Surg Pathol* 1988;12:514–518.
22. Cook PG, Wells IP, McGavin CR. The distribution of pulmonary shadowing in farmer's lung. *Clin Radiol* 1988;39:21–27.
23. Silver SF, Müller NL, Miller RR, Lefcoe MS. Hypersensitivity pneumonitis: evaluation with CT. *Radiology* 1989;173:441–445.
24. Seal RME, Hapke EJ, Thomas GO, et al. The pathology of the acute and chronic stages of farmer's lung. *Thorax* 1968;23:469.
25. Hapke EJ, Seal RME, Thomas GO, Hayes M, Meek JC. Farmer's lung: a clinical, radiographic, functional and serologic correlation of acute and chronic stages. *Thorax* 1968;23:451–468.
26. Hargreave F, Hinson KF, Reid L, Simon G, McCarthy DS. The radiological appearances of allergic alveolitis due to bird sensitivity (bird fancier's lung). *Clin Radiol* 1972;23:1–6.
27. Mindell HJ. Roentgen findings in farmer's lung. *Radiology* 1970;97:341–346.
28. Hansell DM, Moskovic E. High-resolution computed tomography in extrinsic allergic alveolitis. *Clin Radiol* 1991;43:8–12.
29. Remy-Jardin M, Remy J, Wallaert B, Müller NL. Subacute and chronic bird breeder hypersensitivity pneumonitis: sequential evaluation with CT and correlation with lung function tests and bronchoalveolar lavage. *Radiology* 1993;198:111–118.
30. Adler BD, Padley SP, Müller NL, Remy-Jardin M, Remy J. Chronic hypersensitivity pneumonitis: high-resolution CT and radiographic features in 16 patients. *Radiology* 1992;185:91–95.
31. Grenier P, Chevret S, Beigelman C, Brauner MW, Chastang C, Valeyre D. Chronic diffuse infiltrative lung disease: determination of the diagnostic value of clinical data, chest radiography, and CT with Bayesian analysis. *Radiology* 1994;1994:383–390.
32. Buschman DL, Gamsu G, Waldron JA, Klein JS, King TE. Chronic hypersensitivity pneumonitis: use of CT in diagnosis. *AJR* 1992;159:957–960.
33. Lynch DA, Rose CS, Way D, King TE. Hypersensitivity pneumonitis: sensitivity of high-resolution CT in a population-based study. *AJR* 1992;159:469–472.
34. Murch CR, Carr DH. Computed tomography appearances of pulmonary alveolar proteinosis. *Clin Radiol* 1989;40:240–243.
35. Godwin JD, Müller NL, Takasugi JE. Pulmonary alveolar proteinosis: CT findings. *Radiology* 1988;169:609–613.
36. Müller NL, Staples CA, Miller RR, Vedal S, Thurlbeck WM, Ostrow DN. Disease activity in idiopathic pulmonary fibrosis: CT and pathologic correlation. *Radiology* 1987;165:731–734.
37. Hartman TE, Primack SL, Swensen SJ, Hansell D, McGuinness G, Müller NL. Desquamative interstitial pneumonia: thin-section CT findings in 22 patients. *Radiology* 1993;187:787–790.
38. Liebow AA, Steer A, Billingsley JG. Desquamative interstitial pneumonia. *Am J Med* 1965;38:369–404.
39. Farr GH, Harley RA, Hennigan GR. Desquamative interstitial pneumonia: an electron microscopic study. *Am J Pathol* 1970;60:347–370.
40. Colby TV, Carrington CB. Infiltrative lung disease. In: *Pathology of the Lung.* Stuttgart: Thieme Medical; 1988:425–518.
41. Crystal RG, Fulmer JD, Roberts WC, Moss ML, Line BR, Reynolds HY. Idiopathic pulmonary fibrosis: clinical, histologic, radiographic, physiologic, scintigraphic, cytologic, and biochemical aspects. *Ann Intern Med* 1976;85:769–788.
42. Scadding JG, Hinson KFW. Diffuse fibrosing alveolitis (diffuse interstitial fibrosis of the lungs): correlation of histology at biopsy with prognosis. *Thorax* 1967;22:291–304.
43. Dunnill MS. Pulmonary fibrosis. *Histopathology* 1990;16:321–329.
44. Thurlbeck WM, Miller RR, Müller NL, Rosenow EC III. Chronic infiltrative lung disease. In: *Diffuse Diseases of the Lung: A Team Approach.* Philadelphia: Decker; 1991:102–115.
45. Carrington CB, Gaensler EA, Coute RE, Fitzgerald MS, Gupta RG. Natural history and treated course of usual and desquamative interstitial pneumonia. *N Engl J Med* 1978;298:801–809.
46. Gaensler EA, Goff AM, Prowse CM. Desquamative interstitial pneumonia. *N Engl J Med* 1966;274:113–128.
47. Feigin DS, Friedman PJ. Chest radiography in DIP: a review of 37 patients. *AJR* 1980;134:91–99.
48. Vedal S, Welsh EV, Miller RR, Müller NL. Desquamative interstitial pneumonia: computed tomographic findings before and after treatment with corticosteroids. *Chest* 1988;93:215–217.
49. Müller NL, Miller RR, Webb WR, Evans KG, Ostrow DN. Fibrosing alveolitis: CT-pathologic correlation. *Radiology* 1986;160:585–588.
50. Niewoehner DE, Kleinerman J, Rice DB. Pathologic changes in the peripheral airways of young cigarette smokers. *N Engl J Med* 1974;291:755–758.

51. Remy-Jardin M, Remy J, Gosselin B, Becette V, Edme JL. Lung parenchymal changes secondary to cigarette smoking: pathologic-CT correlations. *Radiology* 1993;186:643–651.
52. King TE. Respiratory bronchiolitis-associated interstitial lung disease. *Clin Chest Med* 1993;14:693–698.
53. Myers JL, Veal CF, Shin MS, Katzenstein AA. Respiratory bronchiolitis causing interstitial lung disease: a clinicopathologic study of six cases. *Am Rev Res Dis* 1987;135:880–884.
54. Yousem SA, Colby TV, Gaensler EA. Respiratory bronchiolitis-associated interstitial lung disease and its relationship to desquamative interstitial pneumonia. *Mayo Clin Proc* 1989;64:1373–1380.
55. Gruden JF, Webb WR. CT findings in a proved case of respiratory bronchiolitis. *AJR* 1993;161:44–46.
56. Holt RM, Schmidt RA, Godwin JD, Raghu G. High resolution CT in respiratory bronchiolitis-associated interstitial lung disease. *J Comput Assist Tomogr* 1993;17:46–50.
57. Remy-Jardin M, Remy J, Boulenguez C, Sobaszek A, Edme JL, Furon D. Morphologic effects of cigarette smoking on airways and pulmonary parenchyma in healthy adult volunteers: CT evaluation and correlation with pulmonary function tests. *Radiology* 1993;186:107–115.
58. Rosen SH, Castleman B, Liebow AA. Pulmonary alveolar proteinosis. *N Engl J Med* 1958;258:1123–1144.
59. Sargent EN, Morgan WKC. Silicosis. In: *Induced Disease. Drug, Irradiation, Occupation.* New York: Grune & Stratton; 1980:297–315.
60. Bedrossian CW, Luna MA, Conklin RH, Miller WC. Alveolar proteinosis as a consequence of immunosuppression: a hypothesis based on clinical and pathologic observations. *Hum Pathol* 1980;11(Suppl):527–535.
61. Carnovale R, Zornoza J, Goldman AM, Luna M. Pulmonary alveolar proteinosis: its association with hematologic malignancy and lymphoma. *Radiology* 1977;122:303–306.
62. Davidson JM, MacLeod WM. Pulmonary alveolar proteinosis. *Br J Dis Chest* 1969;63:13–28.
63. Teja K, Cooper PH, Squires JE, Schnatterly PT. Pulmonary alveolar proteinosis in four siblings. *N Engl J Med* 1981;305:1390–1392.
64. Miller RR, Churg AM, Hutcheon M, Lam S. Pulmonary alveolar proteinosis and aluminum dust exposure. *Am Rev Respir Dis* 1984;130:312–315.
65. Kariman K, Kylstra JA, Spock A. Pulmonary alveolar proteinosis: prospective clinical experience in 23 patients for 15 years. *Lung* 1984;162:223–231.
66. Rogers RM, Levin DC, Gray BA, Moseley LW. Physiologic effects of bronchopulmonary lavage in alveolar proteinosis. *Am Rev Respir Dis* 1978;118:255–264.
67. Prakash UBS, Barham SS, Carpenter HA, Dines DE, Marsh HM. Pulmonary alveolar phospholipoproteinosis: experience with 34 cases and a review. *Mayo Clin Proc* 1987;62:499–518.
68. Preger L. Pulmonary alveolar proteinosis. *Radiology* 1969;92:1291–1295.
69. Ramirez RJ. Pulmonary alveolar proteinosis. *AJR* 1964;92:571–577.
70. Genereux GP. CT of acute and chronic distal air space (alveolar) disease. *Semin Roentgenol* 1984;19:211–221.
71. Miller PA, Ravin CE, Walker Smith GJ, Osborne DRS. Pulmonary alveolar proteinosis with interstitial involvement. *AJR* 1981;137:1069–1071.
72. Gaensler EA, Carrington CB. Peripheral opacities in chronic eosinophilic pneumonia: the photographic negative of pulmonary edema. *AJR* 1977;128:1–13.
73. Pearson DJ, Rosenow EC. Chronic eosinophilic pneumonia (Carrington's): a follow-up study. *Mayo Clin Proc* 1978;53:73–78.
74. Dines DE. Chronic eosinophilic pneumonia: a roentgenographic diagnosis [Editorial]. *Mayo Clin Proc* 1978;53:129–130.
75. Jederlinic PJ, Sicilian L, Gaensler EA. Chronic eosinophilic pneumonia: a report of 19 cases and a review of the literature. *Medicine* 1988;67:154–162.
76. Libby DM, Murphy TF, Edwards A, Gray G, King TKC. Chronic eosinophilic pneumonia: an unusual cause of acute respiratory failure. *Am Rev Respir Dis* 1980;122:497–500.
77. Mayo JR, Müller NL, Road J, Sisler J, Lillington G. Chronic eosinophilic pneumonia: CT findings in six cases. *AJR* 1989;153:727–730.
78. Müller NL, Staples CA, Miller RR. Bronchiolitis obliterans organizing pneumonia: CT features in 14 patients. *AJR* 1990;154:983–987.
79. Bartter T, Irwin RS, Nash G, Balikian JP, Hollingsworth HH. Idiopathic bronchiolitis obliterans organizing pneumonia with peripheral infiltrates on chest roentgenogram. *Arch Intern Med* 1989;149:273–279.
80. Müller NL, Guerry-Force ML, Staples CA, et al. Differential diagnosis of bronchiolitis obliterans with organizing pneumonia and usual interstitial pneumonia: clinical, functional, and radiologic findings. *Radiology* 1987;162:151–156.
81. Glazer HS, Levitt RG, Shackelford GD. Peripheral pulmonary infiltrates in sarcoidosis. *Chest* 1984;86:741–744.
82. Epler GR, Colby TV, McLoud TC, et al. Bronchiolitis obliterans organizing pneumonia. *N Engl J Med* 1985;312:152–158.
83. Myers JL, Colby TV. Pathologic manifestations of bronchiolitis, constrictive bronchiolitis, cryptogenic organizing pneumonia and diffuse panbronchiolitis. *Clin Chest Med* 1993;14:611–623.
84. Colby TV, Myers JL. The clinical and histologic spectrum of bronchiolitis obliterans including bronchiolitis obliterans organizing pneumonia (BOOP). *Semin Respir Dis* 1992;13:119–133.
85. Epler GR. Bronchiolitis obliterans organizing pneumonia: definition and clinical features. *Chest* 1992;102(S):2–6.
86. Camus P, Lombard J-N, Perrichon M, et al. Bronchiolitis obliterans-organizing pneumonia in patients taking acebutolol or amiodarone. *Thorax* 1989;44:711–715.
87. Camp M, Mehta JB, Whitson M. Bronchiolitis obliterans and Nocardia asteroides infection of the lung. *Chest* 1987;92:1107–1108.
88. Geddes DM. BOOP and COP. *Thorax* 1991;46:545–547.
89. du Bois RM, Geddes DM. Obliterative bronchiolitis, cryptogenic organizing pneumonitis and bronchiolitis obliterans organizing pneumonia: three names for two different conditions. *Eur Respir J* 1991;4:774–775.
90. Hansell DM. What are bronchiolitis obliterans organizing pneumonia (BOOP) and cryptogenic organizing pneumonia (COP)? *Clin Radiol* 1992;45:369–370.
91. Davison AG, Heard BE, McAllister WC, Turner-Warwick MEH. Cryptogenic organizing pneumonitis. *Q J Med* 1983;52:382–393.
92. King TE. Overview of bronchiolitis. *Clin Chest Med* 1993;14:607–610.
93. Epler GR, Colby TV, McLoud TC, Carrington CG, Gaensler EA. Idiopathic bronchiolitis obliterans with organizing pneumonia. *N Engl J Med* 1985;312:152–159.
94. Chandler PW, Shin MS, Friedman SE, Myers JL, Katzenstein AL. Radiographic manifestations of bronchiolitis obliterans with organizing pneumonia vs. usual interstitial pneumonia. *AJR* 1986;147:899–906.
95. Bouchardy LM, Kuhlman JE, Ball WC, Hruban RH, Askin FB, Siegelman SS. CT findings in bronchiolitis obliterans organizing pneumonia (BOOP) with radiographic, clinical, and histologic correlation. *J Comput Assist Tomogr* 1993;17:352–357.
96. Lee KS, Kullnig P, Hartman TE, Müller NL. Cryptogenic organizing pneumonia: CT findings in 43 patients. *AJR* 1994;162:543–546.
97. Miki Y, Hatabu H, Takahashi M, Sadatoh N, Kuroda Y. Computed tomography of bronchiolitis obliterans. *J Comput Assist Tomogr* 1988;12:512–514.
98. Nishimura K, Itoh H. High-resolution computed tomographic features of bronchiolitis obliterans organizing pneumonia. *Chest* 1992;102:26S–31S.
99. Gruden JF, Webb WR, Warnock M. Centrilobular opacities in the lung on high-resolution CT: diagnostic considerations and pathologic correlation. *AJR* 1994;162:569–574.
100. Joshi RR, Cholankeril JV. Computed tomography in lipoid pneumonia. *J Comput Assist Tomogr* 1985;9:211–213.
101. Hugosson CO, Riff EJ, Moore CC, Akhtar M, Tufenkeji HT.

Lipoid pneumonia in infants: a radiological-pathological study. *Pediatr Radiol* 1991;21:193–197.

102. Lee KS, Müller NL, Hale V, Newell JD Jr, Lynch DA, Im JG. Lipoid pneumonia: CT findings. *J Comput Assist Tomogr* 1995; 19:48–51.

103. Murata K, Itoh H, Todo G, et al. Centrilobular lesions of the lung: demonstration by high-resolution CT and pathologic correlation. *Radiology* 1986;161:641–645.

104. Im JG, Itoh H, Shim YS, et al. Pulmonary tuberculosis: CT findings-early active disease and sequential change with antituberculous therapy. *Radiology* 1993;186:653–660.

105. Murata K, Khan A, Herman PG. Pulmonary parenchymal disease: evaluation with high-resolution CT. *Radiology* 1989;170:629–635.

106. Genereux GP. The Fleischner lecture: computed tomography of diffuse pulmonary disease. *J Thorac Imaging* 1989;4:50–87.

107. Hartman TE, Primack SL, Müller NL, Staples CA. Diagnosis of thoracic complications in AIDS: accuracy of CT. *AJR* 1994; 162:547–553.

108. Primack SL, Müller NL. High-resolution computed tomography in acute diffuse lung disease in the immunocompromised patient. *Radiol Clin North Am* 1994;32:731–744.

109. Murray JF, Mills J. Pulmonary infectious complications of human immunodeficiency virus infection. *Am Rev Res Dis* 1990;141:1356–1372.

110. Miller RF, Mitchell DM. Pneumocystis carinii pneumonia. *Thorax* 1992;47:305–314.

111. Farazio KF, Buehler JW, Chamberland ME, et al. Spectrum of disease in persons with human immunodeficiency virus infections in the United States. *JAMA* 1992;267:1798–1805.

112. Stover DE. Pneumocystis carinii: an update. *Pulm Perspect* 1994;11:3–5.

113. Centers for Disease Control and Prevention. Guidelines for prophylaxis against Pneumocystis carinii pneumonia among persons infected with human immunodeficiency virus. *MMWR* 1992;41(RR-4):1–11.

114. Chien SM, Rawji M, Mintz S, Rachlis A, Chan CK. Changes in hospitalized admission pattern in patients with human immunodeficiency virus in the era of P. carinii prophylaxis. *Chest* 1992;102:1035–1039.

115. Foley NM, Griffiths MH, Miller RF. Histologically atypical Pneumocystis carinii pneumonia. *Thorax* 1993;48:996–1001.

116. Travis WD, Pittaluga S, Lipschik GY, et al. Atypical pathologic manifestations of Pneumocystis carinii pneumonia in the acquired immune deficiency syndrome. *Am J Surg Pathol* 1990; 14:615–625.

117. Suster B, Ackerman M, Orenstein M, Wax MR. Pulmonary manifestations of AIDS: review of 106 episodes. *Radiology* 1987;161:87–93.

118. DeLorenzo LJ, Huang CT, Maguire GP, Stone DJ. Roentgenographic patterns of Pneumocystis carinii pneumonia in 104 patients with AIDS. *Chest* 1987;91:323–327.

119. Naidich DP, Garay SM, Leitman BS, McCauley DI. Radiographic manifestations of pulmonary disease in the acquired immunodeficiency syndrome (AIDS). *Semin Roentgenol* 1987; 22:14–30.

120. Goodman PC. Pneumocystis carinii pneumonia. *J Thorac Imaging* 1991;6:16–21.

121. Goodman PC, Daley C, Minagi H. Spontaneous pneumothorax in AIDS patients with Pneumocystis carinii pneumonia. *AJR* 1986;147:29–31.

122. Sandhu JS, Goodman PC. Pulmonary cysts associated with Pneumocystis carinii pneumonia in patients with AIDS. *Radiology* 1989;173:33–35.

123. Barrio JL, Suarez M, Rodriguez JL, Saldana MJ, Pitchenik AE. Pneumocystis carinii pneumonia presenting as cavitating and noncavitating solitary pulmonary nodules in patients with the acquired immunodeficiency syndrome. *Am Rev Res Dis* 1986;134:1094–1096.

124. Radin DR, Baker EL, Klatt EC, et al. Visceral and nodal calcification in patients with AIDS-related Pneumocystis carinii infection. *AJR* 1990;154:27–31.

125. Wasser LS, Brown E, Talavera W. Miliary PCP in AIDS. *Chest* 1989;96:693–695.

126. Chaffey MH, Klein JS, Gamsu G, Blanc P, Golden JA. Radio-

127. Chow C, Templeton PA, White CS. Lung cysts associated with Pneumocystis carinii pneumonia: radiographic characteristics, natural history, and complications. *AJR* 1993;161:527–531.

128. Naidich DP, Garay SM, Goodman PC, Ryback BJ, Kramer EL. Pulmonary manifestations of AIDS. In: *Radiology of Acquired Immune Deficiency Syndrome*. New York: Raven Press; 1988: 47–77.

129. Kuhlman JE, Kavuru M, Fishman EK, Siegelman SS. Pneumocystis carinii pneumonia: spectrum of parenchymal CT findings. *Radiology* 1990;175:711–714.

130. Bergin CJ, Wirth RL, Berry GJ, Castellino RA. Pneumocystis carinii pneumonia: CT and HRCT observations. *J Comput Assist Tomogr* 1990;14:756–759.

131. McGuinness G, Naidich DP, Garay SM, Leitman BS, McCauley DI. AIDS associated bronchiectasis: CT features. *J Comput Assist Tomogr* 1993;17:260–266.

132. Schinella RA, Clancey C, Fazzini E, Garay S. Pneumocystis carinii as a cause of pulmonary fibrosis. *Am Rev Res Dis* 1986; 133A:180(abst).

133. Kuhlman JE, Knowles MC, Fishman EK, Siegelman SS. Premature bullous pulmonary damage in AIDS: CT diagnosis. *Radiology* 1989;173:23–26.

134. Gurney JW, Bates FT. Pulmonary cystic disease: comparison of Pneumocystis carinii pneumatoceles and bullous emphysema due to intravenous drug abuse. *Radiology* 1989;173: 27–31.

135. Feuerstein I, Archer A, Pluda JM, et al. Thin-walled cavities, cysts, and pneumothorax in Pneumocystis carinii pneumonia: further observations with histopathologic correlation. *Radiology* 1990;174:697–702.

136. Panicek DM. Cystic pulmonary lesions in patients with AIDS [Editorial]. *Radiology* 1989;173:12–14.

137. Huang RM, Naidich DP, Lubat E, Schinella R, Garay SM, McCauley DI. Septic pulmonary emboli: CT-radiographic correlation. *AJR* 1989;153:41–45.

138. Kuhlman JE, Fishman EK, Teigen C. Pulmonary septic emboli: diagnosis with CT. *Radiology* 1990;174:211–213.

139. Brown MJ, Miller RR, Müller NL. Acute lung disease in the immunocompromised host: CT and pathologic examination findings. *Radiology* 1994;190:247–254.

140. Armitage JO. Bone marrow transplantation. *N Engl J Med* 1994;330:827–838.

141. Crawford SE, Hackman RC, Clark JG. Open lung biopsy diagnosis of diffuse pulmonary infiltrates after marrow transplantation. *Chest* 1988;94:949–953.

142. Maurer JR, Tullis E, Grossman RF, Vellend H, Winton TL, Patterson GA. Infectious complications following isolated lung transplantation. *Chest* 1992;101:1056–1059.

143. Herman S, Rappaport D, Weisbrod G, Olscamp G, Patterson G, Cooper J. Single-lung transplantation: imaging features. *Radiology* 1989;170:89–93.

144. O'Donovan P. Imaging of complications of lung transplantation. *Radiographics* 1993;13:787–796.

145. Moore EH, Webb WR, Amend WJC. Pulmonary infections in renal transplantation patients treated with cyclosporin. *Radiology* 1988;167:97–103.

146. Millar AB, Patou GM, Miller RF, et al. Cytomegalovirus in the lungs of patients with AIDS: respiratory pathogen or passenger? *Am Rev Res Dis* 1990;141:1474–1477.

147. Wallace MJ, Hannah J. Cytomegalovirus pneumonitis in patients with AIDS: findings in an autopsy series. *Chest* 1987;92: 198–203.

148. Klatt EC, Shibata D. Cytomegalovirus infection in the acquired immunodeficiency syndrome: clinical and autopsy findings. *Arch Pathol Lab Med* 1988;112:540–544.

149. Miles PR, Baughman RP, Linnemann CC. Cytomegalovirus in the bronchoalveolar lavage fluid in patients with AIDS. *Chest* 1990;97:1072–1076.

150. Hoover DR, Saah AJ, Bacellar H, et al. Clinical manifestations of AIDS in the era of Pneumocystis prophylaxis. *N Engl J Med* 1993;329:1922–1926.

151. Aafedt BC, Halvorsen R, Tylen U, Hertz M. Cytomegalovirus

pneumonia: computed tomography findings. *Can Assoc Radiol J* 1990;41:276–280.

152. Gruden JF, Klein JS, Webb WR. Percutaneous transthoracic needle biopsy in AIDS: analysis in 32 patients. *Radiology* 1993; 189:567–571.

153. McGuinness G, Scholes JV, Garay SM, Leitman BS, McCauley DI, Naidich DP. Cytomegalovirus pneumonitis: spectrum of parenchymal CT findings with pathologic correlation in 21 AIDS patients. *Radiology* 1994;192:451–459.

154. Katzenstein ALA, Myers JL, Mazur MT. Acute interstitial pneumonia: a clinicopathologic, ultrastructural, and cell kinetic study. *Am J Surg Pathol* 1986;10:256–267.

155. Olson J, Colby TV, Elliott CG. Hamman-Rich syndrome revisited. *Mayo Clin Proc* 1990;65:1538–1548.

156. Primack SL, Hartman TE, Ikezoe J, Akira M, Sakatani M, Müller NL. Acute interstitial pneumonia: radiographic and CT findings in nine patients. *Radiology* 1993;188:817–820.

157. Bessis L, Callard P, Gotheil C, Biaggi A, Grenier P. High-resolution CT of parenchymal lung disease: precise correlation with histologic findings. *Radiographics* 1992;12:45–58.

158. Webb WR, Stein MG, Finkbeiner WE, Im JG, Lynch D, Gamsu G. Normal and diseased isolated lungs: high-resolution CT. *Radiology* 1988;166:81–87.

159. Hedlund LW, Vock P, Effmann EL, Lischko MM, Putman CE. Hydrostatic pulmonary edema: an analysis of lung density changes by computed tomography. *Invest Radiol* 1984;19: 254–262.

160. Forster BB, Müller NL, Mayo JR, Okazawa M, Wiggs BJ, Pare PD. High-resolution computed tomography of experimental hydrostatic pulmonary edema. *Chest* 1992;101:1434–1437.

161. Müller-Leisse C, Klosterhalfen B, Hauptmann S, et al. Computed tomography and histologic results in the early stages of endotoxin-injured pig lungs as a model for adult respiratory distress syndrome. *Invest Radiol* 1993;28:39–45.

SEVEN

Diseases Characterized Primarily by Decreased Lung Opacity, Including Cystic Abnormalities, Emphysema, and Bronchiectasis

This disparate group of diseases have in common the presence of focal, multifocal, or diffuse decreased lung opacity, which may be associated with the presence of cysts or abnormal bronchi. These diseases include pulmonary histiocytosis X, lymphangiomyomatosis, different types of emphysema, and airway diseases including bronchiectasis, and diseases primarily affecting small airways, such as bronchiolitis obliterans and panbronchiolitis (1). The appearance of honeycombing and honeycomb cysts are reviewed in Chapters 3 and 4. *Pneumocystis carinii* pneumonia especially in patients with AIDS can also show thin- or thick-walled cysts, and is discussed in Chapter 6.

PULMONARY HISTIOCYTOSIS X (PULMONARY LANGERHANS CELL HISTIOCYTOSIS)

Pulmonary histiocytosis X, also known as Langerhans histiocytosis or eosinophilic granuloma of the lung, is an idiopathic disease characterized in its early stages by granulomatous nodules containing Langerhans histiocytes and eosinophils, which are primarily peribronchial in distribution (2). In its later stages, the cellular granulomas are replaced by fibrosis and the formation of cysts (3,4).

Histiocytosis X (HX) is an uncommon condition. Gaensler et al. (5) found it in only 3.4% of 502 patients who underwent open lung biopsy for chronic, diffuse infiltrative lung disease. The majority of patients with pulmonary histiocytosis X are young or middle-aged adults (average age 32 years) presenting with nonspecific symptoms of cough and dyspnea (3,4). Up to 20%

of patients present with pneumothorax (6). There is a slight male predominance, and over 90% of patients are smokers (2,6–11). A causal relationship between smoking and HX is likely (2).

The radiographic findings consist of reticular, nodular, reticulonodular patterns, and honeycombing, often in combination (6–9,12). Abnormalities are usually bilateral, involving predominantly the middle- and upper-lung zones with relative sparing of the costophrenic angles (6,7). Lung volumes are characteristically normal or increased.

HRCT Findings

The HRCT findings of pulmonary histiocytosis X have been reported by Moore et al. (13), Brauner et al. (14), and Grenier et al. (15). HRCT findings closely mirror the gross pathologic appearances of this disease (Figs. 7-1,7-2). In almost all patients, HRCT demonstrates cystic airspaces, which are usually less than 10 mm in diameter (Fig. 7-2); these cysts are characteristic of HX (13,14,16,17), and were seen in 17 of 18 patients studied by Brauner et al. (14) and all 12 patients studied by Giron et al. (17) (Table 7-1).

On HRCT, the lung cysts have walls that range from being barely perceptible to being several millimeters in thickness. In a study by Grenier et al. (15), 88% of 51 patients with HX showed thin-walled (< 2 mm) cysts on HRCT, while 53% showed thick-walled (> 2 mm) cysts. The presence of distinct walls allows differentiation of these cysts from areas of emphysema that can also be seen in some patients. Although many cysts

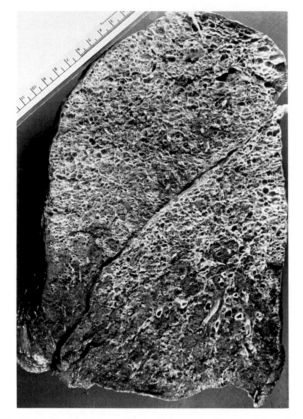

FIG. 7-1. Autopsy specimen from a patient with pulmonary histiocytosis X. Fine cystic spaces predominate in the upper- and mid-lung zones. The lung bases are relatively spared. (From Müller and Miller, ref. 19, with permission.)

TABLE 7-1. HRCT findings in Histiocytosis X[a,b]

1. **Thin-walled Lung Cysts, Some Confluent or with Bizarre Shapes, Usually Less Than 1 cm**
2. ***Nodules, Usually <1–5 mm, Some Centrilobular and Peribronchiolar***
3. ***Upper-lobe Predominance, Costophrenic Angles Spared***
4. Cavitary Nodules
5. Fine Reticular Opacities, Ground-glass Opacity

[a] Most common findings in boldface.
[b] Findings most helpful in differential diagnosis in boldface italics.

...ppear round, they can also have bizarre shapes, being bilobed, clover-leaf shaped, or branching in appearance (Figs. 3-74,3-75,7-2) (13). These unusual shapes are postulated to occur because of fusion of several cysts, or perhaps because the "cysts" sometimes represent ectatic and thick-walled bronchi (13); in the series reported by Brauner et al. (14), "confluent" or "joined cysts" with persisting septations were seen in more than two thirds of patients. An upper-lobe predominance in the size and number of cysts is common (Figs. 3-74,3-75,7-1,7-2). Large cysts or bullae (> 10 mm in diameter) are also seen in more than half of cases; some cysts are larger than 20 mm (14).

In some patients, cysts are the only abnormality visible on HRCT, but in the majority of cases, small nod-

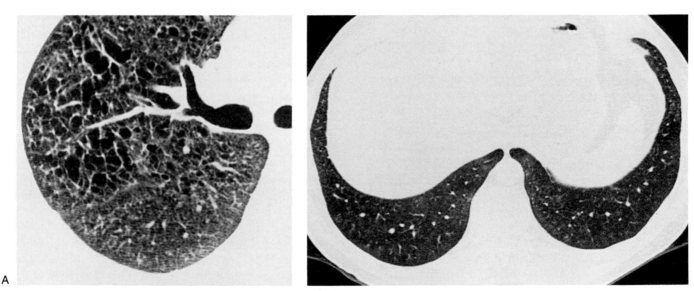

A   B

FIG. 7-2. Cystic pulmonary histiocytosis X in a 37-year-old man. **A:** HRCT at the level of the right upper-lobe bronchus shows cystic airspaces with thin but well-defined walls. Some cysts are confluent or appear irregular in shape. Note the much milder disease in the superior segment of the right lower lobe. **B:** HRCT through the lung bases shows that these are relatively spared. An upper-lobe predominance of abnormalities is characteristic of pulmonary histiocytosis X.

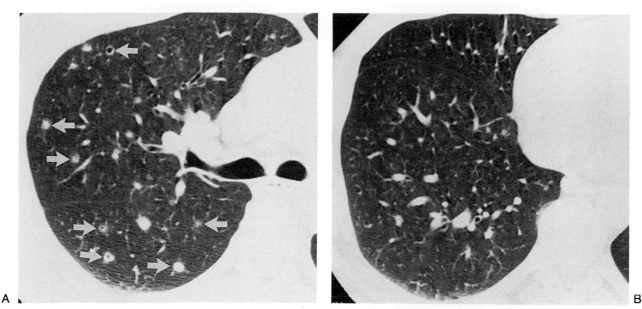

FIG. 7-3. Nodular histiocytosis X in a 30-year-old man. **A:** HRCT at the level of the right upper-lobe bronchus shows several nodules (*arrows*). Some are solid, others are cavitated; some have smooth margins, others have irregular or poorly defined margins. **B:** HRCT through the right lower-lung zone shows relative sparing of the lung bases.

ules (usually < 5 mm in diameter) are also present (Figs. 3-37,7-3) (13,14); nodules were seen in 14 of 18 patients in Brauner's series, and in 14 of 17 patients in Moore's series (13,14). Larger nodules, sometimes exceeding 1 cm, are also seen, but are less common. In the study by Grenier et al. (15), 47% of 51 patients with HX showed nodules < 3 mm in diameter, while 45% showed nodules ranging between 3 mm and 1 cm in diameter, and 24% showed nodules exceeding 1 cm in size. Nodules can vary considerably in number in individual cases, probably depending on the activity of the disease; nodules can be few in number or myriad (13,14). The margins of nodules are often irregular, particularly when there is surrounding cystic or reticular disease. On HRCT, many nodules can be seen to be peribronchial or peribronchiolar, and therefore, centrilobular in location; in this disease, there a tendency for granulomas to form around the bronchioles (14). HRCT may be valuable in directing lung biopsy to areas showing lung nodules (14).

The nodules are usually solid in appearance, but larger nodules (approximately 1 cm in diameter) sometimes show lucent centers, presumably corresponding to small "cavities" (Fig. 7-3) (18). These cavities, however, may sometimes represent the dilated bronchiolar lumen surrounded by granulomas and thickened interstitium (14). In some patients progression of cavitary nodules to cystic lesions has been observed (17). In the study by Grenier et al. (15), 25% of 51 patients with HX showed cavitary nodules.

In many patients with cysts or nodules the intervening lung parenchyma appears normal on HRCT, without evidence of fibrosis or septal thickening (13,14). However, in a small percentage of cases, irregular interfaces (the "interface sign") are present, or a fine reticular network of opacities is visible (Fig. 7-4) (14,17). These fine reticular opacities may correlate with intralobular fibrosis or early cyst formation, or with the progression and confluence of cysts (17). Ground-glass opacity is also sometimes seen, but is not a prominent feature of this disease.

HRCT shows no consistent central or peripheral predominance of lesions (14,15), but in nearly all cases, the lung bases and the costophrenic sulci are relatively spared (13,19). In Brauner's series (14) of 18 patients, 2 had abnormalities localized to the upper lobes and 9 had disease that was predominant in the upper- or mid-lung zones; two patients had diffuse disease, but no patient had disease with a lower-lung predominance. An upper-lobar predominance was reported in 57% of Grenier's 51 patients (15), while a mid-lung or basal predominance was never observed.

Utility of HRCT

HRCT is superior to chest radiographs in demonstrating the morphology and distribution of lung abnormalities in patients with HX (13,14), and in making a specific diagnosis of HX (15). In fact, in many patients

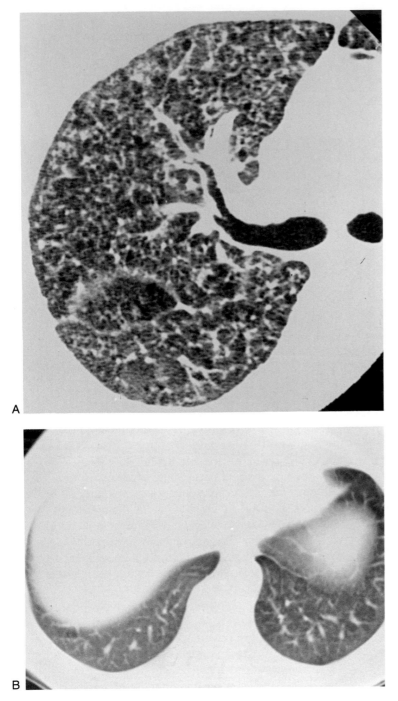

FIG. 7-4. End-stage pulmonary histiocytosis X in a 50-year-old woman. **A:** HRCT at the level of the right upper-lobe bronchus shows extensive fibrosis with small honeycomb cysts. The disease involves the lung diffusely at this level. **B:** Conventional 10-mm collimation CT scan through the lung base is virtually normal.

with HX who have plain radiographic findings of reticular abnormalities, HRCT shows that the plain film findings reflect the presence of numerous superimposed lung cysts. As compared with chest radiographs, HRCT is significantly more sensitive in detecting small and large cysts, and nodules less than 5 mm in diameter (14,15).

HX is not associated with any consistent pattern of pulmonary function test (PFT) abnormalities, although airways obstruction is common (20), and probably related to peribronchial and luminal fibrosis (2). In a study by Moore et al. (13), the extent of disease on HRCT correlated better ($r = -0.71$) with impairment in gas exchange, as assessed by the percent predicted by the carbon monoxide diffusing capacity, than did plain radiographic findings ($r = -0.57$). In another study (20), significant correlation ($r = 0.8$) between HRCT and diffusing capacity was also found. However, no correlation has been shown between CT findings and PFT findings of obstruction (13,20). Air trapping in association with lung cysts has been reported on expiratory HRCT in a patient with HX, despite the absence of evidence of airways obstruction on PFT (21).

In patients who only have nodules on HRCT the differential diagnosis is extensive; differentiation from sarcoidosis, silicosis, metastatic disease, and tuberculosis may be impossible, although the distribution of abnormalities can be valuable. Nodules in HX tend to be centrilobular, while septal, subpleural, and peribronchovascular nodules are typically seen in sarcoidosis, silicosis, and lymphangitic carcinomatosis. On the one hand, sparing of the costophrenic angles should raise the possibility of pulmonary HX, but can be seen in these diseases as well. On the other hand, the cystic changes that are seen in this disease can be easily distinguished from the honeycombing that is seen in end-stage idiopathic pulmonary fibrosis (IPF). Pulmonary HX characteristically involves the upper two thirds of the lungs diffusely, with relative sparing of the costophrenic angles (13,14); IPF and other causes of honeycombing primarily involve the subpleural lung regions and the lung bases (22). Also, in patients with IPF, the honeycomb cysts are surrounded by abnormal parenchyma that show findings of extensive fibrosis, whereas most of the cysts in HX are surrounded by normal lung. Lung volumes are normal or increased in cystic HX, while they are generally reduced in patients with IPF who show honeycombing.

In a woman, cystic changes identical to those seen in histiocytosis X, can be seen in lymphangiomyomatosis or tuberous sclerosis (23–28). However, lymphangiomyomatosis is very rare in men. Furthermore, in lymphangiomyomatosis the lower third of the lungs are usually involved and nodules are rarely seen. The cysts in HX, when adjacent to blood vessels, can mimic the signet-ring sign of bronchiectasis (29). However, distinction from bronchiectasis is straightforward because the cysts in HX lack the characteristic continuity of dilated bronchi seen on contiguous slices in patients with bronchiectasis (13).

LYMPHANGIOMYOMATOSIS

Lymphangiomyomatosis (LAM) is a rare disease characterized by progressive proliferation of spindle cells, resembling immature smooth muscle, in the lung parenchyma and along lymphatic vessels in the chest and abdomen (Fig. 7-5) (30,31). Proliferation of spindle cells along the bronchioles leads to air trapping and the development of emphysema and thin-walled lung cysts (Figs. 7-5,7-6). Rupture of these cysts can result in pneumothorax.

The spindle cell proliferation can also involve the hilar, mediastinal, and extrathoracic lymph nodes, sometimes resulting in dilatation of intrapulmonary lymphatics and the thoracic duct. Involvement of the lymphatics can lead to chylous pleural effusion. Proliferation of cells in the walls of pulmonary veins may cause venous obstruction and lead to pulmonary hemorrhage.

The majority of patients present with dyspnea. Sixty percent develop chylous pleural effusions; 40% develop pneumothorax; and 30% to 40% develop blood-streaked sputum or frank hemoptysis (30–32). Almost all patients die within 10 years of the onset of symptoms. Recently, improved prognosis has been reported following treatment with progesterone or oophorectomy (33,34).

Lymphangiomyomatosis occurs only in women of child-bearing age, usually between 17 and 50 years. However, rarely, it may be seen in postmenopausal women; the oldest patient described was 69 years of

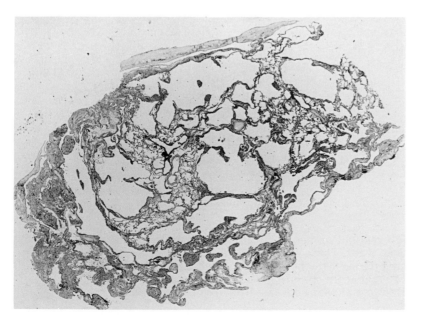

FIG. 7-5. Low-power microscopic view of an open lung biopsy specimen from a patient with LAM. Characteristic cystic spaces with atypical spindle cells lining their walls are seen throughout the specimen.

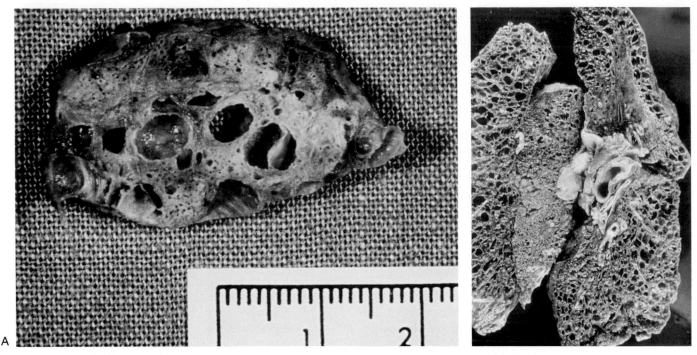

A

B

FIG. 7-6. Lymphangiomyomatosis. **A:** Open lung biopsy specimen shows large cysts. **B:** Whole-lung specimen from a patient with extensive cystic changes. (Case courtesy of Peter Kullnig, M.D., University of Graz, Graz, Austria. A, from Templeton et al., ref. 27, with permission.)

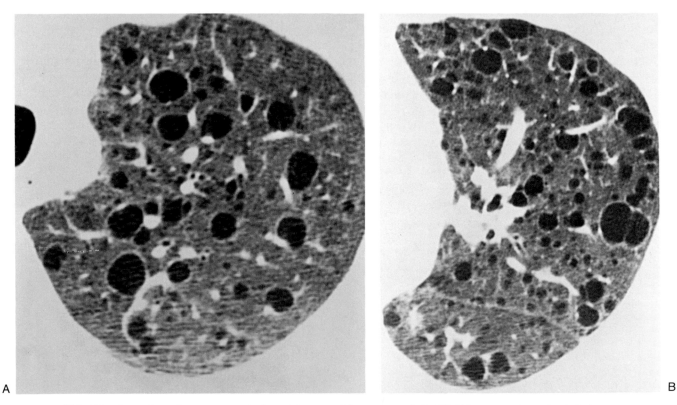

A

B

FIG. 7-7. Lymphangiomyomatosis in a 30-year-old woman. **A,B:** HRCT targeted to the left lung shows multiple cystic airspaces of varying sizes. These have walls ranging from being barely perceptible to 2 mm in thickness. The lung parenchyma between the cystic airspaces is normal. The cysts are primarily round in shape, but some are confluent. As contrasted with histiocytosis X, the upper and lower lobes are involved to a similar degree. (From Templeton et al., ref. 27, with permission.)

TABLE 7-2. *HRCT findings in lymphangiomyomatosis[a,b]*

1. ***Thin-walled Lung Cysts, Some Confluent***
2. ***Diffuse Distribution***
3. Mild Septal Thickening or Ground-glass Opacity
4. Adenopathy
5. Small Nodules
6. *Pleural Effusion*

[a] Most common findings in boldface.
[b] Findings most helpful in differential diagnosis in italics.

age (34). Identical clinical, radiologic, and pathologic pulmonary changes may be seen in about 1% of patients with tuberous sclerosis (Fig. 3-76). Although tuberous sclerosis affects both sexes equally, the pulmonary changes have been described almost exclusively in women.

The plain radiologic manifestations of LAM include reticular, reticulonodular, miliary, and honeycomb patterns (32,35). Lung volumes can be increased in patients with this disease. The radiologic findings may precede, accompany, or postdate other manifestations of the disease such as pneumothorax and chylous pleural effusion. In several patients who were being treated for recurrent pneumothoraces, extensive parenchymal abnormalities have been demonstrated at surgery that were not visible on radiographs (32).

HRCT Findings

On HRCT, patients with LAM characteristically show numerous thin-walled lung cysts, surrounded by relatively normal lung parenchyma (Figs. 3-77,7-7,7-8) (23–28,36–38) (Table 7-2). These cysts usually range from 2 mm to 5 cm in diameter, but can be larger. Their size tends to increase with progression of the disease (28). In patients with mild disease, the cysts usually measure < 5 mm in diameter. In patients with more extensive disease, in which 80% or more of the lung parenchyma is involved, the cysts tend to be larger, most being > 1 cm in diameter. The walls of the lung cysts usually range from being faintly perceptible to 4 mm in thickness (24,28). Irregularly shaped lung cysts, as are seen in patients with HX, are uncommon. Lung cysts seen on HRCT correlate with the presence

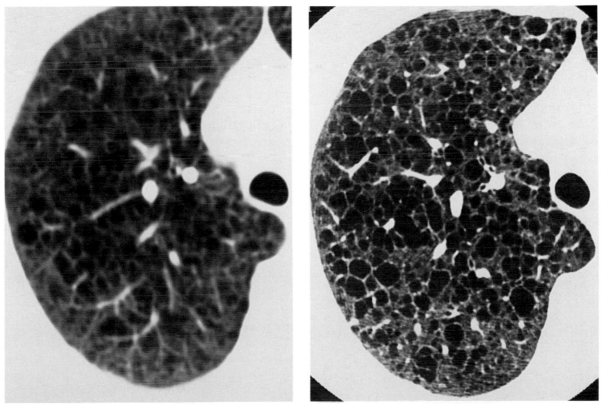

A   B

FIG. 7-8. Lymphangiomyomatosis in a 58-year-old woman. **A:** Conventional 10-mm collimation CT scan through the right upper lobe shows lucent areas. This appearance is similar to that of emphysema. **B:** HRCT demonstrates that the cystic airspaces have well-defined walls allowing easy distinction from emphysema.

of the lung cysts which are common pathologically in this disease; these cysts are partially surrounded by the abnormal spindle cells typical of LAM.

In the majority of patients the cysts are distributed diffusely throughout the lungs, and no lung zone is spared; diffuse lung involvement is seen even in patients with mild disease. In reported series (24,28), there is no evidence of lower-lung zone, or central or peripheral predominance on CT scans. Thus, the HRCT findings do not support the previous impression that the lesions initially have a predominantly basal distribution (31).

In most patients the lung parenchyma between the cysts appears normal on HRCT. In some cases, however, a slight increase in linear interstitial markings (25), interlobular septal thickening (24), or patchy areas of ground-glass opacity (28) are also seen. The latter probably represent areas of pulmonary hemorrhage. Small nodules are occasionally seen, but are not a prominent feature of this disease as they are with histiocytosis X.

Other features of LAM that can be seen on CT include hilar, mediastinal, and retrocrural adenopathy. Adenopathy was visible in 4 of the 7 patients with complete chest CT scans reported by Sherrier et al. (26). Pleural effusions can also be seen, and can be helpful in distinguishing LAM from histiocytosis X.

Utility of HRCT

HRCT is superior to chest radiography in determining the extent and distribution of air cysts in this disease, and it can demonstrate extensive abnormalities in patients with normal radiographic findings (24,26,28). The cystic changes of LAM are also much easier to assess and are better defined on HRCT than on conventional CT (Fig. 7-8). Cysts visible on HRCT were rarely seen on chest radiographs unless larger than 1 cm.

Disease extent as assessed on CT correlates better than do radiographic findings with clinical and functional impairment in patients with lymphangiomyomatosis. The best correlations are observed between the extent of disease on CT, and impairment in gas transfer as assessed by the carbon monoxide diffusing capacity (24,28,38). Significant correlations have also been demonstrated between extent of cystic disease and severity of airways obstruction (24,38). For example in the study by Aberle et al. (38), the correlation between CT scores and both diffusing capacity (DLCO, $r = -0.8, p < 0.017$) and a measure of airways obstruction (FEV$_1$/ FVC%, $r = -0.92, p < 0.002$) were excellent. In the study by Lenoir et al. (24), similar correlations were found.

Cystic airspaces are common in a variety of fibrotic interstitial lung diseases, particularly end-stage idiopathic pulmonary fibrosis (IPF) (22). However, as in patients with histiocytosis X, the different distribution of abnormalities, and the absence of findings of extensive fibrosis in patients with lymphangiomyomatosis allow their differentiation.

Lung cysts very similar to those seen in lymphangiomyomatosis have also been described in patients with pulmonary histiocytosis X (13,14). However, three findings usually allow the differentiation of these two diseases:

1. In many patients with histiocytosis X, a nodular component is also present; this is uncommon with LAM.
2. Irregularly shaped cysts, as are commonly seen in patients with histiocytosis X, are much less frequent with LAM.
3. Histiocytosis X characteristically involves the upper two thirds of the lungs and spares the costophrenic angles, while LAM involves the lungs diffusely (13,14). In some patients, however, the HRCT findings of these two conditions can be identical.

The presence of many small, thin-walled, cystic airspaces scattered throughout both lungs in a young woman is virtually pathognomonic of LAM. However, definitive diagnosis requires open lung biopsy. CT is advantageous in demonstrating parenchymal abnormalities in symptomatic patients with normal or questionably abnormal findings on chest radiographs, thus indicating the need for biopsy. It should be noted, however, that normal findings at CT examination do not rule out parenchymal disease in patients with lymphangiomyomatosis (28).

EMPHYSEMA

Emphysema is defined as a condition of the lung characterized by permanent, abnormal enlargement of airspaces distal to the terminal bronchiole, accompanied by the destruction of their walls (39–41). Previous definitions of emphysema have included the caveat "without obvious fibrosis" (42), but recent observations have established that some degree of fibrosis is not uncommon (39,40).

Emphysema is usually classified into three main subtypes, based on the anatomic distribution of the areas of lung destruction, but the names applied to these subtypes by different investigators often differ (41,43). These subtypes are:

1. proximal acinar, centriacinar, or centrilobular emphysema;

2. panacinar or panlobular emphysema; and
3. distal acinar or paraseptal emphysema.

Although from an anatomic or pathologic point of view, it is most appropriate to refer to these types of emphysema relative to the presence and type of acinar abnormalities (i.e., proximal acinar, panacinar, and distal acinar), from the standpoint of understanding the use of HRCT, it is more appropriate to refer to them relative to the way in which we perceive them at the lobular level (i.e., centrilobular, panlobular, and paraseptal). As indicated in Chapter 2, acini cannot be resolved on HRCT. In the remainder of this chapter, the terms *centrilobular, panlobular, and paraseptal* will be used to describe these these types of emphysema.

Centrilobular emphysema (proximal acinar emphysema, centriacinar emphysema) predominantly affects the respiratory bronchioles in the central portions of acini, and therefore involves the central portion of the lobule. Panlobular emphysema (panacinar emphysema) involves all the components of the acinus more or less uniformly, and therefore involves the entire lobule. Paraseptal (distal acinar emphysema) predominantly involves the alveolar ducts and sacs, with areas of destruction often marginated by interlobular septa.

Centrilobular emphysema usually results from cigarette smoking. It mainly involves the upper-lung zones. In contrast, panlobular emphysema is classically associated with alpha-1-protease inhibitor (alpha-1-antitrypsin) deficiency, although it may also be seen without protease deficiency in smokers, in the elderly, and distal to bronchial and bronchiolar obliteration (42). Paraseptal emphysema can be an isolated phenomenon in young adults, often associated with spontaneous pneumothorax, or can be seen in older patients with centrilobular emphysema (42). In their early stages, these three forms of emphysema can be easily distinguished morphologically. However, as they become more severe, their distinction becomes more difficult.

Bullae can develop in association with any type of emphysema, but are most common with paraseptal or centrilobular emphysema. A bulla, by definition, is a sharply demarcated area of emphysema measuring 1 cm or more in diameter, and possessing a wall < 1 mm in thickness (44). In some patients with emphysema, bullae can become quite large, resulting in significant compromise of respiratory function; this syndrome is sometimes referred to as "bullous emphysema." Bullae have been classified by Reid according to their location and the type of emphysema with which they are associated (45). According to this classification, type 1 bullae are subpleural in location and occur in patients with paraseptal emphysema; type 2 bullae are also subpleural but are associated with generalized emphysema (centrilobular or panlobular); type 3 bullae are associ-

ated with generalized emphysema, but occur within the lung parenchyma rather than in a subpleural location. Irregular air-space enlargement is an additional type of emphysema occurring in patients with pulmonary fibrosis; this form of emphysema is also referred to as paracicatricial or irregular emphysema (42,43).

CT and HRCT Findings

On HRCT, emphysema is characterized by the presence of areas of abnormally low attenuation, which can be easily contrasted with surrounding normal lung parenchyma if sufficiently low-window means (−600 HU to −800 HU) are used (46,47). In most instances, focal areas of emphysema can be easily distinguished from lung cysts or honeycombing; focal areas of emphysema usually lack distinct walls (46,47).

Centrilobular Emphysema

Centrilobular emphysema of mild to moderate degree is characterized on HRCT by the presence of multiple, small round areas of abnormally low attenuation, several millimeters in diameter, distributed throughout the lung, but usually having an upper-lobe predominance. Areas of lucency often appear to be grouped near the centers of secondary pulmonary lobules, surrounding the centrilobular artery branches (Figs. 3-78,3-79,7-9,7-10) (Table 7-3) (46–49). These lucencies correspond to the well-circumscribed centrilobular or centriacinar areas of lung destruction seen pathologically in patients with centrilobular emphysema (46–51). Although the centrilobular location of lucencies cannot always be recognized on CT or HRCT (48,49), the presence of multiple, small areas of emphy-

---

TABLE 7-3. *HRCT findings in emphysema*[a,b]

1. **Focal Areas of Decreased Opacity (Lung Destruction) With or Without Visible Walls**

2. Centrilobular Emphysema—Multiple, Small, Centrilobular Lucencies, Patchy, Predominant Upper-lobe Distribution

3. Panlobular Emphysema—Uniform Destruction of Lobules, Extensive, Predominant Lower-lobe Distribution

4. Paraseptal Emphysema—Subpleural Bullae and Cysts, Visible Walls

5. Irregular Air-space Enlargement—Irregular Areas of Decreased Opacity in Regions of Fibrosis

[a] Most common findings in boldface.
[b] Finding most helpful in differential diagnosis in boldface italics.

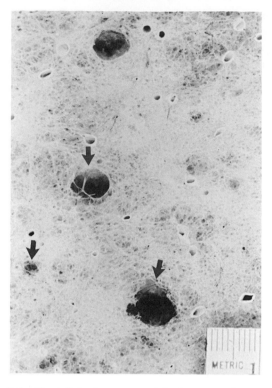

FIG. 7-9. Centrilobular or centriacinar emphysema. A low-power microscopic view of a lung specimen from a patient with mild centrilobular emphysema. Areas of lung destruction measuring 3 to 10 mm in diameter are visible (*arrows*).

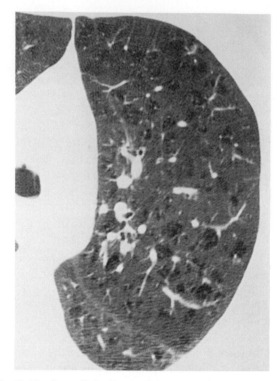

FIG. 7-10. Centrilobular emphysema in a 70-year-old smoker. HRCT at the level of the aortic arch shows localized areas of abnormally low attenuation measuring 2 to 10 mm in diameter, which can be seen to be centrilobular (they surround arteries in the lobular core). The areas of destruction lack recognizable walls.

sema, scattered throughout the lung, is diagnostic of centrilobular emphysema (Figs. 7-10,7-11). In most cases, the areas of low attenuation lack visible walls (Fig. 7-10), although very thin and relatively inconspicuous walls are occasionally seen on HRCT (Fig. 7-11) and are probably related to surrounding fibrosis; it recently has been shown that centrilobular emphysema is commonly associated with some fibrosis (39,40).

With more severe centrilobular emphysema, areas of destruction can become confluent. When this occurs, the centrilobular distribution of abnormalities is no longer recognizable on HRCT (or pathologically); the term *confluent centrilobular emphysema* is sometimes used to describe this occurrence (Fig. 7-12). This appearance can closely mimic the appearance of panlobular emphysema, and a distinction between these is of little clinical significance.

Using HRCT in a study of postmortem lung specimens, Hruban et al. (46) were able to accurately identify centrilobular emphysema, even of mild degree. The correlation between the in vitro CT emphysema score and the pathologic grade was excellent (*r* = 0.91). The ability of HRCT to accurately demonstrate the location and extent of emphysema in lung specimens was also shown by Webb et al. (47).

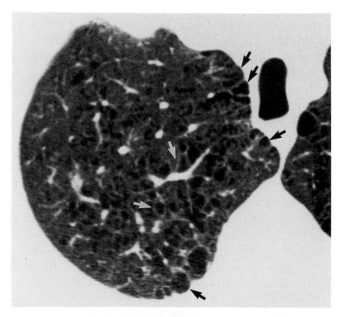

FIG. 7-11. Centrilobular emphysema. Some of the focal areas of lung destruction appear to be outlined by very thin walls (*white arrows*), probably due to fibrosis. Subpleural lucencies (*black arrows*) represent paraseptal emphysema, which can coexist with centrilobular emphysema.

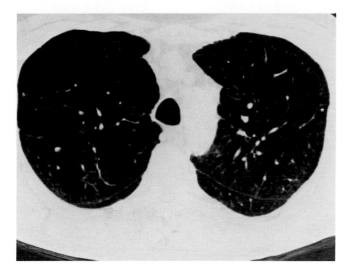

FIG. 7-12. Confluent centrilobular emphysema. Focal areas of centrilobular emphysema are visible on HRCT in the left upper lobe, while in the right upper lobe, areas of emphysema are large and confluent.

While it may be possible to obtain a near one to one correlation between CT and pathologic specimens in vitro, it is not possible to obtain such a good correlation in vivo; minimal emphysema can sometimes be missed by HRCT. Miller et al. (51) found a CT-pathologic correlation of $r = 0.81$ when using 10-mm collimation scans, and a correlation of $r = 0.85$ when using 1.5-mm collimation scans. In this series, 33 of 38 patients had emphysema; out of these 33, 4 patients with mild centrilobular emphysema were interpreted as normal on CT. Kuwano et al. (52) found no significant difference between the HRCT and the pathology scores, in 42 patients with mild to moderate emphysema; correla-

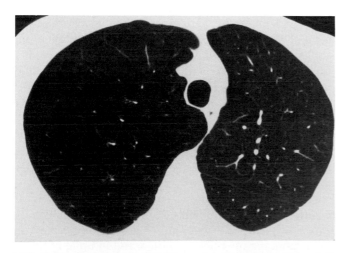

FIG. 7-13. Panlobular emphysema in a patient with a left lung transplant. The emphysematous right lung is relatively large and lucent, and shows fewer and smaller vessels than are visible on the left. This appearance is typical of panlobular emphysema.

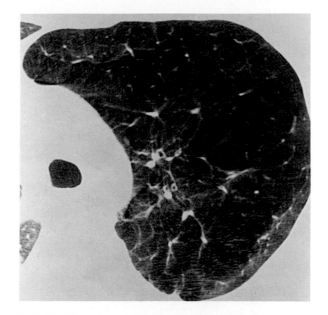

FIG. 7-14. Panlobar emphysema due to alpha-1-antiprotease deficiency in a 50-year-old woman. HRCT at the level of the aortic arch shows marked simplification of the architecture of the pulmonary parenchyma and areas of abnormally low attenuation. The areas of emphysema involve the entire secondary lobule and are easily distinguished from the localized 2- to 10-mm diameter areas of abnormally low attenuation seen in centrilobular emphysema.

tion between the CT scores and the pathology scores in this study was approximately 0.70.

Panlobular Emphysema

Panlobular emphysema is characterized by uniform destruction of the pulmonary lobule, leading to widespread areas of abnormally low attenuation (Figs. 7-13–7-15) (Table 7-3) (49,50). Thurlbeck describes this entity as a ''diffuse 'simplification' of the lung structure with progressive loss of tissue until little remains but the supporting framework of vessels, septa and bronchi'' (43). Pulmonary vessels in the affected lung appear fewer and smaller than normal. Panlobular emphysema is almost always most severe in the lower lobes.

While it may lead to extensive destruction of the lung parenchyma, focal lucencies < 1 cm in diameter, which are characteristically present in mild and moderate centrilobular emphysema, are not seen in panlobular emphysema (Figs. 7-13,7-14). In severe panlobular emphysema, the characteristic appearance of extensive lung destruction and the associated paucity of vascular markings are easily distinguished from normal lung parenchyma (Fig. 7-13). However, mild and even moderately severe panlobular emphysema can be very subtle and difficult to detect radiographically (51).

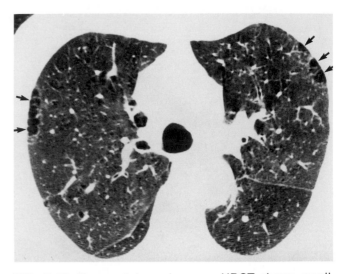

FIG. 7-16. Paraseptal emphysema. HRCT shows small, focal, subpleural lucencies (*arrows*) typical of paraseptal emphysema. These are commonly marginated by visible walls, usually representing interlobular septa. In some patients, areas of emphysema enlarge to form subpleural bullae.

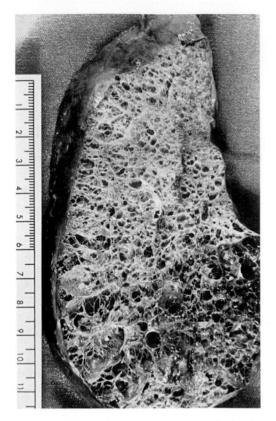

FIG. 7-15. Panlobular emphysema. A pathologic specimen shows diffuse involvement of the parenchyma with "simplification" of lung architecture.

Spouge et al. (53) recently assessed the accuracy of CT in diagnosing and quantifying emphysema in 10 patients with pathologically proven panlobular emphysema and 5 normal controls. They compared the visual assessment and severity of emphysema on CT with pathologic assessment. The correlation between the assessment of extent of panlobular emphysema on CT and the pathologic grade was $r = 0.90$, $p < 0.01$ for conventional CT, and $r = 0.96$, $p < 0.01$ for HRCT. Also, there was significantly less interobserver variation in the grading of emphysema on HRCT than with conventional CT. The observers missed three cases of mild panlobular emphysema on conventional CT and two on HRCT. They concluded that HRCT allows improved correlation with the pathologic score, and decreased interobserver variation than conventional CT in patients with panlobular emphysema.

Paraseptal Emphysema

Paraseptal emphysema is characterized by involvement of the distal part of the secondary lobule and is therefore most striking in a subpleural location (Figs. 3-84,7-11,7-16,7-17). Areas of subpleural paraseptal emphysema often have visible walls, but these walls

are very thin; they often correspond to interlobular septa. As with centrilobular emphysema, some fibrosis may be present. Even mild paraseptal emphysema is easily detected by HRCT (Table 7-3) (51).

When larger than 1 cm in diameter, areas of paraseptal emphysema are most appropriately termed bullae. Subpleural bullae are frequently considered to be a manifestation of paraseptal emphysema although they may be seen in all types of emphysema and as an isolated phenomenon; regardless of the cause of the subpleural bullae, they usually have thin walls which are visible on HRCT.

Lesur et al. (54) has shown that CT may be useful in the early detection of apical subpleural bullae in patients with idiopathic spontaneous pneumothorax. This form of pneumothorax occurs most often in tall young adults (55), and is thought to be due to rupture of a subpleural bulla (54). Out of 20 patients (mean age 27 ± 7 years), CT demonstrated emphysema in 17 with a predominance in the lung apices and in a subpleural location in 16.

Bense et al. (56) has also demonstrated that emphysema is seen on CT in the majority of non-smoking patients with spontaneous pneumothorax. They compared the CT findings in 27 non-smoking patients with spontaneous pneumothorax to the CT findings in 10 healthy subjects who had never smoked. Emphysema was present on CT in 22 of 27 non-smoking patients with spontaneous pneumothorax and in none of the 10 control subjects. The emphysema was present mainly in the periphery of the upper-lung zones, a distribution consistent with paraseptal emphysema. In none of the cases was emphysema detected on a chest radiograph.

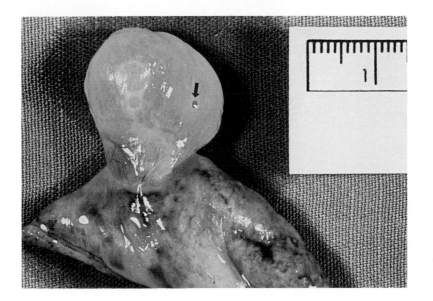

FIG. 7-17. Paraseptal emphysema with a large subpleural bulla. This patient presented with pneumothorax. The small hole in the bulla wall (*arrow*) was presumably the site of air leak.

"Bullous Emphysema"

"Bullous emphysema" does not represent a specific pathologic entity, but refers to the presence of emphysema associated with large bullae; it is generally seen in patients with centrilobular emphysema and/or paraseptal emphysema (Fig. 7-18) (45). A syndrome of bullous emphysema, or "giant bullous emphysema," has been described on the basis of clinical and radiologic features, and is also known as "vanishing lung syndrome," "type 1 bullous disease," or "primary bullous disease of the lung" (57). Giant bullous emphysema is often seen in young men, and is characterized by the presence of large, progressive, upper-lobe bul-

lae, which occupy a significant volume of a hemithorax, and are often asymmetric (Figs. 7-18, 7-19). Arbitrarily, giant bullous emphysema is said to be present if bullae occupy at least one-third of a hemithorax (57). Most patients with giant bullous emphysema are cigarette smokers (58), but this entity may also occur in non-smokers.

In nine patients with giant bullous emphysema reported by Stern et al. (57), the most striking HRCT finding was the presence of multiple large bullae, varying in size from 1 to 20 cm, but usually between 2 and 8 cm in diameter (Figs. 7-18, 7-19). Bullae were visible both in a subpleural location and within the lung parenchyma, but subpleural bullae predominated. Bullae

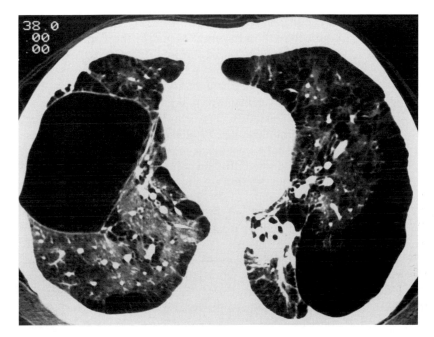

FIG. 7-18. "Bullous emphysema." In this patient, HRCT shows large, bilateral subpleural bullae, associated with areas of paraseptal emphysema (best seen on the right) and centrilobular emphysema (best seen on the left).

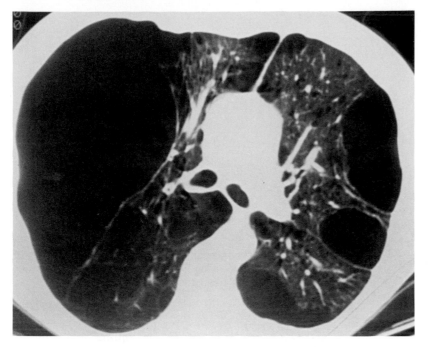

FIG. 7-19. Severe emphysema related to cigarette smoking in a 67-year-old man. Bullae are present bilaterally. Although there is extensive emphysema, the patient improved symptomatically following right bullectomy.

were often asymmetric, with one lung being involved to a greater degree (Fig. 7-19). HRCT better depicted the presence of associated paraseptal and centrilobular emphysema than did chest radiographs. In this study (57), paraseptal emphysema was visible on HRCT in all subjects and was the predominant associated finding; centrilobular emphysema of varying degrees was present in 8 of 9 subjects.

CT has been reported to be of value in the preoperative assessment of patients with bullous emphysema (59–61). In one study (59), CT showed well-defined bullae that were potentially resectable in 23 of 43 patients; 20 patients had bullae in association with generalized emphysema that were not amenable to surgical excision. Surgery is generally impossible if bullae are associated with extensive emphysema. Bullectomy is most effective when localized giant bullae are associated with localized paraseptal emphysema (58).

Irregular Air-Space Enlargement

Irregular air-space enlargement, previously known as irregular or cicatricial emphysema, is commonly found adjacent to localized parenchymal scars, diffuse pulmonary fibrosis, and in the pneumoconioses, particularly progressive massive fibrosis (Fig. 3-54) (62). It is most easily recognized on CT when the associated fibrosis is identified. However, this type of emphysema may also be seen associated with microscopic fibrosis, in which case radiologic distinction between irregular and centrilobular emphysema may be impossible (63).

Utility of HRCT

Standard chest radiography and pulmonary function tests are insensitive for the diagnosis of early emphysema (43,64). As indicated above, HRCT is undoubtedly more sensitive than chest radiographs in diagnosing emphysema and in determining its type and extent; HRCT is also advantageous relative to conventional CT (41,46,50,51,65–68). Furthermore, HRCT has a high specificity for diagnosing emphysema; emphysema is rarely overcalled in normal individuals or in patients with severe hyperinflation due to other causes (69).

In clinical practice HRCT is rarely used in an attempt to diagnose emphysema. Usually, the combination of (i) a smoking history, (ii) a low diffusing capacity, (iii) airways obstruction on pulmonary function tests, and (iv) an abnormal chest radiograph showing large lung volumes is sufficient to make the diagnosis. However, some patients with early emphysema can present with clinical findings more typical of interstitial lung disease or pulmonary vascular disease, namely shortness of breath and low-diffusing capacity, without evidence of airways obstruction on pulmonary function tests (52). In such patients, HRCT can be valuable in detecting the presence of emphysema and excluding an interstitial abnormality. If significant emphysema is found on HRCT, no further workup is necessary; specifically lung biopsy is not needed.

In a study of 470 HRCT examinations (70), there were 47 cases in which emphysema was the dominant or sole parenchymal abnormality. Of these 47, 16 lacked chest radiographic findings of emphysema, and 10 of these 16 had decreased single breath diffusing capacity ($DL_{CO}SB < 80\%$ predicted) without evidence of airways obstruction (FEV_1/FVC and $FEV_1 > 80\%$ predicted). In these patients the severity of emphysema scored on the HRCT correlated closely ($r = 0.8$) with decreasing $DL_{CO}SB$.

As indicated above, HRCT can also be used in the pre-operative assessment of patients undergoing bullectomy (Fig. 7-19). The majority of patients referred for bullectomy have well-demarcated bullae and varying degrees of emphysema (58). Large bullae can compress the remaining lung parenchyma and cause further functional and clinical impairment. CT allows for an assessment not only of the extent of bullous disease but, also the degree of compression and the severity of emphysema in the remaining lung parenchyma (58,60,61,71).

Limitations of CT in the Diagnosis of Emphysema

It should be noted that the CT assessment of emphysema has a number of potential limitations. Thus, although there is good correlation between the CT visual scores and the pathologic scores of emphysema extent, mild emphysema can be missed on HRCT (46,51,52). Furthermore in patients with more severe emphysema, the extent of destruction may be underestimated on CT, because localized areas of destruction, < 5 mm in diameter may be invisible (51). Thus, while CT is undoubtedly the most sensitive method which can be used to diagnose emphysema in vivo, it does not detect the earliest stages of emphysema and it cannot be used to definitely rule out the diagnosis.

The various recent studies that have assessed the accuracy of CT in diagnosing emphysema can be summarized as showing a high sensitivity and specificity, and a good correlation between the CT and pathologic scores of disease extent. However, while there is good correlation between the visual scores and the pathologic scores at a given level, it is extremely difficult to visually estimate the overall amount of lung that is abnormal because of the wide range of volumes represented in the different CT slices. This difficulty may be circumvented by highlighting areas of abnormally low attenuation using a computer program which highlights voxels to create a "density mask" within any desired range. Highlighting all voxels with attenuation values < -910 HU, correlation with pathologic scores has proved comparable to that obtained by visual assessment in 28 patients in one study (72). This method allows objective quantification of the total lung showing emphysema on CT as well as the percent area of lung involved by emphysema relative to total lung area.

Our ability to diagnose emphysema is influenced by scanner type, collimation, window level, window width, inter- and intraobserver variability. Measurements of attenuation can vary, according to scanner type, calibration, kilovoltage, reconstruction algorithm, volume averaging, patient size, location, environment, and size of the area being assessed. In spite of this, once the appropriate attenuation value cut-off is determined, areas of emphysema can be highlighted and objective quantification of emphysematous changes obtained.

BRONCHIECTASIS

Bronchiectasis is defined as localized, irreversible dilatation of the bronchial tree. Although a wide variety of disorders have been associated with bronchiectasis, it most commonly results from acute, chronic, or recurrent infection (Table 7-4) (73–75).

Bronchiectasis can result from chronic or severe bacterial infection, especially with necrotizing infections such as *Staphylococcus*, *Klebsiella*, or *B. pertussis* (75). Granulomatous infections, including those caused by *Mycobacterium tuberculosis* (76), atypical mycobacteria, especially *Mycobacterium avium-intracellulare* (MAC) (77–79), and fungal organisms such as histoplasmosis, are also associated with bronchiectasis. Additionally, bronchiectasis is often present in patients with bronchiolitis obliterans or the Swyer-James syndrome resulting from viral infection.

Bronchiectasis also has recently been identified in AIDS patients in association with a variety of organisms. Although the occurrence of bronchiectasis presumably results from accelerated bronchial wall destruction in severely immunocompromised patients, other mechanisms may be operative, as suggested by the finding of bronchiectasis in AIDS patients both with documented nonspecific and lymphocytic interstitial pneumonitis (80).

Bronchiectasis may occur in association with a variety of genetic abnormalities, especially those with abnormal mucociliary clearance, immune deficiency, or structural abnormalities of the bronchus or bronchial wall (Table 7-4). In addition to cystic fibrosis, causes of bronchiectasis having a genetic basis include alpha-1-antitrypsin deficiency; the dyskinetic cilia syndrome; Young's syndrome; Williams-Campbell syndrome (congenital deficiency of the bronchial cartilage); Mounier-Kuhn syndrome (congenital tracheobronchomegaly); immunodeficiency syndromes, including Bruton's hypogammaglobulinemia, IgA, and combined IgA-IgG subclass deficiencies; and the yellow nail syndrome (yellow nails, lymphedema, and pleural effusions). Although the etiology of bronchiectasis in these

TABLE 7-4. *Bronchiectasis—Associated Diseases and Possible Etiologies*

Condition	Suggested mechanisms
Infection (Bacteria, Mycobacteria, Fungus, Virus)	Impaired mucociliary clearance, disruption of respiratory epithelium, microbial toxins, host-mediated inflammation
Bronchial obstruction	Impaired mucociliary clearance, recurrent infection
Emphysema (Alpha-1-antitrypsin deficiency)	Proteinase-antiproteinase imbalance
Asthma	Airway inflammation, mucous plugging
Allergic bronchopulmonary aspergillosis (ABPA)	Type I and type III immune responses to fungus in airway lumen, mucous plugging
Cystic fibrosis	Abnormal airway epithelial chloride transport, impaired mucous clearance, recurrent infection
Dyskinetic cilia syndrome (Kartagener's syndrome)	Genetic defect, absent or dyskinetic ciliary beating, impaired mucous clearance, recurrent infection
Young's syndrome (Obstructive azoospermia)	Abnormal mucociliary clearance
Immunodeficiency states	Genetic or acquired predisposition to recurrent infection
Yellow nail–lymphedema syndrome	Unknown, lymphatic hypoplasia and sometimes immune deficiency, predisposition to recurrent infection?
Williams-Campbell syndrome	Congenital deficiency of bronchial cartilage, obstruction, impaired mucous clearance, recurrent infection
Tracheobronchomegaly (Mounier-Kuhn syndrome)	Congenital deficiency of membranous and cartilagenous parts of tracheal and bronchial walls, impaired mucous clearance, recurrent infection
Marfan syndrome	Unknown, genetic tissue defect, structural bronchial defect?
Bronchiolitis obliterans (postinfectious, toxic inhalation, lung transplant, etc.)	Bronchial wall inflammation, epithelial damage, recurrent infection in some cases
Chronic fibrosis	Traction bronchiectasis

Modified from Davis and Salzman, ref. 75.

conditions varies (Table 7-4), the presence of bronchial obstruction, abnormal mucociliary clearance, and chronic infection are often present.

Non-infectious diseases which result in airway inflammation and mucous plugging can also result in bronchiectasis. These include allergic bronchopulmonary aspergillosis (81,82) and asthma (83). Bronchiectasis also has been noted to occur in patients with bronchiolitis obliterans, including chronic rejection following heart-lung or lung transplantation (84–90) or bone marrow transplantation, most often as a result of rejection or chronic graft-vs.-host disease (GVHD) (91).

In general, a clinical diagnosis of bronchiectasis is possible only in the most severely affected patients, and even in this setting, differentiation from chronic bronchitis may be problematic (92). Most patients present with purulent sputum production and recurrent pulmonary infections (73,74). Hemoptysis also is frequent, occurring in up to 50% of cases and may be the only clinical finding (74,93,94). Bronchitis, bronchiolitis, or emphysema frequently accompany bronchiectasis and may cause obstructive abnormalities on pulmonary function tests.

Although the incidence of bronchiectasis is generally cited as decreasing in the United States, the true inci-

dence of bronchiectasis has probably been underestimated (95). Documentation of this disease has traditionally relied on bronchography, which is rarely performed, and has not taken into account the significant impact that computed tomography has had on the diagnosis of mild or unsuspected disease.

The radiographic manifestations of bronchiectasis have been well described (96). These include a loss of definition of vascular markings in specific lung segments, presumably secondary to peribronchial fibrosis and volume loss, evidence of bronchial wall thickening, and in more severely affected cases the presence of discrete cystic masses occasionally containing air-fluid levels. It should be emphasized that most of these findings are nonspecific; a definitive diagnosis of bronchiectasis can seldom be made roentgenographically (92).

Bronchographic findings indicative of bronchiectasis include proximal and/or distal bronchial dilatation, pruning or lack of normal tapering of peripheral airways, and luminal-filling defects. Although traditionally considered the "gold standard," the reliability of bronchography in the diagnosis of bronchiectasis has been called into question. Currie et al. in a study of 27 patients with chronic sputum production evaluated bronchographically showed that there was significant interobserver variability when studies were interpreted by two well-trained bronchographers (92). Agreement was only reached in 19 of 27 (70%) of patients and 94 of 448 (21%) of bronchopulmonary segments. Bronchiectasis was further identified in two patients (7%) by one radiologist only. These findings suggest that bronchography may be more limited in its utility than previously thought, and should not be considered an absolute standard for diagnosis.

CT and HRCT Findings

Bronchiectasis results in characteristic abnormalities identifiable on HRCT (Table 7-5) (29). These include bronchial dilatation, bronchial wall thickening, lack of normal bronchial tapering with visibility of airways in the peripheral lung, gross irregularities in airway contour, and mucus or fluid retention in the bronchial lumen. Also, bronchiectasis is often associated with atelectasis in affected lung regions or sometimes air trapping. A diagnosis of bronchiectasis is usually based on a combination of these findings (Table 7-5).

In most patients with bronchiectasis, HRCT findings are similar regardless of the mechanism or cause of disease. However, the HRCT appearances of several diseases associated with bronchiectasis (cystic fibrosis, allergic bronchopulmonary aspergillosis, Williams-Campbell syndrome) are distinct, and are discussed separately below.

Bronchial Dilatation

Since bronchiectasis is defined by the presence of bronchial dilatation, recognition of increased bronchial diameter is key to the CT diagnosis of this abnormality. Unfortunately, to date, no absolute CT criteria of normal bronchial diameter have been determined, and the HRCT diagnosis of bronchial dilatation remains somewhat subjective.

Relating the size of bronchi to the size of adjacent pulmonary artery branches has proven helpful in the diagnosis of bronchiectasis; generally, bronchiectasis is considered to be present when the internal diameter of a bronchus is greater than the diameter of the adjacent pulmonary artery branch (29). The accuracy of this relationship has been validated in a number of studies comparing CT to bronchography in patients with bronchiectasis (97–100). In patients with bronchiectasis, the bronchial diameter is often much larger than the pulmonary artery diameter, a finding which not only reflects the presence of bronchial dilatation, but also some reduction in pulmonary artery size; the abnormal ventilation of lung parenchyma in regions of bronchiectasis results in decreased lung perfusion and a corresponding decrease in pulmonary artery size. The association of a dilated bronchus, with a much

TABLE 7-5. *HRCT findings in bronchiectasis*[a,b]

1. **Bronchial Dilatation**
2. **Bronchial Wall Thickening**
3. **Visibility of Peripheral Airways**
4. **Contour Abnormalities**
   A. Cylindrical Bronchiectasis
      Signet ring sign (vertically oriented bronchi), Tram tracks (horizontally oriented bronchi), Lack of tapering
   B. Varicose Bronchiectasis
      String of Pearls (horizontally oriented bronchi)
   C. Cystic Bronchiectasis
      Cluster or string of cysts (esp. in atelectatic lung), Air-fluid levels
5. **Fluid or Mucus-filled Bronchi**
   Lobular or branching structures due to mucoid impaction, Sharply defined nodules (vertically oriented bronchi), Lack of contrast enhancement
6. Atelectasis

[a] Most common findings in boldface.
[b] Findings most helpful in differential diagnosis in boldface italics.

smaller contiguous pulmonary artery branch, has been termed the *signet-ring sign* (Figs. 3-3, 3-7, 7-20). This sign is quite valuable in recognizing bronchiectasis, and distinguishing it from other cystic lung lesions.

On the other hand, a simple comparison of bronchial and pulmonary artery sizes, can lead to the overdiagnosis of bronchiectasis in some subjects. For example, Lynch et al. (83) compared the internal diameters of lobar, segmental, subsegmental, and smaller bronchi to those of adjacent pulmonary artery branches in 27 normal subjects. Fifty-nine percent of the normal subjects showed at least one bronchus with an internal diameter exceeding that of the adjacent pulmonary artery branch, and 37 (26%) of 142 bronchi assessed in this group showed this finding (83). It must be emphasized that bronchiectasis should not be diagnosed on the basis of increased bronchial diameter alone; bronchial wall thickening is almost always seen in association with bronchial dilatation in patients with bronchiectasis, as are irregularities in bronchial diameter or lack of bronchial tapering. In the normal subjects studied by Lynch et al. (83), bronchial wall thickening was relatively uncommon, and it is unlikely that any of the subjects in this study would have been diagnosed on clinical HRCT studies as having true bronchiectasis.

Furthermore, in this context, it is worth noting that despite potential variability in normal bronchial size, CT measurements of bronchial diameter have proved remarkably consistent (101,102). Desai et al. (101), evaluated both inter- and intraobserver variation in CT measurements of bronchial wall circumference in 61

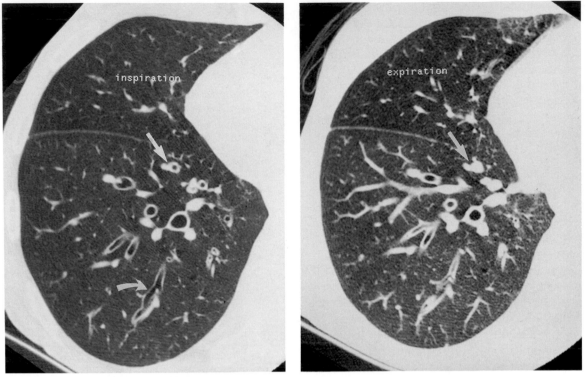

FIG. 7-20. Cylindrical bronchiectasis with bronchial dilatation and wall-thickening. **A:** Target reconstructed HRCT through the right lower lobe in a patient with mild cylindrical bronchiectasis, obtained at full inspiration. Dilated bronchi have a "signet-ring appearance" when sectioned vertically (*straight arrow*) and a "tram-track" appearance when sectioned horizontally (*curved arrow*). Bronchial walls in the lower lobe are considerably thicker than middle-lobe bronchi. **B:** HRCT at the same level following expiration. Note that the bronchial lumens narrow and their walls thicken, rendering identification of disease more difficult.

subsegmental bronchi and found the reproducibility of these measurements sufficiently significant to be clinically useful in demonstrating the progression of bronchiectasis. These findings suggest that in select cases, repeat evaluation may be of value to differentiate subtle cylindrical bronchiectasis from physiologic variations.

Bronchial Wall Thickening

As with bronchial diameter, there are no objective CT criteria as to normal bronchial wall thickness, and this observation is also largely subjective (83). However, since bronchiectasis and bronchial wall thickening are often multifocal rather than diffuse and uniform, a comparison of one lung region to another can be helpful in making this diagnosis. Using consistent window settings is very important in the diagnosis of bronchial wall thickening; bronchial walls can vary significantly in apparent thickness with different CT window settings.

Normal bronchi are visible only in the parahilar regions or middle third of the lung parenchyma. The smallest airways visible using HRCT techniques have a diameter of approximately 2 mm, and a wall thickness of about 0.2 to 0.3 mm (48); airways in the peripheral 2 cm of lung are not normally seen because their walls are too thin (47). Peribronchial fibrosis and bronchial wall thickening in patients with bronchiectasis allows the visualization of small airways in the lung periphery, and this finding can be very helpful in diagnosing the presence of an airway abnormality.

Lack of Bronchial Tapering and Contour Irregularities

Traditionally, bronchiectasis has been classified into three types depending on the severity of bronchial dilatation. These three types are *cylindrical*, *varicose*, and *cystic* (103). Although a distinction between these three types of bronchiectasis is sometimes helpful in diagnosis, and correlates with the severity of both the anatomic and functional abnormality, their differentiation is generally less important clinically than a determination of the extent and distribution of the airway disease. Evaluating the extent of bronchiectasis is particularly important, as surgery is only rarely performed in patients with involvement of multiple lung segments (73,74,104).

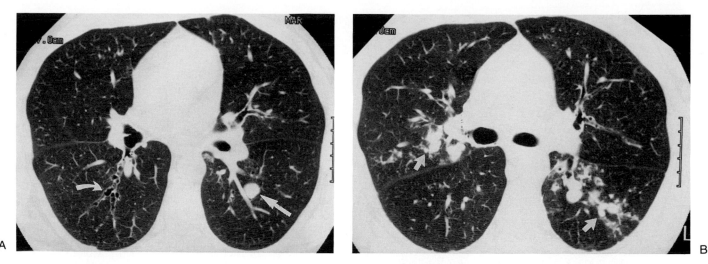

FIG. 7-21. Varicose bronchiectasis in allergic bronchopulmonary aspergillosis. **A:** HRCT at the level of the middle-lobe bronchus in a patient with proven allergic bronchopulmonary aspergillosis. The proximal portion of the superior segmental bronchus of the right lower lobe is dilated and has a distinctly beaded appearance (*curved arrows*). Varicose bronchiectasis can only be diagnosed when involved bronchi course horizontally within the plane of the CT section. The rounded opacity on the left (*straight arrow*) is the result of mucoid impaction within a vertically coursing bronchus. **B:** HRCT in the same patient just below the carina. At this level the predominant finding is mucoid impaction, recognizable as lobulated linear or branching densities extending toward the lung periphery (*arrows*).

Cylindrical Bronchiectasis

Mild, or cylindrical bronchiectasis is diagnosed if the dilated bronchi are of relatively uniform caliber and have roughly parallel walls. The appearance of cylin-

drical bronchiectasis will vary depending on whether the abnormal bronchi have a horizontal or vertical course, relative to the scan plane. When horizontal, bronchi are visualized along their length and are recognizable as branching "tram tracks" which fail to taper

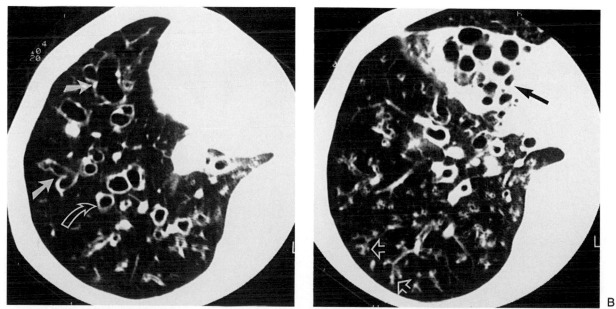

FIG. 7-22. Cystic bronchiectasis. **A,B:** Sequential target reconstructed HRCT sections through the middle and right lower lobe. Markedly dilated airways are apparent diffusely, some obviously branching (*arrows*, A). Numerous signet rings are identifiable as well (*curved open arrow*, A). Note the cluster of cysts appearing within the collapsed middle-lobe arrow in B. A number of fluid-filled airways can be identified peripherally that are clearly centrilobular in distribution (*open arrows*, B); presumably, these represent dilated terminal bronchioles. (From Naidich, ref. 105, with permission.)

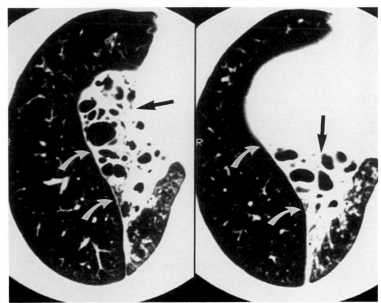

FIG. 7-23. Cystic bronchiectasis. **A,B:** Target reconstructed HRCT images through the right lower-lung field show the characteristic appearance of a "cluster-of-grapes" sign. This sign typically results when bronchiectasis occurs in atelectatic lung. Note that in this case both the middle lobe (*arrow*, A) and the right lower lobe (*arrow*, B) are collapsed, causing marked displacement of the oblique fissure (*curved arrows*, A,B).

as they extend peripherally, and are visible more peripherally than is normal. When cylindrically dilated bronchi are oriented in a vertical direction, they are scanned in cross section and appear as thick-walled, circular lucencies (Fig. 7-20). In most cases, dilated bronchi seen in cross section can be easily distinguished from emphysematous blebs or other causes of lung cysts, by identifying the signet ring sign, and the continuity of the dilated bronchus on adjacent scans.

Varicose Bronchiectasis

With increasingly severe abnormalities of the bronchial wall, bronchi may assume a beaded configuration, referred to as varicose bronchiectasis. This diagnosis can be made consistently only when the involved bronchi course horizontally in the plane of scan (Fig. 7-21). Varicose bronchiectasis is much less frequent than cylindrical bronchiectasis.

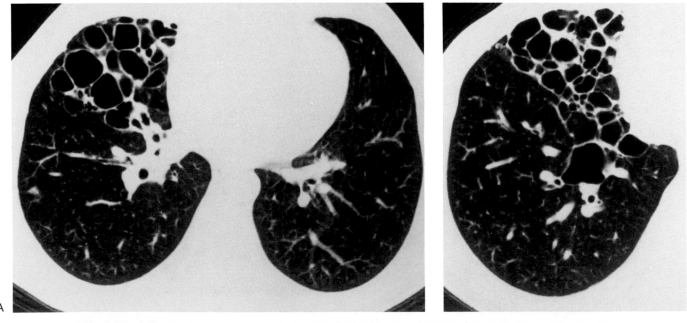

FIG. 7-24. A,B: Cystic bronchiectasis largely limited to the right middle lobe in a patient with a history of tuberculosis.

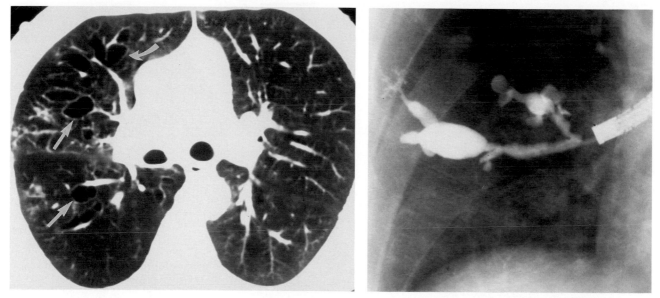

FIG. 7-25. Cystic bronchiectasis with bronchographic correlation. **A:** HRCT through the right upper lobe shows numerous thin-walled cysts (*arrows*). Note that despite their thin walls, many of these cysts lie adjacent to vessels and a few are obviously branching (*curved arrow*). Rarely, bronchiectasis can result in thin-walled cysts which nonetheless still maintain a characteristic anatomic configuration. **B:** Coned-down radiograph after limited bronchography performed through a centrally positioned bronchoscope confirms presence of extensive cystic bronchiectasis. (From McGuinness et al., ref. 113, with permission.)

Cystic Bronchiectasis

With severe, or cystic bronchiectasis, involved airways are "cystic" or "saccular" in appearance, and may extend to the pleural surface (Figs. 7-22–7-25). On HRCT, cystic bronchiectasis may be associated with the presence of (i) air- fluid levels, caused by retained secretions in the dependent portions of the dilated bronchi; (ii) a string of cysts, caused by sectioning irregularly dilated bronchi along their length, or (iii) a cluster of cysts, caused by multiple dilated bronchi lying adjacent to each other. Clusters of cysts are most frequently seen in atelectatic lobes (Figs. 7-22, 7-23), presumably as a result of chronic infection, such as commonly occurs in patients with pulmonary tuberculosis. In general, the dilated airways in patients with cystic bronchiectasis are thick-walled; however, cystic bronchiectasis may also appear thin-walled (Fig. 7-25). Recognition of some combination of dilated bronchi, air-fluid levels, and strings or clusters of cysts should be diagnostic of cystic bronchiectasis (105).

Mucus or Fluid Retention in the Bronchial Lumen

The appearance of fluid- or mucus-filled airways is dependent both on their size and orientation relative to the CT scan plane. Larger fluid-filled airways result in abnormal lobular or branching structures when they lie in the same plane as the CT scan (Figs. 7-21, 7-22, 7-26). Although these may be confused with abnormally

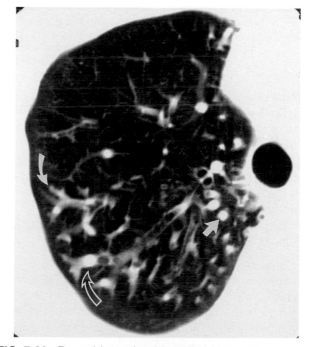

FIG. 7-26. Bronchiectasis with mucoid impaction. Target reconstructed HRCT through the right upper lobe. Mucus-filled airways can be recognized as lobulated linear or branching structures when they course horizontally in the plane of the section (*curved arrows*) or as discrete nodular opacities when they course vertically (*straight arrow*).

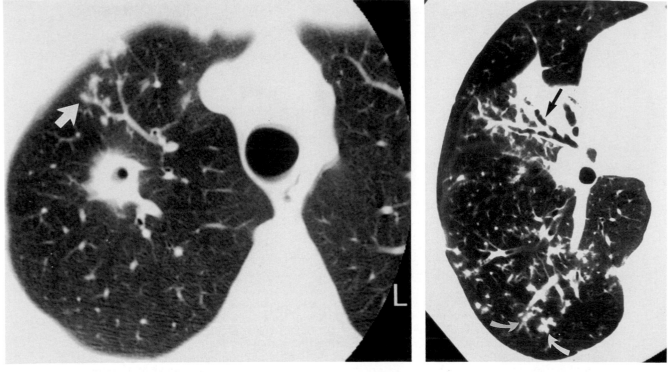

FIG. 7-27. Bronchiectasis associated with endobronchial spread of TB. **A:** Target reconstructed HRCT section through the right upper lobe in a patient with documented active cavitary tuberculosis. Note the presence of a focal cluster of small nodules anterior to the cavity, and adjacent to peripheral pulmonary artery branch (*arrows*). This has been called a "tree-in-bud" appearance and results from mucus or infected material within small peripheral airways. This finding is associated with endobronchial spread of infection. **B:** Target reconstructed HRCT image through the right lung shows marked volume loss and varicose bronchiectasis throughout the middle lobe (*black arrow*). In addition, note the presence of mucous plugging with a "tree-in-bud" appearance in the right lower lobe (*curved arrows*). In the appropriate clinical setting this constellation of findings should suggest the possibility of mycobacterial infection, specifically *Mycobacterium avium-intracellulare* complex (MAC), which was subsequently documented.

dilated vessels, in most cases, the recognition of dilated, fluid-filled airways is simplified by the identification of other areas of bronchiectasis, in which the bronchi are air-filled; these are usually present if carefully sought. In problematic cases, distinction between larger fluid-filled bronchi and dilated blood vessels is easily made by rescanning patients following a bolus of intravenous contrast media.

Dilated mucus-filled airways in the central lung can also result from:

1. Congenital bronchial abnormalities, such as bronchopulmonary sequestration or bronchial atresia (106–108);
2. Focal bronchial inflammation as may be seen in patients with allergic bronchopulmonary aspergillosis (Fig. 7-21); and
3. Central endobronchial obstruction either from tumor or foreign body aspiration.

The use of intravenous contrast media can be helpful in identifying a central tumor mass causing bronchial obstruction and secondary mucoid impaction.

Fluid-filled airways in the peripheral lung are usually identifiable either as branching structures within the center of secondary lobules, aptly described as having a "tree-in-bud" appearance (76), or as ill-defined centrilobular nodules (Figs. 7-22,7-26,7-27). Small fluid-filled airways are easily identified with HRCT, and can be seen in many conditions associated with bronchiectasis. For example, in patients with diffuse panbronchiolitis (109), bronchiolectasis results in small, ring-shaped, round, or branching opacities in the peripheral lung. These opacities correspond to abnormalities of distal airways including terminal and respiratory bronchioles (49,110).

Patients with bronchiectasis of varying causes can show evidence of mosaic perfusion on HRCT, and evidence of air trapping on expiratory scans (111,112). These abnormalities may be related to the presence of either large or small airways obstruction. In one study of 70 patients (111), bronchiectasis was visible in 52% of lobes studied using CT with 3-mm collimation; areas of decreased attenuation (mosaic perfusion) were visible on inspiratory scans in 20% of lobes, and on expira-

TABLE 7-6. *Pitfalls in the HRCT diagnosis of bronchiectasis*

1. Respiratory and/or Cardiac Motion Artifacts
2. Reversible Bronchiectasis (Lung Consolidation or Atelectasis)
3. Pseudobronchiectasis (Cysts, Cavitary Nodules)
4. Traction Bronchiectasis (Pulmonary Fibrosis)
5. Asthma

tion (air trapping) in 34%. Areas of decreased attenuation on expiratory scans were more prevalent in lobes with severe bronchiectasis (59%), or localized bronchiectasis (28%), than in those without bronchiectasis (17%). The presence of decreased attenuation on expiration was also associated with mucous plugging; it was seen in 73% of lobes with large mucous plugs and in 58% of those with centrilobular mucous plugs. There was also a correlation ($r = 0.40$, $p < 0.001$) between the total bronchiectasis extent and severity and the extent of decreased attenuation shown on expiratory CT. In 55 patients who had pulmonary function tests, the extent of expiratory attenuation abnormalities were in-versely related to measures of airways obstruction such as FEV_1 and FEV_1/FVC.

Pitfalls in the Diagnosis of Bronchiectasis

Several potential pitfalls in the diagnosis of bronchiectasis should be avoided (Table 7-6) (113). Transmitted cardiac motion artifacts frequently obscure detail in the left lower lobe, and may lead to an erroneous diagnosis of subtle bronchiectasis (114) (Fig. 7-28). Respiratory motion artifacts cause ghosting that can very closely mimic the appearance of tram-tracks (Figs. 1-15,7-29).

Bronchiectasis is especially difficult to diagnose in patients with concurrent parenchymal consolidation or atelectasis, as CT often discloses dilated peripheral airways that will revert to normal following resolution of the lung disease, so-called reversible bronchiectasis (Fig. 7-30). In these cases, follow-up scans are recommended pending radiographic resolution.

Rarely, the appearance of cavitary nodules in patients either with widespread bronchoalveolar cell carcinoma, cavitary metastases, or even cystic *Pneumocystis carinii* pneumonia or histiocytosis X may mimic

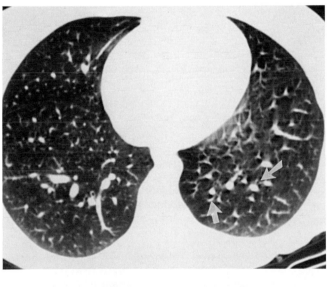

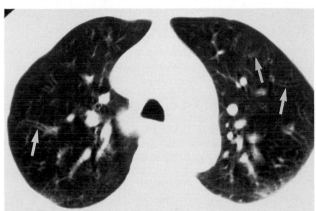

FIG. 7-28. Pseudobronchiectasis. HRCT section through the lung bases in a normal patient. In this case, transmitted cardiac pulsations have caused characteristic stellate artifacts in the left lower lobe that superficially mimic the appearance of bronchiectasis (*arrows*). Note the normal appearance of the lung on the right side by comparison.

FIG. 7-29. Respiratory motion mimicking bronchiectasis. HRCT scan through carina shows typical appearance of a double-vessel sign, simulating diffuse bronchiectasis (*arrows*), caused by respiratory motion. This results in a shift of longitudinally oriented pulmonary vessels causing a pseudo-tramtrack appearance. (From McGuinness et al., ref. 113, with permission.)

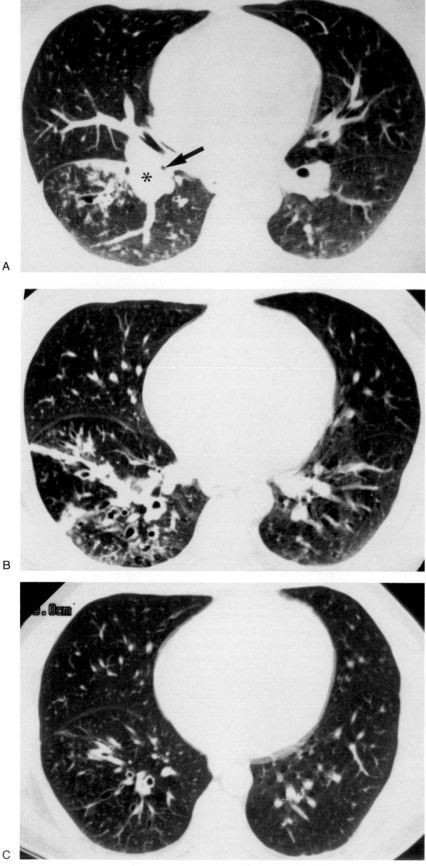

FIG. 7-30. "Reversible bronchiectasis." **A:** HRCT section shows marked narrowing of the right lower-lobe bronchus (*arrow*), with an associated mass in the right hilum (*asterisk*) and apparent bronchiectasis in the right lower lobe. **B:** HRCT section obtained at a lower level, at the same time as A, shows extensive findings of bronchiectasis throughout the lung associated with some focal areas of consolidation. These findings were interpreted as secondary to a partially obstructing proximal tumor. At bronchoscopy the right lower-lobe bronchus proved to be obstructed by aspirated foreign material (cellulose) without tumor. Nodal enlargement proved to be reactive hyperplasia. **C:** HRCT section at the same level as B, obtained 3 months later, shows minimal residual dilatation of the airways. These findings indicate that care should be exercised in diagnosing both the presence and/or severity of bronchiectasis in the presence either of obstruction, atelectasis, or active parenchymal inflammation.

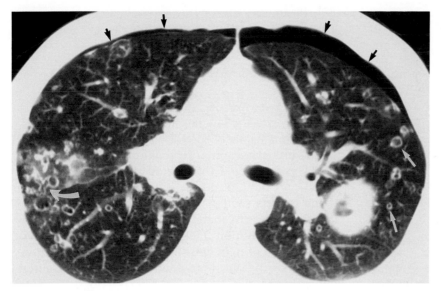

FIG. 7-31. Pseudobronchiectasis in PCP. HRCT scan in a patient with proven *Pneumocystis carinii* pneumonia (PCP) shows typical findings of scattered, variable-sized cysts some of which resemble the "signet ring" sign (*arrows*). In fact, a few dilated peripheral airways can be identified (*curved arrow*), indicating the presence of mild bronchiectasis. Small bilateral pneumothoraces (*black arrows*) presumably have resulted from rupture of subpleural cysts. (From McGuinness et al., ref. 113, with permission.)

the appearance of mild, focal bronchiectasis. This appearance is termed *pseudobronchiectasis* (Figs. 7-31,7-32). In patients with histiocytosis X, characteristically bizarre-shaped cysts are often seen on HRCT, especially in the upper lobes. These may be seen to branch, and suggest the appearance of bronchiectasis (Fig. 7-32). There is some evidence that these cysts are at least partially related to abnormal bronchi.

Bronchiectasis may occur as a component of diffuse fibrotic lung diseases, but does not represent a true airway abnormality and is unassociated with symptoms. In patients with interstitial fibrosis, bronchial dilatation occurs due to fibrous tethering of the bronchial wall, so-called traction bronchiectasis (Fig. 7-33) (115).

Pathologically, patients with asthma show bronchial wall thickening and excess mucus production that can

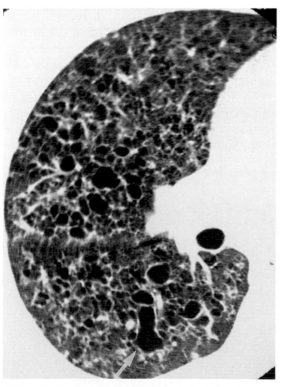

FIG. 7-32. Pseudobronchiectasis in histiocytosis X. Target reconstructed HRCT image through the right mid-lung in a patient with histiocytosis X shows multiple, variably-sized cystic lesions, some with bizarre or branching appearances (*arrow*).

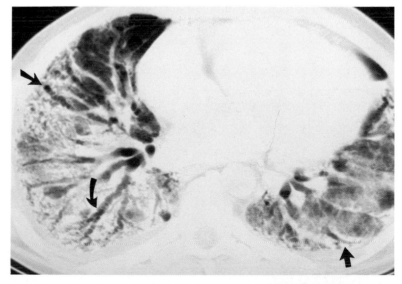

FIG. 7-33. Traction bronchiectasis in interstitial fibrosis. HRCT section through the lower lobes shows evidence both of diffuse parenchymal consolidation and ground-glass opacity associated with numerous dilated, tortuous airways both centrally (*curved arrows*) and peripherally (*straight arrows*). An autopsy performed shortly after this study revealed extensive pulmonary fibrosis and traction bronchiectasis without significant inflammation.

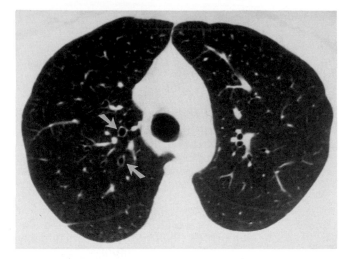

FIG. 7-34. Bronchial dilatation associated with asthma. HRCT section through the upper lobes in an asthmatic shows evidence of proximal bronchial dilatation, especially on the right (*arrows*), with bronchi being larger than adjacent vessels. This finding should be interpreted with caution in an asthmatic as it may be reversible.

result in mucous plugging (116). Recently, the HRCT findings in a group of patients with uncomplicated asthma have been reported (83). In this study (83), bronchi were defined as dilated if their internal diameters exceeded those of accompanying pulmonary arteries. Using this criteria, 77% of asthmatic patients, and 153 (36%) of 429 bronchi assessed in asthmatic patients were considered dilated (Fig. 7-34). Ninety-two percent of the asthmatic patients were also considered to show bronchial wall thickening. As noted by these authors, potential reasons for the appearance of bronchial dilatation include reduction in pulmonary artery diameter, either due to changes in blood volume or local hypoxia, as well as physiologic bronchial dilatation

(83). In another study (81), bronchial dilatation was seen in 15% of patients with asthma.

Utility of HRCT

Although its use was initially controversial, HRCT has emerged as the imaging modality of choice for evaluating bronchiectasis; HRCT has all but eliminated the use of bronchography. Recognition of the value of HCRT has emerged from detailed studies comparing the efficacy of both routine 10-mm and high-resolution 1- and 1.5-mm sections with bronchography.

Initial reports of the CT diagnosis of bronchiectasis utilizing only 10-mm-thick sections provided surprisingly consistent data and showed rather low sensitivities, ranging between 60% and 80%, and specificities between 90% and 100% (97–99,117–119). It became quickly apparent, however, that a significant improvement in diagnostic sensitivity could be achieved by the use of high-resolution 1- and 1.5-mm sections (Fig. 7-35). Grenier et al. (120), utilizing 1.5-mm-thick sections obtained every 10 mm, retrospectively compared CT and bronchography in 44 lungs in 36 patients, and found that CT confirmed the diagnosis of bronchiectasis with a sensitivity of 97% and a specificity of 93%. Young et al. (100) also assessed the reliability of HRCT in the assessment of bronchiectasis, as compared to bronchography, in 259 segmental bronchi from 70 lobes of 27 lungs. HRCT was positive in 87 of 89 segmental bronchi shown to have bronchiectasis (sensitivity 98%). HRCT was negative in 169 of 170 segmental bronchi without bronchiectasis at bronchography (specificity 99%). Similar results have been reported by Giron et al. (121).

Three-millimeter collimation is less accurate than 1- or 1.5-mm collimation in diagnosing bronchiectasis.

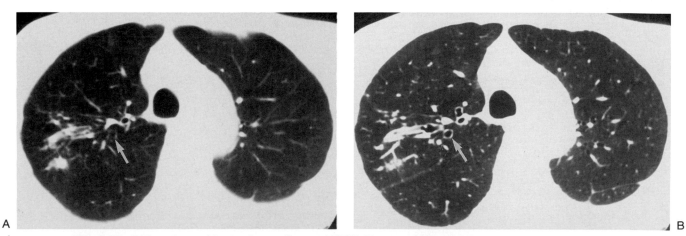

FIG. 7-35. Diffuse bronchiectasis: routine vs. HRCT. Ten-mm (**A**) and 1.5-mm (**B**) sections, respectively, obtained at the same level. Definitive identification of bronchial dilatation (*arrows*) can be made only with HRCT. (From McGuinness et al., ref. 113, with permission.)

Munro et al. (122) reported the accuracy of 3-mm-thick CT in 27 patients evaluated for chronic sputum production, who had bronchography. Overall, the sensitivity of CT was 84% and its specificity was 82%, compared with bronchography. Interestingly, even without the use of high-resolution technique, in five cases the diagnosis of bronchiectasis was made by CT only, including two cases in which bronchial segments were underfilled at bronchography (122).

It should be emphasized that, despite the excellent sensitivity of HRCT, bronchiectasis may be focal and exceedingly subtle on HRCT scans. Cylindrical bronchiectasis, in particular, can be missed on HRCT, especially if care is not taken to obtain images in deep inspiration (120,121,123). Giron et al. (121), in a study of 54 patients with bronchographic evidence of bronchiectasis, found that they missed three cases, all with mild cylindrical bronchiectasis, using 1-mm slices obtained every 10 mm.

Recommended Techniques

Based on the results of reported studies, the following techniques are recommended: In patients in whom there are no specific clinical or radiographic signs to help localize disease, 1- to 1.5-mm high-resolution images should be obtained every 10 mm from the lung apices to bases. Despite the lack of contiguous scanning, this technique allows adequate assessment of the bronchial tree in nearly all cases. Although the routine use of 10-mm sections is not indicated, in select cases, especially those in which mild cylindrical bronchiectasis is suspected, selected 10-mm-thick sections within a limited range of interest may be of value (83).

This approach can be modified to reflect varying clinical presentations. For example, in patients presenting with hemoptysis, it is usually necessary to rule out occult central endobronchial lesions in addition to detecting bronchiectasis. This is best accomplished by obtaining 1- to 1.5-mm- thick sections every 10 mm through the upper-and lower-lung zones, and contiguous 5-mm-thick sections from the carina to the level of the inferior pulmonary veins (94). Utilizing this approach, in a retrospective study of 59 patients evaluated both by CT and fiberoptic bronchoscopy (FOB), CT proved abnormal in all cases in which FOB depicted focal airway pathology (94). Alternatively, when available, helical or spiral scanning can be substituted for the routine 5-mm axial images through the central airways. These have the advantage of eliminating misregistration artifacts as well as allowing high quality 3D and/or multiplanar reconstructions to be performed.

Additional scan techniques have also been advocated. As suggested by Remy-Jardin et al. (124), visualization of bronchiectatic segments may be enhanced by use of 20 degree cranial angulation of the CT gantry. Although unnecessary in most patients, this technique may be of value in equivocal cases, especially for those airways that normally course obliquely, such as the middle lobe and lingular bronchi. Of greater significance is the potential use of low-dose HRCT scans for performing routine follow-up scans in patients with severe chronic disease (125,126). Bhalla et al. (125), evaluating scans obtained using both 70 and 20 mAs showed that high quality HRCT images of bronchiectatic airways could be obtained in patients with cystic fibrosis (Fig. 7-36). These authors proposed replacing routine chest radiographic evaluation with a detailed CT scoring system emphasizing the severity and extent of bronchiectasis, as well as identification and prevalence of mucous plugs and bronchial wall thickening.

More recently, with the advent of electron beam and helical techniques, CT can now be used selectively to evaluate the presence of air-trapping (111,112). This is generally accomplished either by repeatedly acquiring scans at one pre-selected level throughout the respiratory cycle, or as two separate volumetric acquisitions, first in deep inspiration followed by scans obtained through the same region in expiration (127–129) (Fig. 7-20). In either case, the result is a series of dynamic images allowing identification of focal areas of air-trapping as well as changes in the appearance of the airways themselves.

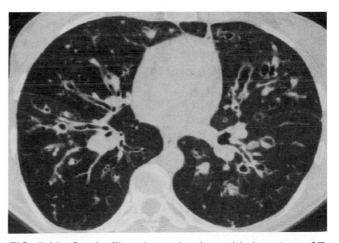

FIG. 7-36. Cystic fibrosis evaluation with low-dose CT. HRCT section through the mid-lung in a patient with diffuse bronchiectasis due to cystic fibrosis. Note that central bronchi are involved to a greater degree than peripheral bronchi. Although cylindrical bronchiectasis predominates, small cystic lucencies are also present, reflecting cystic bronchiectasis or abscess cavities. This 2-sec scan was performed using 120 kVp and 20 mA. In select patients, for whom repeated follow-up CT scans may be indicated, high-quality images can be obtained using a low-dose technique. (Courtesy of Minnie Bhalla, M.D., Massachusetts General Hospital, Boston, Massachusetts.)

TABLE 7-7. *HRCT findings in cystic fibrosis*[a,b]

1. **Bronchiectasis**
   Central bronchi and upper lobes involved in all, Cylindrical or cystic bronchiectasis most common

2. **Bronchial Wall Thickening**
   Central bronchi and upper lobes, Right upper-lobe bronchus usually involved first

3. **Mucous Plugging**

4. Atelectasis

5. Small-airway Abnormalities

6. **Large-lung Volumes**

7. Mosaic perfusion, Air trapping on Expiration

---

[a] Most common findings in boldface.
[b] Findings most helpful in differential diagnosis in boldface italics.

In our experience, most patients studied using HRCT have clinically suspected disease and subtle abnormalities identified on routine radiographs. Symptomatic patients with entirely normal radiographs are the exception. As suggested by Phillips et al. (119), given the high specificity of HRCT findings in patients with documented bronchiectasis, and the unpleasantness and potential risks of bronchography, HRCT is the most appropriate technique for confirming clinically or radiographically suspected disease. In our opinion, bronchography, if utilized at all, should be reserved only for select surgical candidates in whom HRCT has documented segmental or unilateral involvement. The presence of bilateral bronchiectasis shown by HRCT, generally rules out surgery.

Specific Causes of Bronchiectasis

The CT appearances of several diseases associated with bronchiectasis have been described. In many of these, such as hypogammaglobulinemia (130), the appearances of bronchiectasis are as described above. However, a few conditions associated with bronchiectasis have been reported to have distinctive HRCT appearances that can aid in their diagnosis. The most important of these are cystic fibrosis, allergic bronchopulmonary aspergillosis, and nontuberculous mycobacterial infection. Bronchiectasis in association with lung nodules is characteristic of nontuberculous mycobacterial infection resulting from MAC (*Mycobacterium avium-intracellulare* complex), and described in detail in Chapter 5.

Cystic Fibrosis

Cystic fibrosis (CF) is the most common cause of pulmonary insufficiency in the first three decades of life. It results from an autosomal recessive genetic defect in the structure of the "cystic fibrosis transmembrane regulator protein," which leads to abnormal chloride transport across epithelial membranes. The mechanisms by which this leads to lung disease are not entirely understood, but an abnormally low-water content of airway mucus is at least partially responsible, resulting in decreased mucous clearance, mucous plugging of airways, and an increased incidence of bacterial airway infection. Bronchial wall inflammation progressing to secondary bronchiectasis are universal in patients with long-standing disease, and is commonly visible on chest radiographs (131).

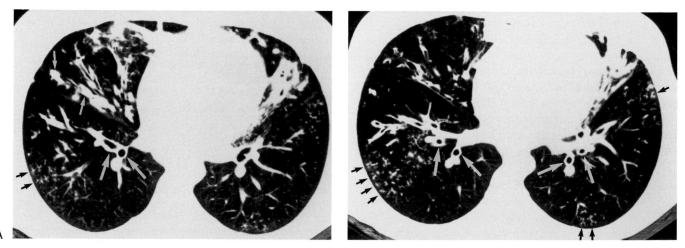

A   B

FIG. 7-37. Cystic fibrosis. HRCT at two levels shows extensive bronchial wall thickening (*large white arrows*); bronchiectasis, which is most evident anteriorly in the middle lobe and lingula; mucous impaction in both large airways (*small white arrows*) and in small airways (*small black arrows*) resulting in a tree-in-bud appearance. Lingular atelectasis is also present. (A from Webb, ref. 1, with permission.)

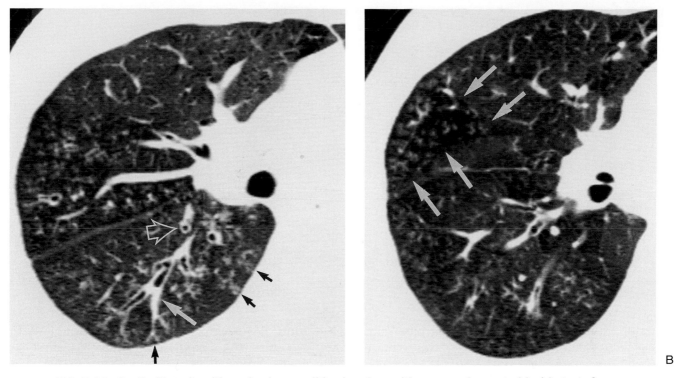

FIG. 7-38. Cystic fibrosis with early abnormalities in a boy with a normal sweat chloride test. **A:** HRCT at the level of the middle and lower lobes shows bronchial wall thickening (*open arrow*), bronchiectasis with mucous impaction (*large arrow*), and small airway impaction with a tree-in-bud appearance. **B:** At a slightly higher level, a region of the right middle lobe (*arrows*) shows extensive bronchiolar impaction with a characteristic tree-in-bud appearance. This region also appears relatively lucent compared to surrounding lung as a result of mosaic perfusion.

HRCT Findings

HRCT findings largely reflect the airway abnormalities typical of this disease. Bronchiectasis is present in all patients with advanced cystic fibrosis who are studied using HRCT (Table 7-7) (132). Proximal or parahilar bronchi are always involved when bronchiectasis is present, and bronchiectasis is limited to these central bronchi in about a third of cases, a finding which is referred to as "central bronchiectasis" (Fig. 7-36). Both the central and peripheral bronchi are abnormal in about two thirds of patients (125,132). All lobes are typically involved, although early in the disease abnormalities are often predominantly upper lobe in distribution, and a right upper-lobe predominance may be present in some patients (125,132–134). Cylindrical bronchiectasis is the most frequent pattern seen, and was visible in 94% of lobes in one study of patients with severe disease (132); 34% of lobes in this study showed cystic bronchiectasis, while varicose bronchiectasis was seen in 11%. In another report, cystic lesions representing cystic bronchiectasis or abscess cavities were present in 8 of 14 (57%) patients (Fig. 7-36) (125).

Bronchial wall and/or peribronchial interstitial thickening is also commonly present in patients with cystic fibrosis (Figs. 7-37,7-38) (135). It is generally more evident than bronchial dilatation in patients who have early disease, and may be seen independent of bronchiectasis (125,133). Thickening of the wall of proximal right upper-lobe bronchi was the earliest abnormal feature visible on HRCT in one study of patients with mild cystic fibrosis (133).

Mucous plugging is also common, evident in 10 of 14 patients in one study, and may be visible in all lobes (Figs. 7-37,7-38) (125,134). Collapse or consolidation can also be seen (125,135). Volume loss was visible in 20% of lobes in patients with advanced disease (Figs. 7-37,7-39) (132).

Branching or nodular centrilobular opacities, which reflect the presence of bronchiolar dilatation with associated mucous impaction, infection, or peribronchiolar inflammation, can be an early sign of disease (Figs. 7-37,7-38) (134). Focal areas of decreased lung opacity, occurred in a geographic fashion, with sharply defined margins, can reflect air trapping or mosaic perfusion (Figs. 7-38,7-39). These can be seen to correspond to pulmonary lobules or subsegments. Areas of decreased

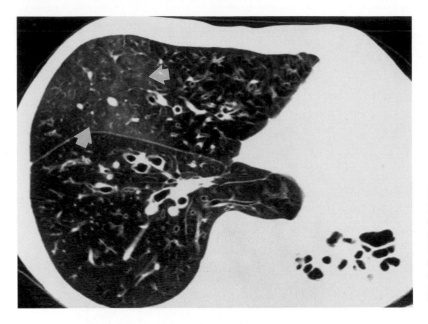

FIG. 7-39. Cystic fibrosis. Atelectasis of the left lung is associated with extensive bronchiectasis. Bronchial wall thickening and bronchiectasis are visible on the right. A region of relatively increased attenuation (*arrows*) anteriorly represents mosaic perfusion. Note that bronchiectasis is not visible in this region, and vessels appear larger than in lucent lung regions. (From Webb, ref. 1, with permission.)

lung opacity sometimes appear to surround mucus-plugged bronchi (Fig. 7-38) (134). Air trapping can be seen on expiratory scans (Fig. 3-96) (112,132).

Lung volumes may appear increased on CT, although this diagnosis is rather subjective and may be better assessed on chest radiographs (132). Cystic or bullous lung lesions can also be visible, and typically predominate in the subpleural regions of the upper lobes (125,132). Hilar or mediastinal lymph node enlargement, and pleural abnormalities can also be seen, largely reflecting chronic infection. Pulmonary artery dilatation resulting from pulmonary hypertension can also be seen in patients with long-standing disease.

Utility of HRCT

HRCT can demonstrate morphologic abnormalities in patients with early CF who are asymptomatic, have normal pulmonary function, and/or have normal chest radiographs. In a study of 38 patients with mild cystic fibrosis who had normal pulmonary function (133), chest radiographs were normal in 17 (45%), showed mild bronchial wall thickening in 17, and mild bronchiectasis in 4 (10%). On HRCT in this group, features of bronchiectasis were present in 77% of all patients, and in 65% of those with normal chest radiographs; only 3 patients had a normal HRCT (133). In another study of HRCT findings in 12 largely asymptomatic pediatric patients with early cystic fibrosis, chest radiographs were normal in 7, while HRCT was normal in only 2. HRCT findings not visible on radiographs included bronchial wall thickening, bronchiectasis, centrilobular small airway abnormalities, and lobular or segmental inhomogeneities representing mosaic perfusion or air trapping (134).

In patients with more advanced disease, HRCT can also show abnormalities not visible on chest radiographs. In a study of 14 patients with CF (125), HRCT was found to be superior to chest radiographs in detecting bronchiectasis and mucous plugging. Of a total of 162 segments assessed, bronchiectasis was detected in 124 segments using HRCT, while only 71 segments were considered to show this finding on chest radiographs. Mucous plugs were detected on HRCT in 38 segments, while they were seen on radiographs in only 4 segments. In a study by Hansell et al. (132), bronchiectasis was considered to be present on HRCT in 124 of 126 lobes; on chest radiographs, only 84 of 102 lung zones were considered to show this finding. Chest radiographs also underestimated the extent of bronchiectasis. Bronchiectasis was considered to be both central and peripheral in only 31% of lung zones on chest radiographs, while a diffuse distribution was seen in 59% of lobes using HRCT.

The routine clinical evaluation of CF makes use of clinical and radiograph-based scoring systems. Several authors have also suggested the use of a HRCT scoring

TABLE 7-8. *HRCT findings in ABPA*[a,b]

1. **Bronchiectasis**
   Central bronchiectasis, cystic in nature
2. **Mucous Plugging**
3. **Atelectasis**
4. Peripheral Consolidation or Ground-glass opacity
5. Mosaic Perfusion, Air Trapping on Expiration

[a] Most common findings in boldface.
[b] Findings most helpful in differential diagnosis in boldface italics.

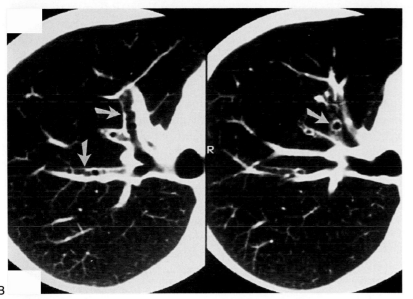

FIG. 7-40. Allergic bronchopulmonary aspergillosis with early changes. **A,B:** Sequential target reconstructed HRCT images through the right upper-lobe bronchus in a patient with allergic bronchopulmonary aspergillosis. The proximal portions of the anterior and posterior segmental bronchi are mildly dilated and have a distinctly beaded, irregular, and varicose appearance (*arrows*, A). Branches of the apical segmental bronchus are also dilated (*arrow*, B). Central bronchiectasis is typical of ABPA.

system (125,136). It is hypothesized that such a scoring system may facilitate the objective evaluation of existing and newly developed therapeutic regimens (125). One scoring system (125), based on an assessment of the degree and extent of bronchiectasis, bronchial wall thickening, mucous plugging, atelectasis, emphysema, and other findings, showed a statistically significant correlation to the percent ratios of FEV_1/FVC (r =0.69, p = 0.006) (125). In another study based on assessment of bronchiectasis and mucous plugging (136), CT scores correlated highly with clinical (r = 0.88, p < 0.0001) and radiographic (r = 0.93, p < 0.0001) scores, and several pulmonary function tests. The best correlation was with bronchiectasis.

Allergic Bronchopulmonary Aspergillosis

Allergic bronchopulmonary aspergillosis (ABPA) is characteristically associated with eosinophilia, symptoms of asthma such as wheezing, and findings of "central" or "proximal" bronchiectasis, mucoid impaction, atelectasis, and sometimes consolidation similar to that seen in patients with eosinophilic pneumonia. ABPA results from both type I and type III (IgE and IgG) immunologic responses to the endobronchial growth of fungal (*Aspergillus*) species. The immune reactions result in central bronchiectasis, which is usually varicose or cystic in appearance (Figs. 7-21,7-40,7-41), and the formation of mucous plugs which contain

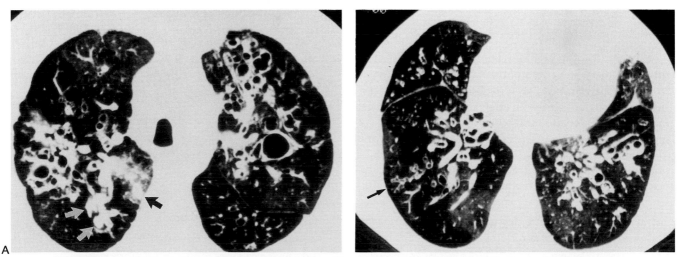

FIG. 7-41. Allergic bronchopulmonary aspergillosis with extensive bronchiectasis. **A:** HRCT scan through the upper lobes shows bilateral cystic bronchiectasis. Mucus-plugged bronchi (*arrows*) are also visible. **B:** HRCT near the lung bases shows extensive bronchiectasis. In some regions, dilated bronchioles (*arrow*) are visible in the lung periphery. Lung attenuation is inhomogeneous as a result of mosaic perfusion.

fungus and inflammatory cells. In four patients with ABPA studied by Kullnig et al. (82), CT revealed central bronchiectasis in all. Other features shown by CT included mucoid impaction (Figs. 7-21,7-41), areas of consolidation, and segmental or subsegmental atelectasis (Table 7-8).

CT may be valuable in the early identification of lung damage in patients with ABPA and thus help in planning treatment (137,138). As in the diagnosis of bronchiectasis, CT is more sensitive than are plain radiographs in detecting abnormalities associated with ABPA. In one study, narrow section (3 mm) CT and plain chest radiography were compared in ten patients with ABPA (137). Bronchiectasis was reported in 31 of 60 lobes on CT scans, but was visible in only 15 lobes on plain chest radiographs; CT was also more sensitive in detecting central bronchiectasis (Fig. 7-40). In another study, CT with 8-mm collimation was compared to bronchography in two pediatric patients with ABPA (138). CT was able to identify 24 of 27 segments that showed central bronchiectasis.

In a study by Neeld et al. (81), the HRCT findings in patients with ABPA were compared to those in patients with uncomplicated asthma. Bronchial dilatation was seen in 41% of lobes in the patients with ABPA, as compared to 15% in the patients with asthma. Small airway abnormalities, with dilatation of mucus- or fluid-filled centrilobular bronchioles, can also be seen on HRCT, resulting in a "tree-in-bud" appearance (Fig. 7-41) (1). Abnormalities of lung attenuation reflecting mosaic perfusion, and air trapping on expiratory CT scans can also be seen (Fig. 7-41). In comparison to patients with cystic fibrosis who often have diffuse cylindrical bronchiectasis, those with ABPA more typically show bronchiectasis that is cystic in appearance (132).

Williams-Campbell Syndrome

Williams-Campbell syndrome is a rare type of cystic bronchiectasis due to defective cartilage in the fourth- to sixth-order bronchi. CT can show areas of central cystic bronchiectasis with distal regions of abnormal lucency, probably related to air trapping. These findings are useful in differentiating Williams-Campbell syndrome from other causes of cystic bronchiectasis (139). Ballooning of central bronchi on inspiration and collapse on expiration has also been reported (140).

BRONCHIOLITIS OBLITERANS (CONSTRICTIVE BRONCHIOLITIS)

Bronchiolitis obliterans (BO), also referred to as obliterative bronchiolitis, or pure bronchiolitis obliterans, is characterized by airflow limitation due to submucosal and peribronchiolar inflammation and fibrosis, primarily involving respiratory bronchioles in the absence of diffuse parenchymal inflammation (141). Recently, it has been suggested that the term *constrictive bronchiolitis* be used instead of bronchiolitis obliterans, and this should be considered a synonym (141,142). Other findings in BO include smooth muscle hyperplasia and bronchiolectasia with inspissated secretions (143). Pulmonary involvement is characteristically patchy and the diagnosis may be difficult to establish even following open lung biopsy (141,144–147).

Bronchiolitis obliterans (constrictive bronchiolitis) represents a nonspecific reaction that may be caused by a variety of insults. Bronchiolitis obliterans may be classified by etiology (142):

1. Post-infectious bronchiolitis obliterans, due to bacterial, mycoplasmal, or viral (especially respiratory syncytial virus, adenovirus, influenza, parainfluenza and cytomegalovirus) infection, or as a sequela of *Pneumocystis carinii* pneumonia (PCP) and/or HIV viral infection in AIDS patients (141,145,148–151);
2. Toxic-fume bronchiolitis obliterans, resulting from exposure to gases such as nitrogen dioxide (silo-filler's lung), sulfur dioxide, ammonia, chlorine, phosgene, and ozone (141,148,152–155);
3. Rarely, bronchiolitis obliterans is idiopathic (143,156).
4. Bronchiolitis obliterans associated with connective tissue diseases, particularly rheumatoid arthritis and polymyositis (141,157–161);
5. Bronchiolitis obliterans associated with drug therapy (penicillamine or gold, for example) (141).
6. Bronchiolitis obliterans as a complication of lung or bone marrow transplantation (84,85,89–91, 162–166).

The radiologic manifestations of the various forms of bronchiolitis obliterans were described by Gosink et al. (148) and have recently been reviewed by McLoud (167). The chest radiograph in bronchiolitis obliterans is often normal. In some patients mild hyperinflation or subtle peripheral attenuation of the vascular markings may be seen (168).

TABLE 7-9. HRCT findings in bronchiolitis obliterans (Constructive Bronchiolitis)[a,b]

1. **Areas of Decreased Lung Opacity, Patchy in Distribution**
2. **Bronchiectasis**
3. **Attenuation of Pulmonary Vessels**
4. *Combination of Findings 1–3*
5. Areas of Consolidation or Increased Lung Opacity
6. Reticulonodular Opacities

---
[a] Most common findings in boldface.
[b] Findings most helpful in differential diagnosis in italics.

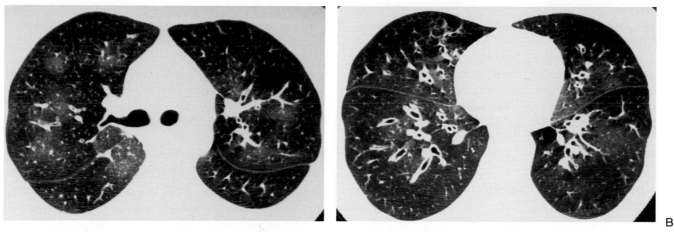

FIG. 7-42. Bronchiolitis obliterans (constrictive bronchiolitis). HRCT sections through the right upper (**A**) and lower (**B**) lobes, in a young woman presenting with progressive dyspnea. Pulmonary function tests disclosed severe obstructive lung disease. Corresponding chest radiograph (not shown) was interpreted as normal. HRCT sections obtained in deep inspiration show geographic areas of low attenuation interspersed with areas of relatively increased opacity. Dilated thick-walled bronchi are easily identified throughout the lower lobes, middle lobe, and lingula. This constellation of clinical and CT findings is characteristic of patients with idiopathic constrictive bronchiolitis (cryptogenic bronchiolitis obliterans). This patient is currently awaiting lung transplantation.

HRCT Findings

The HRCT appearance of bronchiolitis obliterans has been described in a number of studies (Table 7-9) (49,84,88,134,146,147,169–171), and characteristic abnormalities have been reported in patients with both idiopathic and secondary bronchiolitis obliterans (146,147,170,171). HRCT findings are similar regardless of the cause of disease.

The most obvious HRCT finding is that of focal, often sharply defined, areas of decreased lung attenuation associated with vessels of decreased caliber (Fig. 7-42). These changes represent a combination of air-trapping and oligemia, typically occurring in the absence of parenchymal consolidation, and are termed *mosaic perfusion* (147). Bronchiectasis, both central and peripheral, may be present as well (Figs. 3-91, 3-92,7-42). Rarely, 2- to 4-mm-sized centrilobular branching opacities representing inspissated secretions within distal airways, or ill-defined centrilobular opacities, may be the predominant finding (Fig. 3-102) (170,172), but recognizable small airway abnormalities are usually inconspicuous in patients with BO.

Abnormal findings are far more evident on HRCT than on chest radiographs in patients with bronchiolitis obliterans (Figs. 7-42,7-43). For example, in one study

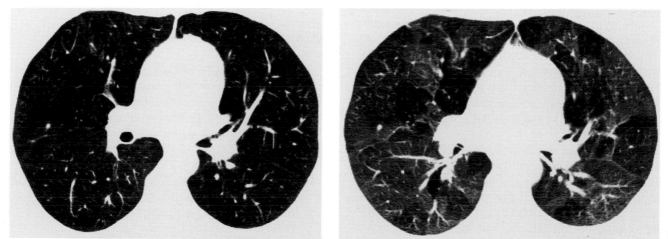

FIG. 7-43. Bronchiolitis obliterans (constrictive bronchiolitis) with air-trapping on expiratory HRCT. **A:** HRCT at full inspiration shows minimal lung inhomogeneity as a result of BO. No bronchiectasis is visible, and the chest radiograph was normal. **B:** On a post-expiratory HRCT, marked lung inhomogeneity is visible as a result of air trapping.

of patients with BO (146), chest radiographs were normal in one third of patients and showed mild hyperinflation and vascular attenuation in the remaining two thirds. CT, on the other hand, showed widespread and conspicuous abnormalities in lung attenuation in nearly 90% of the patients. Interestingly, these CT abnormalities were accentuated on expiration, and air-trapping is commonly visible on expiratory HRCT in patients with BO (Figs. 3-94,3-97,7-43).

Post-infectious Bronchiolitis Obliterans and the Swyer-James Syndrome

Lynch et al. (134) reported the HRCT findings of post-infectious bronchiolitis obliterans in six children. The most striking finding in these patients was the presence of focal areas of decreased lung opacity, which usually had sharp margins. These areas of decreased opacity corresponded to segments or lobules, and the pulmonary vessels within these areas appeared to be reduced in size (Figs. 3-92,3-94). Four of these six had bronchiectasis visible on HRCT (Figs. 7-23,7-27,7-28), and in all four, the abnormal bronchi were in areas of lung showing decreased opacity. It is likely that the areas of decreased opacity represent regions of lung that are poorly ventilated and poorly perfused. Areas of increased lung opacity containing vessels that were normal or large in size were also seen in this series; these areas of increased opacity reflect well-perfused areas of lung or mosaic perfusion.

Bronchiolitis obliterans is a major component of the Swyer-James or MacLeod syndrome (173,174). In patients with Swyer-James syndrome, bronchiolitis obliterans is the result of lower-respiratory tract infection, usually viral, occurring in infancy or early childhood. Damage to the terminal and respiratory bronchioles leads to incomplete development of their alveolar buds. The radiographic hallmark of this syndrome is unilateral hyperlucent lung with reduced lung volume on inspiration and air trapping on expiration. Although previously necessitating confirmation either by bronchography (to demonstrate extensive bronchiectasis), or by arteriography (to demonstrate a small central pulmonary artery and decreased peripheral vascularity) these procedures have been all but obviated by HRCT (Fig. 7-44).

Marti-Bonmati et al. (169) described the CT findings in nine patients with Swyer-James syndrome. On CT, in eight patients, the affected lung showed decreased opacity (Fig. 7-44); in the one remaining patient, the affected lung was very small but of normal attenuation. Lung volume on the affected site was reduced in six patients and normal in three; one patient showed normal lung opacity on chest radiographs but decreased opacity on CT. In all patients the size of the affected

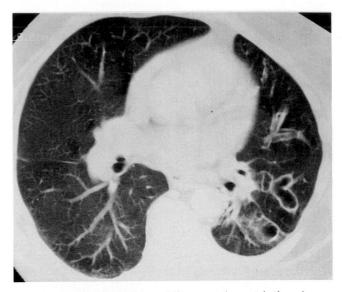

FIG. 7-44. Bronchiolitis obliterans (constrictive bronchiolitis) in the Swyer-James syndrome. On HRCT, the lungs appear asymmetric, with marked volume loss on the left. The left lung appears relatively lucent, with diminished vascular markings, and extensive cystic bronchiectasis. These findings are characteristic of the Swyer-James syndrome. CT scans through the left hilum (not shown) confirmed the presence of a hypoplastic left pulmonary artery. Currently asymptomatic, this patient recalled a history of childhood pneumonia.

lung did not change on CT scans obtained during inspiration and expiration.

All 9 patients had CT findings of bronchiectasis (Fig. 7-44) (169). In each, cylindrical bronchiectasis was present, but 2 also had cystic bronchiectasis and 3 had varicose bronchiectasis. The lower lobes were affected in 8 patients, the middle lobes or lingula in 7, and the upper lobes in 3. Parenchymal abnormalities were present in 8 patients.

Idiopathic Bronchiolitis Obliterans

This entity usually affects middle-aged women and has a relentless downhill course despite steroid therapy. Recently, a more benign course has been described in a limited number of patients with more stable disease, suggesting a wider range of clinical presentations than previously appreciated (143). Sweatman et al. (146) described the CT findings in 15 patients with idiopathic bronchiolitis obliterans. The chest radiograph was normal in 5 patients and showed mild hyperinflation and vascular attenuation in the remaining 10. CT showed widespread abnormalities in 13 (87%) of the 15 patients, consisting of patchy irregular areas of high and low attenuation in variable proportions (Fig. 7-42). These changes were accentuated on expiration.

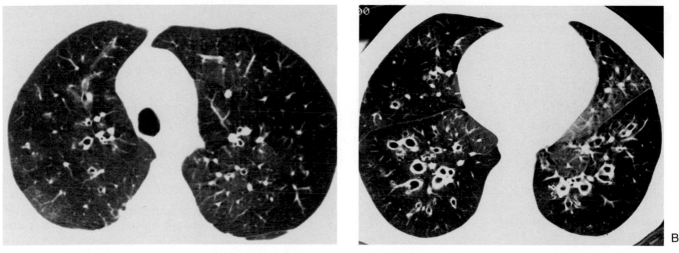

FIG. 7-45. Bronchiolitis obliterans (constrictive bronchiolitis) in a patient with rheumatoid arthritis treated using penicillamine. HRCT at two levels (**A,B**) shows bronchiectasis and patchy lung opacity as a result of air trapping. (B from Webb, ref. 1, with permission.)

Bronchiolitis Obliterans Associated with Rheumatoid Arthritis

The HRCT and expiratory CT findings of 2 patients with rheumatoid arthritis and bronchiolitis obliterans have been reported (175). Both had been treated using penicillamine and gold. Plain film findings were limited to large lung volumes, but HRCT showed similar findings in both patients, with evidence of bronchiectasis and regional lung inhomogeneities (mosaic perfusion) (Fig. 7-45). In both, dynamic expiratory CT showed air trapping on expiratory scans. Among 77 patients with rheumatoid arthritis studied by Remy-Jardin et al. using HRCT, 4 of 16 with bronchiectasis were considered to have BO based on pulmonary function tests (176).

Bronchiolitis Obliterans Associated with Heart-Lung or Lung Transplantation

In patients who have received a heart-lung or single-lung transplantation, bronchiolitis obliterans can occur as the result of chronic rejection (84–89). Although most likely due to immunologically mediated injury of the pulmonary endothelial and bronchial epithelial cells, other etiologies have been implicated, including vascular insufficiency and infection. Rarely if ever occurring less than 3 months following transplantation, bronchiolitis obliterans has been diagnosed as long as 5 years after surgery. As a result of current improvements in therapy for treating early complications, bronchiolitis obliterans has emerged as one of the most important complications of lung transplantation. Occurring in between 25% and 50% of cases, bronchiolitis obliterans represents the primary determinant of long-term survival in most patients.

Histologically, chronic rejection is characterized by submucosal and intraepithelial lymphocytic and histiocytic infiltrates primarily affecting the distal small airways, associated with dense submucosal eosinophilic scar tissue. Intraluminal fibrous plaques also occur leading to both partial and/or complete bronchiolar obstruction (166).

Clinically, the earliest manifestation of chronic rejection is nonproductive cough, which may progress to a cough productive of purulent but sterile sputum. Later, the course is dominated by increasingly severe dyspnea. Pulmonary function tests show progressive obstruction. Although the diagnosis is strongly suggested in patients with a greater than 15% decline in either forced vital capacity (FVC) or forced-expiratory volume in one sec (FEV$_1$) in the absence of other causes of airways obstruction, including bronchospasm or airway (anastomotic) stenosis, these findings are not considered diagnostic; accurate diagnosis requires histologic evaluation in order to exclude the concomitant presence of infection (166). Radiographic findings in these patients are often nonspecific. In most, chronic rejection is associated with a normal-appearing radiograph, or an appearance suggestive of cystic fibrosis with mild to extensive bronchiectasis.

HRCT findings in patients with BO following lung transplantation include both central and peripheral bronchiectasis (Fig. 7-46), focal lucencies, presumably the result of air-trapping and mosaic perfusion, and localized parenchymal consolidation. Skeens et al. (84) described the radiologic findings in 11 patients with bronchiolitis obliterans following heart-lung transplantation. In all patients, the chest radiographs showed parenchymal abnormalities consisting of reticulonodular, nodular, or air-space opacities. Radiographic evidence of central bronchiectasis was present in 9 of the

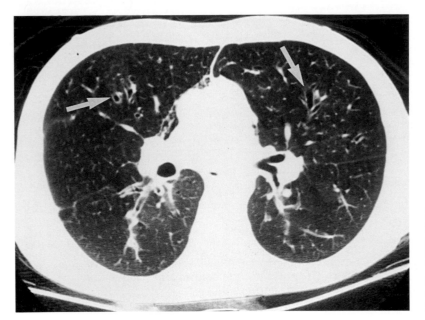

FIG. 7-46. Bronchiolitis obliterans (constrictive bronchiolitis) following heart-lung transplantation. Note that there is moderate dilatation of the central bronchi bilaterally (*arrows*). This may be an early finding in patients with BO. (Case courtesy of Denise Aberle, M.D., University of California Los Angeles Medical Center, Los Angeles, California.)

11 patients. Chest CT scans performed in two patients confirmed the radiographic findings of bronchiectasis by showing dilated airways adjacent to pulmonary arteries. Air trapping can be shown on expiratory HRCT in patients with bronchiolitis obliterans.

Early abnormalities may be more difficult to recognize. In another study of 40 patients with lung transplantation, 14 of whom had chronic rejection and bronchiolitis obliterans, HRCT findings of bronchiectasis had a sensitivity of only 14% in making this diagnosis (177). HRCT had a specificity of 77% in diagnosing rejection, and a positive predictive value of 25%.

Hruban et al. (88) reported the HRCT findings seen in seven lung specimens obtained from patients who had received a heart-lung transplant. The lungs were fixed using a method that allows for direct one-to-one pathologic-radiologic correlation. They examined two lungs from patients with clinical and pathologic evidence of chronic rejection; both lungs showed severe bronchiolitis obliterans associated with bronchiectasis and peribronchial fibrosis. The authors were unable to identify a direct HRCT correlate for bronchiolitis obliterans. However, bronchiectasis with associated peribronchial inflammation and fibrosis, a common finding in lung allograft rejection, was identifiable on HRCT.

Bone Marrow Transplantation

Bronchiolitis obliterans is one of several pulmonary complications of bone marrow transplantation, occurring in about 10% of patients (91). Other complications include infection (bacterial, viral, and fungal, in particular, invasive aspergillosis); pulmonary edema; drug and radiation toxicity; and metastatic tumor. Recently, a syndrome of diffuse pulmonary hemorrhage also has been described occurring within the first 2 weeks following bone marrow transplantation (178). Determining the cause of pulmonary disease in these patients is frequently problematic as biopsies are usually contraindicated due to severe thrombocytopenia.

Bronchiolitis obliterans usually is identified in patients following allogeneic transplants, presumably the result of chronic graft-vs.-host disease (GVHD) (Fig. 7-47) (90,91,162). Histologically, BO (constrictive bronchiolitis) is the predominant abnormality, characterized both by neutrophilic and lymphocytic peribronchiolar inflammation (Fig. 3-102). Importantly, histologic evidence of BOOP/COP (or proliferative bronchiolitis) with extension into alveolar ducts and alveoli is distinctly unusual as a cause of airway obstruction in this population (91). Typically, these patients also have evidence of GVHD involving the skin, liver, and gastrointestinal tract. Patients also frequently have evidence of chronic sinusitis. In fact, bronchiolitis has also been identified in patients following autologous bone marrow transplants, leaving the true etiology of bronchiolitis unexplained (91).

Clinically, patients may present with cough, wheezing, or dyspnea between 1 and 10 months following transplantation (91). Alternatively, evidence of airway obstruction may be present physiologically in otherwise asymptomatic patients. In either setting, the key to diagnosing bronchiolitis in these patients is serial pulmonary function testing (PFT). The hallmark of this disease is a decrease in the FEV_1/FVC ratio of less than 70% predicted, often in association with an increased residual volume (RV). In most institutions, in distinction to patients with lung or heart-lung transplanta-

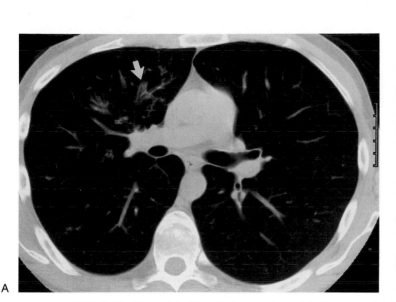
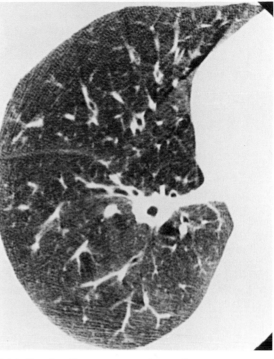

A

B

FIG. 7-47. Bronchiolitis obliterans (constrictive bronchiolitis) following bone marrow transplantation. **A:** HRCT section through the mid-lung shows focal bronchiectasis in the anterior segment of the right upper lobe (*arrow*) associated with marked hyperinflation of the lungs. These findings are consistent with chronic graft-vs.-host disease (GVHD) following allogeneic bone marrow transplantation. **B:** A 37-year-old woman with bronchiolitis obliterans due to graft-vs.-host disease following bone marrow transplant. HRCT at the level of the right inferior pulmonary vein shows mild cylindrical bronchiectasis, and patchy lung opacity as a result of mosaic perfusion. (A, courtesy of Denise Aberle, M.D., University of California Los Angeles Medical Center, Los Angeles, California.)

tions, pulmonary function testing is considered diagnostic even in the absence of histologic verification. Bronchoalveolar lavage is indicated only in those patients who can tolerate this procedure in whom concomitant infection is suspected. Unfortunately, despite aggressive therapy with steroids, bronchodilators, or azathioprine, nearly 50% of patients die from progressive respiratory insufficiency.

Radiographs, in the absence of infection, typically are normal or show only mild hyperinflation, similar to changes identified in other conditions associated with constrictive bronchiolitis. HRCT shows typical findings of BO, with evidence of bronchiectasis, mosaic perfusion, and air trapping (Fig. 7-47). In an early stage, ill-defined peribronchiolar, centrilobular opacities have been identified (Fig. 3-102) (172).

It should be emphasized that constrictive bronchiolitis represents only one of a wide range of potential pulmonary abnormalities that can occur following bone marrow transplantation. Not surprisingly, the range of CT findings that can be identified primarily reflects the patient's clinical status. Graham et al. (90) in a broad-based study of 18 patients with 21 episodes of intratho-

racic complications following allogeneic bone marrow transplantation showed that CT disclosed diagnostically relevant findings not apparent on chest radiographs in over 50% of cases. These included a ground-glass pattern in five patients with early pneumonia; a peripheral distribution of abnormalities including bronchiectasis in four patients with bronchiolitis obliterans and/or eosinophilic lung disease; and cavitating lesions or hemorrhagic infarcts in one case each of *Pneumocystis carinii* pneumonia and invasive aspergillosis, respectively (90). In comparison, a much narrower range of findings has been described when febrile patients only are evaluated. In this setting, CT has been advocated as a noninvasive means for diagnosing invasive fungal infections. Mori et al. (179), in a retrospective study of 33 febrile bone marrow transplant recipients documented 21 episodes of fungal infection. In 20 of 21 of these cases, CT showed nodules most of which proved either cavitary, poorly defined, or had associated characteristic halo signs. In distinction, in nine patients with bacteremia, CT failed to disclose any abnormalities, suggesting that the source of infection was outside the lungs.

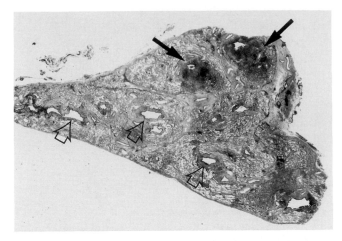

FIG. 7-48. Diffuse panbronchiolitis. Open lung biopsy specimen shows centrilobular peribronchiolar infiltrates of acute and chronic inflammatory cells (*solid arrows*), principally at the level of the respiratory bronchioles, associated with bronchiolar dilatation (*open arrows*). (From Gruden et al., ref. 173, with permission.)

DIFFUSE PANBRONCHIOLITIS

Diffuse panbronchiolitis (DPB) is a unique syndrome described almost exclusively in Asia, especially in Japan and Korea (109,110,141,180,181). This entity typically affects middle-aged men. Patients present with the subacute development of airway obstruction, and in nearly three quarters of patients, there is associated sinusitis. The disease is progressive, marked by frequent episodes of superimposed infection, typically with *Pseudomonas aeroginosa*. In nearly 20% of cases, death occurs within 5 years of the onset of the disease with another 30% dying within 10 years. Current therapy requires long-term low-dose administration of erythromycin.

Histologically, characteristic findings of this disease include centrilobular peribronchiolar infiltrates of acute and chronic inflammatory cells, principally at the level of the respiratory bronchioles, associated with bronchiolar dilatation, and intraluminal inflammatory exudates (Fig. 7-48). A striking accumulation of interstitial foam cells and lymphoid hyperplasia are also commonly seen. This combination of findings has been referred to as the "unit lesion" of panbronchiolitis and is considered unique to this syndrome (141). Although the disease characteristically involves respiratory bronchioles, terminal bronchioles may be involved. In a minority of cases, there is also evidence of peripheral bronchiectasis. Chest radiographs in patients with diffuse panbronchiolitis are nonspecific and usually show small nodular shadows throughout both lungs, and often, increased lung volumes.

HRCT Findings

HRCT findings in patients with diffuse panbronchiolitis have been extensively described (Table 7-10) (109,110,180,181). As initially shown by Akira et al. (109), the most important findings in order of severity are poorly defined centrilobular nodules, centrilobular branching opacities or "tree-in-bud," and branching thick-walled centrilobular lucencies (Figs. 3-35,7-49). As confirmed by Nishimura et al. (110), these findings correspond to, respectively, peribronchiolar inflammation and fibrosis, dilated bronchioles with inflammatory wall thickening and intraluminal secretions, and dilated, air-filled bronchioles (Fig. 7-50) (110). The finding of small, peripheral peribronchiolar nodules is particularly characteristic, resulting in a "tree-in-bud" appearance.

In addition to these findings, patients with diffuse panbronchiolitis usually show evidence of air trapping,

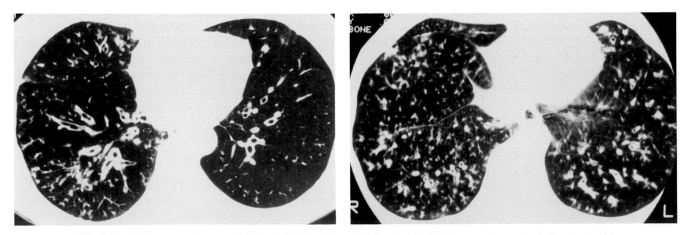

FIG. 7-49. Diffuse panbronchiolitis. HRCT at two levels shows findings of poorly defined centrilobular nodules in the lung periphery, centrilobular branching opacities or "tree-in-bud," and bronchiectasis. (Courtesy of Shin-Ho Kook, M.D., Koryo General Hospital, Seoul, Korea.)

TABLE 7-10. *HRCT findings in diffuse panbronchiolitis[a,b]*

1. **Centrilobular Nodules**
2. **Centrilobular Branching Opacities, Tree-in-Bud**
3. *Dilated, Thick-walled, Centrilobular Bronchioles*
4. Bronchiectasis
5. Large-lung Volumes
6. Peripheral Lung Lucency

[a] Most common findings in boldface.
[b] Findings most helpful in differential diagnosis in boldface italics.

with large lung volumes, and decreased attenuation of peripheral lung parenchyma (110). As documented by Murata et al. (181), in a study comparing positron emission tomography and CT in seven patients with DPB, CT attenuation values were considerably lower in the periphery of the lung as compared with the central por-

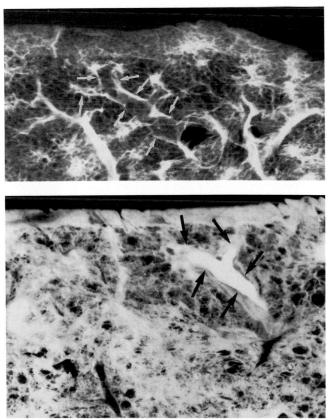

A

B

FIG. 7-50. Diffuse panbronchiolitis. **A:** Radiograph of a 1-mm slice of lung obtained from a patient with panbronchiolitis. A dilated air-filled bronchiole (*arrows*) is visible in the lung periphery, extending to within 5 mm of the pleural surface. **B:** Photomicrograph shows a dilated bronchiole (*arrows*) in the subpleural lung filled with secretions. (Courtesy of Koichi Nishimura, M.D., Chest Disease Research Institute, Kyoto University, Kyoto, Japan. From Nishimura et al., ref. 110, with permission.)

tions, a finding indicative of extensive peripheral air trapping. Such stratified distribution of ventilatory impairment may be considered characteristic of diffuse bronchiolar narrowing.

Utility of HRCT

Although the course of this disease is typically monitored clinically, HRCT may play a role in select cases. As documented by Akira et al. (180), in a study of 19 patients randomly assigned either to therapy with low-dose erythromycin or to follow-up without treatment, centrilobular nodular and branched opacities decreased in number and size in treated patients, suggesting a positive response to therapy. In distinction, among untreated patients, similar densities observed initially were found to have progressed with resultant dilatation of the proximal airways. These findings suggest a potential role for HRCT both for monitoring as well as predicting the outcome of therapy.

It should be noted that the finding of nodular or branching centrilobular opacities may be seen in a number of different diseases in which bronchiolar abnormalities are present (48,172). Linear or branching centrilobular opacities result from bronchiolar dilatation with intraluminal accumulation of mucus, fluid, or pus. As noted previously, this appearance has been termed the "tree-in-bud" appearance, and can be identified in patients with cystic fibrosis (134), endobronchial spread of tuberculosis (76) or nontuberculous mycobacteria, lobular or bronchopneumonia including those with *Pneumocystis carinii* or CMV pneumonia, bronchiectasis of any cause, and other airway diseases that result in the accumulation of mucus or pus within small bronchi. The differential diagnosis of centrilobular opacities is described in detail in Chapter 3.

REFERENCES

1. Webb WR. High-resolution computed tomography of obstructive lung disease. *Radiol Clin North Am* 1994;32:745–757.
2. Travis WD, Borok Z, Roum JH, et al. Pulmonary Langerhans cell granulomatosis (histiocytosis X): a clinicopathologic study of 48 cases. *Am J Surg Pathol* 1993;17:971–986.
3. Marcy TW, Reynolds HY. Pulmonary histiocytosis X. *Lung* 1985;163:129–150.
4. Colby TV, Lombard C. Histiocytosis X in the lung. *Hum Pathol* 1983;14:847–856.
5. Gaensler EA, Carrington CB. Open biopsy for chronic diffuse infiltrative lung disease: clinical, roentgenographic, and physiologic correlations in 502 patients. *Ann Thorac Surg* 1980;30:411–426.
6. Lewis JG. Eosinophilic granuloma and its variants with special reference to lung involvement: a report of 12 patients. *Q J Med* 1964;33:337–359.
7. Lacronique J, Roth C, Battesti JP, Basset F, Chretien J. Chest radiological features of pulmonary histiocytosis X: a report based on 50 adult cases. *Thorax* 1982;37:104–109.
8. Friedman PJ, Liebow AA, Sokoloff J. Eosinophilic granuloma of lung: clinical aspects of primary pulmonary histiocytosis in the adult. *Medicine* 1981;60:385–396.

9. Basset F, Corrin B, Spencer H, et al. Pulmonary histiocytosis X. *Am Rev Respir Dis* 1978;118:811–820.
10. Hance AJ, Basset F, Saumon G, et al. Smoking and interstitial lung disease: the effect of cigarette smoking on the incidence of pulmonary histiocytosis X and sarcoidosis. *Ann N Y Acad Sci* 1986;465:643–656.
11. Winterbauer RH, Dreis DF, Jolly PC. Clinical correlation. In: *Pulmonary Pathology.* New York: Springer-Verlag; 1988: 1148–1151.
12. Prophet D. Primary pulmonary histiocytosis X. *Clin Chest Med* 1982;3:643–653.
13. Moore AD, Godwin JD, Müller NL, et al. Pulmonary histiocytosis X: comparison of radiographic and CT findings. *Radiology* 1989;172:249–254.
14. Brauner MW, Grenier P, Mouelhi MM, Mompoint D, Lenoir S. Pulmonary histiocytosis X: evaluation with high resolution CT. *Radiology* 1989;172:255–258.
15. Grenier P, Valeyre D, Cluzel P, Brauner MW, Lenoir S, Chastang C. Chronic diffuse interstitial lung disease: diagnostic value of chest radiography and high-resolution CT. *Radiology* 1991;179:123–132.
16. Kulwiec EL, Lynch DA, Aguayo SM, Schwarz MI, King TEJ. Imaging of pulmonary histiocytosis X. *Radiographics* 1992;12: 515–526.
17. Giron J, Tawil A, Trussard V, et al. Contribution of high resolution x-ray computed tomography to the diagnosis of pulmonary histiocytosis X: apropos of 12 cases. *Ann Radiol* 1990;33: 31–38.
18. Taylor DB, Joske D, Anderson J, Barry-Walsh C. Cavitating pulmonary nodules in histiocytosis-X: high resolution CT demonstration. *Australas Radiol* 1990;34:253–255.
19. Müller NL, Miller RR. Computed tomography of chronic diffuse infiltrative lung disease: part 2. *Am Rev Respir Dis* 1990; 142:1440–1448.
20. Kelkel E, Pison C, Brambilla E, Ferreti G, Coulomb M, Brambilla C. Value of high resolution tomodensitometry in pulmonary histiocytosis X: radiological, clinical and functional correlations. *Rev Mal Respir* 1992;9:307–311.
21. Stern EJ, Webb WR, Golden JA, Gamsu G. Cystic lung disease associated with eosinophilic granuloma and tuberous sclerosis: air trapping at dynamic ultrafast high-resolution CT. *Radiology* 1992;182:325–329.
22. Müller NL, Miller RR, Webb WR, Evans KG, Ostrow DN. Fibrosing alveolitis: CT-pathologic correlation. *Radiology* 1986;160:585–588.
23. Guhl L. Pulmonary involvement in lymphangioleiomyomatosis: studies using high-resolution computed tomography. *Rofo* 1988;149:576–579.
24. Lenoir S, Grenier P, Brauner MW, et al. Pulmonary lymphangiomyomatosis and tuberous sclerosis: comparison of radiographic and thin-section CT findings. *Radiology* 1990;175: 329–334.
25. Rappaport DC, Weisbrod GL, Herman SJ, Chamberlain DW. Pulmonary lymphangioleiomyomatosis: high-resolution CT findings in four cases. *AJR* 1989;152:961–964.
26. Sherrier RH, Chiles C, Roggli V. Pulmonary lymphangioleiomyomatosis: CT findings. *AJR* 1989;153:937–940.
27. Templeton PA, McLoud TC, Müller NL, Shepard JA, Moore EH. Pulmonary lymphangioleiomyomatosis: CT and pathologic findings. *J Comput Assist Tomogr* 1989;13:54–57.
28. Müller NL, Chiles C, Kullnig P. Pulmonary lymphangiomyomatosis: correlation of CT with radiographic and functional findings. *Radiology* 1990;175:335–339.
29. Naidich DP, McCauley DI, Khouri NF, Stitik FP, Siegelman SS. Computed tomography of bronchiectasis. *J Comput Assist Tomogr* 1982;6:437–444.
30. Colby TV, Carrington CB. Infiltrative lung disease. In: *Pathology of the lung.* Stuttgart: Thieme Medical; 1988:425–518.
31. Corrin B, Liebow AA, Friedman PJ. Pulmonary lymphangiomyomatosis: a review. *Am J Pathol* 1975;79:348–382.
32. Carrington CB, Cugell DW, Gaensler EA, et al. Lymphangioleiomyomatosis: physiologic-pathologic-radiologic correlations. *Am Rev Respir Dis* 1977;116:977–995.
33. Adamson D, Heinrichs WL, Raybin DM, Raffin TA. Successful treatment of pulmonary lymphangiomyomatosis with oophorectomy and progesterone. *Am Rev Respir Dis* 1985;132: 916–921.
34. Braman SS, Mark EJ. A 32-year-old woman with recurrent pneumothorax. Massachusetts General Hospital Case Records, case 24, 1988. *N Engl J Med* 1988;318:1601–1610.
35. Silverstein EF, Ellis K, Wolff M, Jaretzki A. Pulmonary lymphangiomyomatosis. *AJR* 1974;120:120:832–850.
36. Kullnig P, Melzer G, Smolle-Jüttner FM. High-resolutioncomputertomographie des thorax bei lymphangioleiomyomatose und tuberöser sklerose. *Rofo* 1989;151:32–35.
37. Merchant RN, Pearson MG, Rankin RN, Morgan WKC. Computerized tomography in the diagnosis of lymphangioleiomyomatosis. *Am Rev Respir Dis* 1985;131:295–297.
38. Aberle DR, Hansell DM, Brown K, Tashkin DP. Lymphangiomyomatosis: CT, chest radiographic, and functional correlations. *Radiology* 1990;176:381–387.
39. Cardoso WV, Thurlbeck WM. Pathogenesis and terminology of emphysema. *Am J Respir Crit Care Med* 1994;149:1383.
40. Snider GL. Pathogenesis and terminology of emphysema. *Am J Respir Crit Care Med* 1994;149:1382–1383.
41. Thurlbeck WM, Müller NL. Emphysema: definition, imaging, and quantification. *AJR* 1995;163:1017–1025.
42. Snider GL, Kleinerman J, Thurlbeck WM, Bengali ZH. The definition of emphysema: report of a National Heart, Lung, and Blood Institute, Division of Lung Diseases workshop. *Am Rev Respir Dis* 1985;132:182–185.
43. Thurlbeck WM. *Chronic Airflow Obstruction in Lung Disease.* Philadelphia: WB Saunders; 1976:12–30.
44. Tuddenham WJ. Glossary of terms for thoracic radiology: recommendations of the Nomenclature Committee of the Fleischner Society. *AJR* 1984;143:509–517.
45. Thurlbeck WM. Morphology of emphysema and emphysemalike conditions. In: *Chronic Airflow Obstruction in Lung Disease.* Philadelphia: WB Saunders; 1976:96–234.
46. Hruban RH, Meziane MA, Zerhouni EA, et al. High resolution computed tomography of inflation fixed lungs: pathologic-radiologic correlation of centrilobular emphysema. *Am Rev Respir Dis* 1987;136:935–940.
47. Webb WR, Stein MG, Finkbeiner WE, Im JG, Lynch D, Gamsu G. Normal and diseased isolated lungs: high-resolution CT. *Radiology* 1988;166:81–87.
48. Murata K, Itoh H, Todo G, et al. Centrilobular lesions of the lung: demonstration by high-resolution CT and pathologic correlation. *Radiology* 1986;161:641–645.
49. Murata K, Khan A, Herman PG. Pulmonary parenchymal disease: evaluation with high-resolution CT. *Radiology* 1989;170: 629–635.
50. Bergin CJ, Müller NL, Miller RR. CT in the qualitative assessment of emphysema. *J Thorac Imaging* 1986;1:94–103.
51. Miller RR, Müller NL, Vedal S, Morrison NJ, Staples CA. Limitations of computed tomography in the assessment of emphysema. *Am Rev Respir Dis* 1989;139:980–983.
52. Kuwano K, Matsuba K, Ikeda T, et al. The diagnosis of mild emphysema: correlation of computed tomography and pathology scores. *Am Rev Respir Dis* 1990;141:169–178.
53. Spouge D, Mayo JR, Cardoso W, Müller NL. Panacinar emphysema: CT and pathologic correlation. *J Comput Assist Tomogr* 1993;17:710–713.
54. Lesur O, Delorme N, Fromaget JM, Bernadac P, Polu JM. Computed tomography in the etiologic assessment of idiopathic spontaneous pneumothorax. *Chest* 1990;98:341–347.
55. Peters RM, Peters BA, Benirschke SK, Friedman PJ. Chest dimensions in young adults with spontaneous pneumothorax. *Ann Thorac Surg* 1978;25:193–196.
56. Bense L, Lewander R, Eklund G, Hedenstierna G, Wiman LG. Nonsmoking, non-alpha-1-antitrypsin deficiency induced emphysema in nonsmokers with healing spontaneous pneumothorax, identified by computed tomography of the lungs. *Chest* 1993;103:433–438.
57. Stern EJ, Webb WR, Weinacker A, Müller NL. Idiopathic giant bullous emphysema (vanishing lung syndrome): imaging findings in nine patients. *AJR* 1994;162:279–282.

58. Gaensler EA, Jederlinic PJ, FitzGerald MX. Patient work-up for bullectomy. *J Thorac Imaging* 1986;13:75–93.
59. Morgan MD, Denison DM, Strickland B. Value of computed tomography for selecting patients with bullous lung disease for surgery. *Thorax* 1986;41:855–862.
60. Carr DH, Pride NB. Computed tomography in pre-operative assessment of bullous emphysema. *Clin Radiol* 1984;35:43–45.
61. Fiore DW, Biondetti PR, Sartori F, et al. The role of computer tomography in the evaluation of bullous lung disease. *J Comput Assist Tomogr* 1982;6:105–108.
62. Kinsella N, Müller NL, Vedal S, Staples C, Abboud RT, Chan-Yeung M. Emphysema in silicosis: a comparison of smokers with nonsmokers using pulmonary function testing and computed tomography. *Am Rev Respir Dis* 1990;141:1497–1500.
63. Akira M, Higashihara T, Yokoyama K, et al. Radiographic type p pneumoconiosis: high-resolution CT. *Radiology* 1989;171:117–123.
64. Thurlbeck WM, Simon G. Radiographic appearance of the chest in emphysema. *AJR* 1978;130:429–440.
65. Goddard PR, Nicholson EM, Laszlo E, Watt I. Computed tomography in pulmonary emphysema. *Clin Radiol* 1982;33:379–387.
66. Hayhurst MD, MacNee W, Flenley DC, al et. Diagnosis of pulmonary emphysema by computerised tomography. *Lancet* 1984;2:320–322.
67. Foster WL, Pratt PC, Roggli VL, Godwin JD, Halvorsen RA, Putman CE. Centrilobular emphysema: CT-pathologic correlation. *Radiology* 1986;159:27–32.
68. Bergin CJ, Müller NL, Nichols DM, al et. The diagnosis of emphysema: a computed tomographic-pathologic correlation. *Am Rev Respir Dis* 1986;133:541–546.
69. Kinsella M, Müller NL, Staples C, Vedal S, Chan Yeung M. Hyperinflation in asthma and emphysema: assessment by pulmonary function testing and computed tomography. *Chest* 1988;94:286–289.
70. Klein JS, Gamsu G, Webb WR, Golden JA, Müller NL. High-resolution CT diagnosis of emphysema in symptomatic patients with normal chest radiographs and isolated low diffusing capacity. *Radiology* 1992;182:817–821.
71. Morgan MDL, Strickland B. Computed tomography in the assessment of bullous lung disease. *Br J Dis Chest* 1984;78:10–25.
72. Müller NL, Staples CA, Miller RR, Abboud RT. "Density mask": an objective method to quantitate emphysema using computed tomography. *Chest* 1988;94:782–787.
73. Barker AF, Bardana EJ. Bronchiectasis: update on an orphan disease. *Am Rev Res Dis* 1988;137:969–978.
74. Stanford W, Galvin JR. The diagnosis of bronchiectasis. *Clin Chest Med* 1988;9:691–699.
75. Davis AL, Salzman SH. Bronchiectasis. In: Cherniack NS, ed. *Chronic Obstructive Pulmonary Disease*. Philadelphia: WB Saunders; 1991:316–338.
76. Im JG, Itoh H, Shim YS, et al. Pulmonary tuberculosis: CT findings—early active disease and sequential change with antituberculous therapy. *Radiology* 1993;186:653–660.
77. Hartman TE, Swensen SJ, Williams DE. Mycobacterium avium-intracellulare complex: evaluation with CT. *Radiology* 1993;187:23–26.
78. Swensen SJ, Hartman TE, Williams DE. Computed tomography in diagnosis of Mycobacterium avium-intracellulare complex in patients with bronchiectasis. *Chest* 1994;105:49–52.
79. Moore EH. Atypical mycobacterial infection in the lung: CT appearance. *Radiology* 1993;187:777–782.
80. McGuinness G, Naidich DP, Garay SM, Leitman BS, McCauley DI. AIDS associated bronchiectasis: CT features. *J Comput Assist Tomogr* 1993;17:260–266.
81. Neeld DA, Goodman LR, Gurney JW, Greenberger PA, Fink JN. Computerized tomography in the evaluation of allergic bronchopulmonary aspergillosis. *Am Rev Respir Dis* 1990;142:1200–1206.
82. Kullnig P, Pongratz M, Kopp W, Ranner G. Computerized tomography in the diagnosis of allergic bronchopulmonary aspergillosis. *Radiology* 1989;29:228–231.
83. Lynch DA, Newell JD, Tschomper BA, Cink TM, Newman LS, Bethel R. Uncomplicated asthma in adults: comparison of CT appearance of the lungs in asthmatic and healthy subjects. *Radiology* 1993;188:829–833.
84. Skeens JL, Fuhrman CR, Yousem SA. Bronchiolitis obliterans in heart-lung transplantation patients: radiologic findings in 11 patients. *AJR* 1989;153:253–256.
85. O'Donovan P. Imaging of complications of lung transplantation. *Radiographics* 1993;13:787–796.
86. Morrish WF, Herman SJ, Weisbrod GL, Chamberlain DW. Bronchiolitis obliterans after lung transplantation: findings at chest radiography and high-resolution CT. *Radiology* 1991;179:487–490.
87. Lentz D, Bergin CJ, Berry GJ, Stoehr C, Theodore J. Diagnosis of bronchiolitis obliterans in heart-lung transplantation patients: importance of bronchial dilatation on CT. *AJR* 1992;159:463–467.
88. Hruban RH, Ren H, Kuhlman JE, et al. Inflation-fixed lungs: pathologic-radiologic (CT) correlation of lung transplantation. *J Comput Assist Tomogr* 1990;14:329–335.
89. Herman S, Rappaport D, Weisbrod G, Olscamp G, Patterson G, Cooper J. Single-lung transplantation: imaging features. *Radiology* 1989;170:89–93.
90. Graham NJ, Müller NL, Miller RR, Shepherd JD. Intrathoracic complications following allogeneic bone marrow transplantation: CT findings. *Radiology* 1991;181:153–156.
91. Crawford SW, Clark JG. Bronchiolitis associated with bone marrow transplantation. *Clin Chest Med* 1993;14:741–749.
92. Currie DC, Cooke JC, Morgan AD, et al. Interpretation of bronchograms and chest radiographs in patients with chronic sputum production. *Thorax* 1987;42:278–284.
93. Millar A, Boothroyd A, Edwards D, Hetzel M. The role of computed tomography (CT) in the investigation of unexplained hemoptysis. *Resp Med* 1992;86:39–44.
94. Naidich DP, Funt S, Ettenger NA, Arranda C. Hemoptysis: CT-bronchoscopic correlations in 58 cases. *Radiology* 1990;177:357–362.
95. Haponik F, Britt EJ, Smith PL, Bleecker ER. Computed chest tomography in the evaluation of hemoptysis. *Chest* 1987;91:80–85.
96. Gudjberg CE. Roentgenologic diagnosis of bronchiectasis: an analysis of 112 cases. *Acta Radiol* 1955;43:209–226.
97. Joharjy IA, Bashi SA, Abdullah AK. Value of medium-thickness CT in the diagnosis of bronchiectasis. *AJR* 1987;149:1133–1137.
98. Cooke JC, Currie DC, Morgan AD, et al. Role of computed tomography in diagnosis of bronchiectasis. *Thorax* 1987;42:272–277.
99. Silverman PM, Godwin JD. CT/bronchographic correlations in bronchiectasis. *J Comput Assist Tomogr* 1987;11:52–56.
100. Young K, Aspestrand F, Kolbenstvedt A. High resolution CT and bronchography in the assessment of bronchiectasis. *Acta Radiol* 1991;32:439–441.
101. Desai SR, Wells AU, Cheah FK, Cole PJ, Hansell DM. The reproducibility of bronchial circumference measurements using CT. *Br J Radiol* 1994;67:257–262.
102. Seneterre E, Paganin F, Bruel JM, Michel FB, Bousquet J. Measurement of the internal size of bronchi using high resolution computed tomography (HRCT). *Eur Respir J* 1994;7:596–600.
103. Reid LM. Reduction in bronchial subdivision in bronchiectasis. *Thorax* 1950;5:233–236.
104. Annest LS, Kratz JM, Crawford FA. Current results of treatment of bronchiectasis. *J Thorac Cardiovasc Surg* 1982;83:546–550.
105. Naidich DP. High-resolution computed tomography of cystic lung disease. *Semin Roentgenol* 1991;26:151–174.
106. Naidich DP, Rumancik WM, Ettenger NA, et al. Congenital anomalies of the lungs in adults: MR diagnosis. *AJR* 1988;151:13–19.
107. Pugatch RD, Gale ME. Obscure pulmonary masses: bronchial impaction revealed by CT. *AJR* 1983;141:909–914.
108. Rappaport DC, Herman SJ, Weisbrod GL. Congenital bronchopulmonary diseases in adults: CT findings. *AJR* 1994;162:1295–1299.

109. Akira M, Kitatani F, Lee Y-S, et al. Diffuse panbronchiolitis: evaluation with high-resolution CT. *Radiology* 1988;168: 433–438.
110. Nishimura K, Kitaichi M, Izumi T, Itoh H. Diffuse panbronchiolitis: correlation of high-resolution CT and pathologic findings. *Radiology* 1992;184:779–785.
111. Hansell DM, Wells AU, Rubens MB, Cole PJ. Bronchiectasis: functional significance of areas of decreased attenuation at expiratory CT. *Radiology* 1994;193:369–374.
112. Stern EJ, Webb WR, Gamsu G. Dynamic quantitative computed tomography: a predictor of pulmonary function in obstructive lung diseases. *Invest Radiol* 1994;29:564–569.
113. McGuinness G, Naidich DP, Leitman BS, McCauley DI. Bronchiectasis: CT evaluation. *AJR* 1993;160:253–259.
114. Tarver RD, Conces DJ, Godwin JD. Motion artifacts on CT simulate bronchiectasis. *AJR* 1988;151:1117–1119.
115. Westcott JL, Cole SR. Traction bronchiectasis in end-stage pulmonary fibrosis. *Radiology* 1986;161:665–669.
116. Thurlbeck WM. Pathology of chronic airflow obstruction. In: Cherniack NS, ed. *Chronic Obstructive Pulmonary Disease.* Philadelphia: WB Saunders; 1991:3–20.
117. Müller NL, Bergin CJ, Ostrow DN, Nichols DM. Role of computed tomography in the recognition of bronchiectasis. *AJR* 1984;143:971–976.
118. Mootoosamy IM, Reznek RH, Osman J. Assessment of bronchiectasis by computed tomography. *Thorax* 1985;40:920–924.
119. Phillips MS, Williams MP, Flower CDR. How useful is computed tomography in the diagnosis and assessment of bronchiectasis? *Clin Radiol* 1986;37:321–325.
120. Grenier P, Maurice F, Musset D, Menu Y, Nahum H. Bronchiectasis: assessment by thin-section CT. *Radiology* 1986;161: 95–99.
121. Giron J, Skaff F, Maubon A, et al. The value of thin-section CT scans in the diagnosis and staging of bronchiectasis: comparison with bronchography in a series of fifty-four patients. *Ann Radiol* 1988;31:25–33.
122. Munro NC, Cooke JC, Currie DC, Strickland B, Cole PJ. Comparison of thin section computed tomography with bronchography for identifying bronchiectatic segments in patients with chronic sputum production. *Thorax* 1990;45:135–139.
123. Grenier P, Lenoir S, Brauner M. Computed tomographic assessment of bronchiectasis. *Semin Ultrasound CT MR* 1990; 11:430–441.
124. Remy-Jardin M, Remy J. Comparison of vertical and oblique CT in evaluation of the bronchial tree. *J Comput Assist Tomogr* 1988;12:956–962.
125. Bhalla M, Turcios N, Aponte V, et al. Cystic fibrosis: scoring system with thin-section CT. *Radiology* 1991;179:783–788.
126. Zwirewich CV, Mayo JR, Müller NL. Low-dose high-resolution CT of lung parenchyma. *Radiology* 1991;180:413–417.
127. Herold CJ, Brown RH, Mitzner W, Links JM, Hirshman CA, Zerhouni EA. Assessment of pulmonary airway reactivity with high-resolution CT. *Radiology* 1991;181:369–374.
128. Stern EJ, Graham CM, Webb WR, Gamsu G. Normal trachea during forced expiration: dynamic CT measurements. *Radiology* 1993;187:27–31.
129. Stern EJ, Webb WR. Dynamic imaging of lung morphology with ultrafast high-resolution computed tomography. *J Thorac Imaging* 1993;8:273–282.
130. Curtin JJ, Webster AD, Farrant J, Katz D. Bronchiectasis in hypogammaglobulinaemia—a computed tomography assessment. *Clin Radiol* 1991;44:82–84.
131. Friedman PJ. Chest radiographic findings in the adult with cystic fibrosis. *Semin Roentgenol* 1987;22:114–124.
132. Hansell DM, Strickland B. High-resolution computed tomography in pulmonary cystic fibrosis. *Br J Radiol* 1989;62:1–5.
133. Santis G, Hodson ME, Strickland B. High resolution computed tomography in adult cystic fibrosis patients with mild lung disease. *Clin Radiol* 1991;44:20–22.
134. Lynch DA, Brasch RC, Hardy KA, Webb WR. Pediatric pulmonary disease: assessment with high-resolution ultrafast CT. *Radiology* 1990;176:243–248.
135. Taccone A, Romano L, Marzoli A, Girosi D. Computerized tomography in pulmonary cystic fibrosis. *Radiol Med* 1991;82: 79–83.
136. Nathanson I, Conboy K, Murphy S, Afshani E, Kuhn JP. Ultrafast computerized tomography of the chest in cystic fibrosis: a new scoring system. *Pediatr Pulmonol* 1991;11:81–86.
137. Currie DC, Goldman JM, Cole PJ, Strickland B. Comparison of narrow section computed tomography and plain chest radiography in chronic allergic bronchopulmonary aspergillosis. *Clin Radiol* 1987;38:593–596.
138. Shah A, Pant CS, Bhagat R, Panchal N. CT in childhood allergic bronchopulmonary aspergillosis. *Pediatr Radiol* 1992;22: 227–228.
139. Kaneko K, Kudo S, Tashiro M, Kishikawa T, Nakanishi Y, Yamada H. Computed tomography findings in Williams-Campbell syndrome. *J Thorac Imaging* 1991;6:11–13.
140. Watanabe Y, Nishiyama Y, Kanayama H, Enomoto K, Kato K, Takeichi M. Congenital bronchiectasis due to cartilage deficiency: CT demonstration. *J Comput Assist Tomogr* 1987;11: 701–703.
141. Myers JL, Colby TV. Pathologic manifestations of bronchiolitis, constrictive bronchiolitis, cryptogenic organizing pneumonia and diffuse panbronchiolitis. *Clin Chest Med* 1993;14: 611–623.
142. King TE. Overview of bronchiolitis. *Clin Chest Med* 1993;14: 607–610.
143. Kraft M, Mortenson R, Colby TV, Newman L, Waldron J, King T. Cryptogenic constrictive bronchiolitis. *Am Rev Res Dis* 1993;148:1093–1101.
144. Colby TV, Myers JL. The clinical and histologic spectrum of bronchiolitis obliterans including bronchiolitis obliterans organizing pneumonia (BOOP). *Semin Respir Dis* 1992;13: 119–133.
145. Ezri T, Kunichezky S, Eliraz A, Soroker D, Halperin D, Schattner A. Bronchiolitis obliterans—current concepts. *Q J Med* 1994;87:1–10.
146. Sweatman MC, Millar AB, Strickland B, Turner-Warwick M. Computed tomography in adult obliterative bronchiolitis. *Clin Radiol* 1990;41:116–119.
147. Garg K, Lynch DA, Newell JD, King TE Jr. Proliferative and constrictive bronchiolitis: classification and radiologic features. *AJR* 1994;162:803–808.
148. Gosink BB, Friedman PJ, Liebow AA. Bronchiolitis obliterans: roentgenographic-pathologic correlation. *AJR* 1973;117: 816–832.
149. Laraya-Cuasay LR, DeForest A, Huff D, Lischner H, Huang NN. Chronic pulmonary complications of early influenza virus infection in children. *Am Rev Respir Dis* 1977;116:617–625.
150. Nikki P, Meretoja O, Valtonen V, et al. Severe bronchiolitis probably caused by varicella-zoster virus. *Crit Care Med* 1982; 10:344–346.
151. Penn CC, Liu C. Bronchiolitis following infection in adults and children. *Clin Chest Med* 1993;14:645–654.
152. Epler GR, Colby TV. The spectrum of bronchiolitis obliterans. *Chest* 1983;83:161–162.
153. Lowry T, Schuman LM. "Silo-filler's disease"—a syndrome caused by nitrogen dioxide. *JAMA* 1956;162:153–158.
154. Cornelius EA, Betlach EH. Silo-filler's disease. *Radiology* 1960;74:232–235.
155. Charan NB, Myers CG, Lakshminarayan S, Spencer TM. Pulmonary injuries associated with acute sulfur dioxide inhalation. *Am Rev Respir Dis* 1979;119:555–560.
156. St John RC, Dorinsky PM. Cryptogenic bronchiolitis. *Clin Chest Med* 1993;14:667–675.
157. Geddes DM, Corrin B, Brewerton DA, Davies RJ, Turner-Warwick M. Progressive airway obliteration in adults and its association with rheumatoid disease. *Q J Med* 1977;46:427–444.
158. Epler GR, Snider GL, Gaensler EA, Cathcart ES, Fitzgerald MK, Carrington CB. Bronchiolitis and bronchitis in connective tissue disease. *JAMA* 1979;242:528–532.
159. Herzog CA, Miller RR, Hoidal JR. Bronchiolitis and rheumatoid arthritis. *Am Rev Respir Dis* 1979;119:555–560.
160. Schwarz MI, Matthay RA, Sahn SA, et al. Interstitial lung disease in polymyositis and dermatomyositis: an analysis of six cases and review of the literature. *Medicine* 1976;55:89–104.

161. Wells AU, duBois RM. Bronchiolitis in association with connective tissue diseases. *Clin Chest Med* 1993;14:655–666.
162. Ostrow D, Buskard N, Hills RS, Vickars L, Churg A. Bronchiolitis obliterans complicating bone marrow transplantation. *Chest* 1985;87:828–830.
163. Roca J, Granena A, Rodriguez-Roisin J, Alvarez P, Agusti-Vidal A, Rozman C. Fatal airway disease in an adult with chronic graft-versus-host disease. *Thorax* 1982;37:77–78.
164. Stein-Streilen J, Lipscomb MF, Hart DA, Darden A. Graft-versus-host reaction in the lung. *Transplantation* 1981;32:38–44.
165. Burke CM, Theodore J, Dawkins KD, et al. Post transplant obliterative bronchiolitis and other late lung sequelae in human heart-lung transplantation. *Chest* 1984;86:824–829.
166. Paradis I, Yousem S, Griffith B. Airway obstruction and bronchiolitis obliterans after lung transplantation. *Clin Chest Med* 1993;14:751–763.
167. McLoud TC, Epler GR, Colby TV, Gaensler EA, Carrington CB. Bronchiolitis obliterans. *Radiology* 1986;159:1–8.
168. Breatnach E, Kerr I. The radiology of cryptogenic obliterative bronchiolitis. *Clin Radiol* 1982;33:657–661.
169. Marti-Bonmati L, Ruiz PF, Catala F, Mata JM, Calonge E. CT findings in Swyer-James syndrome. *Radiology* 1989;172:477–480.
170. Padley SPG, Adler BD, Hansell DM, Müller NL. Bronchiolitis obliterans: high-resolution CT findings and correlation with pulmonary function tests. *Clin Radiol* 1993;47:236–240.
171. Lynch DA. Imaging of small airways disease. *Clin Chest Med* 1993;14:623–634.
172. Gruden JF, Webb WR, Warnock M. Centrilobular opacities in the lung on high-resolution CT: diagnostic considerations and pathologic correlation. *AJR* 1994;162:569–574.
173. MacLeod EM. Abnormal transradiancy of one lung. *Thorax* 1954;9:147–153.
174. Swyer PR, James GCW. A case of unilateral pulmonary emphysema. *Thorax* 1953;8:133–136.
175. Aquino SL, Webb WR, Golden J. Bronchiolitis obliterans associated with rheumatoid arthritis: findings on HRCT and dynamic expiratory CT. *J Comput Assist Tomogr* 1994;18:555–558.
176. Remy-Jardin M, Remy J, Cortet B, Mauri F, Delcambre B. Lung changes in rheumatoid arthritis: CT findings. *Radiology* 1994;193:375–382.
177. Loubeyre P, Revel D, Delignette A, et al. Bronchiectasis detected with thin-section CT as a predictor of chronic lung allograft rejection. *Radiology* 1995;194:213–216.
178. Witte R, Gurney J, Robbins R, Linder J, Rennard S, Areneson M. Diffuse pulmonary alveolar hemorrhage after bone marrow transplantation: radiographic findings in 39 patients. *AJR* 1991;157:461–464.
179. Mori M, Galvin JR, Barloon TJ, Gingrich RD, Stanford W. Fungal pulmonary infections after bone marrow transplantation: evaluation with radiography and CT. *Radiology* 1991;178:721–726.
180. Akira M, Higashihara T, Sakatani M, Hara H. Diffuse panbronchiolitis: follow-up CT examination. *Radiology* 1993;189:559–562.
181. Murata K, Itoh H, Senda M, et al. Stratified impairment of pulmonary ventilation in "diffuse panbronchiolitis": PET and CT studies. *J Comput Assist Tomogr* 1989;13:48–53.

EIGHT

Clinical Utility of HRCT and Indications for Its Use

The clinical assessment of a patient with suspected diffuse lung disease can be a difficult and perplexing problem. Similar symptoms and, in some cases, chest radiographic findings can result from a variety of acute or chronic lung diseases affecting the lung interstitium, airways, or air spaces. Diffuse infiltrative lung disease (DILD) represents a strikingly heterogeneous group of diseases. Although sarcoidosis and various causes of pulmonary fibrosis account for between one third and one half of all cases of DILD seen in clinical practice, well over a hundred different causes of diffuse infiltrative lung disease have been described (1,2). Similarly, acute diffuse lung diseases in immunocompetent patients or in association with AIDS or other causes of immunosuppression can have a number of infectious or noninfectious causes, and their differentiation on clinical and radiographic findings can be difficult.

Furthermore, diffuse lung diseases are far more common than generally perceived. As estimated in a 1972 Respiratory Diseases Task Force report from the National Institutes of Health, patients with DILD represent as many as 15% of all patients referred to pulmonologists for evaluation (3). More recently, using a population-based registry of 2,936 patients with interstitial lung diseases, Coultas et al. (1) reported the yearly incidence of interstitial disease as 31.5 and 26.1 per 100,000, in men and women, respectively. Also, in a review of autopsy results, these authors found that undiagnosed or preclinical interstitial lung disease was present in 1.8% of all cases (1). Acute diffuse lung diseases are also being seen in increased numbers, at least partially as a result of the AIDS epidemic and the increased use of organ transplantation. For example, *Pneumocystis carinii* pneumonia affects approximately 65% of all HIV-infected patients at some point during the course of their disease, and accounts for nearly 25% of AIDS-related deaths (4–9).

Tests used in diagnosing diffuse lung disease are numerous, with the final diagnosis, or differential diagnosis, often based on a combination of laboratory tests, physiologic studies, radiographic examinations, and invasive procedures, including fiberoptic bronchoscopy with transbronchial biopsy and/or bronchoalveolar lavage, or open lung biopsy. It is in this context that high-resolution CT has assumed an increasingly important role in assessing patients with undiagnosed diffuse lung disease. HRCT should not generally be used by itself in an attempt to diagnose lung disease; it should be part of a comprehensive clinical evaluation, and should be interpreted in light of clinical findings.

In previous chapters, we have reviewed the utility of HRCT in regard to the diagnosis of a number of specific diseases. It is the purpose of this chapter to summarize our current understanding of the clinical utility of HRCT in diagnosing diffuse lung disease and the clinical indications for performing HRCT in patients suspected of having a diffuse abnormality. Special emphasis will be placed on answering the following questions:

1. How sensitive and specific is HRCT for diagnosing diffuse lung disease, both in relation to chest radiographs and conventional CT (CCT)?
2. What is the diagnostic accuracy of HRCT in diagnosing diffuse lung disease, and can HRCT findings be diagnostic of specific disease entities?
3. Is there a role for HRCT in assessing disease activity and prognosis?
4. Of what value is HRCT in planning lung biopsy?

SENSITIVITY AND SPECIFICITY OF HRCT IN THE DIAGNOSIS OF DIFFUSE LUNG DISEASE

Chest radiographs are important in the assessment of patients suspected of having diffuse lung disease; they are inexpensive, readily available, and can display a wide range of abnormalities. In some patients, chest radiographs can provide information which is sufficient for diagnosis and management. Furthermore, in those patients with progressive symptoms for whom prior films are available, radiographs often provide an accurate assessment of the course of disease. It is difficult to imagine a physician evaluating a patient with diffuse lung disease without using chest radiographs in an attempt to detect lung disease, assess its type and extent, and to monitor the effects of treatment.

Nonetheless, it well documented that chest radiographs are limited in both their sensitivity and specificity in patients with diffuse lung disease (Figs. 8-1,8-2) (10--12). For example, in a study by Epler et al. (10) of 458 patients with histologically confirmed diffuse infiltrative lung disease, 44, or nearly 10%, had normal chest radiographs. Similarly, Gaensler and Carrington (11) reported that nearly 16% of patients with pathologic proof of interstitial lung disease had normal chest radiographs. More recently, Padley et al. (12) reviewed the plain radiographs of 86 patients with biopsy-proven diffuse infiltrative lung disease and 14 normal subjects; in keeping with previous reports, 10% of the patients with diffuse infiltrative lung disease were thought to have normal chest radiographs. Chest radiographs are even less sensitive in diagnosing airway abnormalities such as bronchiectasis, with 30% to 50% of patients. with proven bronchiectasis having normal chest films, and in patients with emphysema, radiographs are normal in 20% or more of cases (13–16). Furthermore, it has also been estimated that up to 10% of immunosup-

pressed patients with acute diffuse lung disease have normal radiographs (17).

An equally important limitation of chest radiographs are their susceptibility to over-interpretation—it is easy to overcall the presence of diffuse pulmonary disease on chest radiographs in normal subjects (18). It has been shown that between 10% and 20% of patients with DILD suspected on chest radiographs subsequently prove to have normal lung biopsies (10,11). In the study by Padley et al. (12), 18% of normal subjects were interpreted as having abnormal chest radiographs.

The sensitivity of CT for detecting lung disease has been compared to that of plain radiography in a number of studies; without exception, these have shown that CT, and particularly HRCT, are more sensitive than chest radiography for detecting both acute and chronic diffuse lung diseases (13,19–26). Averaging the results of several recent studies, the sensitivity of HRCT for detecting pulmonary disease is approximately 94%, as compared to 80% for chest radiographs (18).

HRCT has been shown to be more sensitive than chest radiographs in every study of diffuse lung disease in which the two have been compared (Figs. 8-1,8-2) (Table 8-1). Furthermore, it should be noted that the increased sensitivity of HRCT is not achieved at the expense of decreased specificity or diagnostic accuracy (12,27,28). A specificity of 96% for HRCT, as compared to 82% for chest radiographs was reported by Padley et al. (12) in patients with DILD. Similar high sensitivity (97% to 98%) and specificity (93% to

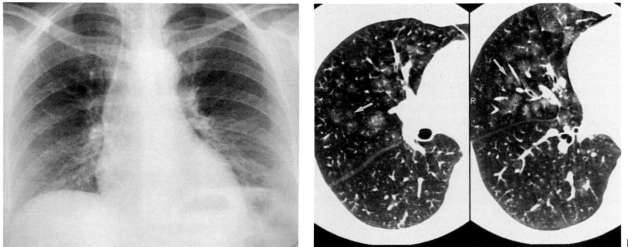

A   B,C

FIG. 8-1. Abnormal HRCT in a patient with a normal chest radiograph. **A:** Posteroanterior radiograph in a patient who presented with recurrent episodes of hemoptysis. No abnormality is visible. **B,C:** Target reconstructed HRCT images through the right lung obtained the same day as the chest radiograph in A show evidence of focal areas of ground-glass opacity, especially in the anterior segment of the right upper lobe and the middle lobe (*arrows*, B,C). At bronchoscopy, no discrete endobronchial lesion was identified although there was extensive blood within the airways on the right side. The HRCT appearance is compatible with the aspiration of blood, identification of which is obviously more apparent with CT than the corresponding radiograph.

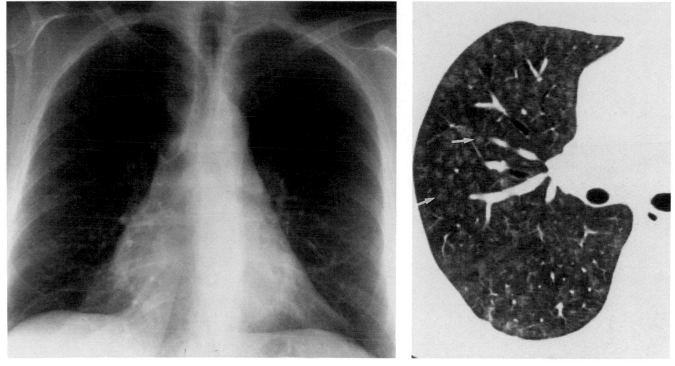

FIG. 8-2. Abnormal HRCT in a patient with a normal chest radiograph. **A:** Chest radiograph in a patient with progressive dyspnea appears normal, even in retrospect. **B:** HRCT through the right mid-lung obtained at the same time as the radiograph in A is distinctly abnormal, showing numerous, ill-defined centrilobular nodules of ground-glass opacity (*arrows*). This appearance is suggestive of hypersensitivity pneumonitis; the patient had a history of exposure to birds.

99%) values have been shown for HRCT in the diagnosis of bronchiectasis (29,30). The accuracy of CT in the diagnosis of pulmonary complications of AIDS was recently assessed by Hartman et al. (31). The CT and HRCT scans of 102 patients who had AIDS and proven thoracic complications were reviewed, along with those of 20 HIV-positive patients without active intrathoracic disease. CT had an average sensitivity greater than 99% in detecting active disease, while its average specificity was 93%. HRCT can further be of value in diagnosing the presence or absence of lung disease in patients who have subtle or questionable plain radiographic findings (Fig. 8-3).

Although HRCT is clearly more sensitive than chest radiographs, its sensitivity in detecting lung disease is not 100%, and a negative HRCT cannot generally be used to rule out lung disease, particularly in patients with DILD. In the largest series reported to date, Padley et al. (12) evaluated HRCT studies in 100 patients, including 86 patients with DILD and 14 normal con-

TABLE 8-1. *Diseases in which CT/HRCT has been shown to be more sensitive than plain radiographs*

Idiopathic Pulmonary Fibrosis (32)	Nontuberculous Mycobacterial Infections (48)
Rheumatoid Lung Disease (33)	Infections in Immunosuppressed Patients (49)
Scleroderma (34)	Septic Embolism (50)
Drug-induced Lung Disease (35)	Hypersensitivity Pneumonitis (19,51)
Radiation-induced Lung Disease (36,37)	Desquamative Interstitial Pneumonitis (52)
Asbestosis (25,26)	Respiratory Bronchiolitis (53,54)
Lymphangitic Spread of Carcinoma (23)	*Pneumocystis carinii* Pneumonia (55)
Hematogenous Metastases (38)	Histiocytosis X (56,57)
Bronchioloalveolar Carcinoma (Diffuse) (39)	Lymphangiomyomatosis (22,58,59)
Sarcoidosis (21,40)	Emphysema (60–62)
Berylliosis (41)	Bronchial Abnormalities and Bronchiectasis (29,30)
Silicosis (42)	Cystic Fibrosis (63,64)
Coal Worker's Pneumoconiosis (43)	Bronchiolitis Obliterans and the Swyer-James Syndrome (65,66)
Tuberculosis (Cavitation, Endobronchial Spread, Miliary) (44–47)	

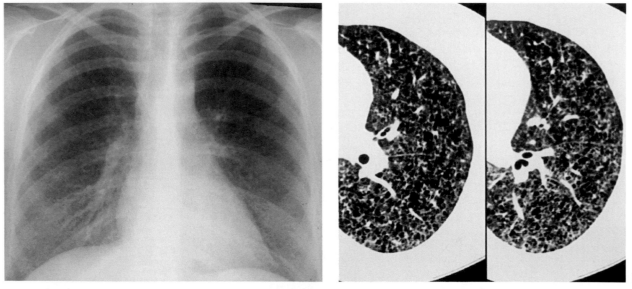

A   B,C

FIG. 8-3. Abnormal HRCT in a patient with questionable radiographic abnormalities. **A:** Routine posteroanterior radiograph in an asymptomatic patient shows a subtle diffuse increase in lung markings difficult to characterize. It would be difficult to say that this radiograph is definitely abnormal. **B,C:** Target reconstructed HRCT images through the left lung show the presence of thin-walled cysts evenly spaced throughout the lungs and associated with a few, small, poorly defined nodules. These findings are characteristic of histiocytosis X. Although the differential diagnosis includes lymphangiomyomatosis, the presence of nodules and the fact that the patient is asymptomatic make this diagnosis much less likely. The diagnosis was subsequently confirmed by transbronchial biopsy.

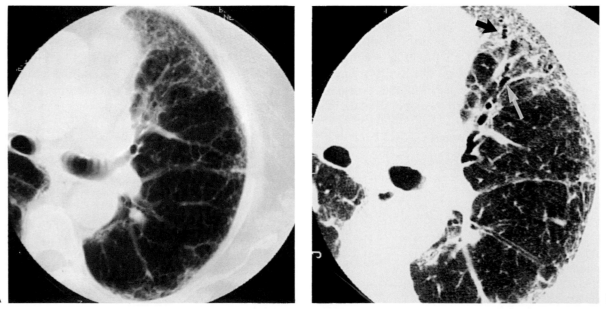

A   B,C

FIG. 8-4. High-resolution CT vs. routine CT in the evaluation of diffuse lung disease. **A,B:** Target reconstructions of routine 10-mm thick (A) and HRCT, 1.5-mm-thick, (B) sections obtained at the same level through the left mid-lung in a patient with biopsy-proven idiopathic pulmonary fibrosis. The presence of reticular opacities is far easier to assess with HRCT. In particular, note the presence of traction bronchiectasis involving the anterior segmental bronchus (*arrows* in B) visible only on the HRCT section.

trols. In this study, although HRCT had very high sensitivity and specificity values, 4% of subjects with biopsy-proven lung disease were interpreted as having a normal HRCT. Similar results in patients with early or subtle DILD have been reported by others (19,67). In a study of 11 patients with histologically proven hypersensitivity pneumonitis, Lynch et al. (19) found that 10 patients had normal chest radiographs, and 6 patients (55%) had a normal HRCT. Among 24 patients and six lungs with pathologic evidence of asbestosis studied by Gamsu et al. (67), 5 had normal HRCT scans.

On the other hand, it has been suggested that HRCT is highly accurate in excluding acute lung disease in patients with immune-deficiency disorders. Hartman et al. (31), in an assessment of HRCT findings in 102 AIDS patients with proven intrathoracic complications and 20 HIV-positive patients without active intratho-

racic disease, found that one observer detected all 102 cases of active disease, while a second observer detected all but one. Similar accuracy in excluding disease has been reported by Mori et al. (49) in a study of 55 pairs of chest radiographs and CT studies obtained in 33 bone marrow transplant patients with fever. On the one hand, these authors found that CT proved a reliable method for detecting fungal infection, with nodules being seen in 20 of 21 cases. On the other hand, a negative CT study suggested that the underlying cause of fever most likely was due to a bacteremia or nonfilamentous fungal infection of nonpulmonary origin (49).

The sensitivity of HRCT has also proven superior to that of conventional CT (CCT) obtained with thicker collimation (Figs. 8-4,8-5) (25,68,69). Remy-Jardin et al. (69) assessed 150 patients using both conventional

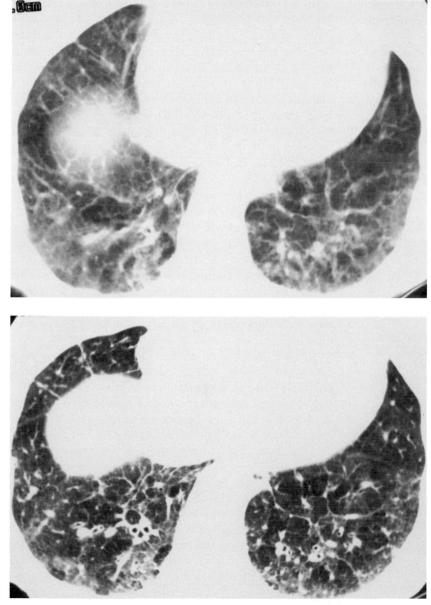

FIG. 8-5. Conventional CT (10-mm collimation) vs. high-resolution CT. Sections at identical levels through the lung bases in a patient with proven lymphangitic carcinomatosis, obtained with 10-mm (**A**) and 1.5-mm (**B**) collimation. Note that identification of fine architectural details, including secondary lobular anatomy and peribronchial infiltration is much better appreciated with high-resolution imaging.

CT (10-mm collimation) and HRCT (1.5-mm collimation), with sections obtained at identical levels; they found that HRCT was clearly superior to CCT in identifying a number of abnormalities, including septal and nonseptal lines, nodular and linear interfaces, small cystic airspaces, bronchiectasis, and pleural thickening. Furthermore, these authors found that reliable identification of ground-glass opacity required the use of HRCT. Conventional CT proved superior to HRCT only in the detection of small nodules, and even here, nearly 15% of small nodules could only be seen using HRCT. Similarly, in a study of patients with asbestosis, Aberle et al. (25) were able to identify subtle parenchymal reticulation on HRCT in 96% of cases, as compared to only 83% of cases with CCT. As another example, studies comparing the accuracy of HRCT to bronchography in diagnosing bronchiectasis (29,30) have found sensitivity values of 97% to 98% and a specificity of 93% to 99%; previous studies of CCT with 10-mm collimation reported sensitivities ranging from 60% to 80% (70,71).

Because of its excellent sensitivity, we consider that HRCT is indicated to detect lung disease in patients with normal or questionable radiographic abnormalities, who have symptoms or pulmonary function findings suggestive of acute or chronic diffuse lung disease (Table 8-2). This includes patients with unexplained dyspnea in whom chronic diffuse infiltrative lung disease is suspected; symptomatic patients with known exposures to inorganic dusts such as silica and asbestos, organic antigens, or drugs; immunosuppressed patients with unexplained dyspnea or fever; patients with unexplained hemoptysis; and patients with dyspnea or other symptoms and suspected airways or obstructive lung disease (18,72).

DIAGNOSTIC ACCURACY OF HRCT

Even in the presence of definite abnormalities, chest radiographs have limited diagnostic accuracy in patients with diffuse lung disease. Because of superimposition of structures and relatively low contrast resolution, it is often difficult to accurately characterize chest radiographic abnormalities (Figs. 8-6,8-7). Although a pattern recognition approach to the diagnosis of lung disease can be helpful in interpreting chest radiographs, it has well-documented limitations, and correlation with histologic findings is often poor (73–75).

In an attempt to improve diagnostic accuracy, McLoud and coworkers (76), employed a semiquantitative approach to the plain film diagnosis of diffuse lung disease based on a modification of the International Labour Office and Union Internationale Contre le Cancer (ILO/UC) classification of plain film abnormalities (76). In an evaluation of 365 patients with open lung biopsy confirmed DILD, these investigators found that their first two diagnostic choices corresponded to the histologic diagnosis in only 50% of patients, improving to only 78% when the first three choices were included. Furthermore, there was only 70% interobserver agreement as to the predominant type of parenchymal abnormality or its extent. These results clearly show how difficult the precise interpretation of chest films can be, even for the experienced observer. Even as seemingly simple a diagnosis as a identification of focal consolidation in patients with clinical evidence of pneumonia is associated with considerable interobserver variation, which furthermore may be independent of level of interpreter expertise (77).

Similar limitations in the diagnostic accuracy of chest radiography have been observed by others (12,27,28). In a study by Mathieson et al. (27), the accuracy of chest radiographs in 118 consecutive patients with chronic diffuse lung disease were assessed; radiographs were assessed independently by three observers who listed their three most likely diagnoses in order of probability, as well as their degree of confidence in these diagnoses. A confident diagnosis was reached radiographically in only 23% of cases; a correct first-choice diagnosis was made in only 57%, and in 73% the correct diagnosis was among the first three choices. In a similarly designed study by Grenier et al. (28) the diagnostic accuracy of chest radiographs determined in 140 consecutive patients with proven diffuse chronic lung disease was 64% for a first-choice diagnosis, and

---

TABLE 8-2. *Indications for the use of HRCT in patients with suspected diffuse lung disease*

Chronic Disease

1. To detect lung disease in patients with normal or questionable radiographic abnormalities, who have symptoms or pulmonary function findings suggestive of diffuse lung disease
2. To make a specific diagnosis, or limit the differential diagnosis, in patients with abnormal chest radiographs, in whom the clinical and radiographic findings are nonspecific, and further evaluation is considered appropriate
3. To assess disease activity, particularly in patients with IPF
4. As a guide for the need or optimal site and type of lung biopsy

Acute Disease

1. To detect lung disease in patients with symptoms of acute lung disease and normal or nondiagnostic chest radiographs, particularly in immunosuppressed patients
2. Patients presenting with hemoptysis
3. As a guide for the need or optimal site for lung biopsy

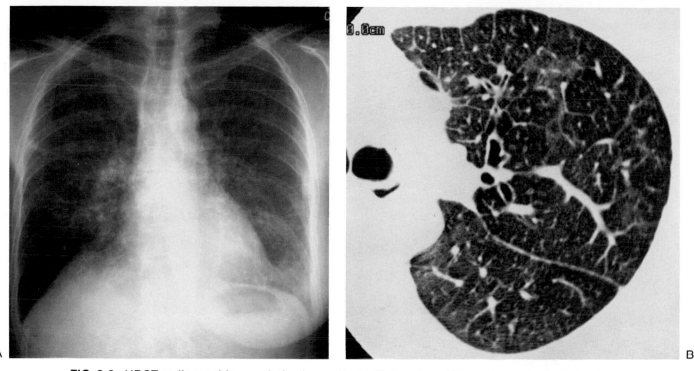

FIG. 8-6. HRCT-radiographic correlation in a patient with lymphangitic carcinomatosis. **A:** Posteroanterior chest radiograph in a middle-aged woman, following a right mastectomy. Increased reticular markings are visible but nonspecific; although these findings could be due to lymphangitic carcinomatosis, their differential diagnosis also includes radiation and/or drug-related pneumonitis, viral pneumonia, and even pulmonary edema. **B:** Targeted HRCT through the left upper lobe shows characteristic findings of lymphangitic carcinomatosis, including slightly nodular interlobular septal thickening.

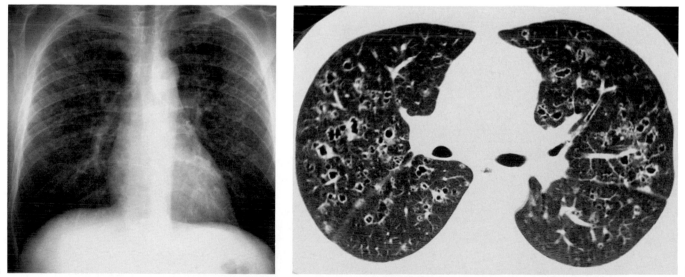

FIG. 8-7. HRCT-radiographic correlation in a patient with Histiocytosis X (Langerhans cell histiocytosis). **A:** Routine posteroanterior radiograph in an asymptomatic young male smoker shows diffuse increased "markings" throughout both lungs with relative sparing of the lung bases. **B:** HRCT through the mid-lungs shows unusually shaped cysts and a few small peripheral nodules, in the absence of reticulation. These findings are characteristic of patients with Langerhans cell histiocytosis, subsequently verified by transbronchial biopsy. In this case HRCT clearly enhances diagnostic accuracy, as compared with the corresponding chest radiograph.

78% if the top three choices were considered. These data substantiate that the accurate radiographic interpretation of DILD represents something of an art, relatively difficult to perform as well as to teach (74).

Given the precision with which HRCT can delineate lung morphology, it is not surprising that there is a close correlation between cross-sectional imaging findings and both gross and, to a lesser degree, microscopic

pathology. To date, close equivalence has been documented for a number of diseases including pulmonary fibrosis of varying causes, asbestosis, sarcoidosis, histiocytosis X (Langerhans cell histiocytosis), hypersensitivity pneumonitis, lymphangitic carcinomatosis, lymphangiomyomatosis, as well as various patterns of bronchiectasis and emphysema (78,79).

Numerous reports have shown that HRCT is signifi-

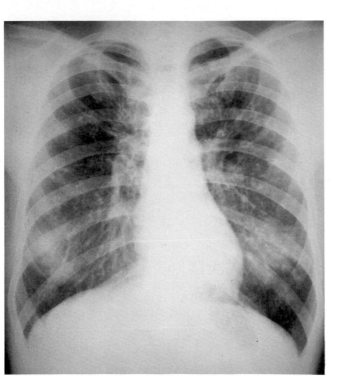

A

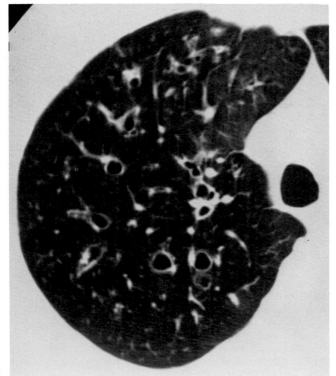

B

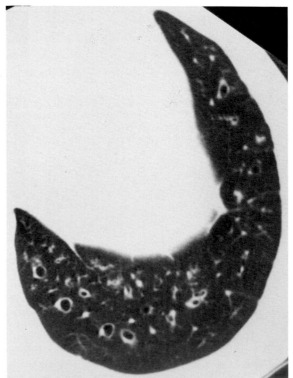

C

FIG. 8-8. HRCT-radiographic correlation in a patient with diffuse bronchiectasis. **A:** Posteroanterior chest radiograph shows nonspecific increased lung markings in both upper lobes, with a suggestion of focal, poorly-defined lucencies in the upper lobes. **B,C:** Targeted HRCT through the right upper lobe (B) and left lower lobe (C), show characteristic findings of bronchiectasis, in the absence of lung fibrosis.

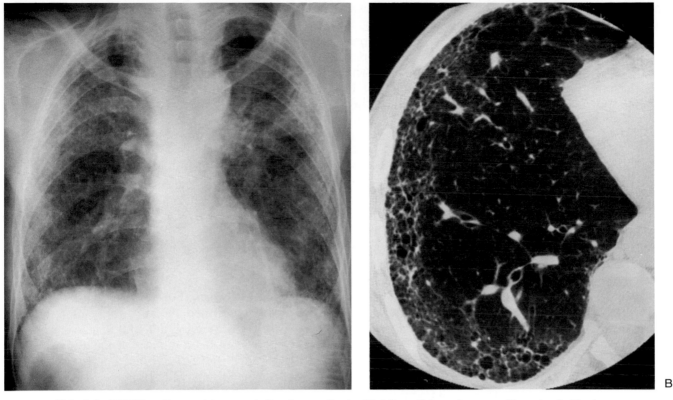

FIG. 8-9. HRCT-radiographic correlation in a patient with idiopathic pulmonary fibrosis. **A:** Posteroanterior radiograph shows diffuse increased reticular markings throughout both lung fields. Although this appearance is suggestive of parenchymal fibrosis, the pattern is nonspecific. **B:** Retrospectively targeted HRCT through the right lower lobe shows characteristic findings of honeycombing, with irregularly thick-walled cystic spaces, mild traction bronchiolectasis, and a strikingly peripheral distribution. Ground-glass opacity and nodules are absent. In this case, HRCT findings strongly mitigate against the need either for transbronchial or open lung biopsy.

cantly more accurate than are plain radiographs in diagnosing both acute and chronic diffuse lung disease, usually allowing a more confident diagnosis, and subject to considerably less interobserver variation in its interpretation (Figs. 8-6–8-9) (12,17,18,27,28,31,69, 80–84). Many of these studies have utilized an approach emphasizing the blinded interpretation of a series of radiographic and CT studies, in which individual observers have listed their first three diagnostic choices in decreasing order of probability, with degrees of confidence in these diagnoses usually expressed on

a three-point scale. Allowing for differences in patient populations, CT technique, and experimental design, these studies consistently show that the accuracy of HRCT in the diagnosis of diffuse lung disease is superior to that of chest radiography (Table 8-3).

In a study reported by Mathieson et al. (27), the accuracies of chest radiographs, and both conventional and high-resolution CT in making specific diagnoses were compared in 118 cases. A confident diagnosis was reached more than twice as often with CT and HRCT than with chest radiographs (49% vs. 23%, respec-

TABLE 8-3. *Comparative accuracy of chest radiographs and HRCT*

Study	Confident first-choice diagnosis		Correct first-choice diagnosis when confident		Correct first-choice diagnosis		Correct diagnosis in first 3 choices	
	CXR	HRCT	CXR	HRCT	CXR	HRCT	CXR	HRCT
Mathieson et al. (27)	23%	49%	77%	93%	57%	72%	73%	89%
Padley et al. (12)	41%	49%	69%	82%	47%	56%	72%	81%
Grenier et al. (28)	—	—	27%	53%	64%	76%	78%	83%
Nishimura et al. (80)	—	—	60%	63%	38%	46%	49%	59%
Average	32%	49%	58%	73%	52%	63%	67%	78%

tively). More importantly, a correct diagnosis was made in 93% of the first-choice CT interpretations, as compared to 77% of the first-choice plain film interpretations ($p < 0.001$). Similar findings have been reported by Padley et al. (12). In this study of 86 patients with DILD, comprising 15 different lung diseases, and 14 normal subjects, a confident diagnosis was reached more often with HRCT (49%) than with chest radiography (41%). Furthermore, the diagnoses were more often correct with HRCT (82%) than with chest radiographs (69%), and were associated with less interobserver disagreement.

The superior diagnostic accuracy of HRCT compared with plain radiographs has also been shown by Grenier et al. (28). In a study of 140 patients with 18 different DILDs, these authors found that the diagnostic accuracy of HRCT was significantly better than chest radiography. A correct first-choice diagnosis was made in 64% of cases with radiographs vs. 76% with HRCT, regardless of the confidence level. When a confident first choice diagnosis was made, HRCT proved accurate in 53% of cases, compared to 27% for chest radiographs ($p < 0.001$). In an attempt to further assess the role of HRCT, these authors also evaluated radiographic and CT findings by ranked stepwise discriminant analysis of five separate groups. These groups included patients with (i) sarcoidosis; (ii) pulmonary fibrosis; (iii) histiocytosis X (Langerhans cell histiocytosis); (iv) silicosis; and (v) miscellaneous diseases. Analyzed in this fashion, the four findings that were most discriminant in distinguishing these groups were visible on HRCT, and included intralobular reticular lines, thin-walled cysts, a peripheral distribution of abnormalities, and traction bronchiectasis. Similarly, 8 of the most discriminant 12 findings were on HRCT.

More recently, Nishimura et al. reported their findings comparing HRCT with plain radiographs in 134 cases of both acute and chronic diffuse lung disease representing 21 different entities, read without history, by 20 different physicians (80). These authors also confirmed the higher diagnostic accuracy of HRCT vs. chest radiographs, although slightly less convincingly than previous authors. Overall, a correct first-choice

diagnosis was made radiographically in 38% of cases vs. 46% using HRCT ($p < 0.01$), while the correct diagnosis was listed among the first three choices in 49% of cases radiographically vs. 59% of cases with HRCT.

Despite the overall similarity of the results of these studies, it should be noted that differences can be identified, especially in the reported accuracies of HRCT in diagnosing specific diseases (Table 8-4). These most likely reflect variations in the populations studied and CT technique. For example, Nishimura et al. (80) included diffuse infectious diseases (endobronchial spread of both tuberculosis and nontuberculous mycobacteria, and mycoplasmal pneumonia) in their study. As noted by the authors themselves, this most probably accounts for the slightly lower accuracy of HRCT in this study as compared to others. Differences in study design also probably account for some differences observed in the diagnostic accuracy of HRCT for specific diseases. For example, while all studies to date have confirmed the superiority of HRCT compared with chest radiography for diagnosing sarcoidosis, this has not been uniformly noted for all DILDs. Differences in the relative accuracies of HRCT vs. chest radiography have been noted for idiopathic pulmonary fibrosis, histiocytosis X, hypersensitivity pneumonitis, and even silicosis (Table 8-4) (27,28, 69,80).

In an attempt to further refine diagnostic accuracy, Grenier et al. used Bayesian analysis to determine the relative value of clinical data, chest radiographs, and HRCT in patients with chronic diffuse infiltrative lung disease (85). For this study, two samples from the same population of patients with 27 different diffuse lung diseases were consecutively assessed: an initial, retrospectively evaluated set of "training" cases ($n = 208$) and a subsequent prospectively evaluated set of "test" cases ($n = 100$) for validation. This approach enabled assignment of diagnostic probabilities based on clinical, radiologic, or CT variables. The results showed that for the test group, an accurate diagnosis could be made in 27% of cases based on clinical data only, increasing to 53% ($p < 0.0001$) with the addition of chest radiographs and to 61% ($p = 0.07$) with the further

TABLE 8-4. *Diseases in which HRCT is advantageous*

Disease	Mathieson et al. (27)	Grenier et al. (28)	Grenier et al. (85)	Nishimura et al. (80)	Padley et al. (12)
Sarcoidosis	X	X	X	X	
UIP	X			X	
Histiocytosis X	X	X	X		X
Hypersensitivity pneumonitis			X	X	
Lymphangitic carcinomatosis	X		X		X
Silicosis	X		X	X	
Alveolar proteinosis				X	X
LAM				X	X
BOOP/COP				X	X

addition of HRCT scans. Assessed for individual diseases, HRCT made the greatest contribution to the diagnosis of sarcoidosis, histiocytosis X (Langerhans cell histiocytosis), hypersensitivity pneumonitis, lymphangitic carcinomatosis, and to a lesser degree silicosis (Table 8-4). Although only minor improvement was seen in the diagnosis of pulmonary fibrosis, as the authors themselves note, this probably reflected a population with advanced disease, as virtually all of these patients presented with diffuse radiographic abnormalities. Not surprisingly, the value of HRCT diminished with less common diseases; 23 (68%) of 34 misdiagnosed patients in this study had diseases classified as "miscellaneous."

Some low-dose HRCT techniques have also been shown to be more accurate than chest radiographs in diagnosing diffuse lung disease (Fig. 8-10). In a study by Lee et al. (83), the diagnostic accuracy of chest radiographs, low-dose HRCT (80 mAs; 120 kVp, 40 mA, 2 sec), and conventional-dose HRCT (340 mAs; 120 kVp, 170 mA, 2 sec) were compared in 10 normal controls and 50 patients with chronic infiltrative lung disease. For each HRCT technique, only three images were used, obtained at the levels of the aortic arch, tracheal carina, and 1-cm above the right hemidiaphragm. A correct first-choice diagnosis was made significantly more often with either HRCT technique than with radiography; the correct diagnosis was made in 65% of cases using radiographs, 74% of cases with low-dose HRCT ($p < 0.02$), and 80% of conventional HRCT ($p < 0.005$). A high-confidence level in making a diagnosis was reached in 42% of radiographic examinations, 61% of the low-dose ($p < 0.01$), and 63% of

the conventional-dose HRCT examinations ($p < 0.005$), which were correct in 92%, 90%, and 96% of the studies, respectively. Although conventional-dose HRCT was more accurate than low-dose HRCT, this difference was not significant, and both techniques were felt to provide quite similar anatomic information (Figs. 1-7,1-8,8-7) (83).

The diagnostic accuracy of HRCT has also been assessed relative to that of CCT. In one study (68), the authors randomly compared three HRCT sections with (i) conventional CT scans obtained at the same three levels and (ii) a complete conventional CT study of the lungs, in 75 patients with proven diffuse lung disease. In each case, observers provided their most likely diagnoses as well as their degrees of confidence. Although there was no real difference in diagnostic accuracy, the highest confidence level in diagnosis (49%) was reached using the three available HRCT sections, as compared with 31% for interpretation based on the corresponding three 10-mm sections and 43% for interpretations based on a complete set of contiguous CCT sections through the thorax. Based on these data, the authors concluded that in patients with diffuse lung disease the correct diagnosis may be suggested by only a limited number of HRCT scans, eliminating the need for a complete conventional CT examination (68).

"Diagnostic" Appearances on HRCT

HRCT is often indicated in patients with an abnormal chest radiograph, when radiographic and clinical findings are nonspecific, and further evaluation is considered appropriate (Table 8-2). In this setting, HRCT findings can often be used to limit the differential diagnosis to a few possibilities, and this can be of considerable value in determining the subsequent diagnostic evaluation. In select cases, HRCT appearances can be diagnostic, or so strongly suggestive that lung biopsy can be avoided. In our judgment, in the appropriate clinical setting there are some diseases in which information derived from HRCT can be sufficiently characteristic to allow a specific or presumptive diagnosis to be made in the absence of histologic verification (Table 8-5).

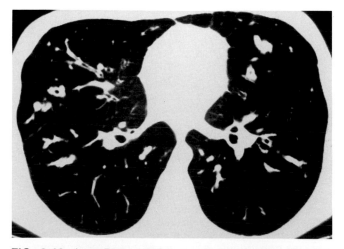

FIG. 8-10. Low-Dose HRCT. A 1.5-mm section through the mid-lungs in a patient with cystic fibrosis and evidence of diffuse bronchiectasis and mucoid impaction. Although this study was performed using 40 mAs, morphologic detail in the lung is comparable to most routine HRCT images. (Courtesy of Minnie Bhalla, M.D., New York University Medical Center, New York, New York.)

TABLE 8-5. *Diseases which can have a "diagnostic" appearance on HRCT*

Hypersensitivity Pneumonitis
Sarcoidosis
Pneumoniosis
Histiocytosis X
Lymphangiomyomatosis
Bronchiectasis
Emphysema
IUP (Honeycombing)

For example, HRCT findings of patchy and centri-lobular ground-glass opacities suggest the diagnosis of hypersensitivity pneumonitis; this diagnosis can usually be confirmed by the clinical history and appropriate serologic tests, precluding lung biopsy (Figs. 8-2,8-11) (86,87). Indeed, in our experience, HRCT findings not infrequently lead to the first suspicion of the diagnosis of hypersensitivity pneumonitis.

It is apparent that in the appropriate clinical setting, classic findings of peribronchovascular and subpleural nodules, especially when associated with central airway abnormalities, should allow a confident diagnosis of sarcoidosis (Fig. 8-12) (20,21,27,85,88–90). Biopsy should be avoidable in most cases.

Likewise, when the HRCT features are highly suggestive of pneumoconiosis and there is a well-documented history of prior occupational exposure, lung biopsy is seldom required. This is especially true of patients with silica and asbestos exposure (67).

In our experience, HRCT can also prove diagnostic in patients with lymphangiomyomatosis, histiocytosis X (Langerhans cell histiocytosis) (Fig. 8-7), and lymphangitic carcinomatosis (Fig. 8-6) provided the HRCT shows characteristic abnormalities, and in the appropriate clinical settings (13,27,28,78,79,85,88). HRCT can also allow a confident diagnosis of both bronchiectasis and emphysema (Fig. 8-8).

HRCT findings have been shown to be highly accurate in making a diagnosis of IPF or other causes of UIP (Fig. 8-9) (81,91,92). As shown by Tung et al., in a study of 86 patients, including 41 with IPF and 45 with various other diffuse lung diseases, HRCT accurately identified 88% of patients with IPF. Based on these data, these authors have gone so far as to suggest that the typical HRCT appearance is "virtually pathognomonic" (91). Although no doubt an exaggeration, HRCT clearly may be of value in identifying patients likely to have IPF, or other causes of UIP, and honeycombing who present with radiographic evidence of nonspecific reticulation. Even more importantly, in the majority of patients who present with clinical features of idiopathic pulmonary fibrosis, the presence of predominantly subpleural and basal distribution of fibrosis on HRCT can be sufficiently characteristic to obviate biopsy, especially in those patients in which HRCT shows no evidence suggesting disease activity (Fig. 8-9) (93,94).

As documented by Primack et al., HRCT is even of value in differentiating among the various causes of end-stage lung disease. In this study of 61 consecutive patients, observers made a correct first-choice diagnosis in an average of 87% of cases, including 100% of cases with silicosis and histiocytosis X, 90% of patients with asbestosis, and 88% of patients with usual interstitial pneumonia (81). Conventional wisdom to the contrary (95), these data strongly suggest that open lung biopsy may be unnecessary in order to distinguish some causes of diffuse pulmonary fibrosis.

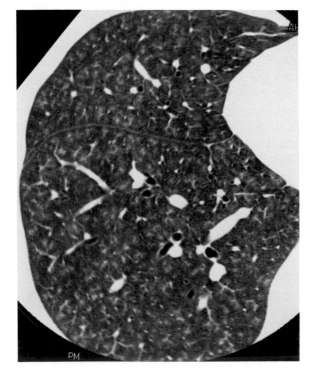

FIG. 8-11. Hypersensitivity pneumonitis with suggestive HRCT findings. Retrospectively targeted HRCT through the right middle and lower lobes shows a pattern of poorly defined centrilobular nodules evenly distributed throughout the lungs, in the absence of reticular changes or ground-glass opacity. Although this pattern can be seen in a number of diseases, it is most characteristic of subacute hypersensitivity pneumonitis. In this case, the patient was scanned prior to bronchoscopy for evaluation of otherwise nonspecific infiltrates on chest radiographs (not shown). Based on the HRCT findings, a specific diagnosis of hypersensitivity pneumonitis was suggested, leading to the appropriate diagnosis without a necessity for histologic confirmation.

ASSESSMENT OF DISEASE ACTIVITY AND PROGNOSIS WITH HRCT

In addition to being more sensitive, specific, and accurate than chest radiographs, HRCT may also play a critical role in the evaluation of disease activity in patients with diffuse lung disease. Available data suggest that, in certain cases, HRCT may be used to determine the presence or absence, and extent, of reversible (acute or active) lung disease as compared to irreversible (fibrotic) lung disease. Furthermore, because HRCT may accurately identify subtle "active" lung disease, it can be used to follow patients who are being treated, in order to monitor the success or failure of the treatment that is being employed (40,96–99).

Although a number of HRCT findings have been described as being indicative of active or reversible lung disease in patients with different disease entities (Table 8-6), most attention has focused on the potential significance of ground-glass opacity in patients with chronic diffuse infiltrative lung disease (100). To date, this find-

ing has been reported in a wide range of diffuse infiltrative lung diseases, including idiopathic pulmonary fibrosis and other causes of UIP, desquamative interstitial pneumonitis (Figs. 4-14,4-15,6-8,6-9,8-13), lymphocytic interstitial pneumonitis (Fig. 4-1), sarcoidosis (Fig. 5-16), hypersensitivity pneumonitis Figs. 8-2,8-11), alveolar proteinosis, bronchiolitis obliterans organizing pneumonia, respiratory bronchiolitis (Fig. 6-10), and chronic eosinophilic pneumonia (100). Ground-glass opacity also has been described in patients with neoplasms, in particular bronchioloalveolar carcinoma as well as a wide variety of acute lung processes, such as acute interstitial pneumonia (Fig. 6-39), bacterial (Fig. 8-9), fungal, viral (Figs. 6-36,6-37), and *Pneumocystis carinii* infections (Figs. 6-26,6-27), pulmonary hemorrhage syndromes (Fig. 3-57), and congestive heart failure and other causes of pulmonary edema. Ground-glass opacity has even been described in such unusual diseases as extramedullary hematopoesis and in patients with metastatic pulmonary calcification (101,102).

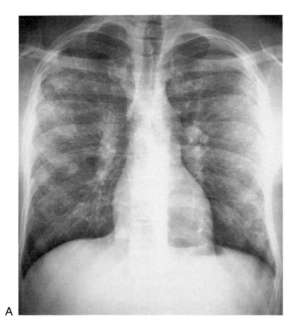

A

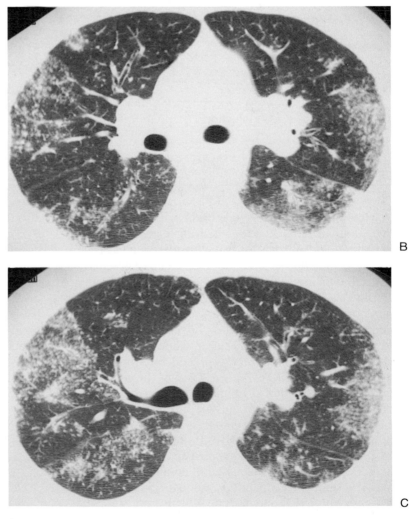

B

C

FIG. 8-12. Sarcoidosis with diagnostic HRCT findings. **A:** Posteroanterior radiograph in an asymptomatic 20-year-old man shows symmetric bilateral hilar and mediastinal lymphadenopathy associated with bilateral, ill-defined reticulonodular opacities. **B,C:** HRCT through the mid- and upper-lung fields, respectively, confirms the presence of diffuse, poorly defined parenchymal nodules, clustered in a predominantly peribronchovascular distribution. In this case, the combination of clinical, radiographic, and HRCT findings were sufficiently characteristic to warrant empiric therapy without the need for biopsy confirmation.

TABLE 8-6. *HRCT findings and histologic abnormalities associated with active diffuse lung disease*

Diagnosis	HRCT findings	Histologic findings
Usual Interstitial Pneumonia (UIP) in IPF, Scleroderma, Rheumatoid Lung Disease, etc.	Ground-glass opacity	Alveolar septal inflammation; intra-alveolar histiocytes; fibrosis
Desquamative Interstitial Pneumonia (DIP)	Ground-glass opacity	Alveolar macrophages; interstitial inflammatory infiltrate
Lymphocytic Interstitial Pneumonia (LIP)	Ground-glass opacity	Mature lymphocytic and plasma cell infiltrates
Bronchiolitis obliterans organizing pneumonia (BOOP/COP)	Consolidation, ground-glass opacity, nodules	Alveolar septal inflammation; alveolar cellular desquamation
Sarcoidosis, Berylliosis	Nodules, less often ground-glass opacity	Numerous small granulomas
Hypersensitivity Pneumonitis	Ground-glass opacity	Alveolitis, poorly defined granulomas, cellular bronchiolitis
Alveolar proteinosis	Ground-glass opacity, septal thickening	Intra-alveolar and septal lipo-protein
Acute Interstitial Pneumonia	Ground-glass opacity, consolidation	Interstitial inflammatory exudate; edema; diffuse alveolar damage
Pneumocystis carinii pneumonia	Ground-glass opacity	Alveolar inflammatory exudate, alveolar septal thickening
Eosinophilic pneumonia	Consolidation, ground-glass opacity	Eosinophilic interstitial infiltrate; alveolar eosinophils and histiocytes
Respiratory bronchiolitis	Ground-glass opacity, centrilobular nodules	Pigment-containing alveolar macrophages
Tuberculosis	Small nodules, centrilobular opacities, tree-in-bud, consolidation	Miliary spread, endobronchial spread of infection, pneumonia
Nontuberculous mycobacterial infection	Bronchiectasis, centrilobular opacities, tree-in-bud	Chronic infection, endobronchial spread of infection
Cytomegalovirus (CMV) Infection	Ground-glass opacity, consolidation, reticulation	Diffuse alveolar damage, interlobular and intralobular thickening
Histiocytosis X	Nodules	Granulomas containing Langerhans histiocytes and eosinophils

Although ground-glass opacity is a nonspecific finding, and can reflect various histologic abnormalities, in patients with chronic diffuse infiltrative lung disease, ground-glass opacity often represents active parenchymal inflammation (Table 8-6). As reported by Remy-Jardin et al. (93), in a study of 26 patients with DILD in whom histologic correlation was obtained, biopsies demonstrated that ground-glass opacity corresponded to inflammation in 24 (65%) cases, while in 8 additional cases (22%), inflammation was present but fibrosis predominated; in only 5 (13%), was fibrosis the sole histologic finding. Similarly, Leung et al. in a study of 22 patients with a variety of chronic infiltrative lung diseases and evidence of ground-glass opacity either as a predominant or exclusive HRCT finding showed that 18 (82%) had potentially active disease identified on lung biopsy (103). As discussed in detail in Chapters 3 and 4, ground-glass opacity is a nonspecific finding in patients with DILD and does not always represent "alveolitis" or lung inflammation. Ground-glass opacity may also be seen in the presence of interstitial fibrosis and without disease activity (100,103). In order to strongly suggest that ground-glass opacity indicates active disease, this finding should generally be unassociated with HRCT findings of fibrosis (93,103).

In general, HRCT is indicated in the assessment of disease activity in patients with chronic diffuse lung disease, and in the detection of active disease in some patients with suspected acute lung disease and normal or nonspecific chest radiographs (Table 8-2). In patients with chronic lung disease, the assessment of disease activity is most clearly indicated in patients with idiopathic pulmonary fibrosis (IPF) or other causes of usual interstitial pneumonia (UIP). Its utility in demonstrating HRCT findings of active disease in other chronic diseases, including sarcoidosis and hypersensitivity pneumonitis, remains to be established (Table 8-6).

Disease Activity in IPF and UIP

To date, the significance of ground-glass opacity as a potential marker of disease activity has been most thoroughly evaluated in patients with idiopathic pul-

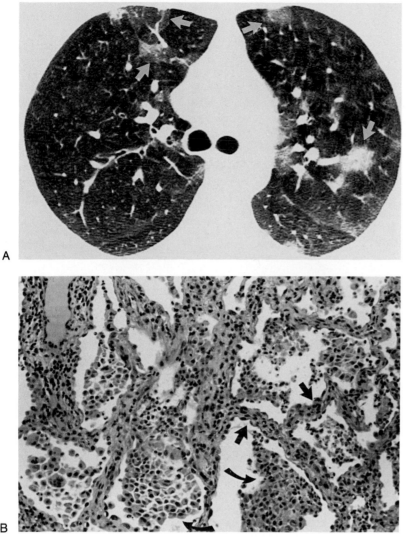

FIG. 8-13. Ground-glass opacification; HRCT pathologic correlation. **A:** HRCT at the level of the carina in a 40-year-old man with desquamative interstitial pneumonitis and marked disease activity. HRCT shows patchy bilateral areas of ground-glass opacity (*arrows*) highly suggestive of active alveolitis. **B:** Corresponding histologic section from an open lung biopsy obtained in this same patient demonstrates alveolar septal inflammation (*straight arrows*) and intra-alveolar histiocytes (*curved arrows*) characteristic of active alveolitis. The combination of alveolar septal inflammation and intra-alveolar histiocytes account for the air-space opacification seen on CT.

monary fibrosis (IPF); this disease is relatively common, and its clinical course is notoriously difficult to predict (96,104–107). Traditional methods of assessing disease activity, including transbronchial biopsy and/or bronchoalveolar lavage, chest radiographs, gallium scintigraphy, and pulmonary function testing have all proven unreliable indicators both of disease activity and prognosis in patients with IPF. As a consequence, open lung biopsy has remained the "gold standard" both for the diagnosis of IPF as well as assessment of disease activity (95).

In patients with IPF, a significant correlation has been found between the presence of HRCT findings of ground-glass opacity and pathologic findings of active inflammation (104,108), the development of pulmonary fibrosis, the patient's prognosis (94,96,99,105,106), and the likelihood of response to therapy (96,99,107).

In the largest study to date of HRCT findings in patients with IPF, Wells et al. (94) found that the presence of ground-glass opacity and its extent, relative to findings of fibrosis, was related to prognosis and likelihood

of response to treatment. In this study, CT abnormalities were interpreted as predominantly ground-glass opacity (group 1), mixed ground-glass and reticular opacities (group 2), or predominantly reticular opacities (group 3). Four-year survival was highest in patients with predominant ground-glass opacity, and higher in patients with mixed opacities than in those with reticular abnormalities, independent of the duration of symptoms, or severity of pulmonary function abnormalities ($p < 0.001$). Similarly, response to therapy in previously untreated patients was significantly greater in patients with predominant ground-glass opacity, and greater in group 2 than in group 3 (94). It is important to note that the HRCT findings reported in patients with desquamative interstitial pneumonia (DIP) bear a striking resemblance to those of the group 1 patients described by Wells et al. in their assessment of IPF (Fig. 8-13) (52,94); DIP typically responds well to treatment, and has a relatively good prognosis.

These cumulative data suggest that HRCT should play a decisive role both in the diagnosis and assessment of disease activity in patients with suspected IPF prior to biopsy and treatment. By differentiating between patients with a predominantly ground-glass pattern of abnormality and those with a predominantly fibrotic pattern as represented by traction bronchiectasis, bronchiolectasis, and/or honeycombing, HRCT can be used to identify those patients most likely to respond to therapy, without the need for histologic confirmation. Although not as thoroughly documented, it is apparent that HRCT can also provide an accurate, noninvasive method for following the course of patients receiving therapy. Furthermore, in patients with predominant HRCT findings of fibrosis and

honeycombing, it can be suggested with confidence that the likelihood of active disease or a response to therapy is low, and that lung biopsy is unlikely to yield significant information (Fig. 8-9).

It should be emphasized that these conclusions primarily pertain to patients with idiopathic pulmonary fibrosis. The role of HRCT in assessing prognosis in other diseases associated with lung fibrosis remains to be evaluated. Although findings similar to those described in patients with IPF also have been identified in patients with parenchymal fibrosis secondary to systemic sclerosis (scleroderma), for example, including close correlation between HRCT abnormalities and

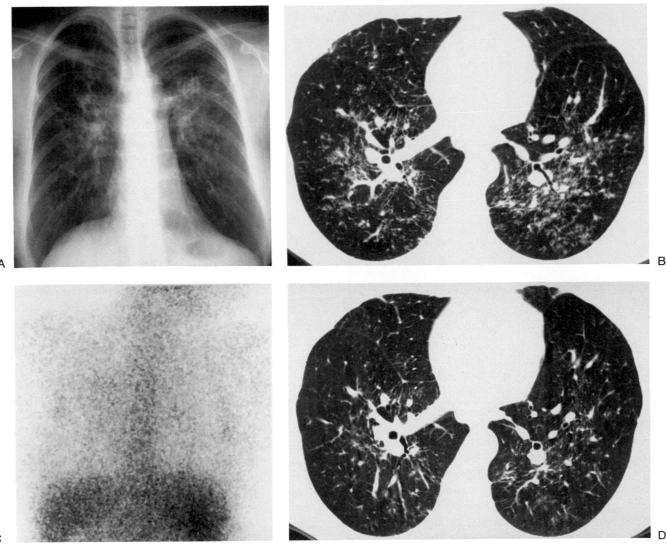

FIG. 8-14. Disease activity in sarcoidosis. **A:** Posteroanterior chest radiograph shows findings of stage 3 sarcoidosis. **B:** HRCT through the lower lobes obtained at the same time as the chest radiograph shows poorly defined peribronchovascular nodules typical of sarcoidosis and the presence of granulomas. **C:** Anteroposterior scintigraphic image obtained 48 hours after administration of ^{67}Ga citrate shows scant evidence of abnormal activity. **D:** HRCT obtained at the same level as B following 6 weeks of steroid therapy. Note that there is a marked reduction in the number of nodules identifiable in both lungs. This change is consistent with regression of parenchymal granulomas.

findings at bronchoalveolar lavage and biopsy, the prognostic significance of these findings is less certain (106,109).

The significance of HRCT findings in assessing disease activity has also been shown in patients with hypersensitivity pneumonitis (51). Those patients in whom the primary CT abnormalities included diffuse small ill-defined nodules, ground-glass opacity, and focal air-trapping in the absence of diffuse reticulation and/or honeycombing uniformly improved following cessation of exposure, while those with a predominantly fibrotic pattern showed little if any change.

Disease Activity in Sarcoidosis

HRCT has been used to assess disease activity as well as the likelihood of response to therapy in patients with sarcoidosis (40,97,110–112). In most series of patients with sarcoidosis, the main HRCT determinant of disease activity has been the presence and, to a lesser degree, the extent and distribution of small nodules. The finding of ground-glass opacity has proved to be of lesser diagnostic or prognostic significance (112); although ground-glass opacity has been identified in a small subset of patients with sarcoidosis, in most cases this finding probably results from conglomerates of small nodules below the resolution of HRCT (110). Generally speaking, nodules and areas of parenchymal consolidation or ground-glass opacity decrease or disappear following treatment; in distinction, little if any change can usually be identified after treatment in patients showing parenchymal reticulation, cystic airspaces, and/or architectural distortion on HRCT (Figs. 5-19,8-14) (40,97).

Unfortunately, despite this distinction between reversible and irreversible HRCT findings in patients with sarcoidosis, the utility of HRCT in patient management has yet to be clearly defined. Unlike patients with idiopathic pulmonary fibrosis, in most patients with sarcoidosis, a combination of clinical, radiographic, scintigraphic, and/or bronchoscopic findings are usually adequate for successful diagnosis and management (113). Furthermore, in a recent study, Remy-Jardin et al. (112) did not find a significant correlation between the presence of nodules on HRCT and disease activity as measured by serum angiotensin converting enzyme activity and/or lymphocytosis at bronchoalveolar lavage (112). However, it must be pointed out that these measures of disease activity do not necessarily reflect the activity of sarcoid granulomas in the lung (110). In this study (112), only the profusion of septal lines correlated with serum angiotensin converting enzyme activity and/or lymphocytosis at bronchoalveolar lavage, and the authors concluded that HRCT findings were of no value in predicting the evolution of lung changes over time. Given the seemingly contradictory results of this study and those reported previously, it is apparent that a definitive conclusion regarding the role of HRCT in assessing disease activity in patients with sarcoidosis will have to await further evaluation.

Acute Lung Diseases

In addition to assessing disease activity in patients with chronic diffuse infiltrative lung diseases, HRCT has also proved to be of value in assessing disease activity in patients with acute lung diseases, especially those associated with infection (Fig. 8-15). Clinically, this has been most useful in the evaluation of immunocompromised patients, and particularly those patients with AIDS. As shown by Hartman et al. in a review of CT scans from 102 AIDS patients with intrathoracic

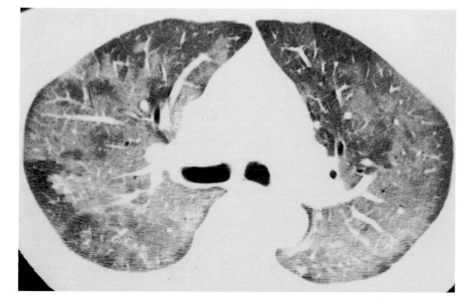

FIG. 8-15. Ground-glass opacity in acute lung disease. HRCT at the level of the carina in a febrile patient with mycoplasmal pneumonia. HRCT shows a pattern of diffuse ground-glass opacity. In this case, these changes are primarily the result of diffuse air-space disease.

abnormalities and 20 HIV-positive patients without intrathoracic disease, acute disease was correctly diagnosed in more than 99% of cases (31). In patients with acute lung disease, ground-glass opacity has been shown to accurately reflect the presence of air-space consolidation, especially in patients with pneumonia due to such organisms as *Pneumocystis carinii* although other findings can also be indicative of active infectious disease (17,31,55,114–116).

HRCT may play a pivotal role in assessing disease activity in patients with mycobacterial infections with or without a history of immune compromise. Im et al. evaluated sequential HRCT scans before and after antituberculous chemotherapy in a total of 26 patients with documented active tuberculosis (44). On HRCT examination the most common findings was the presence of centrilobular nodules and/or linear branching structures (''tree-in-bud'') corresponding pathologically to the presence of small airways filled with infected material; in virtually all cases, sequential studies showed these opacities to be reversible within 5 months after the start of treatment. Furthermore, in 11 of 12 patients with recent reactivation, HRCT accurately differentiated old fibrotic lesions from new active ones (44). Based on this data, the authors concluded that HRCT was a reliable method for determining disease activity in patients with mycobacterial infection.

Despite HRCT findings, definitive diagnosis and treatment of mycobacterial infection in most cases still requires that organisms be cultured. Although HRCT is not routinely recommended for evaluating patients with suspected tuberculosis, it may provide the initial clue to the diagnosis, especially in patients with AIDS. As reported by Bissuel et al. (117) in a retrospective study of 57 HIV-infected patients presenting with fever of unknown origin, CT examination proved to be the one test that contributed most to the diagnosis of mycobacterial infection by disclosing otherwise unsuspected adenopathy in 7 (38%) of 18 scans performed.

DETERMINATION OF LUNG BIOPSY SITE AND TYPE

Among the many indications for using HRCT, perhaps the most important is as a potential guide for lung biopsy (Table 8-2). Many ''diffuse'' lung diseases are quite patchy in distribution, with areas of abnormal lung frequently interspersed among relatively normal areas of lung parenchyma. Furthermore, both active and fibrotic disease can be present in the same lung (94,95,106). In order to establish a specific diagnosis and assess the clinical significance of the abnormalities present, it is critically important to selectively sample those portions of the lung that are abnormal and most likely to be active. This can be accomplished by using

HRCT. Also, as a direct consequence of its ability to visualize, characterize, and determine the distribution of parenchymal disease, HRCT also provides a unique insight into the likely efficacy of transbronchial (TBBx) or open lung biopsy (via thoracotomy or video-assisted thoracoscopy) in patients with either acute or chronic diffuse lung disease.

Lung Biopsy in Chronic Infiltrative Lung Disease

To date, there is little consensus as to the best method for establishing a diagnosis in patients with suspected DILD (118). Available methods include fiberoptic bronchoscopy either with transbronchial biopsy and/or bronchoalveolar lavage, or open lung biopsy.

Although transbronchial biopsy (TBBx) is frequently used in an attempt to diagnose diffuse lung disease, the limitations of TBBx for establishing the etiology of diffuse pulmonary disease have been well documented. In a classic study, Wall et al. showed that TBBx was diagnostic in only 20 (38%) of 53 patients presenting with radiographic evidence of diffuse lung disease (119). In the remaining 33 cases, transbronchial biopsies were reported either as normal or nonspecific, whereas open lung biopsies resulted in specific diagnoses in 92%. Similar results have been reported by Wilson et al. (120) in a study of 127 patients with a variety of parenchymal abnormalities. They found that TBBx allowed a ''specific'' diagnosis in only 52% of patients with diffuse infiltrative processes. Also, diagnoses suggested by transbronchial biopsy may bear little relationship to diagnoses subsequently made on open biopsy (119), and a nonspecific transbronchial biopsy diagnosis, such as ''interstitial pneumonia'' or ''interstitial fibrosis'' should be considered as potentially misleading (95).

In patients with chronic diffuse lung disease, transbronchial biopsy is most accurate in patients with sarcoidosis or lymphangitic carcinomatosis (119); these entities preferentially involve peribronchial tissues and therefore are most accessible to transbronchial biopsy (Fig. 8-16) (89,119). Although the accuracy of transbronchial biopsy has improved over the past decade, especially in establishing such diagnoses as Langerhans cell histiocytosis, pulmonary alveolar proteinosis, eosinophilic lung disease, Goodpasture's syndrome, and Wegener's granulomatosis, these entities represent a distinct minority of cases (1,121). More importantly, there has been little improvement in the ability of TBBx or bronchoalveolar lavage to assess patients with pulmonary fibrosis (95).

Open lung biopsy (OLBx) is often diagnostic, with accuracies greater than 90% generally reported (11,119,122), but this procedure is also subject to sampling error, as biopsies taken from a small region of

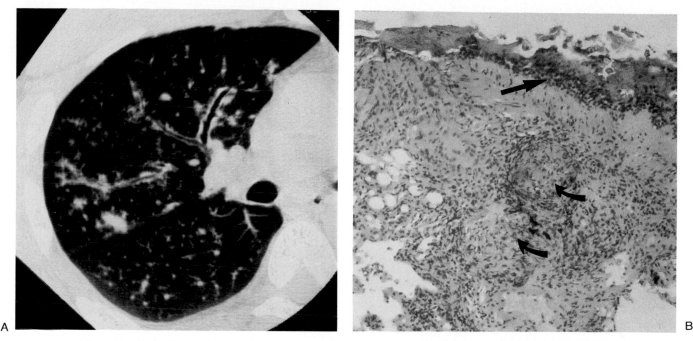

FIG. 8-16. HRCT/bronchoscopic correlation in sarcoidosis. **A:** Retrospectively targeted HRCT through the right upper lobe shows peribronchial nodules associated with narrowing and irregular thickening of bronchial walls. This appearance is characteristic of sarcoidosis. **B:** Photomicrograph of a specimen obtained following transbronchial biopsy clearly shows the intimate relationship between the bronchial mucosa (*straight arrow*) and noncaseating granulomata (*curved arrows*). Not surprisingly, transbronchial biopsies are most accurate in diseases such as sarcoid or lymphangitic carcinomatosis that preferentially involve the bronchial wall. These entities also produce characteristic changes easily identified with HRCT.

lung may not reflect the state of the diseased lung as a whole. This is most important when attempts are made to assess disease activity in patients with diffuse fibrotic lung diseases such as idiopathic pulmonary fibrosis or collagen vascular disease (95). It has been emphasized that the role of the surgeon at the time of open lung biopsy is to obtain representative tissue, while avoiding areas of extensive honeycombing (11). However, this may be difficult, especially in patients with idiopathic pulmonary fibrosis, owing to the predominantly subpleural distribution of the fibrosis. Furthermore, as shown by Newman et al. (123), the routine practice of obtaining lingular biopsies may lead to nonspecific findings in patients with patchy disease, and the lingula may not be a valid biopsy site when compared to biopsy material obtained simultaneously from two other lung segments.

Given the limitations of both transbronchial and open biopsy techniques, it is not surprising that HRCT has emerged as an important tool for assessing patients with suspected DILD prior to lung biopsy. HRCT is of considerable value in determining the most appropriate sites for biopsy (82). As already noted, diffuse pulmonary disease is frequently non-uniform or patchy in distribution, and HRCT can be used to target the lung regions most likely to be active and, therefore, most likely to be diagnostic (Fig. 8-10). Also, using HRCT,

areas of end-stage honeycombing can be avoided. Second, HRCT can play a decisive role in selecting among transbronchial biopsy, lavage and/or open lung biopsy as the most efficacious method for obtaining a histologic diagnosis. Of particular value is the identification of peribronchial abnormalities, as characteristically occur in patients with sarcoidosis (20,21,28,111,124) and lymphangitic carcinomatosis (27,125,126). As shown by Lenique et al., the demonstration of abnormal airways in patients with sarcoidosis clearly correlates with the likelihood of obtaining a histologic diagnosis (Fig. 8-16) (89). In this study, HRCT findings were compared both with the macroscopic or visual appearance of the airways during fiberoptic bronchoscopy as well as the results of both endo- and transbronchial biopsies; bronchial abnormalities were present in 39 (65%) of 60 patients (89). There was particularly good correlation between HRCT findings and biopsy results—of 39 patients with evidence of bronchial wall thickening on HRCT, biopsies showed typical granulomatous changes in 31 (80%) (Fig. 8-16). Still more convincingly, 13 (93%) of 14 patients with HRCT evidence of bronchial luminal abnormalities had positive biopsies. As reliance was placed almost exclusively on the use of endobronchial instead of transbronchial biopsies to establish the diagnosis in this study, it is likely that a histologic diagnosis would have been still more common if transbronchial biopsies had been routinely employed.

Not surprisingly, HRCT has proved far more efficacious than chest radiographs in predicting the likely efficacy of TBBx for diagnosing DILD. Mathieson et al. (27) compared the accuracy of plain radiographs and CT in determining whether transbronchial biopsy or open lung biopsy would be most appropriate in patients with chronic infiltrative lung disease. Using CT, three observers correctly predicted that a transbronchial biopsy would be necessary for diagnosis in 87% of patients in which this was appropriate. They correctly predicted the need for open lung biopsy in 99% of cases. By comparison, plain radiographs proved significantly less valuable ($p < 0.001$).

Recently, video-assisted thoracoscopic lung biopsy (VAT) has gained acceptance as an alternate to thoracotomy for performing an open lung biopsy. As most

studies confirm equivalent diagnostic accuracy, VAT may be the preferred method given lower cost and morbidity compared with thoracotomy (122). Because the operator's field of view is rather limited when performing this procedure, HRCT has proven extremely helpful in directing the surgeon to the most appropriate biopsy site. Additionally, using CT guidance, needle localization of the biopsy site may be performed prior to the procedure. Although this technique has been described primarily as a localization technique for resection of lung nodules (127,128), it has proved equally applicable to the biopsy of diffuse lung disease.

Lung Biopsy in Acute Lung Disease

In addition to evaluating specific diffuse chronic infiltrative lung diseases prior to biopsy, HRCT also plays a complementary role to fiberoptic bronchos-

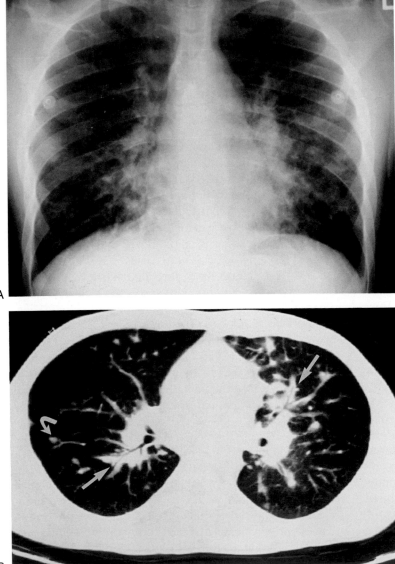

FIG. 8-17. HRCT diagnosis of Kaposi's sarcoma. **A:** Posteroanterior radiograph shows bilateral perihilar nodular infiltrates in a patient with AIDS. There is also a suggestion of mediastinal adenopathy in the region of the aorticopulmonary window. These findings are nonspecific. **B:** HRCT section through the hila shows bilateral peribronchial infiltrates emanating from the hila (*arrows*) associated with a few peripheral, perivascular nodules (*curved arrow*). This appearance is characteristic of intraparenchymal KS especially in patients with previously documented cutaneous involvement.

copy in the assessment of patients with acute diffuse lung disease. Although bronchoalveolar lavage and transbronchial biopsy are generally more accurate in diagnosing acute lung disease than chronic lung disease, there is still considerable controversy concerning appropriate guidelines for the use of these techniques (129,130).

It cannot be overemphasized that meaningful evaluation of the role of both HRCT and fiberoptic bronchoscopy must take into account the clinical and in particular the immune status of patients being evaluated (82). HRCT has been shown to play an especially important potential role in the prebronchoscopic assessment of immunocompromised patients. As documented by Janzen et al., in a retrospective study evaluating 33 consecutive immunocompromised non-AIDS patients (including 20 bone marrow transplant patients) presenting with acute pulmonary disease with both HRCT and bronchoscopy (82), bronchoscopy provided a specific diagnosis in 17 (52%) of 33 patients. Significantly, bronchoscopy proved diagnostic more often in patients with HRCT disease involving the central vs. the peripheral third of the lungs (70% vs. 23%, $p = 0.02$). Results also proved more diagnostic in patients with infectious vs. noninfectious disease (71% vs. 17%, $p < 0.005$). Based on these findings the authors concluded that HRCT should precede bronchoscopy in immunocompromised patients in order to determine optimal sites for biopsy as well as predict likely results of bronchoscopy.

Similar studies have also concluded a role for HRCT in evaluating bone marrow transplant patients (49,131). Mori et al. in a study of 33 febrile bone marrow recipients found that CT showed nodules in 20 of 21 episodes of documented fungal infection but none in nine bacteremic episodes (49). From this data, the authors concluded that CT studies showing the presence of nodules in this population could be taken as presumptive evidence of fungal infection warranting empiric therapy without the need for bronchoscopy. In a similar prospective study of 36 symptomatic episodes in 33 bone marrow transplant patients, Barloon et al. reported that in comparison with plain radiographs, HRCT resulted in a change of management in a total of 11 (50%) of 22 patients, including establishing the need for bronchoscopy and/or open lung biopsy in 6 patients (131).

HRCT may also play a role in the prebronchoscopic assessment of symptomatic patients with AIDS. As reported by Hartman et al., in an assessment of 102 patients with AIDS and 20 HIV-positive patients without active intrathoracic disease, HRCT proved especially accurate in the confident diagnosis of *Pneumocystis carinii* pneumonia (94%) and Kaposi's sarcoma (90%) (Fig. 8-17) (31). Furthermore, in this same population, HRCT proved 93% accurate in excluding active thoracic disease.

Of even greater potential clinical utility is the potential role of HRCT in evaluating patients presenting with hemoptysis (132–134). The role of bronchoscopy in the evaluation of patients presenting with hemoptysis has proved controversial (135,136). In fact, the etiology of hemoptysis most often proves elusive; nearly 50% of cases remain undiagnosed despite radiographic and bronchoscopic evaluation (135,137). In most reported series to date, HRCT has proved of greatest value in identifying bronchiectasis as a cause of hemoptysis (133,134,137). As shown by McGuinness et al. (137), in a prospective study of 57 consecutive patients presenting with hemoptysis evaluated both with CT and FOB, CT identified all cancers; furthermore, the overall diagnostic yield of bronchoscopy was documented to be less than CT (47% compared with 61%, respectively). CT proved especially valuable in diagnosing bronchiectasis, present in 25% of cases.

REFERENCES

1. Coultas DB, Zumwalt RE, Black WC, Sobonys RE. The epidemiology of interstitial lung diseases. *Am J Respir Crit Care Med* 1994;150:967–972.
2. DeRemee RA. Diffuse interstitial pulmonary disease from the perspective of the clinician. *Chest* 1987;92:1068–1073.
3. U.S. Department of Health, Education and Welfare. *Respiratory Diseases Task Force: Report of Problems, Research, Approaches, and Needs.* Washington, D.C.: U.S. Government Printing Office; 1976.
4. Murray JF, Mills J. Pulmonary infectious complications of human immunodeficiency virus infection. *Am Rev Resp Dis* 1990;141:1356–1372.
5. Miller RF, Mitchell DM. Pneumocystis carinii pneumonia. *Thorax* 1992;47:305–314.
6. Farazio KF, Buehler JW, Chamberland ME, et al. Spectrum of disease in persons with human immunodeficiency virus infections in the United States. *JAMA* 1992;267:1798–1805.
7. Stover DE. Pneumocystis carinii: an update. *Pulmon Perspect* 1994;11:3–5.
8. Centers for Disease Control and Prevention. Guidelines for prophylaxis against Pneumocystis carinii pneumonia among persons infected with human immunodeficiency virus. *MMWR* 1992;41(RR-4):1–11.
9. Chien SM, Rawji M, Mintz S, Rachlis A, Chan CK. Changes in hospitalized admission pattern in patients with human immunodeficiency virus in the era of P. carinii prophylaxis. *Chest* 1992;102:1035–1039.
10. Epler GR, McLoud TC, Gaensler EA, Mikus JP, Carrington CB. Normal chest roentgenograms in chronic diffuse infiltrative lung disease. *N Engl J Med* 1978;298:801–809.
11. Gaensler EA, Carrington CB. Open biopsy for chronic diffuse infiltrative lung disease: clinical, roentgenographic, and physiologic correlations in 502 patients. *Ann Thorac Surg* 1980;30:411–426.
12. Padley SPG, Hansell DM, Flower CDR, Jennings P. Comparative accuracy of high resolution computed tomography and chest radiography in the diagnosis of chronic diffuse infiltrative lung disease. *Clin Radiol* 1991;44:222–226.
13. Müller NL. Clinical value of high-resolution CT in chronic diffuse lung disease. *AJR* 1991;157:1163–1170.
14. Thurlbeck WM, Simon G. Radiographic appearance of the chest in emphysema. *AJR* 1978;130:429–440.
15. Pratt PC. Role of conventional chest radiography in diagnosis and exclusion of emphysema. *Am J Med* 1987;82:998–1006.
16. Burki NK. Roentgenologic diagnosis of emphysema: accurate or not? *Chest* 1989;95:1178–1179.

17. Primack SL, Müller NL. High-resolution computed tomography in acute diffuse lung disease in the immunocompromised patient. *Radiol Clin North Am* 1994;32:731–744.
18. Padley SPG, Adler B, Müller NL. High-resolution computed tomography of the chest: current indications. *J Thorac Imaging* 1993;8:189–199.
19. Lynch DA, Rose CS, Way D, King TE. Hypersensitivity pneumonitis: sensitivity of high-resolution CT in a population-based study. *AJR* 1992;159:469–472.
20. Brauner MW, Grenier P, Mompoint D, Lenoir S, de Cremoux H. Pulmonary sarcoidosis: evaluation with high-resolution CT. *Radiology* 1989;172:467–471.
21. Müller NL, Kullnig P, Miller RR. The CT findings of pulmonary sarcoidosis: analysis of 25 patients. *AJR* 1989;152:1179–1182.
22. Müller NL, Chiles C, Kullnig P. Pulmonary lymphangiomyomatosis: correlation of CT with radiographic and functional findings. *Radiology* 1990;175:335–339.
23. Stein MG, Mayo J, Müller N, Aberle DR, Webb WR, Gamsu G. Pulmonary lymphangitic spread of carcinoma: appearance on CT scans. *Radiology* 1987;162:371–375.
24. Strickland B, Strickland NH. The value of high definition, narrow section computed tomography in fibrosing alveolitis. *Clin Radiol* 1988;39:589–594.
25. Aberle DR, Gamsu G, Ray CS, Feuerstein IM. Asbestos-related pleural and parenchymal fibrosis: detection with high-resolution CT. *Radiology* 1988;166:729–734.
26. Staples CA, Gamsu G, Ray CS, Webb WR. High resolution computed tomography and lung function in asbestos-exposed workers with normal chest radiographs. *Am Rev Respir Dis* 1989;139:1502–1508.
27. Mathieson JR, Mayo JR, Staples CA, Müller NL. Chronic diffuse infiltrative lung disease: comparison of diagnostic accuracy of CT and chest radiography. *Radiology* 1989;171:111–116.
28. Grenier P, Valeyre D, Cluzel P, Brauner MW, Lenoir S, Chastang C. Chronic diffuse interstitial lung disease: diagnostic value of chest radiography and high-resolution CT. *Radiology* 1991;179:123–132.
29. Grenier P, Maurice F, Musset D, Menu Y, Nahum H. Bronchiectasis: assessment by thin-section CT. *Radiology* 1986;161:95–99.
30. Young K, Aspestrand F, Kolbenstvedt A. High resolution CT and bronchography in the assessment of bronchiectasis. *Acta Radiol* 1991;32:439–441.
31. Hartman TE, Primack SL, Müller NL, Staples CA. Diagnosis of thoracic complications in AIDS: accuracy of CT. *AJR* 1994;162:547–553.
32. Staples CA, Müller NL, Vedal S, Abboud R, Ostrow D, Miller RR. Usual interstitial pneumonia: correlation of CT with clinical, functional, and radiologic findings. *Radiology* 1987;162:377–381.
33. Fujii M, Adachi S, Shimizu T, Hirota S, Sako M, Kono M. Interstitial lung disease in rheumatoid arthritis: assessment with high-resolution computed tomography. *J Thorac Imaging* 1993;8:54–62.
34. Schurawitzki H, Stiglbauer R, Graninger W, et al. Interstitial lung disease in progressive systemic sclerosis: high-resolution CT versus radiography. *Radiology* 1990;176:755–759.
35. Padley SPG, Adler B, Hansell DM, Müller NL. High-resolution computed tomography of drug-induced lung disease. *Clin Radiol* 1992;46:232–236.
36. Bell J, McGivern D, Bullimore J, Hill J, Davies ER, Goddard P. Diagnostic imaging of post-irradiation changes in the chest. *Clin Radiol* 1988;39:109–119.
37. Ikezoe J, Takashima S, Morimoto S, et al. CT appearance of acute radiation-induced injury in the lung. *AJR* 1988;150:765–770.
38. Peuchot M, Libshitz HI. Pulmonary metastatic disease: radiologic-surgical correlation. *Radiology* 1987;164:719–722.
39. Metzger RA, Multhern CB, Arger PH, Coleman BG, Epstein DM, Gefter WB. CT differentiation of solitary from diffuse bronchioloalveolar carcinoma. *J Comput Assist Tomogr* 1981;5:830–833.
40. Brauner MW, Lenoir S, Grenier P, Cluzel P, Battesti JP, Valeyre D. Pulmonary sarcoidosis: CT assessment of lesion reversibility. *Radiology* 1992;182:349–354.
41. Newman LS, Buschman DL, Newell JD, Lynch DL. Beryllium disease: assessment with CT. *Radiology* 1994;190:835–840.
42. Bégin R, Ostiguy G, Fillion R, Colman N. Computed tomography scan in the early detection of silicosis. *Am Rev Respir Dis* 1991;3:1.
43. Remy-Jardin M, Degreef JM, Beuscart R, Voisin C, Remy J. Coal worker's pneumoconiosis: CT assessment in exposed workers and correlation with radiographic findings. *Radiology* 1990;177:363–371.
44. Im JG, Itoh H, Shim YS, et al. Pulmonary tuberculosis: CT findings-early active disease and sequential change with antituberculous therapy. *Radiology* 1993;186:653–660.
45. McGuinness G, Naidich DP, Jagirdar J, Leitman B, McCauley DI. High resolution CT findings in miliary lung disease. *J Comput Assist Tomogr* 1992;16:384–390.
46. Naidich DP, McCauley DI, Leitman BS, Genieser NB, Hulnick DH. Computed tomography of pulmonary tuberculosis. In: Siegelman SS, ed. *Contemporary Issues in Computed Tomography*. New York: Churchill Livingstone; 1984:175–217.
47. Kuhlman JE, Deutsch JH, Fishman EK, Siegelman SS. CT features of thoracic mycobacterial disease. *Radiographics* 1990;10:413–431.
48. Hartman TE, Swensen SJ, Williams DE. Mycobacterium avium-intracellulare complex: evaluation with CT. *Radiology* 1993;187:23–26.
49. Mori M, Galvin JR, Barloon TJ, Gingrich RD, Stanford W. Fungal pulmonary infections after bone marrow transplantation: evaluation with radiography and CT. *Radiology* 1991;178:721–726.
50. Huang RM, Naidich DP, Lubat E, Schinella R, Garay SM, McCauley DI. Septic pulmonary emboli: CT-radiographic correlation. *AJR* 1989;153:41–45.
51. Remy-Jardin M, Remy J, Wallaert B, Müller NL. Subacute and chronic bird breeder hypersensitivity pneumonitis: sequential evaluation with CT and correlation with lung function tests and bronchoalveolar lavage. *Radiology* 1993;198:111–118.
52. Hartman TE, Primack SL, Swensen SJ, Hansell D, McGuinness G, Müller NL. Desquamative interstitial pneumonia: thin-section CT findings in 22 patients. *Radiology* 1993;187:787–790.
53. Gruden JF, Webb WR. CT findings in a proved case of respiratory bronchiolitis. *AJR* 1993;161:44–46.
54. Holt RM, Schmidt RA, Godwin JD, Raghu G. High resolution CT in respiratory bronchiolitis-associated interstitial lung disease. *J Comput Assist Tomogr* 1993;17:46–50.
55. Bergin CJ, Wirth RL, Berry GJ, Castellino RA. Pneumocystis carinii pneumonia: CT and HRCT observations. *J Comput Assist Tomogr* 1990;14:756–759.
56. Moore AD, Godwin JD, Müller NL, et al. Pulmonary histiocytosis X: comparison of radiographic and CT findings. *Radiology* 1989;172:249–254.
57. Brauner MW, Grenier P, Mouelhi MM, Mompoint D, Lenoir S. Pulmonary histiocytosis X: evaluation with high resolution CT. *Radiology* 1989;172:255–258.
58. Lenoir S, Grenier P, Brauner MW, et al. Pulmonary lymphangiomyomatosis and tuberous sclerosis: comparison of radiographic and thin-section CT findings. *Radiology* 1990;175:329–334.
59. Sherrier RH, Chiles C, Roggli V. Pulmonary lymphangioleiomyomatosis: CT findings. *AJR* 1989;153:937–940.
60. Miller RR, Müller NL, Vedal S, Morrison NJ, Staples CA. Limitations of computed tomography in the assessment of emphysema. *Am Rev Respir Dis* 1989;139:980–983.
61. Thurlbeck WM, Müller NL. Emphysema: definition, imaging, and quantification. *AJR* 1995;163:1017–1025.
62. Klein JS, Gamsu G, Webb WR, Golden JA, Müller NL. High-resolution CT diagnosis of emphysema in symptomatic patients with normal chest radiographs and isolated low diffusing capacity. *Radiology* 1992;182:817–821.
63. Santis G, Hodson ME, Strickland B. High resolution computed tomography in adult cystic fibrosis patients with mild lung disease. *Clin Radiol* 1991;44:20–22.

64. Lynch DA, Brasch RC, Hardy KA, Webb WR. Pediatric pulmonary disease: assessment with high-resolution ultrafast CT. *Radiology* 1990;176:243–248.

65. Sweatman MC, Millar AB, Strickland B, Turner-Warwick M. Computed tomography in adult obliterative bronchiolitis. *Clin Radiol* 1990;41:116–119.

66. Marti-Bonmati L, Ruiz PF, Catala F, Mata JM, Calonge E. CT findings in Swyer-James syndrome. *Radiology* 1989;172:477–480.

67. Gamsu G, Salmon CJ, Warnock ML, Blanc PD. CT quantification of interstitial fibrosis in patients with asbestosis: a comparison of two methods. *AJR* 1995;164:63–68.

68. Leung AN, Staples CA, Müller NL. Chronic diffuse infiltrative lung disease: comparison of diagnostic accuracy of high-resolution and conventional CT. *AJR* 1991;157:693–696.

69. Remy-Jardin M, Remy J, Deffontaines C, Duhamel A. Assessment of diffuse infiltrative lung disease: comparison of conventional CT and high-resolution CT. *Radiology* 1991;181:157–162.

70. Silverman PM, Godwin JD. CT/bronchographic correlations in bronchiectasis. *J Comput Assist Tomogr* 1987;11:52–56.

71. Müller NL, Bergin CJ, Ostrow DN, Nichols DM. Role of computed tomography in the recognition of bronchiectasis. *AJR* 1984;143:971–976.

72. Webb WR. High-resolution computed tomography of obstructive lung disease. *Radiol Clin North Am* 1994;32:745–757.

73. Heitzman ER. Pattern recognition in pulmonary radiology. In: *The Lung: Radiologic-Pathologic Correlations*, 2nd ed. St. Louis: CV Mosby; 1984:70–105.

74. Felson B. A new look at pattern recognition of diffuse pulmonary disease. *AJR* 1979;133:183–189.

75. Genereux GP. Pattern recognition in diffuse lung disease: a review of theory and practice. *Med Radiogr Photog* 1985;61:2–31.

76. McLoud TC, Carrington CB, Gaensler EA. Diffuse infiltrative lung disease: a new scheme for description. *Radiology* 1983;149:353–363.

77. Young M, Marrie TJ. Interobserver variability in the interpretation of chest roentgenograms of patients with possible pneumonia. *Arch Intern Med* 1994;154:2729–2732.

78. Müller NL, Miller RR. Computed tomography of chronic diffuse infiltrative lung disease: part 1. *Am Rev Respir Dis* 1990;142:1206–1215.

79. Müller NL, Miller RR. Computed tomography of chronic diffuse infiltrative lung disease: part 2. *Am Rev Respir Dis* 1990;142:1440–1448.

80. Nishimura K, Izumi T, Kitaichi M, Nagai S, Itoh H. The diagnostic accuracy of high-resolution computed tomography in diffuse infiltrative lung diseases. *Chest* 1993;104:1149–1155.

81. Primack SL, Hartman TE, Hansell DM, Müller NL. End-stage lung disease: CT findings in 61 patients. *Radiology* 1993;189:681–686.

82. Janzen DL, Padley SP, Adler BD, Müller NL. Acute pulmonary complications in immunocompromised non-AIDS patients: comparison of diagnostic accuracy of CT and chest radiography. *Clin Radiol* 1993;47:159–165.

83. Lee KS, Primack SL, Staples CA, Mayo JR, Aldrich JE, Müller NL. Chronic infiltrative lung disease: comparison of diagnostic accuracies of radiography and low- and conventional-dose thin-section CT. *Radiology* 1994;191:669–673.

84. Aberle DL. HRCT in acute diffuse lung disease. *J Thorac Imaging* 1993;8:200–212.

85. Grenier P, Chevret S, Beigelman C, Brauner MW, Chastang C, Valeyre D. Chronic diffuse infiltrative lung disease: determination of the diagnostic value of clinical data, chest radiography, and CT with Bayesian analysis. *Radiology* 1994;1994:383–390.

86. Buschman DL, Gamsu G, Waldron JA, Klein JS, King TE. Chronic hypersensitivity pneumonitis: use of CT in diagnosis. *AJR* 1992;159:957–960.

87. Rose C, King TE. Controversies in hypersensitivity pneumonitis [Editorial]. *Am Rev Resp Dis* 1992;145:1–2.

88. Bergin CJ, Coblentz CL, Chiles C, Bell DY, Castellino RA. Chronic lung diseases: specific diagnosis using CT. *AJR* 1989;152:1183–1188.

89. Lenique F, Brauner MW, Grenier P, Battesti JP, Loiseau A, Valeyre D. CT assessment of bronchi in sarcoidosis: endoscopic and pathologic correlations. *Radiology* 1995;194:419–423.

90. Lynch DA, Webb WR, Gamsu G, Stulbarg M, Golden J. Computed tomography in pulmonary sarcoidosis. *J Comput Assist Tomogr* 1989;13:405–410.

91. Tung KT, Wells AU, Rubens MB, Kirk JM, du Bois RM, Hansell DM. Accuracy of the typical computed tomographic appearances of fibrosing alveolitis. *Thorax* 1993;48:334–338.

92. Al-Jarad N, Strickland B, Pearson MC, Rubens MB, Rudd RM. High-resolution computed tomographic assessment of asbestosis and cryptogenic fibrosing alveolitis: a comparative study. *Thorax* 1992;47:645–650.

93. Remy-Jardin M, Giraud F, Remy J, Copin MC, Gosselin B, Duhamel A. Importance of ground-glass attenuation in chronic diffuse infiltrative lung disease: pathologic-CT correlation. *Radiology* 1993;189:693–698.

94. Wells AU, Hansell DM, Rubens MB, Cullinan P, Black CM, du Bois RM. The predictive value of appearances of thin-section computed tomography in fibrosing alveolitis. *Am Rev Respir Dis* 1993;148:1076–1082.

95. Raghu G. Idiopathic pulmonary fibrosis. A rational clinical approach. *Chest* 1987;92:148–154.

96. Terriff BA, Kwan SY, Chan-Yeung MM, Müller NL. Fibrosing alveolitis: chest radiography and CT as predictors of clinical and functional impairment at follow-up in 26 patients. *Radiology* 1992;184:445–449.

97. Murdoch J, Müller NL. Pulmonary sarcoidosis: changes on follow-up CT examinations. *AJR* 1992;159:473–477.

98. Akira M, Higashihara T, Sakatani M, Hara H. Diffuse panbronchiolitis: follow-up CT examination. *Radiology* 1993;189:559–562.

99. Lee JS, Im JG, Ahn JM, Kim YM, Han MC. Fibrosing alveolitis: prognostic implication of ground-glass attenuation at high-resolution CT. *Radiology* 1992;184:415–454.

100. Remy-Jardin M, Remy J, Giraud F, Wattinne L, Gosselin B. Computed tomography assessment of ground-glass opacity: semiology and significance. *J Thorac Imaging* 1993;8:249–264.

101. Wyatt SH, Fishman EK. Diffuse pulmonary extramedullary hematopoiesis in a patient with myelofibrosis: CT findings. *J Comput Assist Tomogr* 1994;18:815–817.

102. Greenberg S, Suster B. Metastatic pulmonary calcifications: appearance on high resolution CT. *J Comput Assist Tomogr* 1994;18:497–499.

103. Leung AN, Miller RR, Müller NL. Parenchymal opacification in chronic infiltrative lung diseases: CT-pathologic correlation. *Radiology* 1993;188:209–214.

104. Müller NL, Staples CA, Miller RR, Vedal S, Thurlbeck WM, Ostrow DN. Disease activity in idiopathic pulmonary fibrosis: CT and pathologic correlation. *Radiology* 1987;165:731–734.

105. Wells AU, Rubens MB, du Bois RM, Hansell DM. Serial CT in fibrosing alveolitis: prognostic significance of the initial pattern. *AJR* 1993;161:1159–1165.

106. Wells AU, Hansell DM, Corrin B, et al. High resolution computed tomography as a predictor of lung histology in systemic sclerosis. *Thorax* 1992;47:508–512.

107. Akira M, Sakatani M, Ueda E. Idiopathic pulmonary fibrosis: progression of honeycombing at thin-section CT. *Radiology* 1993;189:687–691.

108. Nishimura K, Kitaichi M, Izumi T, Nagai S, Itoh H. Usual interstitial pneumonia: histologic correlation with high-resolution CT. *Radiology* 1992;182:337–342.

109. Wells AU, Hansell DM, Rubens MB, Cullinan P, Haslam PL, Black CM, Du Bois RM. Fibrosing alveolitis in systemic sclerosis. bronchoalveolar lavage findings in relation to computed tomographic appearance. *Am J Respir Crit Care Med* 1994;150:462–468.

110. Müller NL, Miller RR. Ground-glass attenuation, nodules, alveolitis, and sarcoid granulomas [Editorial]. *Radiology* 1993;189:31–32.

111. Bergin CJ, Bell DY, Coblentz CL, et al. Sarcoidosis: correlation of pulmonary parenchymal pattern at CT with results of pulmonary function tests. *Radiology* 1989;171:619–624.
112. Remy-Jardin M, Giraud F, Remy J, Wattinne L, Wallaert B, Duhamel A. Pulmonary sarcoidosis: role of CT in the evaluation of disease activity and functional impairment and in prognosis assessment. *Radiology* 1994;191:675–680.
113. Austin JHM. Pulmonary sarcoidosis: what are we learning from CT? *Radiology* 1989;171:603–604.
114. Naidich DP, Garay SM, Goodman PC, Ryback BJ, Kramer EL. Pulmonary manifestations of AIDS. In: *Radiology of Acquired Immune Deficiency Syndrome*. New York: Raven Press; 1988: 47–77.
115. Kuhlman JE, Kavuru M, Fishman EK, Siegelman SS. Pneumocystis carinii pneumonia: spectrum of parenchymal CT findings. *Radiology* 1990;175:711–714.
116. McGuinness G, Scholes JV, Garay SM, Leitman BS, McCauley DI, Naidich DP. Cytomegalovirus pneumonitis: spectrum of parenchymal CT findings with pathologic correlation in 21 AIDS patients. *Radiology* 1994;192:451–459.
117. Bissuel F, Leport C. Perronne C, Longeut P, Vilde JL. Fever of unknown origin in HIV-infected patients: a critical analysis of a retrospective series of 57 cases. *J Int Med* 1994;236: 529–535.
118. Smith CM, Moser KM. Management of interstitial lung disease. State of the art. *Chest* 1989;95:676–678.
119. Wall CP, Gaensler EA, Carrington CB, Hayes JA. Comparison of transbronchial and open biopsies in chronic infiltrative lung diseases. *Am Rev Respir Dis* 1981;123:280–285.
120. Wilson RK, Fechner RE, Greenberg SD, Estrada R, Stevens PM. Clinical implications of a "nonspecific" transbronchial biopsy. *Am J Med* 1978;65:252–256.
121. Shure D. Transbronchial biopsy and needle aspiration. *Chest* 1989;95:1130–1138.
122. Bensard DD, McIntyre RC Jr, Waring BJ, Simon JS. Comparison of video thoracoscopic lung biopsy to open lung biopsy in the diagnosis of interstitial lung disease. *Chest* 1993;103: 765–770.
123. Newman SL, Michel RP, Wang NS. Lingular biopsy: is it representative? *Am Rev Resp Dis* 1985;132:1084–1086.
124. Nishimura K, Itoh H, Kitaichi M, Nagai S, Izumi T. Pulmonary sarcoidosis: correlation of CT and histopathologic findings. *Radiology* 1993;189:105–109.
125. Munk PL, Müller NL, Miller RR, Ostrow DN. Pulmonary lymphangitic carcinomatosis: CT and pathologic findings. *Radiology* 1988;166:705–709.
126. Johkoh T, Ikezoe J, Tomiyama N, et al. CT findings in lymphangitic carcinomatosis of the lung: correlation with histologic findings and pulmonary function tests. *AJR* 1992;158: 1217–1222.
127. Templeton PA, Krasna M. Localization of pulmonary nodules for thoracoscopic resection: use of needle/wire breast biopsy system. *AJR* 1993;160:761–762.
128. Shah RM, Spirn PW, Salazar AM, et al. Localization of peripheral pulmonary nodules for thoracoscopic excision: value of CT-guided wire placement. *AJR* 1993;161:279–283.
129. Schluger NW, Rom WN. Current approaches to the diagnosis of active pulmonary tuberculosis. *Am J Respir Crit Care Med* 1994;149:264–267.
130. Tu JV, Biem J, Detsky AS. Bronchoscopy versus empirical therapy in HIV-infected patients with presumptive Pneumocystis carinii pneumonia. *Am Rev Resp Dis* 1993;148:370–377.
131. Barloon TJ, Galvin JR, Mori M, Stanford W, Gingrich RD. High-resolution ultrafast chest CT in the clinical management of febrile bone marrow transplant patients with normal or nonspecific chest roentgenograms. *Chest* 1991;99:928–933.
132. Naidich DP, Funt S, Ettenger NA, Arranda C. Hemoptysis: CT-bronchoscopic correlations in 58 cases. *Radiology* 1990; 177:357–362.
133. Millar A, Boothroyd A, Edwards D, Hetzel M. The role of computed tomography (CT) in the investigation of unexplained hemoptysis. *Resp Med* 1992;86:39–44.
134. Set PAK, Flower CDR, Smith IE, Cahn AP, Twentyman OP, Shneerson JM. Hemoptysis: comparative study of the role of CT and fiberoptic bronchoscopy. *Radiology* 1993;189:677–680.
135. Poe RH, Levy PC, Israel RH, Ortiz CR, Kallay MC. Use of fiberoptic bronchoscopy in the diagnosis of bronchogenic carcinoma. A study in patients with idiopathic pleural effusions. *Chest* 1994;105:1663–1667.
136. Rohwedder JJ. Enticements for fruitless bronchoscopy [Editorial]. *Chest* 1989;96:708–710.
137. McGuinness G, Beacher JR, Harkin TJ, Garay SM, Rom WN, Naidich DP. Hemoptysis. High-resolution CT/bronchoscopic correlation. *Chest* 1994;105:982–983.

NINE

An Illustrated Glossary of HRCT Terms

As a quick reference, and as an aid to understanding the nomenclature used in this book, we have listed the definitions of a number of useful HRCT terms and their significance, and have provided illustrations of their typical appearances. As throughout this book, we have attempted to define HRCT terms relative to their specific anatomic correlates. Nonspecific and nonanatomic terms, and purely descriptive terms, have been avoided except in situations where the findings themselves are nonspecific, and cannot be related to particular anatomic abnormalities, or when the nonspecific descriptive term is particularly helpful in understanding and recognizing the abnormal finding. Of course, the specific terms we have chosen reflect our personal preferences (1).

ACINUS. A unit of lung structure distal to a terminal bronchiole and supplied by first-order respiratory bronchioles. An acinus is the largest lung unit in which all airways participate in gas exchange. Acini average about 7 to 8 mm in diameter in adults and range from 6 to 10 mm in diameter (Fig. 9-29) (2–5). Acini are not visible on HRCT in normal subjects, although acinar arteries can sometimes be seen. Secondary pulmonary lobules are comprised of a varying number of acini, ranging from 3 to 24 (6).
Equivalent. Pulmonary acinus.

ACINAR SHADOW (ACINAR NODULE). See *Air-space nodule*.

AIR-SPACE CONSOLIDATION. See *Consolidation*.

AIR-SPACE NODULE. A small nodular opacity, ranging from a few millimeters to 1 centimeter in diameter, which can be seen in patients with air-space diseases. It represents a focal area of peribronchiolar inflammation or air-space consolidation (7–10). Air-space nodules are typically ill-defined and often appear centrilobular in location (Fig. 9-1).

However, HRCT findings are unreliable in distinguishing small nodules which are primarily air-space in origin from those which are primarily interstitial; thus, a description of the size, appearance, and distribution of nodules is usually more appropriate when interpreting HRCT. See *Centrilobular; nodule*.
Equivalents. acinar shadow, acinar nodule.

AIR TRAPPING. Abnormal retention of gas within a lung or lung units following expiration. It is diagnosa-

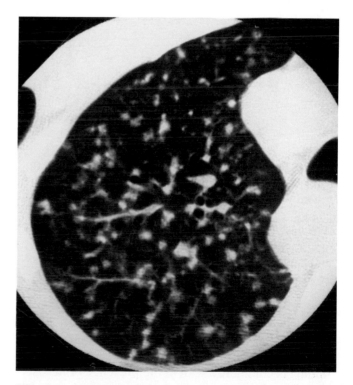

FIG. 9-1. Air-space nodules. In this patient with endobronchial spread of tuberculosis, small, ill-defined, centrilobular nodules reflect the presence of peribronchiolar inflammation and consolidation. As is typical of centrilobular nodules, some are associated with small arteries, and many are centered 5 to 10 mm from the pleural surfaces.

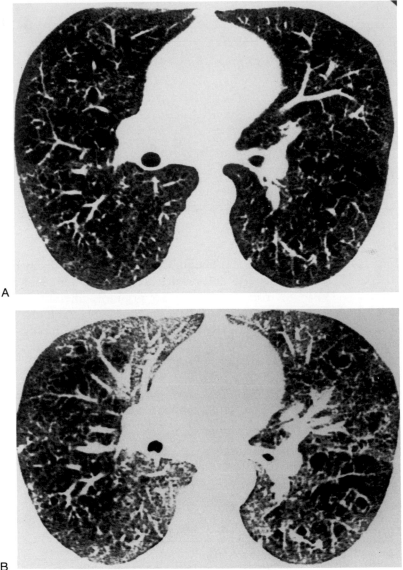

FIG. 9-2. Air trapping on expiratory HRCT. **A:** Inspiratory scan in a patient with histiocytosis X obtained as part of a dynamic expiratory HRCT. Some cystic lesions are visible, but lung parenchyma is relatively homogeneous in attenuation. **B:** On an expiratory scan, some lung regions remain lucent as a result of air trapping, while more normal lung regions increase in attenuation. (From Stern et al., ref. 69, with permission.)

ble if lung parenchyma remains lucent on post-expiratory CT, shows a less than normal increase in attenuation following expiration, or shows little change in cross-sectional area (Fig. 9-2) (11–13). Air trapping cannot be diagnosed on inspiratory scans; lung inhomogeneity on inspiratory scans in patients with airways disease should be referred to preferably as *mosaic perfusion*.

ARCHITECTURAL DISTORTION. Abnormal displacement of pulmonary structures including bronchi, vessels, fissures, and interlobular septa, resulting in a distorted appearance of lung anatomy. This finding is commonly seen in the presence of fibrosis or volume loss.

BLEB. A gas-containing space within the visceral pleura (14). Radiologically, this term is sometimes used to describe a focal thin-walled lucency, contig-

uous with the pleura, usually at the lung apex. However, a distinction between bleb and bulla is of little practical significance and is seldom justified. On HRCT, a bleb and bulla cannot be distinguished, and the term *bulla* is usually preferred (14).

BRONCHIECTASIS. Localized or diffuse, irreversible bronchial dilatation, usually resulting from chronic infection, airway obstruction by tumor, stricture, impacted material, inherited bronchial abnormalities, or fibrosis (see *traction bronchiectasis*). Although the definition of this term indicates that abnormalities must be irreversible, this is difficult to establish in the absence of serial examinations, and is not required for diagnosis. Bronchiectasis can be classified into three types (cylindrical, varicose, and cystic) depending on the appearances of the abnormal bronchi (Figs. 9-3,9-4,9-10B,9-30,9-34). Although bronchial dilatation is the primary feature of

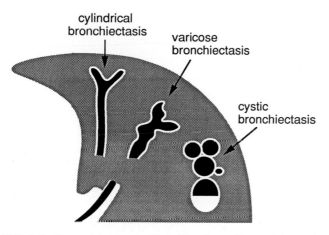

FIG. 9-3. Bronchiectasis. Classification of bronchiectasis based on morphology and HRCT appearance.

bronchiectasis, bronchial wall thickening, fluid retention within the bronchi, and small airway abnormalities are also commonly visible on HRCT.

BRONCHIOLAR IMPACTION. See *bronchiolectasis* and *tree-in-bud.*

BRONCHIOLE. Small airways which lack cartilage in their walls. The largest bronchioles measure about 3 mm in diameter and have walls about 0.3 mm in thickness.

BRONCHIOLECTASIS. Dilatation of bronchioles. Bronchiolectasis can occur as a result of airways disease (Fig. 9-4), or in the presence of lung fibrosis (see *traction bronchiolectasis*). Dilated bronchioles can be air-filled or fluid-filled. Dilated fluid-filled bronchioles are often described using the terms

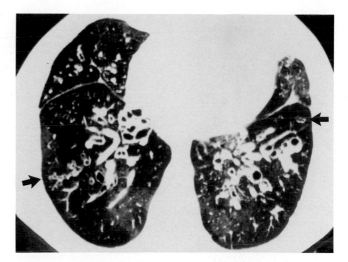

FIG. 9-4. Bronchiolectasis. In a patient with allergic bronchopulmonary aspergillosis, there is extensive bronchiectasis bilaterally, manifested by bronchial dilatation and bronchial wall thickening. Dilated air-filled bronchioles in the peripheral lung (*arrows*) reflect bronchiolectasis. Also note lung inhomogeneity due to mosaic perfusion.

bronchiolar impaction or *tree-in-bud* (15,16), or may be visible as centrilobular nodular opacities.

BRONCHOVASCULAR BUNDLE. See *peribronchovascular interstitium.*

BULLA. A sharply demarcated area of emphysema, measuring 1 cm or more in diameter, and possessing a wall less than 1 mm in thickness (Figs. 9-5,9-12,9-24) (14). To make the diagnosis of a bulla on HRCT, other areas of emphysema should also be visible. Subpleural bullae are commonly the result of paraseptal emphysema (17,18).

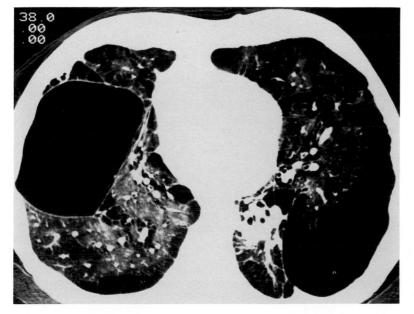

FIG. 9-5. Bulla. Large thin-walled subpleural bullae are visible bilaterally, in association with centrilobular emphysema. Because of the predominance of bullae in this patient, the term "bullous emphysema" could be used to describe this appearance.

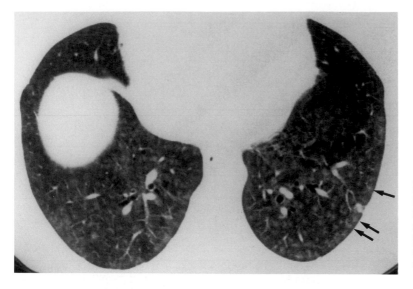

FIG. 9-6. Centrilobular nodules. Centrilobular nodules (*arrows*) of ground-glass opacity in a patient with hypersensitivity pneumonitis. The nodules can be localized to the centrilobular region because of their relationship to centrilobular arteries. The nodules appear to be centered 5 to 10 mm from the pleural surface.

BULLOUS EMPHYSEMA. Emphysema in which bulla are the predominant feature (Fig. 9-5) (19).

CENTRILOBULAR. An adjective describing a structure (e.g., centrilobular bronchiole), HRCT finding (e.g., centrilobular nodule), or disease process which involves the center of the lobule or *lobular core*. It is also used to describe abnormal findings seen in relation to centrilobular structures such as bronchioles or small arteries, but cannot be precisely localized to the centers of lobules (Figs. 9-1,9-6,9-22). On HRCT, a centrilobular abnormality can appear as an opacity or lucency centered within the lobule or as a group of opacities or lucencies surrounding centrilobular arteries (15). It can reflect interstitial fibrosis or inflammation, air-space consolidation, or airways disease.
Equivalents. Lobular core, peribronchiolar, perivascular.

CENTRILOBULAR EMPHYSEMA. Emphysema which predominantly affects the respiratory bronchioles in the center of acini, and therefore predominantly involves the central portion of secondary lobules (17,18). Common in the upper lobes; common in smokers. Usually visible on HRCT as multifocal areas of lucency that lack visible walls, although thin walls can sometimes be seen (Figs. 9-5,9-7,9-12). Occasionally the lucencies can be seen to surround the centrilobular artery.
Equivalents. Proximal acinar emphysema, centriacinar emphysema.

CENTRILOBULAR INTERSTITIUM. The peripheral, centrilobular extension of the peribronchovascular interstitium. Part of the "axial fiber network" described by Weibel (3).
Equivalents. Centrilobular peribronchovascular interstitium; axial interstitium (14).

CENTRILOBULAR INTERSTITIAL THICKENING. Thickening of the centrilobular peribronchovascular interstitium which surrounds centrilobular bronchioles and vessels. It is usually distinguished from peribronchovascular interstitial thickening because of its different HRCT appearance and differential diagnosis. It is recognizable by an increase in prominence of centrilobular structures.

CONGLOMERATE MASS. A large opacity that often surrounds and encompasses bronchi and vessels, usually in the central or parahilar lung (Fig. 9-8). It often represents a mass of fibrous tissue. It is

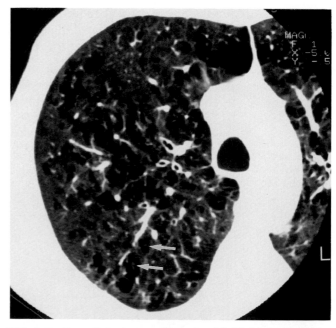

FIG. 9-7. Centrilobular emphysema. Multiple areas of low attenuation without distinct walls are visible bilaterally. Some of the areas of emphysema (*arrows*) surround visible centrilobular arteries.

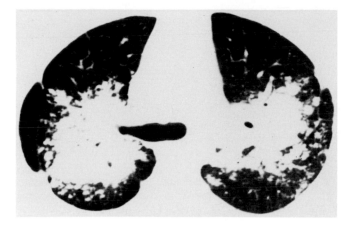

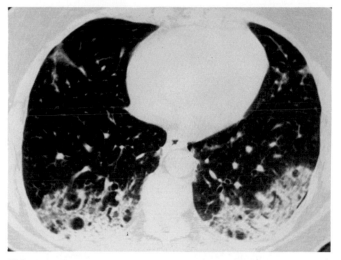

FIG. 9-8. Conglomerate mass. Bilateral upper lobe masses obscuring the parahilar vessels in a patient with active sarcoidosis. Air-bronchograms are visible within the masses. These conglomerate masses reflect a multitude of confluent granulomas. This appearance could also be referred to as consolidation.

FIG. 9-9. Consolidation. A patient with bronchiolitis obliterans organizing pneumonia shows bilateral consolidation. Pulmonary vessels are invisible in the densest areas, and air-bronchograms are visible.

most common in silicosis (Fig. 9-20), coal worker's pneumoconiosis, and sarcoidosis (Figs. 9-8,9-34).

Equivalent in pneumoconiosis patients. "Complicated pneumoconiosis," "progressive massive fibrosis."

CONSOLIDATION. An increase in lung opacity, discernable on plain radiographs or HRCT, that results in obscuration of underlying vessels (Figs. 9-8,9-9). This finding usually indicates the replacement of alveolar air, or filling of air-spaces by fluid, cells, or other material (9), but can also be seen with exten-

sive interstitial disease. Differentiate from "ground-glass opacity," in which underlying vessels are not obscured by increased lung opacity.

Equivalents. Air-space consolidation, air-space opacification, air-space attenuation.

CYST. A nonspecific term describing the presence of a thin-walled (usually < 3 mm), well-defined and circumscribed, air- or fluid-containing lesion, 1 cm or more in diameter (Fig. 9-10) (1,14). On HRCT, the

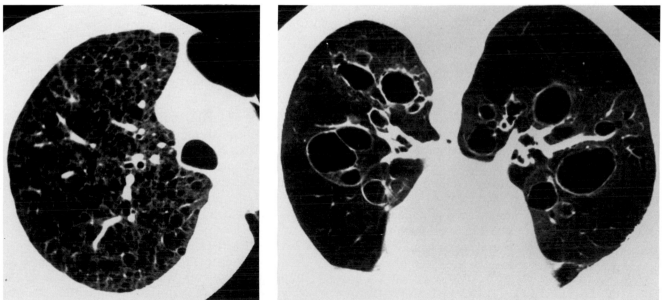

A   B

FIG. 9-10. Cysts. **A:** Multiple lung cysts in a patient with lymphangiomyomatosis. The low attenuation air-filled cysts are marginated by thin walls. **B:** Lung cysts in this patient probably reflect cystic bronchiectasis. Although the cysts are thin-walled, thick-walled bronchi are visible centrally. Bronchiolitis obliterans was also present in this patient, manifested by decreased lung attenuation and hypovascularity.

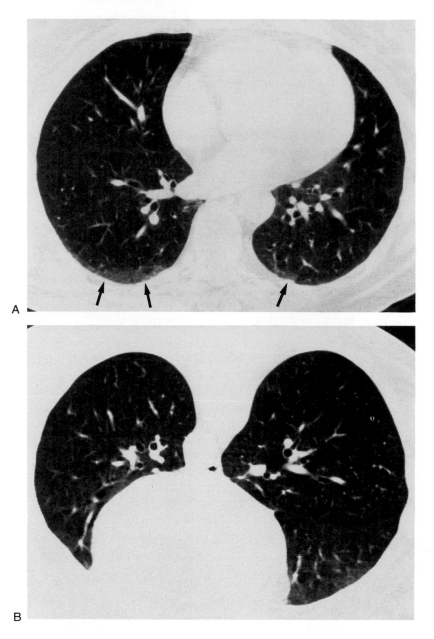

FIG. 9-11. Dependent opacity. **A:** Ill-defined opacities (*arrows*) are visible in the posterior lungs, more evident on the right than the left. **B:** At the same level, with the patient positioned prone, the posterior lungs appear normal.

term cyst is usually used to refer to an air-containing lesion, or air-filled cyst. Air-filled cysts are commonly seen in patients with histiocytosis X and lymphangiomyomatosis (20–24), but can be seen in other diseases as well. Honeycombing also results in the presence of cysts. The term cyst can be used to describe the dilated bronchi seen in patients with cystic bronchiectasis (Fig. 9-10B), although the latter term is preferred. This term is not usually used to refer to focal lucencies associated with emphysema.

DEPENDENT OPACITY ("DEPENDENT DENSITY"). An ill-defined subpleural opacity ranging from a few millimeters to a centimeter or more in thickness, which is only visible in dependent lung regions, and disappears when the lung region is nondependent (Fig. 9-11). It is usually visible in the pos-

terior lung when the subject is supine and disappears in the prone position. Although the term "dependent density" has been extensively used (25), "opacity" is generally preferred to "density" (14). Distinguish from a *subpleural line* (Fig. 9-32), which is usually thin and sharply defined, visible in nondependent lung, and usually indicates fibrosis.

DYNAMIC EXPIRATORY HRCT. HRCT scans performed during expiration in order to diagnose air trapping in patients with obstructive lung disease (Fig. 9-2) (11,26). Performed using either electron-beam (ultrafast) or spiral (helical) CT.
Equivalent. Dynamic ultrafast high-resolution CT.

EMPHYSEMA. Permanent, abnormal enlargement of airspaces distal to the terminal bronchiole, accom-

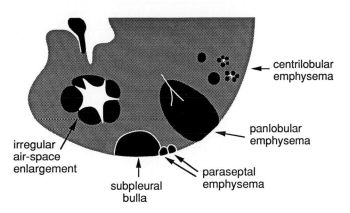

centrilobular
emphysema

panlobular
emphysema

paraseptal
emphysema

subpleural
bulla

irregular
air-space
enlargement

FIG. 9-12. Emphysema. Morphologic classification.

panied by the destruction of their walls (27,28). Previous definitions of emphysema have included the caveat "without obvious fibrosis" (17), but recent observations have established that some fibrosis is not uncommon (27,28). Visible on HRCT as areas of low attenuation, with or without visible walls, and classified morphologically relative to the pulmonary lobule as centrilobular, panlobular, or paraseptal (Fig. 9-12) (29,30). Also see *bulla* (Fig. 9-5), *bullous emphysema, centrilobular emphysema* (Fig. 9-7), *irregular air-space enlargement* (Fig. 9-20), *panlobular emphysema* (Fig. 9-23), and *paraseptal emphysema* (Fig. 9-24).

END-STAGE LUNG. The final stage in progression of a lung disease, usually characterized by fibrosis, alveolar dissolution, bronchiolectasis, and disruption of normal lung architecture. Generally speaking, end-stage lung is considered to be present in patients who have morphologic evidence of honeycombing, extensive cystic changes, or conglomerate fibrosis (31–34). See *Honeycombing.*

EXPIRATORY HRCT. HRCT scans performed during or following expiration in order to diagnose air trapping in patients with obstructive lung disease (Fig. 9-2) (11,26). Scans can be obtained following expiration, can be gated to spirometry (35,36), or can be obtained dynamically during forced expiration (see *dynamic expiratory HRCT*).

"GROUND-GLASS" OPACITY. A hazy increase in lung opacity on HRCT which is not associated with obscuration of underlying vessels and can therefore be differentiated from air-space consolidation (Fig. 9-13). This finding is nonspecific and can reflect the presence of minimal interstitial thickening, air-space filling, or a combination of both (10,37–39). In many different diseases, and to varying degrees, this finding suggests an active or acute disease (38,39). Ground-glass opacity visible on CT scans obtained

with thick collimation (> 5 mm) is much less specific because of volume averaging, and it has been recommended that this term be applied to HRCT only (39). Ground-glass opacity can be diffuse, patchy, or nodular (Fig. 9-6). Whenever possible, it should be distinguished from *MOSAIC PERFUSION*, which can have a similar appearance.

HIGH-RESOLUTION CT (HRCT). A CT technique which attempts to optimize spatial resolution in visu-

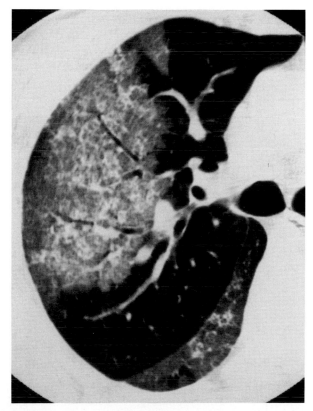

FIG. 9-13. "Ground-glass" opacity. In a patient with pulmonary hemorrhage, focal areas of increased attenuation represent ground-glass opacity. Note that vessels are visible within the area of increased opacity. Air-bronchograms are visible.

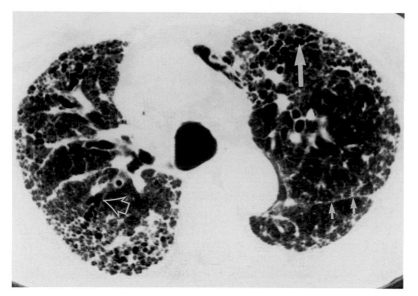

FIG. 9-14. Honeycombing. In a 73-year-old man with end-stage idiopathic pulmonary fibrosis, honeycombing is visible predominantly in the subpleural lung regions (*large arrow*). The cystic airspaces show clearly definable walls, and adjacent cysts tend to share walls. Also note irregular interfaces at the pleural surfaces, traction bronchiectasis (*open arrow*), interlobular interstitial thickening, and subpleural interstitial thickening (*small arrows*) adjoining the left major fissure.

alizing lung parenchyma. The use of thin sections (e.g., 1- to 2-mm collimation) and a high-spatial frequency (sharp) reconstruction algorithm are essential (40), but other modifications of CT technique also can enhance spatial resolution. This term is preferable to "thin-section CT," which takes into account only one technical modification.

HONEYCOMBING. Cystic spaces ranging from several millimeters to several centimeters in diameter, characterized by thick, clearly definable fibrous walls, which are typically lined by bronchiolar epithelium. It results from, and is associated with, pulmonary fibrosis. The cystic airspaces of honeycombing commonly share walls, are predominantly subpleural, and occur in several layers (Figs. 9-14, 9-15).

Equivalents. End-stage lung, honeycomb lung (41, 42), honeycomb cysts.

INTERFACE SIGN. The presence of irregular interfaces at the edges of pulmonary parenchymal structures such as vessels or bronchi, or at the pleural surfaces of lung (Figs. 9-14, 9-15) (37, 43). A nonspe-

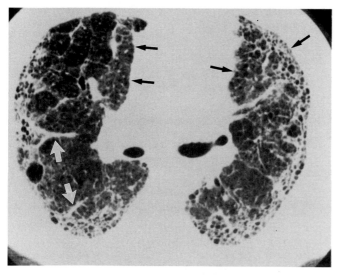

FIG. 9-15. The interface sign. In this patient with pulmonary fibrosis and honeycombing, irregular interfaces at the edges of pulmonary vessels (*white arrows*) and bronchi, and at the pleural surfaces (*black arrows*), are indicative of the interface sign. As in this patient, it is not necessary to rely on this sign for diagnosis, as other abnormalities (e.g., honeycombing) are also evident.

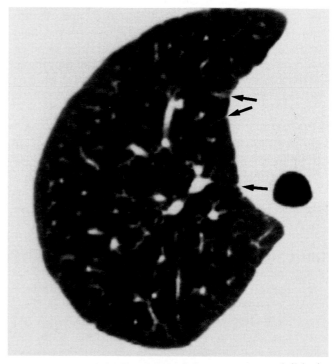

FIG. 9-16. Interlobular septa. A few septa are visible in this normal subject. These are most evident along the mediastinal pleural surface (*arrows*).

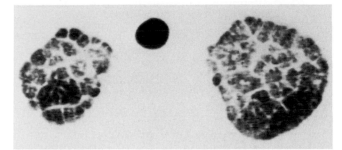

FIG. 9-17. Interlobular septal thickening. Marked thickening of septa is present in the upper lobes of this patient with lymphangitic spread of carcinoma.

cific finding usually indicative of interstitial thickening. Other more specific HRCT abnormalities are always or almost always visible, and a diagnosis of disease should rarely be based on this finding.

INTERLOBULAR SEPTUM. A connective tissue septum that marginates part of a secondary pulmonary lobule, and contains pulmonary veins and lymphatics. It represents an inward extension of the "peripheral interstitium" described by Weibel (3), which extends over the surface of the lung beneath the visceral pleura. Septa measure about 100μ (0.1 mm) in thickness, and are occasionally visible in normal subjects (Fig. 9-16).
Equivalent. Septum.

INTERLOBULAR SEPTAL THICKENING. Abnormal thickening of interlobular septa usually resulting from fibrosis, edema, or infiltration by cells or other materials (Figs. 9-17,9-25,9-34). Thickening can be smooth, nodular, or irregular.
Equivalents. Septal thickening; septal lines.

INTERSTITIAL NODULE. A small nodule, ranging from a few mm to 1 cm in diameter, that is predominantly interstitial in location. This term should generally be avoided in interpreting HRCT, as HRCT findings are unreliable in making this diagnosis. However, interstitial nodules are often well-defined, and can be seen when quite small (Fig. 9-18). See *Nodule*.

INTERSTITIUM. The fibrous supporting structure of the lung.

INTRALOBULAR INTERSTITIUM. The interstitial network, excluding the interlobular septa, that supports structures of the pulmonary lobule. It is not normally visible, but can be seen on HRCT when abnormally thickened. This term refers primarily to the fine network of very thin connective tissue fibers within the alveolar walls [the "septal fibers" described by Weibel (2,3) or the "parenchymal" interstitium (14)].

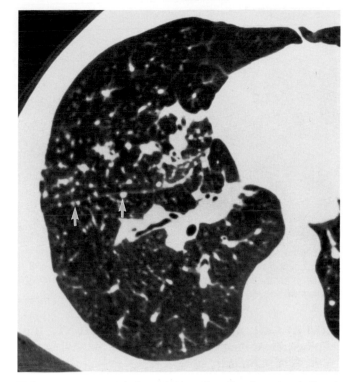

FIG. 9-18. Interstitial nodules. Small, sharply defined nodules (*arrows*) in a patient with sarcoidosis are primarily interstitial in origin. In this patient, nodules show a perilymphatic distribution, being predominantly subpleural (*arrows*), septal, and peribronchovascular.

INTRALOBULAR INTERSTITIAL THICKENING. Thickening of the intralobular interstitium, resulting in a fine reticular, or "mesh-like" appearance to the lung parenchyma (Fig. 9-19) may be an early sign of lung fibrosis.
Equivalent. Intralobular lines (29).

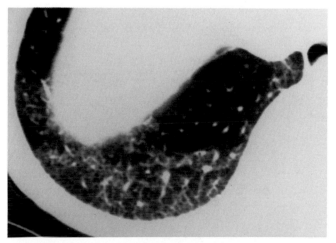

FIG. 9-19. Intralobular interstitial thickening. In this patient with pulmonary fibrosis, a fine reticular pattern visible posteriorly reflects intralobular interstitial thickening. Note the presence of irregular interfaces at the posterior pleural surface.

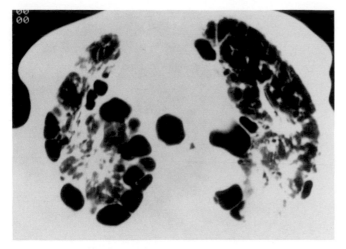

FIG. 9-20. Irregular air-space enlargement. In this patient with silicosis and progressive massive fibrosis, areas of emphysema adjacent to the fibrotic masses reflect irregular air-space enlargement or "irregular emphysema."

IRREGULAR AIR-SPACE ENLARGEMENT. Emphysema or lung destruction that occurs adjacent to areas of pulmonary fibrosis (Figs. 9- 12,9-20) (17,18). **Equivalent.** Paracicatricial or irregular emphysema.

LOBULAR CORE. The central portion of a secondary lobule (44) containing the pulmonary artery and bronchiolar branches which supply the lobule, as

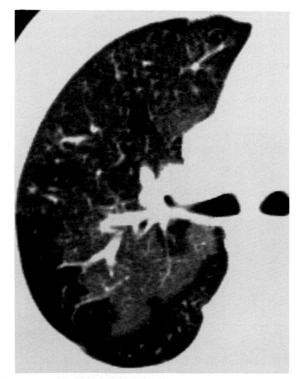

FIG. 9-21. Mosaic perfusion. In a child with bronchiolitis obliterans, focal regions of lucency reflect airway obstruction and decreased perfusion. Vessels in the lucent regions appear smaller, a characteristic finding.

well as supporting peribronchovascular or "axial" connective tissue (3).
Equivalent. Centrilobular region, peribronchiolar region.

LOBULE. See *secondary pulmonary lobule*.

LOW-DOSE HIGH-RESOLUTION CT. A HRCT technique in which radiation dose is reduced by using reduced milliamperes (mA). This technique results in some decrease in resolution and diagnostic accuracy, and is most suitable for screening or follow-up of patients. Appropriate technical factors for low-dose HRCT are 120 kVp and 40–80 mAs (45,46).

LUNG CYST. See *cyst*.

MOSAIC PERFUSION. Regional differences in lung perfusion that result in visible attenuation differences on HRCT. This finding can reflect vascular obstruction or abnormal ventilation, but is most

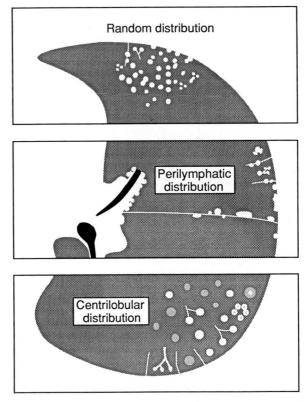

FIG. 9-22. Nodules. Nodules with a random distribution can be seen in relation to small vessels, interlobular septa, and the pleural surfaces, but appear to be diffuse and uniformly distributed. Perilymphatic nodules predominate in the parahilar peribronchovascular regions, the centrilobular regions, and in relation to interlobular septa and the pleural surfaces. Centrilobular nodules are widely distributed mimicking the appearance of random nodules, but spare the pleural surfaces and interlobular septa.

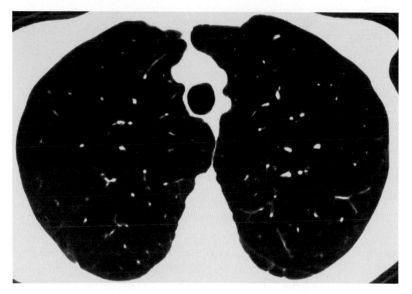

FIG. 9-23. Panlobular emphysema. Emphysema that more or less uniformly involves the pulmonary lobule is termed panlobular. As in this patient, HRCT usually shows large regions of lucency, and a paucity of vascular markings.

common with airways disease (1). Vessels in the lucent regions of lung characteristically appear smaller than in denser lung regions (Figs. 9-4,9-21).

Equivalent. Mosaic oligemia (47).

NODULE. A focal, rounded opacity of varying size, which can be well-defined or ill-defined. In this book, nodules have been classified on the basis of their size as small (< 1 cm) or large (> 1 cm). "Micronodule" is used by some authors to describe nodules < 3 mm in diameter (48), < 5 mm in diameter, or < 7 mm in diameter (49–51), but we have avoided this term. Nodules are also classified as well-defined or ill-defined, and by location (e.g., random, perilymphatic, centrilobular) (Figs. 9-1,9-6,9-18,9-22). The terms "air-space nodule" and "interstitial nodule" should generally be avoided; air-space and interstitial nodules can be difficult to distinguish on HRCT.

OPACIFICATION. A term indicating an increase in lung attenuation, as in "parenchymal opacification" (38,52). Opacification can represent ground-glass opacity or consolidation. It is not usually used to refer to increased lung attenuation reflecting mosaic perfusion.

OPACITY. A term indicating a focal increase in lung attenuation. It can indicate the presence of air-space consolidation or ground-glass opacity.

PANLOBULAR EMPHYSEMA. Emphysema that more or less uniformly involves all the components of the acinus, and therefore involves the entire lobule (17,18). It predominates in the lower lobes, and is classically associated with alpha-1-protease inhibitor (alpha-1-antitrypsin) deficiency. HRCT usually shows large regions of increased lucency, a paucity

of vascular markings, and is usually unassociated with focal lucencies or bullae (Figs. 9-12,9-23).

Equivalent. Panacinar emphysema.

PARASEPTAL EMPHYSEMA. Emphysema which predominantly involves the alveolar ducts and sacs (17,18). It is typically subpleural in location, and is commonly associated with subpleural bullae (Figs. 9-12,9-24). It can be seen as an isolated abnormality, and may be associated with spontaneous pneumo-

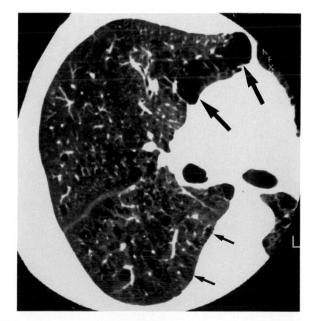

FIG. 9-24. Paraseptal emphysema. In this patient with centrilobular emphysema, subpleural lucencies (*small arrows*) represent paraseptal emphysema. These areas of emphysema may be marginated by interlobular septa. When larger than 1 cm, areas of paraseptal emphysema are called bullae (*large arrows*).

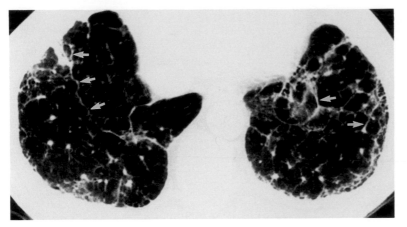

FIG. 9-25. Parenchymal bands. In a 66-year-old patient with asbestosis, interlobular septal thickening is associated with numerous (*small arrows*) parenchymal bands.

thorax. It is commonly associated with centrilobular emphysema (Fig. 9-24).

Equivalent. Distal acinar emphysema.

PARENCHYMAL BAND. The term parenchymal band has been used to describe linear opacities, from 2 to 5 cm in length, which can be seen in patients with pulmonary fibrosis or other causes of interstitial thickening (25,53); these have also been described as "long lines" (54). They are often peripheral and generally contact the pleural surface. Parenchymal bands can represent contiguous thickened interlobular septa, peribronchovascular fibrosis, coarse scars, or atelectasis associated with lung or pleural fibrosis (Figs. 9-25,9-36) (55,56). They are most common in patients with asbestosis and sarcoidosis.

PERIBRONCHOVASCULAR INTERSTITIUM. The strong connective tissue sheath which encloses the bronchi and hilar vessels, and extends from the level of the pulmonary hila into the peripheral lung. Part of the "axial fiber network" described by Weibel (3).

Equivalents. Axial interstitium; bronchovascular interstitium (14), bronchovascular bundle.

PERIBRONCHOVASCULAR INTERSTITIAL THICKENING. Thickening of the peribronchovascular interstitium which surrounds the parahilar bronchi and vessels (10,54,57,58). This is recognizable by an apparent thickening of the bronchial wall, and an apparent increase in size or nodular appearance of the pulmonary arteries (Fig. 9-26) (57). This term is generally used to describe interstitial thickening in relation to relatively large airways. In a centrilobular

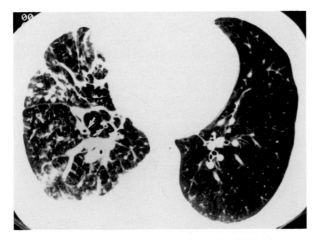

FIG. 9-26. Peribronchovascular interstitial thickening. In a patient with unilateral lymphangitic carcinomatosis, smooth peribronchovascular interstitial thickening is visible in the right middle and lower lobes. The bronchial walls (*arrows*) appear thicker than on the left and vessels in the right lower zone appear larger than left-sided vessels. Subpleural interstitial thickening is present on the right, making the right major fissure appear thickened.

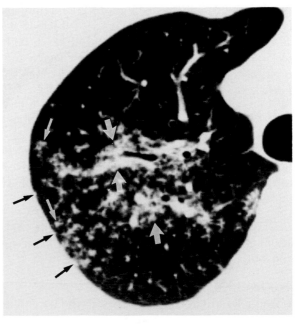

FIG. 9-27. Perilymphatic nodules. In this patient with sarcoidosis, nodules predominate in the peribronchovascular regions (*large white arrows*), subpleural regions (*black arrows*), and in the centrilobular regions (*small white arrow*).

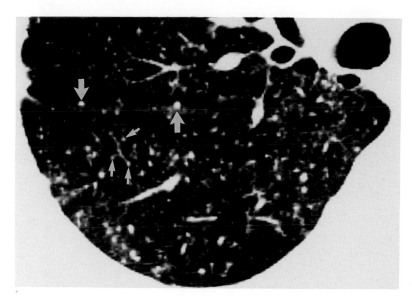

FIG. 9-28. Random nodules. A patient with miliary mycobacterial disease shows numerous, widely distributed, small nodules. Some are visible in relation to small vessels (*small arrows*) and the pleural surfaces (*large arrows*).

location, peribronchovascular interstitial thickening is usually referred to as *centrilobular interstitial thickening* on HRCT, and is recognized by increased prominence of the centrilobular arteries or bronchioles. It can be irregular, smooth (Fig. 9-26), or nodular (Fig. 9-27), and represent fibrosis or interstitial infiltration, as in lymphangitic spread of carcinoma or sarcoidosis.

Equivalents. "peribronchial cuffing," thickening of the bronchovascular bundle.

PERILYMPHATIC. A term which refers to a distribution of abnormalities (e.g., nodules) corresponding to the location of lymphatics in the lung (49,59). Nodules which predominate in relation to the parahilar peribronchovascular interstitium, the centrilobular interstitium, interlobular septa, and in a subpleural location are typical of a perilymphatic distribution (Figs. 9-22,9-27), and are most commonly seen in patients with sarcoidosis, silicosis and coal worker's pneumoconiosis, and lymphangitic spread of carcinoma (49,59).

PNEUMATOCELE. A thin-walled, gas-filled cystic space within the lung, usually occurring in association with acute pneumonia, and almost invariably transient (14). Pneumatoceles have an appearance similar to lung cyst or bulla on HRCT and cannot be distinguished on the basis of HRCT findings. However, the association of such an abnormality with acute pneumonia would suggest the presence of a pneumatocele.

PSEUDOPLAQUE. A grouping of small subpleural nodules, several millimeters thick, that together form a sessile, subpleural opacity which mimics the appearance of an asbestos-related parietal pleural plaque (49). Most common in sarcoidosis (Fig. 9-27) and silicosis.

PULMONARY LOBULE. See *secondary pulmonary lobule.*

RANDOM DISTRIBUTION. A term referring to a random distribution of abnormalities relative to structures of the secondary lobule. A random distribution is often seen in metastatic neoplasm, miliary tuberculosis, and miliary fungal infections, although nodules in histiocytosis X and silicosis can also show this distribution. Nodules appear to be diffuse, but can be seen in relation to interlobular septa, the pleural surfaces, and small vessels (Figs. 9-22,9-28).

RESPIRATORY BRONCHIOLE. The largest bronchiole with alveoli arising from its walls. Thus, the largest bronchiole that participates in gas exchange. An acinus is supplied by one or more respiratory bronchioles.

SECONDARY PULMONARY LOBULE. This term is defined differently by Miller and Reid (Fig. 9-29).

1. According to Miller (2,60), the smallest unit of lung structure marginated by connective tissue septa (2,60). Secondary pulmonary lobules are variably delineated by interlobular septa containing veins and lymphatics, and are supplied by arterial and bronchiolar branches in the lobular core. Using this definition, a secondary pulmonary lobule is usually made up of a dozen or fewer acini, appears irregularly polyhedral in shape, and measures approximately 1 to 2.5 cm on each side (2–6). Miller's

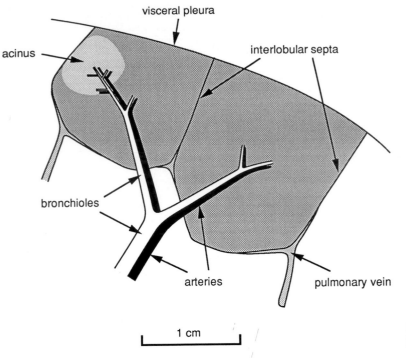

FIG. 9-29. Secondary pulmonary lobule. According to Miller's definition.

definition is most appropriate to interpretation of HRCT, because interlobular septa, core arteries, and septal veins can be seen using this technique.

2. According to Reid, the unit of lung supplied by any bronchiole which gives off 3 to 5 terminal bronchioles (44,61,62); these lobules are about 1 cm in diameter and contain 3 to 5 acini. This definition does not necessarily describe lung units equivalent to secondary lobules as defined by Miller or marginated by interlobular septa (6,61). Reid's definition is most appropriate to interpretation of bronchograms.

Equivalents. Lobule, secondary lobule, pulmonary lobule.

SEPTUM. See *interlobular septum*.

SIGNET-RING SIGN. A ring shadow (representing a dilated, thick-walled bronchus) associated with a small, soft-tissue opacity (the adjacent pulmonary artery), which has the appearance of a ''signet-ring'' (Fig. 9-30). Diagnostic of bronchiectasis (63,64). **Distinguish from** *peribronchovascular interstitial thickening* or ''peribronchial cuffing,'' in which the bronchus is not dilated.

SUBPLEURAL INTERSTITIUM. The interstitial fiber network which lies beneath the visceral pleura and envelopes the lung in a fibrous sac. It extends over the surface of the lung and in relation to the interlobar fissures. Along with the interlobular septa, the subpleural interstitium represents a portion of the ''peripheral fiber system'' described by Weibel (3).

SUBPLEURAL INTERSTITIAL THICKENING. Abnormal thickening of the subpleural interstitium. Most easily seen on HRCT adjacent to the fissures, giving the appearance of thickening of the fissures (Fig. 9-31). Commonly associated with interlobular septal thickening. Subpleural interstitial thickening is preferred to ''fissural thickening.''

SUBPLEURAL LINE. A thin, curvilinear opacity a few millimeters or less in thickness, usually less than

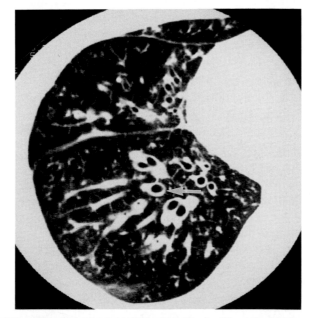

FIG. 9-30. Signet-ring sign. A patient with cylindric bronchiectasis shows several examples of the signet ring sign (*arrow*) in the right lower lobe.

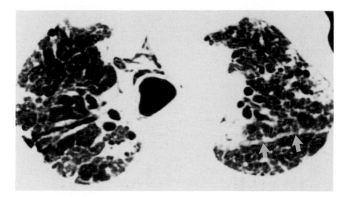

FIG. 9-31. Subpleural interstitial thickening. Apparent thickening of the left major fissure (*arrows*) in this patient with pulmonary fibrosis represents subpleural interstitial thickening. An incidental pneumomediastinum is also present.

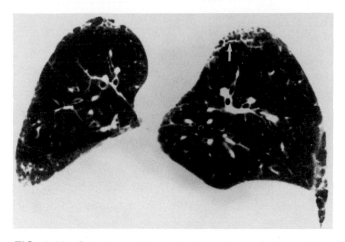

FIG. 9-32. Subpleural line. An irregular subpleural line (*arrow*) is visible on the right on a prone scan in a patient with rheumatoid arthritis, pulmonary fibrosis, and early honeycombing.

1 cm from the pleural surface, and paralleling the pleura (Fig. 9-32) (65,66). This is a nonspecific term, and may be used to describe dependent opacity, dependent and transient atelectasis, or fibrosis. A subpleural line that persists when nondependent often reflects fibrosis or honeycombing, and other findings of fibrosis will usually be visible. **Distinguish from** *dependent opacity* which is a normal finding.

TARGETED RECONSTRUCTION. Reconstruction of the CT image using a smaller field of view than used to scan the entire chest in order to reduce the image pixel size and increase spatial resolution (40,67). **Equivalent.** Target-reconstructed HRCT.

TERMINAL BRONCHIOLE. The last purely conducting airway, which does not participate in gas exchange. Approximately 0.7 mm in diameter, it gives rise to respiratory bronchioles.

TRACTION BRONCHIECTASIS. Bronchial dilatation and irregularity occurring in patients with pulmonary fibrosis, because of traction by fibrous tissue on the bronchial wall (Fig. 9-33) (29,68). Visible on HRCT as bronchiectasis that is commonly irregular in contour. The term *traction bronchiolectasis* applies to intralobular bronchioles, and is usually diagnosed if dilated airways are visible in the lung periphery.

TRACTION BRONCHIOLECTASIS. See *bronchiolectasis.*

TREE-IN-BUD. Bronchiolar dilatation and filling by mucus, pus, or fluid, resembling a branching tree, and usually somewhat nodular in appearance (16). Usually visible in the lung periphery, this finding is indicative of airways disease, and is particularly common in endo-

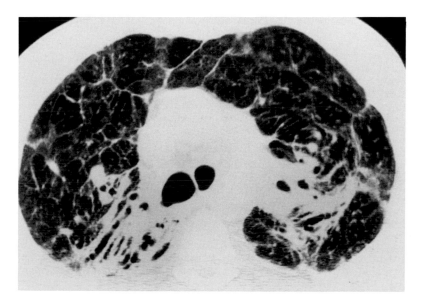

FIG. 9-33. Traction bronchiectasis. In a patient with end-stage sarcoidosis, dilated bronchi are associated with parahilar conglomerate masses of fibrosis. Also note septal thickening and parenchymal bands anteriorly.

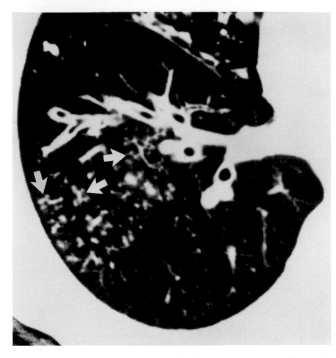

FIG. 9-34. Tree-in-bud. A patient with cystic fibrosis shows numerous examples of "tree-in-bud." Several of these are indicated by *arrows*. This appearance reflects the presence of dilated, branching, mucus-filled bronchioles. Also noted is central bronchial wall thickening.

bronchial spread of infection (TB), cystic fibrosis, diffuse panbronchiolitis, and chronic airways infection (Fig. 9-34) (15).

REFERENCES

1. Webb WR, Müller NL, Naidich DP. Standardized terms for high-resolution computed tomography of the lung: a proposed glossary. *J Thorac Imaging* 1993;8:167–185.
2. Weibel ER, Taylor CR. Design and structure of the human lung. In: *Pulmonary Diseases and Disorders*. New York: McGraw-Hill; 1988:11–60.
3. Weibel ER. Looking into the lung: what can it tell us? *AJR* 1979; 133:1021–1031.
4. Raskin SP. The pulmonary acinus: historical notes. *Radiology* 1982;144:31–34.
5. Osborne DR, Effmann EL, Hedlund LW. Postnatal growth and size of the pulmonary acinus and secondary lobule in man. *AJR* 1983;140:449–454.
6. Itoh H, Murata K, Konishi J, Nishimura K, Kitaichi M, Izumi T. Diffuse lung disease: pathologic basis for the high-resolution computed tomography findings. *J Thorac Imaging* 1993;8: 176–188.
7. Murata K, Itoh H, Todo G, et al. Centrilobular lesions of the lung: demonstration by high-resolution CT and pathologic correlation. *Radiology* 1986;161:641–645.
8. Murata K, Herman PG, Khan A, Todo G, Pipman Y, Luber JM. Intralobular distribution of oleic acid-induced pulmonary edema in the pig: evaluation by high-resolution CT. *Invest Radiol* 1989; 24:647–653.
9. Naidich DP, Zerhouni EA, Hutchins GM, Genieser NB, McCauley DI, Siegelman SS. Computed tomography of the pulmonary parenchyma: part 1. distal air-space disease. *J Thorac Imaging* 1985;1:39–53.
10. Webb WR. High-resolution CT of the lung parenchyma. *Radiol Clin North Am* 1989;27:1085–1097.
11. Stern EJ, Webb WR, Gamsu G. Dynamic quantitative computed tomography: a predictor of pulmonary function in obstructive lung diseases. *Invest Radiol* 1994;29:564–569.
12. Webb WR. High-resolution computed tomography of obstructive lung disease. *Radiol Clin North Am* 1994;32:745–757.
13. Webb WR, Stern EJ, Kanth N, Gamsu G. Dynamic pulmonary CT: findings in normal adult men. *Radiology* 1993;186:117–124.
14. Tuddenham WJ. Glossary of terms for thoracic radiology: recommendations of the Nomenclature Committee of the Fleischner Society. *AJR* 1984;143:509–517.
15. Gruden JF, Webb WR, Warnock M. Centrilobular opacities in the lung on high-resolution CT: diagnostic considerations and pathologic correlation. *AJR* 1994;162:569–574.
16. Im JG, Itoh H, Shim YS, et al. Pulmonary tuberculosis: CT findings-early active disease and sequential change with antituberculous therapy. *Radiology* 1993;186:653–660.
17. Snider GL, Kleinerman J, Thurlbeck WM, Bengali ZH. The definition of emphysema: report of a National Heart, Lung, and Blood Institute, Division of Lung Diseases workshop. *Am Rev Respir Dis* 1985;132:182–185.
18. Thurlbeck WM. *Chronic Airflow Obstruction in Lung Disease.* Philadelphia: WB Saunders; 1976:12–30.
19. Stern EJ, Webb WR, Weinacker A, Müller NL. Idiopathic giant bullous emphysema (vanishing lung syndrome): imaging findings in nine patients. *AJR* 1994;162:279–282.
20. Brauner MW, Grenier P, Mouelhi MM, Mompoint D, Lenoir S. Pulmonary histiocytosis X: evaluation with high resolution CT. *Radiology* 1989;172:255–258.
21. Moore AD, Godwin JD, Müller NL, et al. Pulmonary histiocytosis X: comparison of radiographic and CT findings. *Radiology* 1989;172:249–254.
22. Aberle DR, Hansell DM, Brown K, Tashkin DP. Lymphangiomyomatosis: CT, chest radiographic, and functional correlations. *Radiology* 1990;176:381–387.
23. Lenoir S, Grenier P, Brauner MW, et al. Pulmonary lymphangiomyomatosis and tuberous sclerosis: comparison of radiographic and thin-section CT findings. *Radiology* 1990;175: 329–334.
24. Müller NL, Chiles C, Kullnig P. Pulmonary lymphangiomyomatosis: correlation of CT with radiographic and functional findings. *Radiology* 1990;175:335–339.
25. Aberle DR, Gamsu G, Ray CS, Feuerstein IM. Asbestos-related pleural and parenchymal fibrosis: detection with high-resolution CT. *Radiology* 1988;166:729–734.
26. Stern EJ, Webb WR. Dynamic imaging of lung morphology with ultrafast high-resolution computed tomography. *J Thorac Imaging* 1993;8:273–282.
27. Cardoso WV, Thurlbeck WM. Pathogenesis and terminology of emphysema. *Am J Respir Crit Care Med* 1994;149:1383.
28. Snider GL. Pathogenesis and terminology of emphysema. *Am J Respir Crit Care Med* 1994;149:1382–1383.
29. Webb WR, Stein MG, Finkbeiner WE, Im JG, Lynch D, Gamsu G. Normal and diseased isolated lungs: high-resolution CT. *Radiology* 1988;166:81–87.
30. Naidich DP. High-resolution computed tomography of cystic lung disease. *Semin Roentgenol* 1991;26:151–174.
31. Hogg JC. Benjamin Felson lecture. Chronic interstitial lung disease of unknown cause: a new classification based on pathogenesis. *AJR* 1991;156:225–233.
32. Genereux GP. The end-stage lung: pathogenesis, pathology, and radiology. *Radiology* 1975;116:279–289.
33. Snider GL. Interstitial pulmonary fibrosis. *Chest* 1986; 89(Suppl):115–121.
34. Fulmer JD, Crystal RG. Interstitial lung disease. *Curr Pulmonol* 1979;1:1–65.
35. Kalender WA, Rienmuller R, Seissler W, Behr J, Welke M, Fichte H. Measurement of pulmonary parenchymal attenuation: use of spirometric gating with quantitative CT. *Radiology* 1990; 175:265–268.
36. Kalender WA, Fichte H, Bautz W, Skalej M. Semiautomatic evaluation procedures for quantitative CT of the lung. *J Comput Assist Tomogr* 1991;15:248–255.

37. Zerhouni EA, Naidich DP, Stitik FP, Khouri NF, Siegelman SS. Computed tomography of the pulmonary parenchyma: part 2. interstitial disease. *J Thorac Imaging* 1985;1:54–64.
38. Leung AN, Miller RR, Müller NL. Parenchymal opacification in chronic infiltrative lung diseases: CT-pathologic correlation. *Radiology* 1993;188:209–214.
39. Remy-Jardin M, Giraud F, Remy J, Copin MC, Gosselin B, Duhamel A. Importance of ground-glass attenuation in chronic diffuse infiltrative lung disease: pathologic-CT correlation. *Radiology* 1993;189:693–698.
40. Mayo JR, Webb WR, Gould R, et al. High-resolution CT of the lungs: an optimal approach. *Radiology* 1987;163:507–510.
41. Genereux GP. The Fleischner lecture: computed tomography of diffuse pulmonary disease. *J Thorac Imaging* 1989;4:50–87.
42. Primack SL, Hartman TE, Hansell DM, Müller NL. End-stage lung disease: CT findings in 61 patients. *Radiology* 1993;189:681–686.
43. Zerhouni E. Computed tomography of the pulmonary parenchyma: an overview. *Chest* 1989;95:901–907.
44. Heitzman ER, Markarian B, Berger I, Dailey E. The secondary pulmonary lobule: a practical concept for interpretation of radiographs. I. Roentgen anatomy of the normal secondary pulmonary lobule. *Radiology* 1969;93:508–513.
45. Zwirewich CV, Mayo JR, Müller NL. Low-dose high-resolution CT of lung parenchyma. *Radiology* 1991;180:413–417.
46. Lee KS, Primack SL, Staples CA, Mayo JR, Aldrich JE, Müller NL. Chronic infiltrative lung disease: comparison of diagnostic accuracies of radiography and low- and conventional-dose thin-section CT. *Radiology* 1994;191:669–673.
47. Martin KW, Sagel SS, Siegel BA. Mosaic oligemia simulating pulmonary infiltrates on CT. *AJR* 1986;147:670–673.
48. Grenier P, Valeyre D, Cluzel P, Brauner MW, Lenoir S, Chastang C. Chronic diffuse interstitial lung disease: diagnostic value of chest radiography and high-resolution CT. *Radiology* 1991;179:123–132.
49. Remy-Jardin M, Beuscart R, Sault MC, Marquette CH, Remy J. Subpleural micronodules in diffuse infiltrative lung diseases: evaluation with thin-section CT scans. *Radiology* 1990;177:133–139.
50. Remy-Jardin M, Remy J, Deffontaines C, Duhamel A. Assessment of diffuse infiltrative lung disease: comparison of conventional CT and high-resolution CT. *Radiology* 1991;181:157–162.
51. Remy-Jardin M, Remy J, Wallaert B, Müller NL. Subacute and chronic bird breeder hypersensitivity pneumonitis: sequential evaluation with CT and correlation with lung function tests and bronchoalveolar lavage. *Radiology* 1993;198:111–118.
52. Müller NL, Staples CA, Miller RR, Vedal S, Thurlbeck WM, Ostrow DN. Disease activity in idiopathic pulmonary fibrosis: CT and pathologic correlation. *Radiology* 1987;165:731–734.
53. Aberle DR, Gamsu G, Ray CS. High-resolution CT of benign asbestos-related diseases: clinical and radiographic correlation. *AJR* 1988;151:883–891.
54. Stein MG, Mayo J, Müller N, Aberle DR, Webb WR, Gamsu G. Pulmonary lymphangitic spread of carcinoma: appearance on CT scans. *Radiology* 1987;162:371–375.
55. Akira M, Yamamoto S, Yokoyama K, et al. Asbestosis: high-resolution CT-pathologic correlation. *Radiology* 1990;176:389–394.
56. Lynch DA, Gamsu G, Ray CS, Aberle DR. Asbestos-related focal lung masses: manifestations on conventional and high-resolution CT scans. *Radiology* 1988;169:603–607.
57. Munk PL, Müller NL, Miller RR, Ostrow DN. Pulmonary lymphangitic carcinomatosis: CT and pathologic findings. *Radiology* 1988;166:705–709.
58. Bergin CJ, Müller NL. CT in the diagnosis of interstitial lung disease. *AJR* 1985;145:505–510.
59. Colby TV. Anatomic distribution and histopathologic patterns in interstitial lung disease. In: Schwarz MI, King TE Jr, eds. *Interstitial Lung Disease*. St. Louis: Mosby Year Book; 1993:59–77.
60. Miller WS. *The Lung*. Springfield: Charles C Thomas; 1947:203.
61. Reid L. The secondary pulmonary lobule in the adult human lung, with special reference to its appearance in bronchograms. *Thorax* 1958;13:110–115.
62. Reid L, Simon G. The peripheral pattern in the normal bronchogram and its relation to peripheral pulmonary anatomy. *Thorax* 1958;13:103–109.
63. Naidich DP, McCauley DI, Khouri NF, Stitik FP, Siegelman SS. Computed tomography of bronchiectasis. *J Comput Assist Tomogr* 1982;6:437–444.
64. Grenier P, Maurice F, Musset D, Menu Y, Nahum H. Bronchiectasis: assessment by thin-section CT. *Radiology* 1986;161:95–99.
65. Yoshimura H, Hatakeyama M, Otsuji H, et al. Pulmonary asbestosis: CT study of subpleural curvilinear shadow. work in progress. *Radiology* 1986;158:653–658.
66. Arai K, Takashima T, Matsui O, Kadoya M, Kamimura R. Transient subpleural curvilinear shadow caused by pulmonary congestion. *J Comput Assist Tomogr* 1990;14:87–88.
67. Murata K, Khan A, Herman PG. Pulmonary parenchymal disease: evaluation with high-resolution CT. *Radiology* 1989;170:629–635.
68. Westcott JL, Cole SR. Traction bronchiectasis in end-stage pulmonary fibrosis. *Radiology* 1986;161:665–669.
69. Stern EJ, Webb WR, Golden JA, Gamsu G. Cystic lung disease associated with eosinophilic granuloma and tuberous sclerosis: air trapping at dynamic ultrafast high-resolution CT. *Radiology* 1992;182:325–329.

Subject Index

ISBN 0-7817-0217-8

9 780781 702171